Toxicology: Advanced Concepts

Toxicology: Advanced Concepts

Editor: Braylon Holden

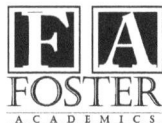

FA
FOSTER
A C A D E M I C S

www.fosteracademics.com

www.fosteracademics.com

FA
FOSTER
ACADEMICS

Cataloging-in-Publication Data

Toxicology : advanced concepts / edited by Braylon Holden.
    p. cm.
Includes bibliographical references and index.
ISBN 978-1-63242-514-0
1. Toxicology. 2. Toxicity testing--In vitro. 3. Toxicity testing--In vivo. 4. Medicine. I. Holden, Braylon.
RA1216 .T69 2017
615.9--dc23

© Foster Academics, 2017

Foster Academics,
118-35 Queens Blvd., Suite 400,
Forest Hills, NY 11375, USA

ISBN 978-1-63242-514-0 (Hardback)

Printed and bound in the United States of America.

Contents

Preface

This book was inspired by the evolution of our times; to answer the curiosity of inquisitive minds. Many developments have occurred across the globe in the recent past which has transformed the progress in the field.

Toxicology researches the effect of chemicals on living beings. Treatment and assessment are fundamental aspects of toxicology. It has many branches ranging from forensic and legal toxicology to ecotoxicology. This book is a valuable compilation of topics, ranging from the basic to the most complex advancements in this field. It presents the complex subject of toxicology in a comprehensive manner. With state-of-the-art inputs by acclaimed experts of this field, this book targets students and professionals. Through this book, we attempt to further enlighten the readers about the new concepts in this field.

This book was developed from a mere concept to drafts to chapters and finally compiled together as a complete text to benefit the readers across all nations. To ensure the quality of the content we instilled two significant steps in our procedure. The first was to appoint an editorial team that would verify the data and statistics provided in the book and also select the most appropriate and valuable contributions from the plentiful contributions we received from authors worldwide. The next step was to appoint an expert of the topic as the Editor-in-Chief, who would head the project and finally make the necessary amendments and modifications to make the text reader-friendly. I was then commissioned to examine all the material to present the topics in the most comprehensible and productive format.

I would like to take this opportunity to thank all the contributing authors who were supportive enough to contribute their time and knowledge to this project. I also wish to convey my regards to my family who have been extremely supportive during the entire project.

Editor

A Bayesian Meta-Analysis of Multiple Treatment Comparisons of Systemic Regimens for Advanced Pancreatic Cancer

Kelvin Chan[1,2]*, Keya Shah[1], Kelly Lien[1], Doug Coyle[3], Henry Lam[1], Yoo-Joung Ko[1]

1 Sunnybrook Odette Cancer Centre, University of Toronto, Toronto, ON, Canada, **2** Division of Biostatistics, Dalla Lana School of Public Health, University of Toronto, Toronto, ON, Canada, **3** University of Ottawa, Ottawa, ON, Canada

Abstract

Background: For advanced pancreatic cancer, many regimens have been compared with gemcitabine (G) as the standard arm in randomized controlled trials. Few regimens have been directly compared with each other in randomized controlled trials and the relative efficacy and safety among them remains unclear.

Methods: A systematic review was performed through MEDLINE, EMBASE, Cochrane Central Register of Controlled Trials, and ASCO meeting abstracts up to May 2013 to identify randomized controlled trials that included advanced pancreatic cancer comparing the following regimens: G, G+5-fluorouracil, G+ capecitabine, G+S1, G+ cisplatin, G+ oxaliplatin, G+ erlotinib, G+ nab-paclitaxel, and FOLFIRINOX. Overall survival and progression-free survival with 95% credible regions were extracted using the Parmar method. A Bayesian multiple treatment comparisons was performed to compare all regimens simultaneously.

Results: Twenty-two studies were identified and 16 were included in the meta-analysis. Median overall survival, progression free survival, and response rates for G arms from all trials were similar, suggesting no significant clinical heterogeneity. For overall survival, the mixed treatment comparisons found that the probability that FOLFIRINOX was the best regimen was 83%, while it was 11% for G+ nab-paclitaxel and 3% for G+ S1 and G+ erlotinib, respectively. The overall survival hazard ratio for FOLFIRINOX versus G+ nab-paclitaxel was 0.79 [0.50–1.24], with no obvious difference in toxicities. The hazard ratios from direct pairwise comparisons were consistent with the mixed treatment comparisons results.

Conclusions: FOLFIRINOX appeared to be the best regimen for advanced pancreatic cancer probabilistically, with a trend towards improvement in survival when compared with other regimens by indirect comparisons.

Editor: Jonathan R. Brody, Thomas Jefferson University, United States of America

Funding: The authors have no support or funding to report.

Competing Interests: Keya Shah has read the journal's policy and the authors of this manuscript have the following competing interests: Yoo-Joung Ko declared that he received research support and honoraria from Sanofi-Aventis, and Celgene; however, he has no stock ownership. The remaining authors have no competing interests to declare.

* Email: kelvin.chan@sunnybrook.ca

Introduction

Pancreatic cancer is the 4th leading cause of cancer death in the United States and 5th in the United Kingdom [1,2] with most cases being categorized as either metastatic or locally advanced at first presentation [3]. As potentially curative surgical resection can be performed in only 15–20% of pancreatic cancer patients [4], the treatment goal for the majority of these patients is palliative in nature. For more than 15 years, the current standard of care for advanced disease has been chemotherapy with gemcitabine alone (G), after it was shown in a phase III randomized control trial (RCT) to offer greater symptom relief with a modest 1-year survival advantage (18% versus 2%) when compared to 5-fluorouracil [5]. Since then, a number of phase II and III RCTs have attempted to improve the gemcitabine anti-tumour activity

through gemcitabine-based combinations with cytotoxic and/or targeted agents such as capecitabine, oxaliplatin, erlotinib, and cisplatin [6–10]. Recent trials have also compared gemcitabine alone to gemcitabine plus nab-paclitaxel (GnP), and a combination regimen without gemcitabine consisting of folinic acid, fluorouracil, irinotecan hydrochloride and oxaliplatin (FOLFIRINOX) [11,12]. The trial of G versus GnP found statistically significant hazard ratios (HRs) for overall survival (OS) in favour of the GnP combination. The safety analysis found that serious life-threatening toxicity was not increased with GnP and that adverse events were acceptable and manageable. Thus, the authors concluded that GnP may be considered as a new standard of treatment for advanced pancreatic cancer [11]. In the FOLFIRINOX trial, survival was significantly better in the FOLFIRINOX group, but with an increased occurrence of adverse events. The study concluded that FOLFIRINOX should also be considered as a first-line option for advanced pancreatic cancer patients; however, due to safety concerns, it should be reserved for patients younger than 75 years of age and with a good performance status [12]. No currently ongoing trials directly compare GnP and FOLFIRINOX. While the addition of these two chemotherapy regimens and their improvement in survival represent significant recent progress over gemcitabine monotherapy, the most effective chemotherapy strategy in clinical practice remains to be determined.

As direct comparison of combination therapies has been tested mostly against single agent gemcitabine as the control arm in most clinical trials, the relative effectiveness of the various regimens remains unclear. In these instances, multiple treatment comparisons (MTC) can be used to synthesize evidence from RCTs using both direct (head-to-head) and indirect (using a common comparator) comparisons [13]. MTC are valuable tools that are frequently employed by healthcare decision makers such as the National Institute for Health and Clinical Excellence and the Canadian Agency for Drugs and Technologies in Health, where their usage is gaining widespread acceptance [14,15].

The aim of this study was to perform Bayesian MTC in order to determine the most effective treatment for advanced pancreatic cancer, taking into account the efficacy and safety profiles of each regimen. Through our analysis, we were able to achieve this goal.

Methods

Literature Search

We conducted a systematic literature review through the MEDLINE, EMBASE, and Cochrane Centre Register of Controlled Trials databases, as well as ASCO meeting abstracts up to and including May 23, 2013. Trials were limited to first-line treatment in pancreatic cancer or adenocarcinoma patients. Studies were limited to randomized controlled trials (RCTs) that used one of the following chemotherapy regimens: G, G + fluorouracil (GF), G + capecitabine (GCap), G + S1 (GS), G + cisplatin (GCis), G + oxaliplatin (GOx), G + erlotinib (GE), GnP, and FOLFIRINOX. These regimens were determined a priori by the authors, as they are clinically the most commonly considered treatments for advanced pancreatic cancer with prior studies suggesting possible benefits to patients. The outcomes of interest included OS, progression-free survival (PFS), and grade 3/4 toxicities. RCTs that did not include patients with advanced pancreatic cancer were excluded. Non-randomized trials and those concerning other malignancies, such as neuroendocrine tumours or lymphoma, were excluded. Trials comparing radiotherapy, hormonal, or gene therapy, and those comparing chemotherapy to no treatment (best supportive care) were excluded. No language restrictions were imposed. The articles that were not freely available to us were requested from the authors.

Screening

Two independent authors reviewed the literature search results and included studies that met the prespecified eligibility criteria. When reports overlapped or were duplicated, we retained the study with the most recent data that could be used in the meta-analysis. Discrepancies were resolved by consensus or by a third author. Our review has been reported using the PRISMA reporting guidelines (Checklist S1).

Data Abstraction and Analysis

Data recorded included the following: first author, publication year, study location, regimens being compared, number of patients randomized to each treatment arm, median age of patients, percentage of patients with performance status of ECOG 0, 1, or 2 and the percentage of patients with locally advanced or advanced disease respectively was recorded (Appendix S1 and S2). The treatments were sorted into categories based on the regimen: G, GF, GCap, GS, GCis, GOx, GE, GnP, and FOLFIRINOX. Risk of bias assessment was performed using the Cochrane risk of bias tool [16].

The data extracted from each study included the following: OS, PFS, objective response rate (ObRR), and the occurrence of adverse events (febrile neutropenia, neuropathy, fatigue, and diarrhea) for all the chemotherapy regimens. If median values for PFS and OS were available, they were also recorded. If the HRs for OS and PFS were detailed in the publication, they were extracted directly, along with 95% confidence intervals (CIs) from Cox regression. Otherwise, HRs were calculated using the methods outlined by Parmar et al [17]. A two-tailed $p<0.05$ value was recorded whenever available to determine whether a statistically significant difference was detected between the two regimens being compared. Two independent authors extracted data and discrepancies were reviewed by a third author to reach consensus.

Statistical Analysis

We first made pairwise comparisons of regimens from the trials based on direct evidence only. We then performed MTC in a Bayesian model. The MTC combined direct and indirect evidence for specific pairwise comparisons and allowed data across a range of regimens to be compared in a simple network. Bayesian methods combine likelihoods, as a function of the parameters with a prior probability distribution based on previous knowledge, to obtain a posterior probability distribution of the parameters [18]. The posterior probabilities provide a straightforward way to calculate the most effective treatment in the absence of head-to-head trials. By plotting the posterior densities of the direct, indirect, and network estimates, direct and indirect evidence can be combined to provide a network estimate and a single effect size. This effect size has increased precision than that of any one type of evidence alone. The Bayesian approach has undergone significant development in recent years and is able to monitor convergence in posterior distribution and reflect the uncertainty in estimating heterogeneity, offering significant improvements over the frequentist random-effects model, which cannot estimate that uncertainty. In more complex networks, especially those involving multi-armed trials, Bayesian approaches are more developed and more accessible than their frequentist counterparts [18,19].

Analyses were done using Bayesian Markov Chain Monte-Carlo (MCMC) sampling in WinBUGS, version 1.4.3 and reported according to the Quality of Reporting of Meta-analyses (QUOROM) and International Society for Pharmacoeconomics and Outcomes Research (ISPOR) guidelines. In WinBUGS, 3 chains were fit with 40,000 burn-ins and 40,000 iterations each. Assessment of convergence was done using model diagnostics, such as trace plots and the Brooks-Gelman-Rubin statistic [20]. Model fit was determined based on the residual deviance and deviance information criterion (DIC) for each outcome measure. The random effects model was used for OS, PFS, and ObRR because the residual deviance was less than the number of unconstrained data points and the deviance information criterion for each of these outcome measures favoured this model over the fixed effects model. Fixed effects were used in reporting toxicities

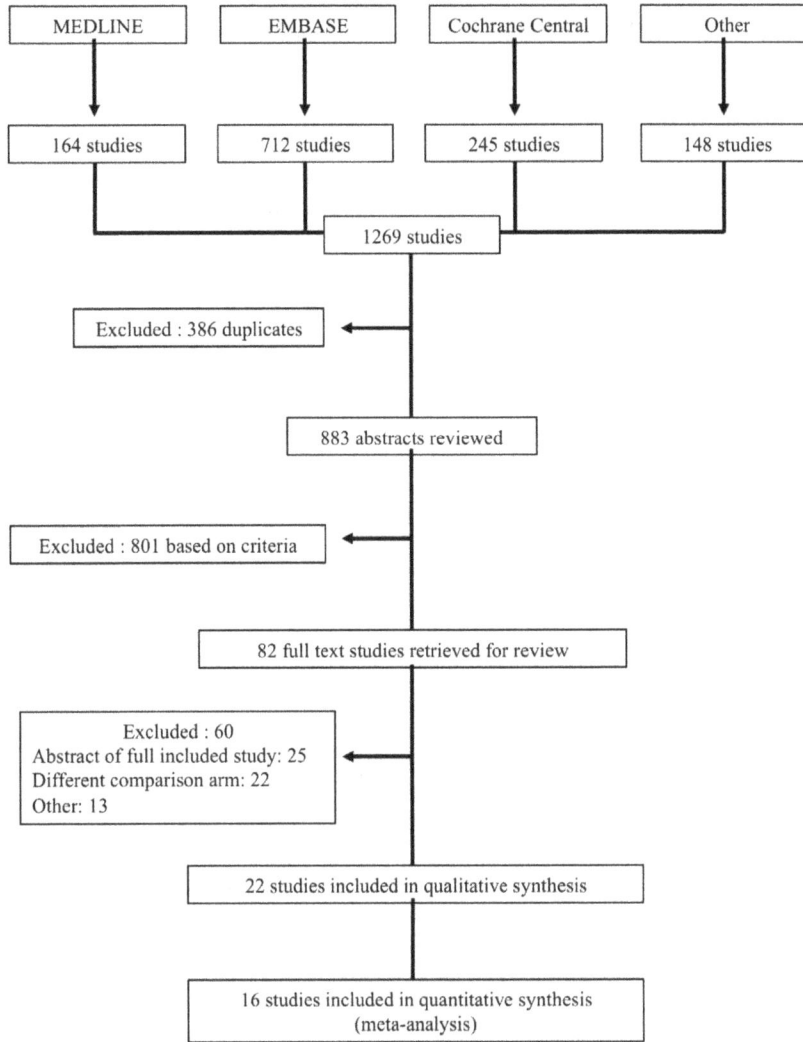

Figure 1. PRISMA Flow diagram of included and excluded trials identified from the literature search. There were 13 studies that were excluded after full text review for "other" reasons. The reasons are as follows: 4 were secondary analyses, 2 were quality of life studies, 2 were pooled analyses, 1 study was not randomized, 1 was a review, 1 was a tumour marker study, 1 was a safety analysis, and 1 study was excluded because it was retrospective.

because the residual deviance and DIC favoured this model. We used the following non-informative prior distributions: uniform (0,2) for standard deviation of the random effects model and normal (0, tau = 0.0001) for log[HR]s. Non-informative priors were used because this allowed the trial data to inform the results, rather than letting strong priors dictate the results.

The primary endpoint was OS and the secondary endpoints were PFS and ObRR. OS and PFS were summarized as log[HR], ObRR and toxicities were summarized as log[Odds Ratio]. Effect sizes are described with 95% credible regions (CRs), since "credible" is a more appropriate term than "confidence" when conducting Bayesian MTC. Consistency between direct and indirect evidence was assessed by comparing direct pairwise comparison estimates to the results generated in the MTC. Probability of each regimen being the best among all regimens were computed by ranking the relative efficacies of all regimens in each iteration and then calculating the proportion of each regimen being ranked first across all iterations [21]. In order to assess the comparability of included studies, between-study heterogeneity

was estimated and reported using the I^2 statistic; the value of I^2 lies between 0% and 100%, where 0% indicates no observed heterogeneity and larger values show increasing heterogeneity [17].

Based on the HR results of the MTC, we attempted to project the survival of patients receiving each of the regimens and compared the results to the median OS of G. Projected median OS was calculated using a median OS of 5.65 months for G as reported by Buris et al [5]. Survival was estimated based on the MTC results and the methods presented by Altman and Andersen [22].

Results

Literature Search Results

Figure 1 shows a flow diagram of the selection process for the studies included in our meta-analysis. 1269 studies were identified from the literature search, 386 studies were excluded because they were duplicates, and 801 were excluded after the abstracts were reviewed based on the prespecified criteria. Of the 82 studies that

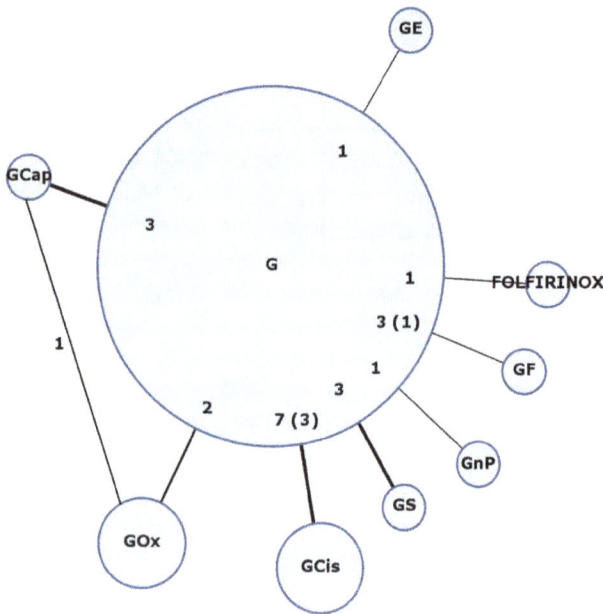

Figure 2. Treatment strategy network. Numbers represent the number of studies comparing the linked regimens; brackets represent the number included in the quantitative analysis.

underwent full text review, 25 were excluded because they were an abstract of a full-included study, 22 had a different comparison arm, 4 were secondary analyses, 2 were quality of life studies, 2 were pooled analyses, 1 study was not randomized, 1 was a review, 1 was a tumour marker study, 1 was a safety analysis, and 1 study was excluded because it was retrospective. Twenty-two studies were identified to be included in this review [6–12,23–38]. 16 studies, involving 5488 randomized patients contained sufficient data to be included in the quantitative synthesis (meta-analysis). The studies included in the meta-analysis consisted of 15 manuscripts and 1 ASCO meeting abstract, which was subsequently published as a full manuscript [38]. The subsequent publication was reviewed and the results were verified and found to be identical to the results reported in the original abstract [11,38].

Study Quality

A summary of the risk of bias for each included study can be found in Appendices S14 and S15. All included studies were randomized and 12 out of the 16 studies followed intention-to-treat analysis for the primary endpoint, thus minimizing selection bias and attrition bias, respectively. Only one study had blinding of patients or personnel. Although blinding of outcome assessors was not explicitly indicated, 13 studies had OS as the primary endpoint, which would not be influenced by the outcome assessor. Therefore there is a low risk of detection bias in these studies. Allocation concealment was not mentioned in any of the studies, so some potential selection bias may be present.

Trial Characteristics

The chemotherapy regimens used in the included studies were G vs. GF (three studies), G vs. GCap (three studies), G vs. GS (three studies), G vs. GCis (seven studies), G vs. GOx (two studies), G vs. GE (one study), G vs. FOLFIRINOX (one study), GCap + GOx (one study), and G + GnP (one study). The treatment strategy network is shown in Figure 2. All trials included in the

meta-analysis reported median PFS and OS. There was no significant clinical heterogeneity between the studies based on the patient characteristics and outcomes in the G reference arm (median PFS = 3 to 4 months, median OS = 6 to 7 months) (Appendix S3).

Comparison of Regimens

The outcomes assessed in all the trials were OS, PFS, ObRR, and number of toxicity-related adverse events. Of the 16 trials that compared different regimens, seven found statistically significant differences in OS based on direct evidence only (Figure 3). These seven studies compared G alone to a different treatment arm. Direct comparisons detected statistically significant improvements in OS with GnP versus G (HR = 0.72, [95% CR 0.62–0.84]), GCap versus G (HR = 0.86, [0.75–0.98]), GE versus G (HR = 0.82, [0.69–0.97]), FOLFIRINOX versus G (HR = 0.57, [0.45–0.72]), GOx versus G (HR = 0.87, [0.76–0.98]), and GS versus G (HR = 0.80, [0.66 to 0.96]). These results can be seen in Figure 3. Statistical heterogeneity ($I^2 > 35\%$) was found only for the comparisons of GCis versus G (seven studies, $I^2 = 64\%$) and GF versus G (three studies, $I^2 = 62\%$) for OS. The direct comparisons for PFS with I^2 values are shown in Appendix S4.

Through our Bayesian MTC, HR comparisons were made of OS (Figure 4) and PFS (Appendix S5) to compare all the regimens simultaneously. The results of the MTC were similar to the results seen in direct pairwise comparisons (Appendix S9). For OS, the results of the Bayesian MTC found that the probability that FOLFIRINOX was the best regimen was 83%, while it was 11% for GnP and 3% for GS and GE, respectively. For PFS, the Bayesian MTC found an 80% probability that FOLFIRINOX was the best regimen. Figure 5 shows the probabilities of each treatment regimen being the best in terms of OS. The probabilities for PFS can be seen in Appendix S6.

The next best regimens according to the calculated probabilities are GnP, GE, and GS. The OS HR for FOLFIRINOX versus GS was 0.72 [0.48–1.11], FOLFIRINOX versus GnP was 0.79 [0.50–1.24], and FOLFIRINOX versus GE was 0.70 [0.44–1.10], where HRs are given with 95% CRs. The PFS HR for FOLFIRINOX versus GS was 0.78 [0.47–1.40], FOLFIRINOX versus GnP was 0.68 [0.37–1.27], and FOLFIRINOX versus GE was 0.61 [0.33–1.15].

Projected survivals were estimated comparing each regimen to G. The projected median OS ranged from 5.8 months for GCis and 9.9 months for FOLFIRINOX (see Table 1). The number needed to treat (NNT) at 6 months and 1 year relative to G have been shown in Table 1. The NNT at 1 year ranges from 5 for FOLFIRINOX to 146 for GCis. These estimates will be helpful in clinical decision-making and providing information to patients.

Odds ratio (OR) comparisons were made of ObRR (Appendix S7) to compare all the regimens simultaneously. The Bayesian MTC found a 58% probability that FOLFIRINOX is the best regimen in terms of ObRR, while it was 33% and 8% for GnP and GS respectively. The ObRR HR [95% CR] for FOLFIRINOX versus GnP is 1.59 [0.74–2.94]. The probabilities that each treatment regimen is the best in terms of ObRR are shown in Appendix S8.

The toxicity-related adverse events assessed in this study were febrile neutropenia and grade 3/4 fatigue, neuropathy, and diarrhea, as these are the most clinically relevant treatment related toxicities. ORs with 95% CRs were reported for each comparison with sufficient direct evidence available to make network estimates (Appendices S10, S11, S12, and S13). Based on cross-trial comparisons, there was no obvious difference in toxicities for

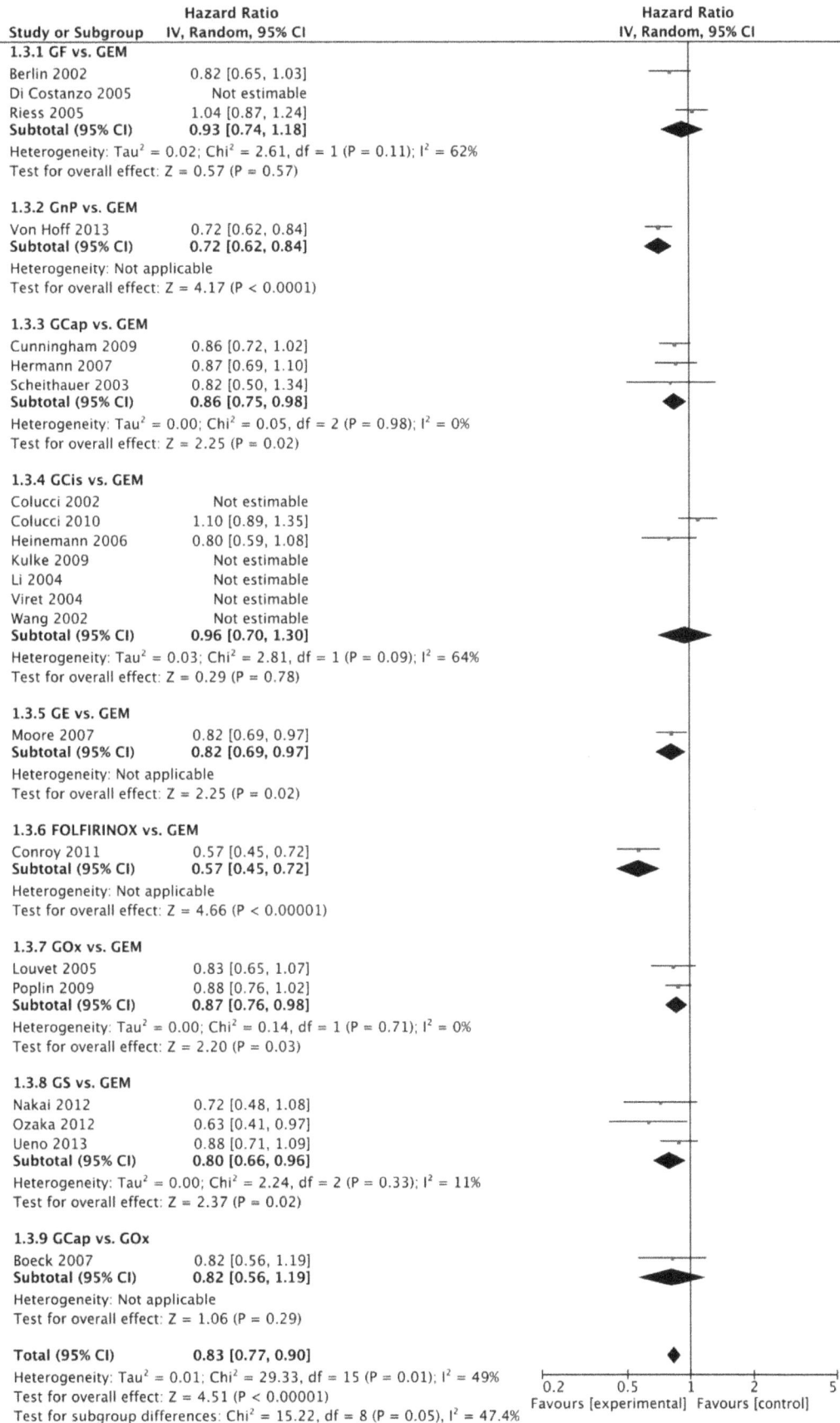

Study or Subgroup	Hazard Ratio IV, Random, 95% CI	Hazard Ratio IV, Random, 95% CI
1.3.1 GF vs. GEM		
Berlin 2002	0.82 [0.65, 1.03]	
Di Costanzo 2005	Not estimable	
Riess 2005	1.04 [0.87, 1.24]	
Subtotal (95% CI)	**0.93 [0.74, 1.18]**	
Heterogeneity: Tau² = 0.02; Chi² = 2.61, df = 1 (P = 0.11); I² = 62%		
Test for overall effect: Z = 0.57 (P = 0.57)		
1.3.2 GnP vs. GEM		
Von Hoff 2013	0.72 [0.62, 0.84]	
Subtotal (95% CI)	**0.72 [0.62, 0.84]**	
Heterogeneity: Not applicable		
Test for overall effect: Z = 4.17 (P < 0.0001)		
1.3.3 GCap vs. GEM		
Cunningham 2009	0.86 [0.72, 1.02]	
Hermann 2007	0.87 [0.69, 1.10]	
Scheithauer 2003	0.82 [0.50, 1.34]	
Subtotal (95% CI)	**0.86 [0.75, 0.98]**	
Heterogeneity: Tau² = 0.00; Chi² = 0.05, df = 2 (P = 0.98); I² = 0%		
Test for overall effect: Z = 2.25 (P = 0.02)		
1.3.4 GCis vs. GEM		
Colucci 2002	Not estimable	
Colucci 2010	1.10 [0.89, 1.35]	
Heinemann 2006	0.80 [0.59, 1.08]	
Kulke 2009	Not estimable	
Li 2004	Not estimable	
Viret 2004	Not estimable	
Wang 2002	Not estimable	
Subtotal (95% CI)	**0.96 [0.70, 1.30]**	
Heterogeneity: Tau² = 0.03; Chi² = 2.81, df = 1 (P = 0.09); I² = 64%		
Test for overall effect: Z = 0.29 (P = 0.78)		
1.3.5 GE vs. GEM		
Moore 2007	0.82 [0.69, 0.97]	
Subtotal (95% CI)	**0.82 [0.69, 0.97]**	
Heterogeneity: Not applicable		
Test for overall effect: Z = 2.25 (P = 0.02)		
1.3.6 FOLFIRINOX vs. GEM		
Conroy 2011	0.57 [0.45, 0.72]	
Subtotal (95% CI)	**0.57 [0.45, 0.72]**	
Heterogeneity: Not applicable		
Test for overall effect: Z = 4.66 (P < 0.00001)		
1.3.7 GOx vs. GEM		
Louvet 2005	0.83 [0.65, 1.07]	
Poplin 2009	0.88 [0.76, 1.02]	
Subtotal (95% CI)	**0.87 [0.76, 0.98]**	
Heterogeneity: Tau² = 0.00; Chi² = 0.14, df = 1 (P = 0.71); I² = 0%		
Test for overall effect: Z = 2.20 (P = 0.03)		
1.3.8 GS vs. GEM		
Nakai 2012	0.72 [0.48, 1.08]	
Ozaka 2012	0.63 [0.41, 0.97]	
Ueno 2013	0.88 [0.71, 1.09]	
Subtotal (95% CI)	**0.80 [0.66, 0.96]**	
Heterogeneity: Tau² = 0.00; Chi² = 2.24, df = 2 (P = 0.33); I² = 11%		
Test for overall effect: Z = 2.37 (P = 0.02)		
1.3.9 GCap vs. GOx		
Boeck 2007	0.82 [0.56, 1.19]	
Subtotal (95% CI)	**0.82 [0.56, 1.19]**	
Heterogeneity: Not applicable		
Test for overall effect: Z = 1.06 (P = 0.29)		
Total (95% CI)	**0.83 [0.77, 0.90]**	
Heterogeneity: Tau² = 0.01; Chi² = 29.33, df = 15 (P = 0.01); I² = 49%		
Test for overall effect: Z = 4.51 (P < 0.00001)		
Test for subgroup differences: Chi² = 15.22, df = 8 (P = 0.05), I² = 47.4%		

0.2   0.5   1   2   5
Favours [experimental] Favours [control]

Figure 3. Forest plot of direct comparisons between the regimens. Forest plot showing hazard ratio comparisons with 95% CI for overall survival (OS) from meta-analyses of direct comparisons between different combinations of gemcitabine (GEM), gemcitabine + fluorouracil (GF), gemcitabine + nab-paclitaxel (GnP), gemcitabine + capecitabine (GCap), gemcitabine + cisplatin (GCis), gemcitabine + erlotinib (GE), FOLFIRINOX, gemcitabine + oxaliplatin (GOx), and G + S1 (GS). I^2 values indicate statistical heterogeneity, where 0% indicates no observed heterogeneity and larger values show increasing heterogeneity (17).

FOLFIRINOX and GnP. The raw numbers of toxicities from each included study can be found in Appendix S3.

When comparing the direct pairwise comparisons to the results generated from the MTC, we found that the results are consistent (Appendix S9).

Discussion

Key Findings and Implications

Based on the analysis of both the direct evidence and MTC, FOLFIRINOX had the highest probability of being the best regimen in terms of both OS (83%) and PFS (80%). In our study, selected comparisons of FOLFIRINOX with the regimens that had the next highest probabilities were also conducted. These results provide further evidence, albeit indirect, that FOLFIR-INOX may be the most effective regimen in the treatment of advanced pancreatic cancer. Although this meta-analysis allows for network comparisons of FOLFIRINOX with other chemotherapy regimens, further large prospective trials with FOLFIR-INOX and the other regimens, especially GnP, would ideally be performed to confirm these results.

For over the past 15 years, gemcitabine monotherapy has been the standard of care in many countries for the treatment of metastatic pancreatic cancer based on its modest clinical efficacy. Although the tumor response rate and survival benefit of gemcitabine is modest, its favorable toxicity profile and ease of administration has led to its wide spread and continued use. Many

studies have attempted to improve on the efficacy of gemcitabine by adding either another chemotherapeutic agent or a targeted agent. However, the vast majority of the phase III studies conducted in this setting have been remarkably negative with the exception of the addition of erlotinib and more recently, nab-paclitaxel [38,39]. Although the gemcitabine and erlotinib study demonstrated a statistically significant overall survival benefit in favour of the combination, the modest improvement in survival and higher toxicity likely influenced a more broad adoption of this regimen.

In addition, a population-based study conducted in 2012 examined the tolerance and effectiveness of FOLFIRINOX at three institutions [40]. The median PFS and OS reported in this study were 7.5 and 13.5 months respectively [40]. The PFS and OS from this study were actually higher than those from the pivotal randomized trial by Conroy et al [12]. However, this may be attributed to the fact that the population-based study included patients with all stages of pancreatic cancer, while the Conroy study enrolled only those with metastatic disease [12,40]. With respect to adverse events, the observed rate of febrile neutropenia in the population-based study was 4.9%, which is similar to the rate observed in the Conroy study (5.4%), which suggests that the results of the clinical trial may be generalizable to an uncontrolled setting. This population-based study concluded that FOLFIR-INOX was clinically effective in the treatment of advanced pancreatic adenocarcinoma and that the toxicity profile of the regimen does not outweigh the benefits in terms of ObRR and

Control	Experimental								
Treatment	G	GF	GCap	GOx	GCis	FOLFIRINOX	GE	GS	GnP
G		0.94 0.75 – 1.18	0.83 0.67 – 1.02	0.88 0.73 – 1.09	0.98 0.75 – 1.24	0.57 0.40 – 0.80	0.82 0.60 – 1.11	0.79 0.62 – 0.98	0.72 0.53 – 0.97
GF	1.06 0.85 – 1.34		0.88 0.65 – 1.20	0.94 0.70 – 1.30	1.04 0.73 – 1.44	0.60 0.40 – 0.92	0.87 0.60 – 1.28	0.84 0.60 – 1.14	0.76 0.54 – 1.12
GCap	1.20 0.98 – 1.48	1.14 0.83 – 1.54		1.07 0.83 – 1.39	1.18 0.85 – 1.60	0.69 0.46 – 1.03	0.99 0.69 – 1.43	0.96 0.69 – 1.27	0.87 0.61 – 1.25
GOx	1.13 0.92 – 1.38	1.07 0.77 – 1.43	0.94 0.72 – 1.20		1.10 0.78 – 1.50	0.64 0.43 – 0.95	0.93 0.64 – 1.33	0.90 0.64 – 1.19	0.82 0.56 – 1.16
GCis	1.03 0.81 – 1.33	0.97 0.70 – 1.36	0.85 0.63 – 1.18	0.91 0.67 – 1.28		0.58 0.39 – 0.90	0.84 0.57 – 1.27	0.81 0.58 – 1.12	0.74 0.51 – 1.10
FOLFIRINOX	1.75 1.24 – 2.48	1.66 1.09 – 2.48	1.45 0.97 – 2.16	1.55 1.05 – 2.33	1.71 1.11 – 2.59		1.44 0.91 – 2.28	1.39 0.90 – 2.07	1.27 0.80 – 1.99
GE	1.22 0.90 – 1.65	1.15 0.79 – 1.66	1.01 0.70 – 1.45	1.08 0.75 – 1.57	1.19 0.79 – 1.74	0.70 0.44 – 1.10		0.97 0.65 – 1.38	0.88 0.58 – 1.34
GS	1.26 1.02 – 1.62	1.19 0.87 – 1.66	1.05 0.79 – 1.44	1.11 0.84 – 1.55	1.23 0.89 – 1.73	0.72 0.48 – 1.11	1.27 0.78 – 2.24		0.91 0.64 – 1.35
GNP	1.39 1.03 – 1.87	1.31 0.89 – 1.89	1.15 0.80 – 1.64	1.23 0.87 – 1.77	1.35 0.91 – 1.96	0.79 0.50 – 1.24	1.12 0.61 – 2.05	0.88 0.50 – 1.41	

Figure 4. Hazard ratio comparisons of overall survival (OS) from mixed treatment comparisons. Median values given with 95% credible regions. Hazard ratios (HRs) expressed as experimental vs. control. G, gemcitabine; GF, gemcitabine + fluorouracil; GCap, gemcitabine + capecitabine; GOx, gemcitabine + oxaliplatin; GCis, gemcitabine + cisplatin; FOLFIRINOX; GE, gemcitabine + erlotinib; GS, gemcitabine + S1; GnP, gemcitabine + nab-paclitaxel.

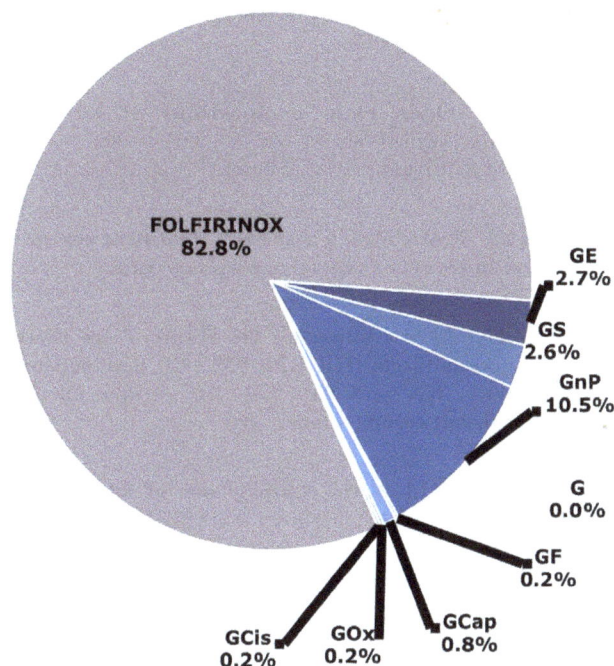

Figure 5. Probabilities that each treatment regimen is the best based on overall survival (OS). G, gemcitabine; GF, gemcitabine + fluorouracil; GCap, gemcitabine + capecitabine; GOx, gemcitabine + oxaliplatin; GCis, gemcitabine + cisplatin; FOLFIRINOX; GE, gemcitabine + erlotinib; GS, gemcitabine + S1; GnP, gemcitabine + nab-paclitaxel.

survival [12,40]. Although FOLFIRINOX demonstrates the best overall survival, progression-free survival, and objective response rate as per the large Phase III Trial [12], it is important to note that this regimen has a higher toxicity profile. When comparing the safety profiles of FOLFIRINOX and GnP from two separate clinical trials, the rate of febrile neutropenia in patients treated with FOLFIRINOX was 5.4% [12], while it was 3% in the GnP group [11]. G-CSF was administered in 42.5% of patients receiving FOLFIRINOX [11] and in 26% of patients receiving GnP [12]. In addition, it is important to note that the FOLFIRINOX study excluded patients older than 75 years of

age and those with an ECOG performance status of 2. Therefore, FOLFIRINOX may be more challenging to prescribe in elderly or frail patients and caution should be taken in these cases. Ongoing prospective population-based studies are being performed to assess the efficacy and safety of FOLFIRINOX outside of clinical trials, which will provide further real life experience of the regimen. In addition, no population-based studies conducted to evaluate the survival benefit and toxicity of GnP so further research should be done in order to compare FOLFIRINOX with GnP in clinical practice.

Strengths and Limitations

There are a number of strengths of the current MTC. For example, a comprehensive and robust search strategy was used, with data being extracted by two authors independently to ensure accuracy. Although MTC allow indirect comparisons to be made, these indirect estimates may be influenced by potential biases and uncertainties. Multiple-treatment comparison meta-analysis should be interpreted with caution and specifically, the underlying assumptions of homogeneity and consistency of studies across the network should be carefully scrutinized. In our study, heterogeneity between studies was indeed assessed and reported using I^2 values. Although some heterogeneity was noted in the comparisons of GCis versus G and GF versus G, all studies in included in the meta-analysis were comparable in terms of patient characteristics and outcomes in the G reference arm (median PFS = 3–4 months, median OS = 6–7 months). The HRs from direct pairwise comparisons and the MTC were also compared and found to be consistent (Appendix S9). A limitation of our analysis was the small number of studies included which is a reflection of the landscape of the medical evidence. For many of the comparisons, data was extracted from only one trial so any biases or limitations from that study were more likely to affect the conclusions drawn from the MTC. Another limitation of this method is that it is based on published group data, rather than individual patient information. Individual patient data may allow for more patterns to be seen in terms of risk factors, however, it would still remain difficult to make strong inferences in such a complex network of treatments.

Both the FOLFIRINOX and nab-paclitaxel trials included only those patients with metastatic pancreatic cancer in contrast to the other gemcitabine combination studies, which enrolled both metastatic and locally advanced pancreatic patients. One of the

Table 1. Comparisons of each regimen with Gemcitabine (G).

Regimen Name	OS Hazard Ratio when compared with G	Projected Median OS (months)*	NNT at 6 months when compared with G	NNT at 1 year when compared with G
FOLFIRINOX	0.57	9.9	6	5
G + nab-paclitaxel	0.72	7.8	9	9
G + S1	0.79	7.2	12	12
G + erlotinib	0.82	6.9	15	14
G + capecitabine	0.83	6.8	16	15
G + oxaliplatin	0.88	6.4	23	23
G + fluorouracil	0.94	6.0	46	47
G + cisplatin	0.98	5.8	141	146
G	—	5.65	—	—

Footnotes: Hazard ratios when comparing each regimen with Gemcitabine (G), projected median overall survival (OS), number needed to treat (NNT) at 6 months and 1 year when compared with G. Projected median OS was calculated using a median OS of 5.65 months as reported by Buris et al (5). Survival and NNT was estimated based on the mixed treatment comparisons results and the method by Altman and Andersen (22).

reasons behind this shift in patient profile of advanced pancreatic studies were the recommendations of a group of experts convened in 2009 by the National Cancer Institute in the United States based on the well described differences in survival between those with locally advanced and metastatic disease. Unfortunately, this difference in patient population across the trials included in our study could not be accounted for. However, given that the inclusion of locally advanced patients tends to magnify the overall and progression free survival, we do not expect this difference in the patients included in the studies to significantly influence our observed results.

As RCTs directly comparing FOLFIRINOX and GnP, or other existing regimens are unlikely to be conducted in advanced pancreatic cancer in the future due to both commercial and scientific reasons, indirect comparisons such as ours may represent the best possible level of evidence as to which regimen is best. Such indirect evidence may still in fact be informative in terms of both clinical and policy decision-making.

Conclusions

Our meta-analysis reviewed and analyzed the existing high-quality evidence for treating advanced pancreatic cancer in an MTC, which help synthesize evidence and may inform decision-making in the absence of direct pairwise comparisons. Based on our MTC, FOLFIRINOX appears to be the most effective regimen, however, direct pairwise comparisons are warranted to definitively address. Existing uncertainties of the relative effectiveness of FOLFIRINOX, as well as the potential toxicities and long-term effects suggest that further clinical trials and longitudinal studies are needed.

Supporting Information

Appendix S1 Summary table of trial characteristics included in systematic review and quantitative synthesis.

Appendix S2 Studies identified through the literature search. The geographic location of the institution of the primary investigator is described in the case where no study location was specified.

Appendix S3 Extracted data for PFS, OS, ObRR, and side effects (febrile neutropenia, neuropathy, fatigue, diarrhea) for each relevant reference arms from the studies included in this review.

Appendix S4 Forest plot showing hazard ratio comparisons with 95% CI for PFS from meta-analyses of direct comparisons between various systemic regimens for advanced pancreatic cancer.

Appendix S5 Hazard ratio comparisons of PFS from network meta-analysis. Median values given with 95% credible regions. HR expressed as experimental vs. control.

Appendix S6 Probabilities that each treatment regimen is the best based on PFS.

Appendix S7 Odds ratio comparisons of objective response rate. Median values given with 95% credible regions. HR expressed as experimental vs. control.

Appendix S8 Probabilities that each treatment regimen is the best in terms of objective response rate.

Appendix S9 Table comparing OS results from direct pairwise comparisons (HR with 95% CI) and network meta-analysis (HR with 95% CR) for various chemotherapy regimen comparisons.

Appendix S10 Odds ratio comparisons of febrile neutropenia rates. Median values given with 95% credible regions. HR expressed as experimental vs. control.

Appendix S11 Odds ratio comparisons of grade 3 or 4 neuropathy rates. Median values given with 95% credible regions. HR expressed as experimental vs. control.

Appendix S12 Odds ratio comparisons of grade 3 or 4 fatigue rates. Median values given with 95% credible regions. HR expressed as experimental vs. control.

Appendix S13 Odds ratio comparisons of grade 3 or 4 diarrhea rates. Median values given with 95% credible regions. HR expressed as experimental vs. control.

Appendix S14 Risk of bias graph for all included trials.

Appendix S15 Risk of bias summary for all included trials.

Checklist S1 Completed PRISMA Checklist for reporting a systematic review and/or meta-analysis.

Acknowledgments

Chris Cameron and Dr. Sharon Straus for their guidance on Bayesian statistical analysis and comments on the manuscript. **Previous Presentations of the Manuscript**: Presented in part in the poster discussion at the Annual Meeting of the American Society of Clinical Oncology 2013, Chicago, USA.

Author Contributions

Conceived and designed the experiments: KC YK DC. Performed the experiments: KC KL KS HL YK. Analyzed the data: KC KL KS. Wrote the paper: KC KS KL HL YK. Revised the manuscript: DC.

References

1. American Cancer Society (2013) Cancer facts and figures 2013. Available: http://www.cancer.org/acs/groups/content/@epidemiologysurveilance/documents/document/acspc-036845.pdf Accessed 2013 July 30.

2. Office for National Statistics (2011) Cancer Survival in England patients diagnosed 2005–2009 followed up to 2010. Available: http://www.ons.gov.uk/ons/rel/cancer-unit/cancer-survival/2005-2009-followed-up-to-2010/stb-cancer-survival-2005-09-and-followed-up-to-2010.html Accessed 2014 July 4.

3. Warsame R, Grothey A (2012) Treatment options for advanced pancreatic cancer: A review. Expert Rev Anticancer Ther 12: 1327–36.
4. Li D, Xie K, Wolff R, Abbruzzese JL (2004) Pancreatic cancer. Lancet 363: 1049–57.
5. Burris HA 3rd, Moore MJ, Andersen J, Green MR, Rothenberg ML, et al. (1997) Improvements in survival and clinical benefit with gemcitabine as first-line therapy for patients with advanced pancreas cancer: a randomized trial. J Clin Oncol 15: 2403–13.
6. Herrmann R, Bodoky G, Ruhstaller T, Glimelius B, Bajetta E, et al. (2007) Gemcitabine plus capecitabine compared with gemcitabine alone in advanced pancreatic cancer: a randomized, multicenter, phase III trial of the Swiss Group for Clinical Cancer Research and the Central European Cooperative Oncology Group. J Clin Oncol 25: 2212–7.
7. Cunningham D, Chau I, Stocken DD, Valle JW, Smith D, et al. (2009) Phase III randomized comparison of gemcitabine versus gemcitabine plus capecitabine in patients with advanced pancreatic cancer. J Clin Oncol 27: 5513–8.
8. Moore MJ, Goldstein D, Hamm J, Figer A, Hecht JR, et al. (2007) Erlotinib plus gemcitabine compared with gemcitabine alone in patients with advanced pancreatic cancer: a phase III trial of the National Cancer Institute of Canada Clinical Trials Group. J Clin Oncol 25: 1960–6.
9. Boeck S, Hoehler T, Seipelt G, Mahlberg R, Wein A, et al. (2008) Capecitabine plus oxaliplatin (CapOx) versus capecitabine plus gemcitabine (CapGem) versus gemcitabine plus oxaliplatin (mGemOx): final results of a multicenter randomized phase II trial in advanced pancreatic cancer. Ann Oncol 19: 340–7.
10. Heinemann V, Quietzsch D, Gieseler F, Gonnermann M, Schonekas H, et al. (2006) Randomized phase III trial of gemcitabine plus cisplatin compared with gemcitabine alone in advanced pancreatic cancer. J Clin Oncol 24: 3946–52.
11. Von Hoff DD, Ervin TJ, Arena FP, Chiorean EG, Infante JR, et al. (2012) Randomized phase III study of weekly *nab*-paclitaxel plus gemcitabine versus gemcitabine alone in patients with metastatic adenocarcinoma of the pancreas (MPACT). J Clin Oncol suppl 34: abstract LBA148.
12. Conroy T, Desseigne F, Ychou M, Bouche O, Guimbaud R, et al. (2011) FOLFIRINOX versus gemcitabine for metastatic pancreatic cancer. N Engl J Med 364: 1817–25.
13. Li T, Puhan MA, Vedula SS, Singh S, Dickersin K (2011) Network meta-analysis-highly attractive but more methodological research is needed. BMC Med 9: 79.
14. Wells GA, Sultan SA, Chen L, Khan M, Coyle D (2009) Indirect Evidence: indirect treatment comparisons in meta-analysis. Ottawa: Canadian Agency for Drugs and Technologies in Health. Available: http://www.cadth.ca/en/products/health-technology-assessment/publication/884 Accessed 2014 July 4.
15. (2008) Erlotinib for the treatment of non-small-cell lung cancer. London: National Institute for Health and Clinical Excellence. Available: http://www.nice.org.uk/Guidance/TA162 Accessed 2014 July 4.
16. Higgins JP, Altman DG (2008) Assessing risk of bias in included studies. In: Higgins JPT, Green S, editors. Cochrane handbook for systematic reviews of interventions. Wiley. pp. 187–241.
17. Parmar MK, Torri V, Stewart L (1998) Extracting summary statistics to perform meta-analyses of the published literature for survival endpoints. Stat Med 17: 2815–34.
18. Sutton AJ, Abrams KR (2001) Bayesian methods in meta-analysis and evidence synthesis. Stat Methods Med Res 10: 277–303.
19. Higgins JP, Thompson SG, Deeks JJ, Altman DG (2003) Measuring inconsistency in meta-analyses. BMJ 327: 557–60.
20. Ntzoufras I (2009) Bayesian modeling using WinBUGS. New York: Wiley. 220 p.
21. Hoglin DC, Hawkins N, Jansen JP, Scott DA, Itzler R, et al. (2011) Conducting Indirect-Treatment-Comparison and Network-Meta-Analysis Studies: Report of the ISPOR Task Force on Indirect Treatment Comparisons Good Research Practices –Part 2. Value Health 14: 429–437.
22. Altman DG, Andersen PK (1999) Calculating the number needed to treat for trials where the outcome is time to an event. BMJ 319: 1492–1495.
23. Berlin JD, Catalano P, Thomas JP, Kugler JW, Haller DG, et al. (2002) Phase III study of gemcitabine in combination with fluorouracil versus gemcitabine alone in patients with advanced pancreatic carcinoma: Eastern Cooperative Oncology Group Trial E2297. J Clin Oncol 20: 3270–5.
24. Colucci G, Giuliani F, Gebbia V, Biglietto M, Rabitti P, et al. (2002) Gemcitabine alone or with cisplatin for the treatment of patients with locally advanced and/or metastatic pancreatic carcinoma: a prospective, randomized phase III study of the Gruppo Oncologia dell'Italia Meridionale. Cancer 94: 902–10.
25. Colucci G, Labianca R, Di Costanzo F, Gebbia V, Carteni G, et al. (2010) Randomized phase III trial of gemcitabine plus cisplatin compared with single-agent gemcitabine as first-line treatment of patients with advanced pancreatic cancer: the GIP-1 study. J Clin Oncol 28: 1645–51.
26. Di Costanzo F, Carlini P, Doni L, Massidda B, Mattioli R, et al. (2005) Gemcitabine with or without continuous infusion 5-FU in advanced pancreatic cancer: a randomised phase II trial of the Italian oncology group for clinical research (GOIRC). Br J Cancer 93: 185–9.
27. Kulke MH, Tempero MA, Niedzwiecki D, Hollis DR, Kindler HL et al. (2009) Randomized phase II study of gemcitabine administered at a fixed dose rate or in combination with cisplatin, docetaxel, or irinotecan in patients with metastatic pancreatic cancer: CALGB 89904. J Clin Oncol 27: 5506–12.
28. Li CP, Chao Y (2004) A prospective randomized trial of gemcitabine alone or gemcitabine plus cisplatin in the treatment of metastatic pancreatic cancer. J Clin Oncol, 2004 ASCO Annual Meeting Proceedings (Post-Meeting Edition) 22: Abstract 4144.
29. Louvet C, Labianca R, Hammel P, Lledo G, Zampino MG, et al. (2005) Gemcitabine in combination with oxaliplatin compared with gemcitabine alone in locally advanced or metastatic pancreatic cancer: results of a GERCOR and GISCAD phase III trial. J Clin Oncol 23: 3509–16.
30. Nakai Y, Isayama H, Sasaki T, Sasahira N, Tsujino T, et al. (2012) A multicentre randomised phase II trial of gemcitabine alone vs gemcitabine and S-1 combination therapy in advanced pancreatic cancer: GEMSAP study. Br J Cancer 106: 1934–9.
31. Ozaka M, Matsumura Y, Ishii H, Omuro Y, Itoi T, et al. (2012) Randomized phase II study of gemcitabine and S-1 combination versus gemcitabine alone in the treatment of unresectable advanced pancreatic cancer (Japan Clinical Cancer Research Organization PC-01 study). Cancer Chemother Pharmacol 69: 1197–204.
32. Poplin E, Feng Y, Berlin J, Rothenberg ML, Hochster H, et al. (2009) Phase III, randomized study of gemcitabine and oxaliplatin versus gemcitabine (fixed-dose rate infusion) compared with gemcitabine (30-minute infusion) in patients with pancreatic carcinoma E6201: a trial of the Eastern Cooperative Oncology Group. J Clin Oncol 27: 3778–85.
33. Riess A, Niedergethmann HM, Molk ISM, Hammer C, Zippel K, et al. (2005) A Randomised, Prospective, Multicenter, Phase III trial of Gemcitabine, 5-Fluorouracil (5-FU), Folinic Acid vs. Gemcitabine alone in Patients with Advanced Pancreatic Cancer. J Clin Oncol, 2005 ASCO Annual Meeting Proceedings 23: Abstract 4009.
34. Scheithauer W, Schull B, Ulrich-Pur H, Schmid K, Raderer M, et al. (2003) Biweekly high-dose gemcitabine alone or in combination with capecitabine in patients with metastatic pancreatic adenocarcinoma: a randomized phase II trial. Ann Oncol 14: 97–104.
35. Ueno H, Ioka T, Ikeda M, Ohkawa S, Yanagimoto H, et al. (2013) Randomized phase III study of gemcitabine plus S-1, S-1 alone, or gemcitabine alone in patients with locally advanced and metastatic pancreatic cancer in Japan and Taiwan: GEST study. J Clin Oncol 31: 1640–8.
36. Viret F, Ychou M, Lepille D, Mineur L, Navarro F, et al. (2004) Gemcitabine in combination with cisplatin (GP) versus gemcitabine (G) alone in the treatment of locally advanced or metastatic pancreatic cancer: Final results of a multicenter randomized phase II study. J Clin Oncol, 2004 ASCO Annual Meeting Proceedings 22: Abstract 4118.
37. Wang X, Ni Q, Jin M, Li Z, Wu Y, et al. (2002) Gemcitabine or gemcitabine plus cisplatin for in 42 patients with locally advanced or metastatic pancreatic cancer. Zhonghua zhong liu za zhi. Chinese journal of oncology 24: 404–7.
38. Von Hoff DD, Ervin T, Arena FP, Chiorean EG, Infante J, et al. (2013) Increased survival in pancreatic cancer with nab-paclitaxel plus gemcitabine. N Engl J Med 369: 1691–703.
39. Philip PA, Mooney M, Jaffe D, Eckhardt G, Moore M, et al. (2009) Consensus Report of the National Cancer Institute Clinical Trials Planning Meeting on a Pancreas Cancer Treatment. J Clin Oncology 27: 5660–9.
40. Peddi PF, Lubner S, McWilliams R, Tan BR, Picus J, et al. (2012) Multi-institutional experience with FOLFIRINOX in pancreatic adenocarcinoma. JOP 13: 497–501.

2

Synergism between Basic Asp49 and Lys49 Phospholipase A$_2$ Myotoxins of Viperid Snake Venom *In Vitro* and *In Vivo*

Diana Mora-Obando[1], Julián Fernández[1], Cesare Montecucco[2], José María Gutiérrez[1], Bruno Lomonte[1]*

1 Instituto Clodomiro Picado, Facultad de Microbiología, Universidad de Costa Rica, San José, Costa Rica, **2** Department of Biomedical Sciences, University of Padova, Padova, Italy

Abstract

Two subtypes of phospholipases A$_2$ (PLA$_2$s) with the ability to induce myonecrosis, 'Asp49' and 'Lys49' myotoxins, often coexist in viperid snake venoms. Since the latter lack catalytic activity, two different mechanisms are involved in their myotoxicity. A synergism between Asp49 and Lys49 myotoxins from *Bothrops asper* was previously observed *in vitro*, enhancing Ca^{2+} entry and cell death when acting together upon C2C12 myotubes. These observations are extended for the first time *in vivo*, by demonstrating a clear enhancement of myonecrosis by the combined action of these two toxins in mice. In addition, novel aspects of their synergism were revealed using myotubes. Proportions of Asp49 myotoxin as low as 0.1% of the Lys49 myotoxin are sufficient to enhance cytotoxicity of the latter, but not the opposite. Sublytic amounts of Asp49 myotoxin also enhanced cytotoxicity of a synthetic peptide encompassing the toxic region of Lys49 myotoxin. Asp49 myotoxin rendered myotubes more susceptible to osmotic lysis, whereas Lys49 myotoxin did not. In contrast to myotoxic Asp49 PLA$_2$, an acidic non-toxic PLA$_2$ from the same venom did not markedly synergize with Lys49 myotoxin, revealing a functional difference between basic and acidic PLA$_2$ enzymes. It is suggested that Asp49 myotoxins synergize with Lys49 myotoxins by virtue of their PLA$_2$ activity. In addition to the membrane-destabilizing effect of this activity, Asp49 myotoxins may generate anionic patches of hydrolytic reaction products, facilitating electrostatic interactions with Lys49 myotoxins. These data provide new evidence for the evolutionary adaptive value of the two subtypes of PLA$_2$ myotoxins acting synergistically in viperid venoms.

Editor: Chi Zhang, University of Texas Southwestern Medical Center, United States of America

Funding: Funding support by the Graduate Studies Program, Universidad de Costa Rica; International Centre for Genetic Engineering and Biotechnology, Italy (CRP/COS13-01); and Vicerrectoria de Investigacion, Universidad de Costa Rica (741-B4-100). The funders had no role in study design, data collection and analysis, decision to publish, or preparation of the manuscript.

* Email: bruno.lomonte@ucr.ac.cr

Introduction

Phospholipases A$_2$ (PLA$_2$s) are widespread enzymes in snake venoms, where they play major toxic roles in the immobilization and/or killing of prey [1,2]. Among their diverse activities, myotoxicity is a clinically relevant effect which may lead to severe tissue damage and associated sequelae in envenomings [3–5]. Two divergent ancestral PLA$_2$ genes representing the group I and group II scaffolds, respectively, were recruited and expressed in the venom gland secretions of Elapidae and Viperidae [6]. Through a process of accelerated evolution [7], these genes accumulated mutations that converted their corresponding non-toxic proteins into potent toxins, most notably displaying neurotoxicity and/or myotoxicity. The independent emergence of such toxic activities in these two lineages of advanced snakes illustrates a case of convergent evolution [8,9]. A growing body of knowledge has been gathered on the characterization of PLA$_2$ toxins, but the structural bases for their toxicity and precise modes of action

remain only partially understood, thus leaving opened a number of challenging questions [10].

In the venoms of viperid snakes, two subtypes of myotoxic PLA$_2$s can be found, commonly referred to as 'Asp49' and 'Lys49' variants. The latter, first described in the venom of *Agkistrodon piscivorus piscivorus* [11] and then isolated from many viperid venoms [9], present the substitution of Asp49 by Lys49, a critical change in the catalytic center of the molecule which, together with key amino acid substitutions located in the calcium-binding loop, precludes catalysis [12–14]. Therefore, in sharp contrast with their Asp49 PLA$_2$ counterparts, the Lys49 myotoxins are enzymatically-inactive PLA$_2$ homologues, or 'PLA$_2$-like' proteins [13,15–18].

Notwithstanding their difference in catalytic activity, both Lys49 and Asp49 PLA$_2$ variants display myotoxicity *in vivo* [4,19–21]. The Asp49 PLA$_2$s depend on their enzymatic activity to induce skeletal muscle damage, since their catalytic inactivation by covalently modifying His48 with *p*-bromophenacyl bromide results in the loss of myotoxicity [22–24]. Furthermore, the toxic effects of

Asp49 PLA$_2$s on myogenic cells in culture can be mimicked by the products of their hydrolytic activity, i.e. fatty acids and lysophospholipids [25], and hydrolysis of muscle phospholipids of the external monolayer of the sarcolemma by these enzymes has been demonstrated in myotubes in culture as well as in injected mouse muscles [26]. On the other hand, the catalytic-independent mechanism by which Lys49 PLA$_2$ homologues induce myonecrosis, has been shown to depend on a cluster of amino acids at their C-terminal region which directly affect the integrity of the sarcolemma [9,18,27–32].

The venom of *Bothrops asper*, the snake species causing the majority of envenomings in Central America [33], contains multiple Asp49 and Lys49 myotoxin isoforms [34] as well as a non-myotoxic, acidic Asp49 PLA$_2$ [35]. In a previous study, a synergistic action between purified Asp49 and Lys49 myotoxins was observed *in vitro*, whereby these two proteins induced a more pronounced Ca^{2+} entry and cell death by acting together, rather than individually [25]. The present work extends these observations by exploring for the first time whether the same phenomenon occurs *in vivo*, and characterizes in further detail relevant features of this synergistic action using an *in vitro* model.

Materials and Methods

Isolation of phospholipases A$_2$ from *Bothrops asper* venom

Snake venom was collected from specimens kept at the Serpentarium of Instituto Clodomiro Picado, under authorization of the University of Costa Rica. Pooled venom of *Bothrops asper* from the Pacific versant of Costa Rica was fractionated as previously described, to obtain myotoxin II (Lys49; UniProt accession P24605; [36,37]), a mixture of myotoxins I/III (Asp49; P20474; [24,38]), and an acidic BaspPLA$_2$-II (non-myotoxic, Asp49; P86389; [35]). Fractionation steps included ion-exchange chromatography followed by semi-preparative reverse-phase HPLC on a C$_8$ support. Purity was assessed by nano-electrospray mass spectrometry in a QTrap-3200 instrument (ABSciex) operated in positive ion-enhanced multicharge mode, as described [24]. The lack of contaminating Asp49 PLA$_2$s in the Lys49 myotoxin II preparation was evaluated by assaying PLA$_2$ activity using the synthetic substrate 4-nitro-3-octanoyloxybenzoic acid [39]. Conversely, the lack of contaminating Lys49 myotoxins in the basic Asp49 PLA$_2$ myotoxin preparation was ascertained by automated N-terminal amino acid sequencing using a PPSQ-33A

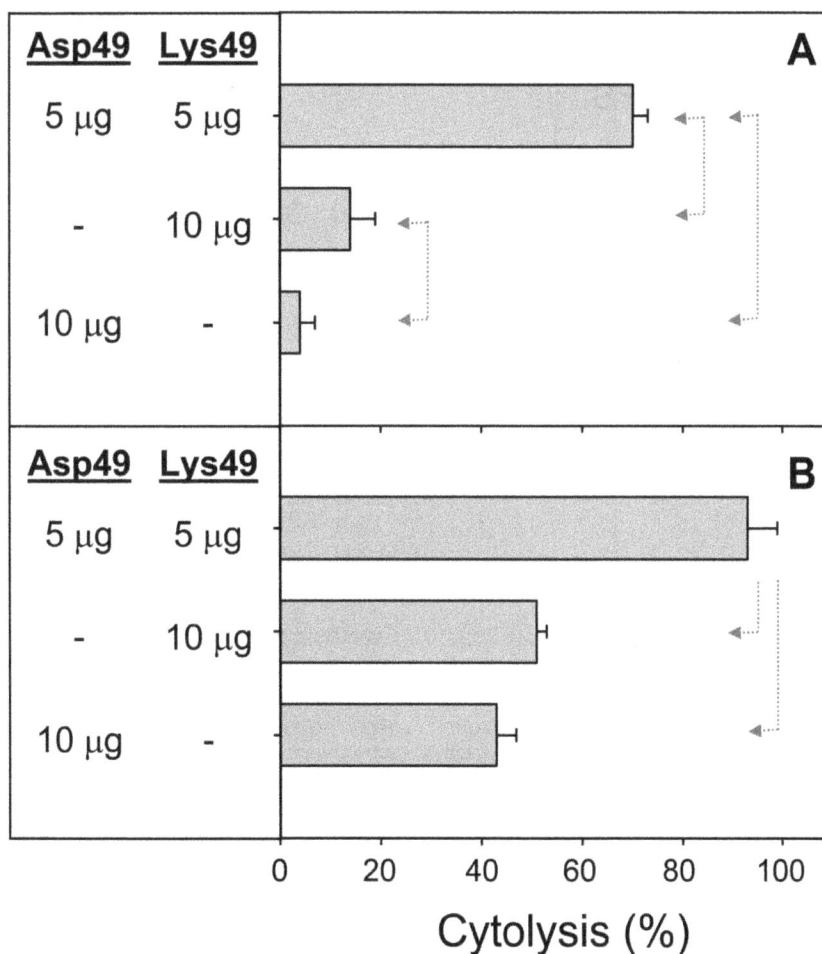

Figure 1. Cytotoxic activity of Asp49 and Lys49 myotoxins from *Bothrops asper*, alone or in combination, upon C2C12 myoblasts (A) or myotubes (B). The indicated amounts of toxins were added in a total volume of 150 µL. Cytolysis was determined by the release of lactate dehydrogenase to the medium 3 h after exposure of the cells to the toxins, as described in Materials and Methods. Reference values of 0 and 100% cytolysis were established using medium or 0.1% Triton X-100 in medium, respectively. Each bar represents mean ± SD of triplicate cell cultures. Statistically significant differences (p<0.05) between two groups are indicated by dotted arrow lines.

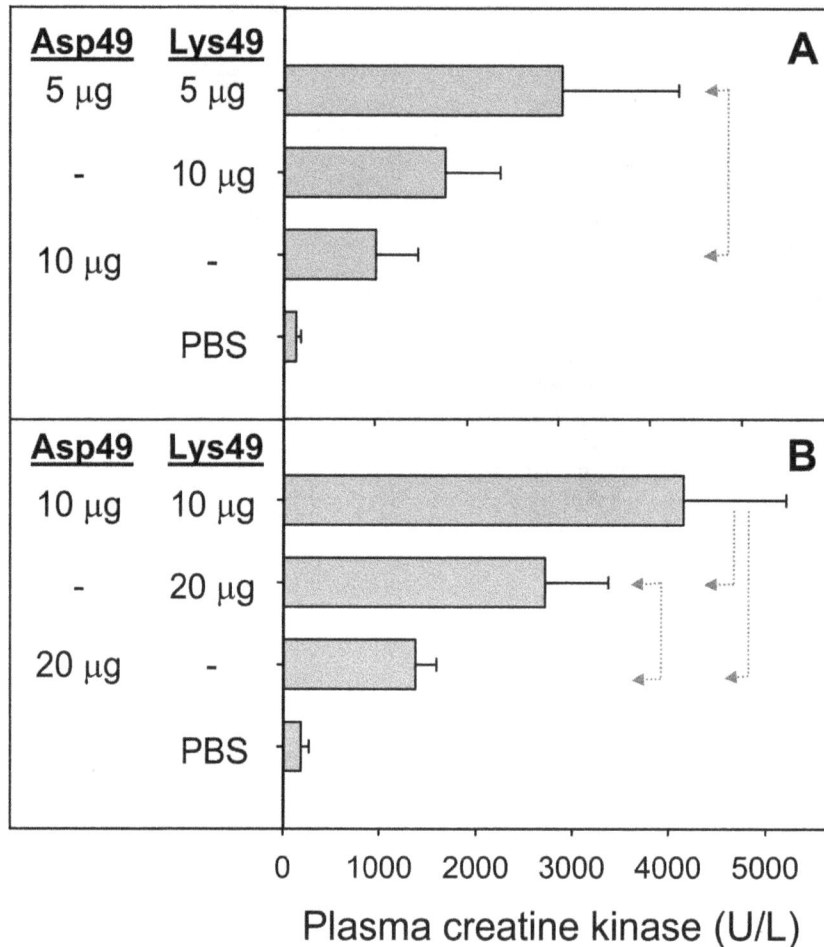

Figure 2. Myotoxic activity of Asp49 and Lys49 myotoxins from *Bothrops asper*, alone or in combination, injected by intramuscular route in CD-1 mice. Plasma creatine kinase activity was determined 3 h after injection of the indicated amounts of toxins. Control mice received only vehicle (PBS). Each bar represents mean ± SD of five animals. Statistically significant differences (p<0.05) between two groups are indicated by dotted arrow lines. Synergistic action is shown at a total dose of 10 µg in (A) or 20 µg in (B), respectively.

instrument (Shimadzu Biotech), to confirm the absence of a Leucine signal in the fifth cycle [24].

Asp49 PLA₂ myotoxin inactivation by *p*-bromophenacyl bromide

Three mg of the Asp49 myotoxin were dissolved in 1 mL of 0.1 M Tris, 0.7 mM EDTA, pH 8.0 buffer. Then, 125 µL of *p*-bromophenacyl bromide (*p*-BPB; 1.5 mg/mL in ethanol; Sigma Chemical Co.) were added and incubated at room temperature (20–25°C) for 24 h [22]. Excess *p*-BPB and salts were eliminated by RP-HPLC on a semi-preparative C$_8$ column, as described [24]. The protein was collected and finally dried by vacuum centrifugation at 45°C. Enzymatic inactivation was determined on the 4-nitro-3-octanoyloxybenzoic acid substrate in comparison to a control sample of the toxin which was processed identically but omitting the *p*-BPB reagent [24].

Synthetic peptide of *B. asper* myotoxin II

A synthetic peptide from the C-terminal region of *B. asper* myotoxin II, corresponding to the sequence 115–129 (KKYR-YYLKPLCKK; p$^{115-129}$), was obtained from a commercial provider (Peptide 2.0, Inc.). The peptide was synthesized with native endings by Fmoc chemistry, and its molecular mass was in

agreement with the expected value. Its purity level was at least 95% by RP-HPLC analysis. This 13-mer peptide has been shown to reproduce, albeit with a lower potency, the cytolytic effect of myotoxin II *in vitro* [27,29].

Cytotoxic activity

Cytolysis was determined on the murine myogenic cell line C2C12 (ATCC-CRL1772) using a lactate dehydrogenase release assay, as previously described [40]. Cells were grown at subconfluent densities in 25 cm^2 bottles using Dulbecco's modified Eagle's medium supplemented with 10% fetal calf serum (DMEM, 10% FCS), and after detachment by trypsin, they were seeded in 96-well plates for cytotoxicity assays. These were performed either at the myoblast stage in near-confluent cell monolayers, or after their differentiation to fused myotubes in DMEM 1% FCS during 4–6 additional days. In brief, different amounts of toxins, alone or in combination, dissolved in 150 µL of assay medium (DMEM, 1% FCS) were added to the cells immediately after removal of their medium, and incubated for 3 h at 37°C. Then, an aliquot of cell supernatant (60 µL) was collected from each well and the lactate dehydrogenase (LDH) activity was quantified by a UV kinetic assay (LDH-BR Cromatest, Linear Chemicals). Controls for 0 and 100% cytotoxicity consisted of assay medium, and 0.1%

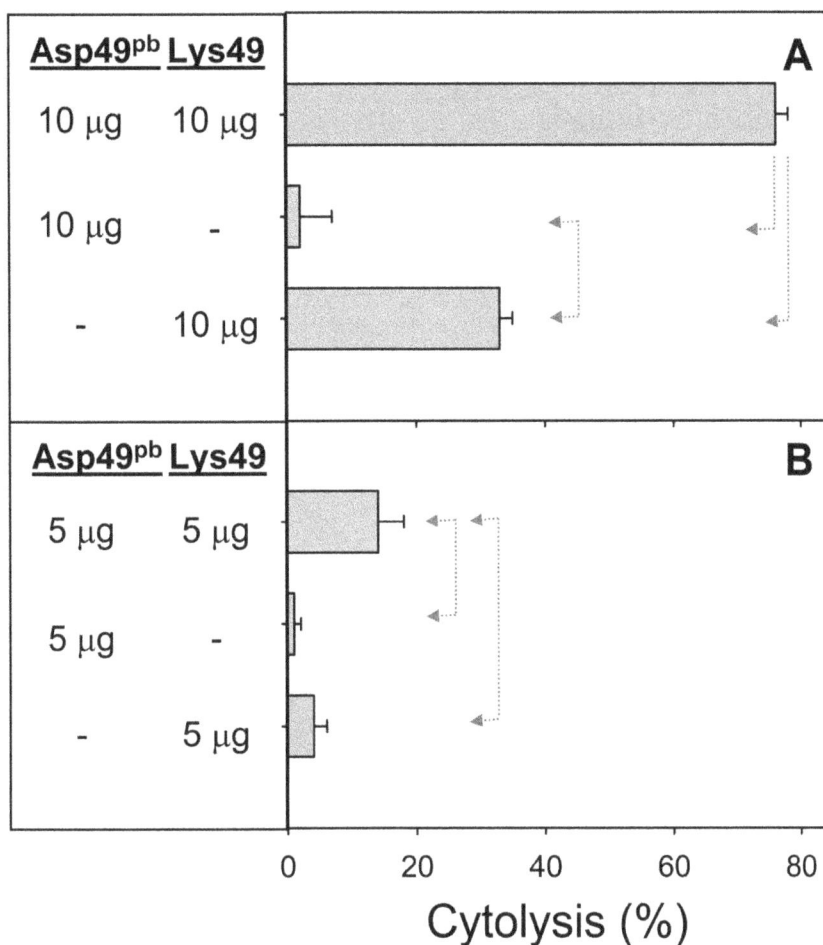

Figure 3. Cytotoxic activity of _p_-bromophenacyl bromide-modified Asp49 myotoxin (Asp49^{pb}) and Lys49 myotoxin, alone or in combination at 10 µg (A) or 5 µg (B), upon C2C12 myotubes. The indicated amounts of toxins were added in a total volume of 150 µL. Cytolysis was determined by the release of lactate dehydrogenase to the medium, 3 h after exposure of the cells to the toxins. Each bar represents mean ± SD of triplicate cell cultures. Statistically significant differences (p<0.05) between two groups are indicated by dotted arrow lines.

Triton X-100 diluted in assay medium, respectively. All samples were assayed in triplicate wells.

Myotoxic activity

Myotoxic activity was determined in CD-1 mice of 18 to 20 g of body weight, using five animals per group. These _in vivo_ assays were kept to a minimum, and followed protocols authorized by the Institutional Committee for the Use and Care of Animals (CICUA; #132-13), University of Costa Rica. Mice were housed in cages for groups of 4–6, and provided food and water _ad libitum_. Different amounts of the toxins, alone or in combination, dissolved in 50 µL of phosphate-buffered saline (PBS; 0.12 M NaCl, 0.04 M sodium phosphate buffer, pH 7.2), were injected into the gastrocnemius muscle [36]. A control group of mice received an identical injection of PBS. After 3 h, blood was collected from the tip of the tail into a heparinized capillary and centrifuged. The plasma creatine kinase (CK) activity, expressed in U/L, was determined using a UV kinetic assay (CK-Nac, Biocon Diagnostik). Mice were sacrificed by CO_2 inhalation, at the end of the experiment.

Statistical analysis

ANOVA was used for the comparison of mean values from more than two groups, followed by Tukey-Kramer tests, with a statistical significance of p<0.05. Calculations were performed with the aid of the Instat (GraphPad) software.

Results

The cytolytic effect of Asp49 and Lys49 myotoxins, when added alone or in combination to cultures of the C2C12 cell line at the myoblast or myotube stages, is shown in Fig. 1. A higher effect of these toxins was observed in myotubes than in myoblasts, and this difference was more conspicuous in the case of the Asp49 myotoxin, which was extremely weak against myoblasts (Fig. 1A). In both stages of cell differentiation, the combination of the myotoxins induced a significantly higher cytotoxicity in comparison to the effect of either toxin alone (Fig. 1). The observed effect was clearly synergistic and not just additive. Following these _in vitro_ findings, experiments were performed in mice to determine whether synergism also occurs in mature skeletal muscle, under conditions that mimic envenomings. Results revealed a clear enhancement of myotoxicity, as judged by the higher release of creatine kinase from damaged muscle to the

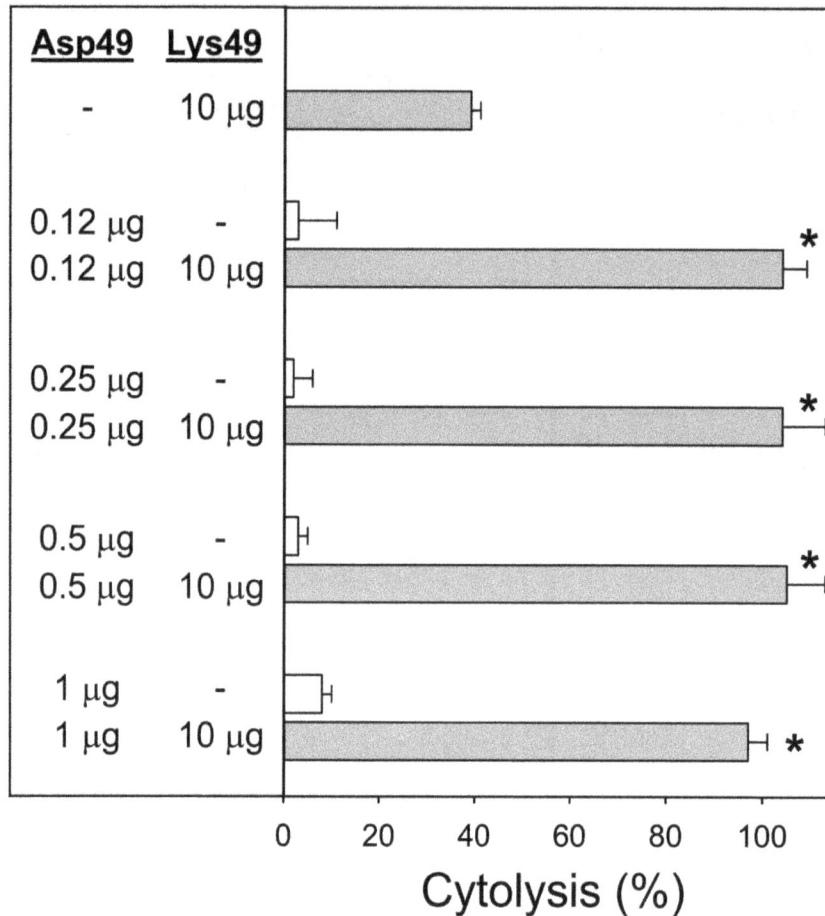

Figure 4. Cytotoxic activity of a fixed amount of Lys49 myotoxin, alone or in combination with low amounts of Asp49 myotoxin, upon C2C12 myotubes. The indicated amounts of toxins were added in a total volume of 150 μL. Cytolysis was determined by the release of lactate dehydrogenase to the medium, 3 h after exposure of the cells to the toxins. Each bar represents mean ± SD of triplicate cell cultures. All values from cultures where the Lys49 myotoxin was added together with Asp49 myotoxin were significantly different (p<0.05) from the value of cultures exposed only to Lys49 myotoxin (indicated by asterisks).

plasma, when the Asp49 and Lys49 toxins acted in combination (Fig. 2). When injected individually, the myotoxic effect of the Lys49 myotoxin was significantly higher than that of the Asp49 myotoxin at the dose of 20 μg (Fig. 2B), although at 10 μg (Fig. 2A) this same trend did not reach statistical significance.

The role of enzymatic activity of the Asp49 myotoxin in the synergistic effect was studied by using a p-BPB-treated enzyme. This protein incorporated a single molecule of the alkylating agent, as confirmed by mass spectrometry, and its catalytic activity was inactivated by 97% in comparison to the untreated enzyme [24]. As shown in Fig. 3, the cytolytic action of the p-BPB-treated Asp49 myotoxin alone was negligible, as expected. However, the combined action of this protein and the Lys49 myotoxin caused a significant enhancement of the cytotoxic effect (Fig. 3). Since the p-PBP-treated Asp49 protein had a residual enzymatic activity of 3%, further experiments were designed to determine whether the synergistic effect observed in Fig. 3 could be due to this low residual catalytic action or, alternatively, depended on a non-catalytic mechanism of the Asp49 myotoxin. Therefore, low amounts of native Asp49 myotoxin, within a range comparable to the proportion of enzymatically-active protein remaining in the p-PBP-treated toxin, were combined with a fixed amount of Lys49 myotoxin (Fig. 4). Results showed that Asp49 myotoxin amounts

as low as 0.12 μg (representing 1.2% in proportion to the Lys49 myotoxin), efficiently enhanced the cytotoxicity of the final mixture. Importantly, these low amounts of Asp49 myotoxin were essentially non-toxic when added alone to the myotube cultures (Fig. 4). Further titration of the effect of Asp49 myotoxin in this assay showed that the minimal amount of enzyme capable of inducing synergism was 0.012 μg. The reverse combination, i.e. addition of low quantities of Lys49 myotoxin to a fixed amount of Asp49 myotoxin (Fig. 5) did not enhance toxicity, thus revealing the directionality of the synergistic mechanism.

Since results indicated that the Asp49 myotoxin, even in low amounts, enhanced the toxicity of the Lys49 myotoxin, an experiment was performed to determine whether this synergy was dependent on the time lapse when a low amount of the enzyme was in contact with myotubes, before the addition of the Lys49 myotoxin. The Asp49 enzyme was incubated with the cells for the time periods indicated in Fig. 6 (0, 15, 30, or 60 min) and, after five washings of the cell cultures, the Lys49 myotoxin was added. A significant enhancement in cytotoxicity was recorded at all time periods of cell exposure to the Asp49 myotoxin and, remarkably, even when the Asp49 enzyme was added and the cultures were immediately washed (Fig. 6).

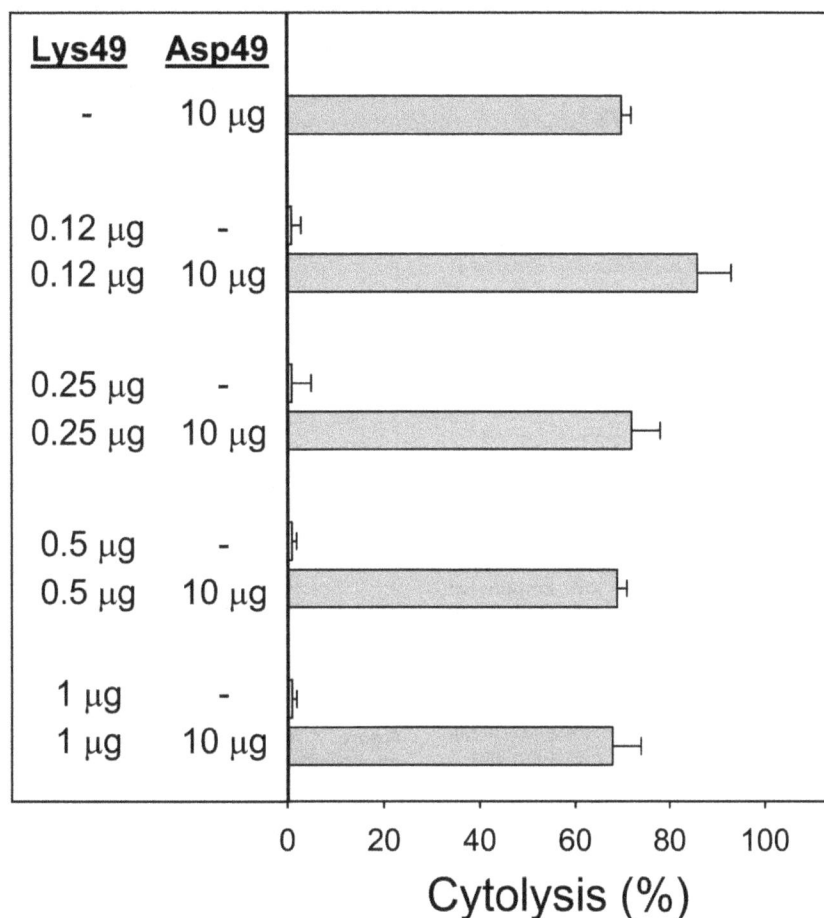

Figure 5. Cytotoxic activity of a fixed amount of Asp49 myotoxin, alone or in combination with low amounts of Lys49 myotoxin, upon C2C12 myotubes. The indicated amounts of toxins were added in a total volume of 150 µL. Cytolysis was determined by the release of lactate dehydrogenase to the medium, 3 h after exposure of the cells to the toxins. Each bar represents mean ± SD of triplicate cell cultures. None of the values from cultures where the Asp49 myotoxin was added together with Lys49 myotoxin were significantly different from the value of cultures exposed only to Asp49 myotoxin.

Since *B. asper* venom also contains non-myotoxic Asp49 PLA$_2$s whose role in venom's toxicity is uncertain [35], the effect of a non-myotoxic, acidic-type PLA$_2$ on the cytotoxic activity of Lys49 myotoxin was investigated in the same assay system, as shown in Fig. 7. As expected, the acidic Asp49 enzyme alone was not cytotoxic. The combination of this enzyme with the Lys49 myotoxin caused a significant, although only modest increase at 5 µg, but at 10 µg was unable to significantly enhance cytotoxicity of Lys49 myotoxin (Fig. 7).

The synergistic effect of a low amount of Asp49 myotoxin toward the cytolytic action of the synthetic peptide p$^{115-129}$ of the Lys49 myotoxin was evaluated. As presented in Fig. 8, the cytotoxicity induced by this short peptide was markedly enhanced by acting in combination with the Asp49 enzyme.

Finally, the cytotoxic action of Asp49 and Lys49 myotoxins was tested under conditions of osmotic imbalance of the cells. Culture medium was rendered hypotonic by the addition of varying proportions of purified water (8:2, 9:1, or 10:1 water:medium), and cytolysis was determined in the absence or presence of the toxins. As shown in Fig. 9A, myotubes exposed to a low amount of Asp49 myotoxin became significantly more susceptible to the deleterious action of the hypotonic media, at 8:2 and 9:1 water:medium proportions. At the 10:0 proportion (100% water), the high

cytolysis in the control cells did not allow the assessment of the effect of myotoxin. In contrast, when the same experiment was performed with Lys49 myotoxin, it revealed that this protein does not alter the susceptibility of myotubes exposed to hypotonic conditions, since similar values of cytolysis were observed in the absence or in the presence of the toxin (Fig. 9B).

Discussion

The venoms of many viperid snake species contain variable combinations of PLA$_2$s, often including acidic and basic variants, and among the latter, Asp49 and Lys49 myotoxin subtypes [1,2,41]. Phylogenetic analyses indicate that the myotoxic Lys49 PLA$_2$ homologues diverged from ancestral, group II Asp49 PLA$_2$s before the separation of Viperinae and Crotalinae [42–46]. Intriguingly, however, a comprehensive examination of the bioactivities displayed by myotoxic Asp49 and Lys49 variants does not provide evident clues on the possible evolutionary advantages conferred by the emergence of the latter, since both types of myotoxins share similar toxicological profiles and often coexist in viperid venoms [41]. Nevertheless, the abundance and common occurrence of these coexisting myotoxins in many viperid species strongly suggest that they provided an important adaptive value in this family of snakes. Several speculative hypotheses have

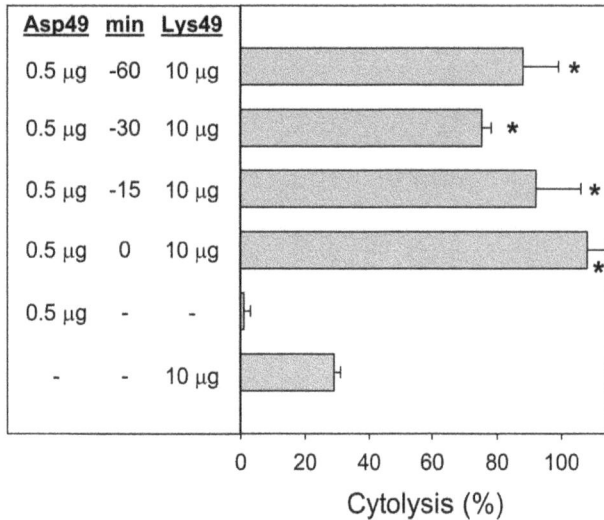

Figure 6. Cytotoxic activity of a fixed amount of Lys49 myotoxin, alone or in combination with a low amount of Asp49 myotoxin. In this experiment, Asp49 myotoxin was first incubated for variable periods of time with C2C12 myotubes, and then washed five times, before the addition of Lys49 myotoxin. The indicated amounts of toxins were added in a total volume of 150 µL. Cytolysis was determined by the release of lactate dehydrogenase to the medium 3 h after exposure of the cells to the toxins. Each bar represents mean ± SD of triplicate cell cultures. All values from cultures where the Lys49 myotoxin was added together with Asp49 myotoxin were significantly different (p<0.05) from the value of cultures exposed only to Lys49 myotoxin (indicated by asterisks).

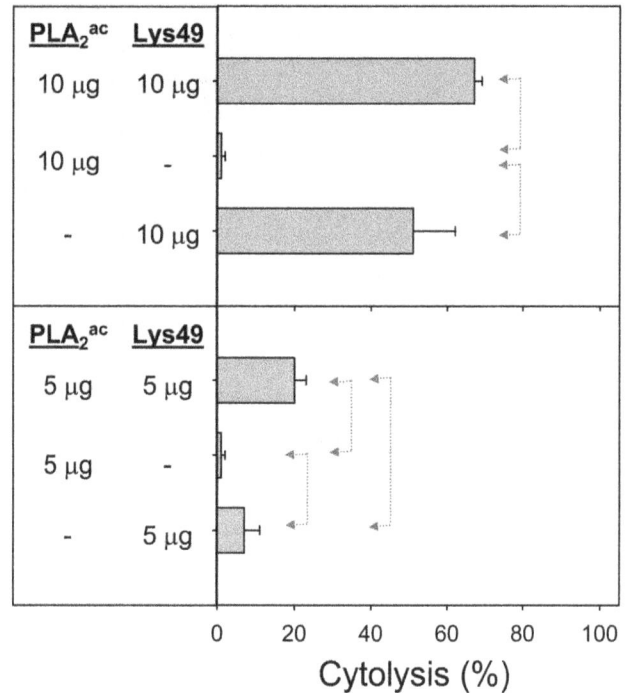

Figure 7. Cytotoxic activity of *Bothrops asper* acidic Asp49 phospholipase A$_2$ (PLA$_2$^{ac}) and Lys49 myotoxin, alone or in combination, upon C2C12 myotubes. The indicated amounts of toxins were added in a total volume of 150 µL. Cytolysis was determined by the release of lactate dehydrogenase to the medium, 3 h after exposure of the cells to the toxins. Each bar represents mean ± SD of triplicate cell cultures. Statistically significant differences (p< 0.05) between two groups are indicated by dotted arrow lines.

been proposed to envisage their possible biological significance and adaptive value, one of them being synergism [41]. A synergistic action upon myogenic cells in culture was first described by Cintra-Francischinelli et al. [25] using the C2C12 cell line as a target for Asp49 and Lys49 myotoxins isolated from the venom of *B. asper*. The present study extends such observations by demonstrating the *in vivo* synergism between these two toxin subtypes in the induction of myonecrosis, and provides further insights into the mechanisms of this synergistic effect.

In agreement with previous studies [47], a higher susceptibility of myotubes over myoblasts to the cytotoxic action of the myotoxins was observed. Also, myoblasts were more resistant to the Asp49 than to the Lys49 myotoxin, as previously noted by Cintra-Francischinelli et al. [25]. In agreement with their study, a cytotoxic synergism between the two toxins was confirmed at both stages of cell differentiation, i.e. myoblasts and myotubes. In order to determine whether these *in vitro* observations would also apply to the biologically-relevant target of myotoxins, i.e. skeletal muscle, similar experiments were conducted in mice. Results demonstrate, for the first time *in vivo*, a clear enhancement of myotoxicity by the combined action of Asp49 and Lys49 myotoxins in comparison to the effect of either protein alone. Therefore, these *in vivo* results add new evidence for the adaptive value of the emergence of two subtypes of PLA$_2$ myotoxins in viperid venoms, conferring a selective advantage in the light of the high energetic costs of venom protein synthesis [48,49].

The *in vivo* synergism hereby shown helps to clarify previous observations in the study of viperid PLA$_2$ myotoxins, in which crude venoms have generally been found to induce stronger myonecrosis than their isolated myotoxins [50]. Although the contribution to muscle damage of other toxin types in crude

venoms (for example hemorrhagic metalloproteinases that promote myonecrosis as a consequence of ischemia [51]) cannot be excluded, the combined action of Asp49 and Lys49 myotoxins in crude venoms may explain the higher magnitude of myonecrosis

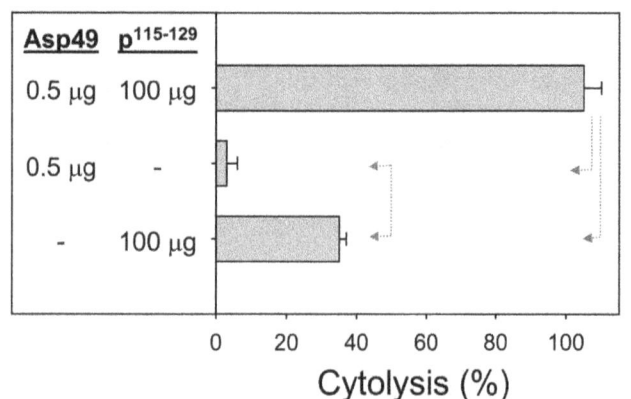

Figure 8. Cytotoxic activity of Asp49 myotoxin and the synthetic C-terminal peptide p115–129 of Lys49 myotoxin II from *Bothrops asper*, alone or in combination, upon C2C12 myotubes. The indicated amounts of toxin or synthetic peptide were added in a total volume of 150 µL. Cytolysis was determined by the release of lactate dehydrogenase to the medium, 3 h after exposure of the cells to the toxins. Each bar represents mean ± SD of triplicate cell cultures. Statistically significant differences (p<0.05) between two groups are indicated by dotted arrow lines.

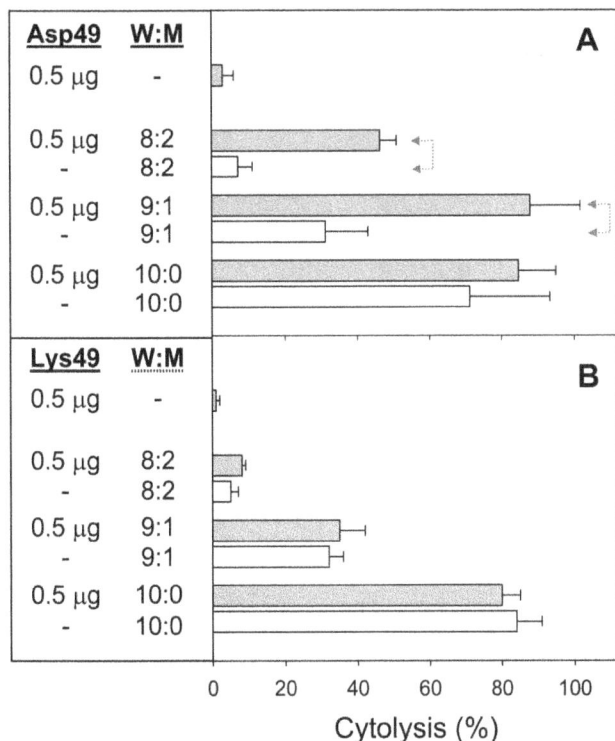

Figure 9. Cytotoxic activity of Asp49 and Lys49 myotoxins upon C2C12 myotubes under conditions of osmotic imbalance. Myotubes were grown and differentiated as described in Methods, and then the toxins (0.5 µg) were added to cultures using medium that contained the indicated proportion of water (gray bars). (**A**) Asp49 myotoxin, (**B**) Lys49 myotoxin. Control cultures exposed to the same medium conditions, in the absence of toxin, were tested in parallel (empty bars). Cytolysis was determined by the release of lactate dehydrogenase to the medium after 3 h. Each bar represents mean ± SD of triplicate cell cultures. Statistically significant differences (p<0.05) between two groups are indicated by dotted arrow lines.

observed in comparison to experiments analyzing isolated myotoxins. Also noteworthy, the extent of muscle damage induced by the Lys49 myotoxin was higher than that caused by the Asp49 myotoxin. This result is in agreement with the proposal that Lys49 PLA$_2$ homologues in viperids provided an adaptive value due to their increased myotoxic potency, as discussed by Kihara et al. [52]. From the biological standpoint, an enhanced capacity to induce acute muscle damage might contribute to a more efficient digestion of the abundant muscle mass characteristic of mammalian prey [41].

In order to determine whether the synergistic mechanism depends on the PLA$_2$ activity of Asp49 myotoxins, this enzyme was inactivated by p-BPB [22,24]. As expected, the modified enzyme essentially lost its cytotoxic effect upon myotubes, but surprisingly, still enhanced the cytotoxic action of the Lys49 myotoxin. This prompted us to evaluate the residual catalytic activity of the p-BPB-treated protein, which revealed a low, but detectable hydrolysis of the 4-nitro-3-octanoyloxybenzoic acid substrate, estimated at the level of 3% of the unmodified toxin. On this basis, it was hypothesized that such low residual catalytic activity could either be sufficient for the occurrence of synergism, or, alternatively, the synergistic action recorded for the p-BPB-modified enzyme would be caused by a catalytically-independent mechanism. To address this point, the synergism was subsequently tested with low amounts of the Asp49 PLA$_2$, mimicking the

proportion of the corresponding residual enzymatic activity of the p-BPB-treated myotoxin. Results confirmed that these minute amounts of the Asp49 PLA$_2$, in sublytic concentrations *per se*, are able to enhance the cytolytic effect of the Lys49 myotoxin. Therefore, the mechanism of synergism can be attributed to the enzymatic action of the Asp49 PLA$_2$, rather than a catalytically-independent activity. A similar conclusion was reached by Cintra-Francischinelli et al. [25] by observing that, in the absence of external Ca^{2+}, the Asp49 myotoxin was unable to synergize with the Lys49 myotoxin due to the requirement of this ion for enzymatic activity. Moreover, the present observations underscore that even a very low enzymatic activity of Asp49 myotoxins is enough for the observed synergism. The directionality of this 'micro-synergism' was determined to be an enhancement of the Lys49 myotoxin toxicity by the Asp49 enzyme, and not the converse, since low quantities of the Lys49 myotoxin did not increase the toxic action of the Asp49 enzyme.

Using this experimental model of 'micro-synergism', additional aspects of the mechanisms involved were explored. Since the enhancing action of the Asp49 enzyme was found to depend on its catalytic activity, an experiment was designed to evaluate the effect of time by which cells were exposed to the enzyme, then washed, and finally exposed to the Lys49 myotoxin. The addition of a low amount of the Asp49 PLA$_2$, independently of the time of contact with the cells, and even when washing was performed immediately after toxin addition, led to a similar cytotoxic outcome. One possibility to explain these findings would be that the enzyme binds rapidly and tightly to the cell membrane interface, and is not removed by gentle washing, thus continuing its enzymatic phospholipid hydrolysis. The assessment of this hypothesis awaits experiments on the binding of myotoxins to myotubes.

Considering that the venom of *B. asper* contains, in addition to basic PLA$_2$s, an acidic Asp49 PLA$_2$ enzyme which is devoid of myotoxicity (BaspPLA$_2$-II [35]), it was of interest to evaluate whether this enzyme would be able to synergize with the basic Lys49 myotoxin. In agreement with its previous characterization, this acidic PLA$_2$ did not induce cytotoxicity *per se*. Interestingly, this acidic PLA$_2$ did not induce the marked synergistic effect observed with the basic Asp49 PLA$_2$. Only a minor increase in cytotoxicity was observed when using 5 µg of the enzyme, and twice this amount did not result in a statistically significant difference of toxicity in comparison to the Lys49 myotoxin alone. This result is noteworthy because the acidic enzyme displays a higher catalytic activity than the Asp49 myotoxin [35]. This suggests that the acidic enzyme might be unable to hydrolyze the membrane phospholipids of myotubes, which in turn would explain both its lack of toxicity and its inability to synergize effectively with Lys49 myotoxin in this model. This hypothesis awaits the study of phospholipid hydrolysis in the membranes of myotubes and muscle cells by using highly sensitive methodologies such as mass spectrometry [26]. Hence, the role of this non-cytotoxic acidic PLA$_2$ in the overall toxicity of the venom of *B. asper*, if any, remains uncertain.

A key question arising from the present and previous studies on the synergism between Asp49 PLA$_2$ and Lys49 myotoxins concerns how does the enzymatic activity of the former enhance the toxicity of the latter. To the best of our knowledge, the first evidence of a synergism between these two myotoxin subtypes was reported by Shen and Cho [53], who demonstrated that an Asp49 PLA$_2$ from *A. p. piscivorus* venom enhanced the liposome-permeabilizing effect of a Lys49 PLA$_2$ homologue isolated from the same source. These authors proposed that the Asp49 enzyme would generate anionic patches of hydrolytic reaction products on the surface of the liposomes, which in turn would facilitate the

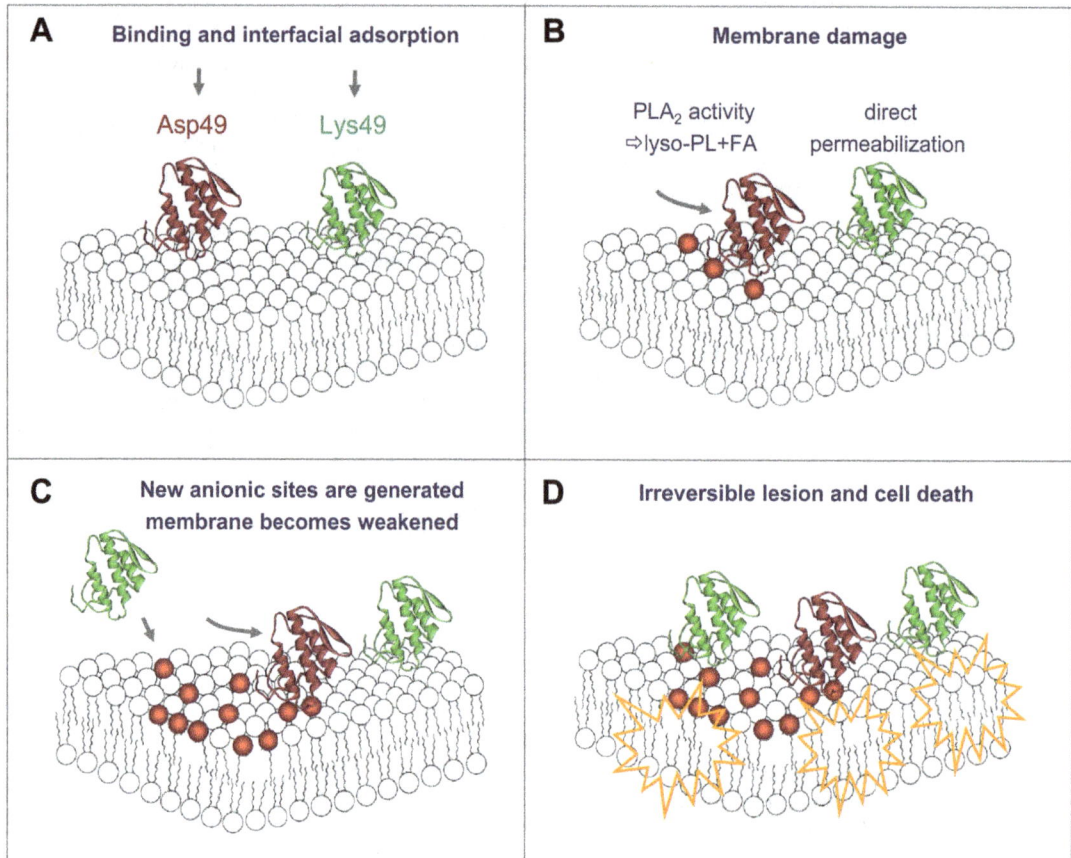

Figure 10. Cartoon representation of the hypothetical synergistic mechanism involved in the membrane-damaging activity of Asp49 and Lys49 myotoxins. Toxins bind to the muscle cell membrane (A), although acceptor moieties for this event are unknown. Each toxin type by its own has the ability to induce cytotoxicity *in vitro* or myonecrosis *in vivo* through membrane damage. Asp49 myotoxins destabilize the membrane by the enzymatic hydrolysis of phospholipids (PL) and consequent production of lyso-PL and fatty acids (FA), whereas Lys49 myotoxins exert a direct permeabilization mechanism via their C-terminal region (B). When acting in combination, FA produced by the Asp49 myotoxin generate new anionic sites (red spheres) that facilitate the binding of Lys49 myotoxin through electrostatic interactions (C). The membrane becomes more unstable due to PL hydrolysis *per se*, and to the accumulation of the reaction products (lysoPL and FA). As a result of these combined actions of Asp49 and Lys49 myotoxins, membrane damage is enhanced and the cell becomes irreversibly damaged (D). Note that the toxin cartoons are represented as monomers for simplicity, although these toxins actually occur as homodimers. Cartoons are not drawn to scale, and the orientation of the toxins interacting with the membrane is only for illustrative purposes.

electrostatic interaction with the Lys49 protein, and the consequent permeabilization of the vesicle by the non-enzymatic, bilayer penetrating mechanism of the latter [53]. A second, non-mutually exclusive explanation for the synergistic mechanism was proposed [25], whereby the products of phospholipid hydrolysis generated by the Asp49 myotoxin would enhance the toxicity of the Lys49 myotoxin by rendering the cell membrane more unstable, based on the observation that a mixture of lysophospholipids and fatty acids can mimic *per se* the membrane-damaging effects of Asp49 myotoxin.

In the present study, two further observations shed light into the possible mechanisms of the synergy here characterized. First, the bioactive C-terminal synthetic peptide of the Lys49 myotoxin, $p^{115-129}$, reproduced the synergy phenomenon observed with the parent protein, i.e. the concomitant addition of a low amount of Asp49 PLA$_2$ and peptide resulted in a significant enhancement of myotube cell lysis. Since this peptide is highly cationic [27], this finding (as well as results with the parent Lys49 myotoxin) would be compatible with the hypothesis that proposed the generation of new anionic sites by the Asp49 enzyme [53], thus facilitating the electrostatic interaction of the peptide or the toxin with the

membrane [54,55], and ultimately its permeabilization [8,25,56]. However, the higher cytotoxic effect of the peptide when acting in synergy with the Asp49 myotoxin might as well be explained by the weakening of membrane stability caused by the catalytic action of the enzyme and by the generation of fatty acids and lysophospholipids. Thus, results of this experiment would be compatible with both mechanisms. The hypothesis of a general membrane-destabilizing effect caused by phospholipid hydrolysis and generation of products that alter its biophysical properties [25] is hereby experimentally supported. It was hypothesized that, if the myotube cell membrane becomes more unstable due to the enzymatic action of Asp49 PLA$_2$, it would be less capable of resisting a non-specific stress such as osmotic imbalance. Results confirmed this assumption, showing that myotubes were significantly more susceptible to the cytolysis induced by hypotonic media if they were exposed to minute amounts of Asp49 PLA$_2$ myotoxin. In contrast, myotubes exposed to equivalent amounts of Lys49 myotoxin were equally susceptible to lysis in such hypotonic media, as in the absence of toxin. Taken together, these experiments indicate that the enhancing mechanism for the toxicity of Lys49 myotoxins exerted by Asp49 PLA$_2$ myotoxin involves at least the weakening of cell membrane integrity by the latter. On the other hand, the possibility of the generation of new anionic sites by the accumulation of products of catalysis in the membrane remains to be tested, but clearly, both mechanisms would rely on the enzymatic activity of the Asp49 PLA$_2$ myotoxin (Fig. 10).

The synergistic mechanism hereby characterized contributes to rationalize the evolutionary advantage for the emergence of two different subtypes of PLA$_2$ myotoxins in the venom of many viperids, which are known to use two contrasting molecular mechanisms that lead to the same outcome: skeletal muscle necrosis. The synergy between Asp49 and Lys49 myotoxins represents at least one advantageous feature for the snakes, but additional mechanisms of adaptive value for these toxins may also exist [41], for example in their possible functional interactions with other snake venom components [57,58]. On a more general ground, our findings stress the need to study the action of snake venoms from a holistic perspective, i.e. by analyzing not only the action of purified toxins, but also the interaction of different components in the context of the complexity of snakebite envenoming.

Acknowledgments

The valuable contribution of Juan Manuel Ureña and Wan-Chih Tsai in various aspects of this work is gratefully acknowledged. This study was performed in partial fulfillment of the M.Sc degree of D. Mora-Obando at the University of Costa Rica.

Author Contributions

Conceived and designed the experiments: BL DMO. Performed the experiments: DMO. Analyzed the data: DMO JF CM JMG BL. Contributed reagents/materials/analysis tools: JF. Contributed to the writing of the manuscript: BL JMG CM.

References

1. Kini RM (1997) Venom Phospholipase A$_2$ Enzymes. Structure, Function, and Mechanisms. John Wiley & Sons, Chichester, 511.
2. Kini RM (2003) Excitement ahead: structure, function and mechanism of snake venom phospholipase A$_2$ enzymes. Toxicon 42: 827–840.
3. Harris JB, Cullen MJ (1990) Muscle necrosis caused by snake venoms and toxins. Electron Microsc Rev 3: 183–211.
4. Gutiérrez JM, Ownby CL (2003) Skeletal muscle degeneration induced by venom phospholipases A$_2$: insights into the mechanisms of local and systemic myotoxicity. Toxicon 42: 915–931.
5. Warrell DA (2010) Snakebite. Lancet 375, 77–88.
6. Fry BG, Wüster W (2004) Assembling an arsenal: origin and evolution of the snake venom proteome inferred from phylogenetic analysis of toxin sequences. Mol Biol Evol 21: 870–883.
7. Nakashima KI, Nobuhisa I, Deshimaru M, Nakai M, Ogawa T, et al. (1995) Accelerated evolution in the protein-coding regions is universal in crotalinae snake venom gland phospholipase A$_2$ isozyme genes. Proc Natl Acad Sci USA 92: 5605–5609.
8. Lomonte B, Gutiérrez JM (2011) Phospholipases A$_2$ from Viperidae snake venoms: how do they induce skeletal muscle damage? Acta Chim Slovenica 58: 647–659.
9. Lomonte B, Rangel J (2012) Snake venom Lys49 myotoxins: from phospholipases A$_2$ to non-enzymatic membrane disruptors. Toxicon 60: 520–530.
10. Gutiérrez JM, Lomonte B (2013) Phospholipases A$_2$: unveiling the secrets of a functionally versatile group of snake venom toxins. Toxicon 62: 27–39.
11. Maraganore JM, Merutka G, Cho W, Welches W, Kézdy FJ, et al. (1984) A new class of phospholipases A$_2$ with lysine in place of aspartate 49. J Biol Chem 259: 13839–13843.
12. Arni RK, Ward RJ (1996) Phospholipase A$_2$ - a structural review. Toxicon 34: 827–841.
13. Petan T, Križaj I, Pungerčar J (2007) Restoration of enzymatic activity in a Ser-49 phospholipase A$_2$ homologue decreases its Ca^{2+}-independent membrane-damaging activity and increases its toxicity. Biochemistry 46: 12795–12809.
14. Fernandes CAH, Marchi-Salvador DP, Salvador GM, Silva MCO, Costa TR, et al. (2010) Comparison between apo and complexed structures of bothropstoxin-I reveals the role of Lys122 and Ca2+-binding loop region for the catalytically inactive Lys49-PLA$_2$s. J Structural Biol 171: 31–43.
15. Scott DL, Achari A, Vidal JC, Sigler PB (1992) Crystallographic and biochemical studies of the (inactive) Lys-49 phospholipase A$_2$ from the venom of *Agkistrodon piscivorus piscivorus*. J Biol Chem 267: 22645–22657.
16. Ward RJ, Chioato L, de Oliveira AHC, Ruller R, Sá JM (2002) Active-site mutagenesis of a Lys49-phospholipase A$_2$: biological and membrane-disrupting activities in the absence of catalysis. Biochem J 362: 89–96.
17. Lomonte B, Angulo Y, Calderón L (2003) An overview of Lysine-49 phospholipase A$_2$ myotoxins from crotalid snake venoms and their structural determinants of myotoxic action. Toxicon 42: 885–901.
18. dos Santos JI, Fernandes CAH, Magro AJ, Fontes MRM (2009) The intriguing phospholipases A$_2$ homologues: relevant structural features on myotoxicity and catalytic inactivity. Prot Peptide Lett 16: 887–893.
19. Gutiérrez JM, Lomonte B (1995) Phospholipase A$_2$ myotoxins from *Bothrops* snake venoms. Toxicon 33: 1405–1424.
20. Gutiérrez JM, Lomonte B (1997) Phospholipase A$_2$ myotoxins from Bothrops snake venoms. In: Kini RM (Ed), Venom phospholipase A$_2$ enzymes: structure, function, and mechanism. John Wiley & Sons, England, 321–352.
21. Montecucco C, Gutiérrez JM, Lomonte B (2008) Cellular pathology induced by snake venom phospholipase A$_2$ myotoxins and neurotoxins: common aspects of their mechanisms of action. Cell Mol Life Sci 65: 2897–2912.
22. Díaz-Oreiro C, Gutiérrez JM (1997) Chemical modification of histidine and lysine residues of myotoxic phospholipases A$_2$ isolated from *Bothrops asper* and

Bothrops godmani snake venoms: effects on enzymatic and pharmacological properties. Toxicon 35: 241–252.
23. Soares AM, Giglio JR (2003) Chemical modifications of phospholipases A$_2$ from snake venoms: effects on catalytic and pharmacological properties. Toxicon 42: 855–868.
24. Mora-Obando D, Díaz-Oreiro C, Angulo Y, Gutiérrez JM, Lomonte B (2014) Role of enzymatic activity in muscle damage and cytotoxicity induced by *Bothrops asper* Asp49 phospholipase A$_2$ myotoxins: are there additional effector mechanisms involved? Peer J (in press). dx.doi.org/10.7717/peerj.569.
25. Cintra-Francischinelli M, Pizzo P, Rodrigues-Simioni L, Ponce-Soto L, Rossetto O, et al. (2009) Calcium imaging of muscle cells treated with snake myotoxins reveals toxin synergism and presence of receptors. Cell Mol Life Sci 66: 1718–1728.
26. Fernández J, Caccin P, Koster G, Lomonte B, Gutiérrez JM, et al. (2013) Muscle phospholipid hydrolysis by *Bothrops asper* Asp49 and Lys49 phospholipase A$_2$ myotoxins - distinct mechanisms of action. FEBS J 280: 3878–3886.
27. Lomonte B, Moreno E, Tarkowski A, Hanson LÅ, Maccarana M (1994) Neutralizing interaction between heparins and myotoxin II, a Lys-49 phospholipase A$_2$ from *Bothrops asper* snake venom. Identification of a heparin-binding and cytolytic toxin region by the use of synthetic peptides and molecular modeling. J Biol Chem 269: 29867–29873.
28. Lomonte B, Angulo Y, Santamaría C (2003) Comparative study of synthetic peptides corresponding to region 115–129 in Lys49 myotoxic phospholipases A$_2$ from snake venoms. Toxicon 42: 307–312.
29. Núñez CE, Angulo Y, Lomonte B (2001) Identification of the myotoxic site of the Lys49 phospholipase A$_2$ from *Agkistrodon piscivorus piscivorus* snake venom: synthetic C-terminal peptides from Lys49, but not from Asp49 myotoxins, exert membrane-damaging activities. Toxicon 39: 1587–1594.
30. Chioato L, de Oliveira AHC, Ruller R, Sá JM, Ward RJ (2002) Distinct sites for myotoxic and membrane-damaging activities in the C-terminal region of a Lys49-phospholipase A$_2$. Biochem J 366: 971–976.
31. Chioato L, Ward RJ (2003) Mapping structural determinants of biological activities in snake venom phospholipases A$_2$ by sequence analysis and site directed mutagenesis. Toxicon 42, 869–883.
32. Cintra-Francischinelli M, Pizzo P, Angulo Y, Gutiérrez JM, Montecucco C, et al. (2010) The C-terminal region of a Lys49 myotoxin mediates Ca^{2+} influx in C2C12 myotubes. Toxicon 55: 590–596.
33. Gutiérrez JM (1995) Clinical toxicology of snakebite in Central America. In: Handbook of Clinical Toxicology of Animal Venoms and Poisons (Meier J, White J, eds), 645–665. CRC Press, Boca Ratón.
34. Angulo Y, Lomonte B (2009) Biochemistry and toxicology of toxins purified from the venom of the snake *Bothrops asper*. Toxicon 54: 949–957.
35. Fernández J, Gutiérrez JM, Angulo Y, Sanz L, Juárez P, et al. (2010) Isolation of an acidic phospholipase A$_2$ from the venom of the snake *Bothrops asper* of Costa Rica: Biochemical and toxicological characterization. Biochimie 92: 273–283.
36. Lomonte B, Gutiérrez JM (1989) A new muscle damaging toxin, myotoxin II, from the venom of the snake *Bothrops asper* (terciopelo). Toxicon 27: 725–733.
37. Francis B, Gutiérrez JM, Lomonte B, Kaiser II (1991) Myotoxin II from *Bothrops asper* (Terciopelo) venom is a lysine-49 phospholipase A$_2$. Archs Biochem Biophys 284: 352–359.
38. Kaiser II, Gutierrez JM, Plummer D, Aird SD, Odell GV (1990) The amino acid sequence of a myotoxic phospholipase from the venom of *Bothrops asper*. Archs Biochem Biophys 278: 319–325.
39. Holzer M, Mackessy SP (1996) An aqueous endpoint assay of snake venom phospholipase A$_2$. Toxicon 34: 1149–1155.
40. Lomonte B, Angulo Y, Rufini S, Cho W, Giglio JR, et al. (1999) Comparative study of the cytolytic activity of myotoxic phospholipases A$_2$ on mouse

endothelial (tEnd) and skeletal muscle (C2C12) cells *in vitro*. Toxicon 37: 145–158.

41. Lomonte B, Angulo Y, Sasa M, Gutiérrez JM (2009) The phospholipase A_2 homologues of snake venoms: biological activities and their possible adaptive roles. Prot Peptide Lett 16: 860–876.

42. Moura-da-Silva AM, Paine MJI, Diniz MRV, Theakston RDG, Crampton JM (1995) The molecular cloning of a phospholipase A_2 from *Bothrops jararacussu* snake venom: evolution of venom group II phospholipase A_2's may imply gene duplications. J Mol Evol 41: 174–179.

43. Tsai IH, Chen YH, Wang YM, Tu MC, Tu AT (2001) Purification, sequencing, and phylogenetic analyses of novel Lys-49 phospholipases A_2 from the venoms of rattlesnakes and other pit vipers. Archs Biochem Biophys 394: 236–244.

44. Angulo Y, Olamendi-Portugal T, Alape-Girón A, Possani LD, Lomonte B (2002) Structural characterization and phylogenetic relationships of myotoxin II from *Atropoides (Bothrops) nummifer* snake venom, a Lys49 phospholipase A_2 homologue. Int J Biochem Cell Biol 34: 1268–1278.

45. Lynch VJ (2007) Inventing an arsenal: adaptive evolution and neofunctionalization of snake venom phospholipase A_2 genes. BMC Evolut Biol 7: 2, doi:10.1186/1471-2148-7-2.

46. dos Santos JI, Cintra-Francischinelli M, Borges RJ, Fernandes CAH, Pizzo P, et al., (2010) Structural, functional, and bioinformatics studies reveal a new snake venom homologue phospholipase A_2 class. Proteins 79: 61–78.

47. Angulo Y, Lomonte B (2005) Differential susceptibility of C2C12 myoblasts and myotubes to group II phospholipase A_2 myotoxins from crotalid snake venoms. Cell Biochem Funct 23: 307–313.

48. McCue MD (2006) Cost of producing venom in three North American pitviper species. Copeia 2006: 818–825.

49. Morgenstern D, King GF (2013) The venom optimization hypothesis revisited. Toxicon 63: 120–128.

50. Gutiérrez JM, Ownby CL, Odell GV (1984) Isolation of a myotoxin from *Bothrops asper* venom: partial characterization and action on skeletal muscle. Toxicon 22: 115–128.

51. Gutiérrez JM, Romero M, Núñez J, Chaves F, Borkow G, et al., (1995) Skeletal muscle necrosis and regeneration after injection of BaH1, a hemorrhagic metalloproteinase isolated from the venom of the snake *Bothrops asper* (terciopelo). Exp Mol Pathol 62: 28–41.

52. Kihara H, Uchikawa R, Hattori S, Ohno M (1992) Myotoxicity and physiological effects of three *Trimeresurus flavoviridis* phospholipases A_2. Biochem Int 28: 895–903.

53. Shen Z, Cho W (1995) Membrane leakage induced by synergetic action of Lys-49 and Asp-49 *Agkistrodon piscivorus piscivorus* phospholipases A_2: implications in their pharmacological activities. Int J Biochem Cell Biol 27: 1009–1013.

54. Díaz C, Gutiérrez JM, Lomonte B, Gené JA (1991) The effect of myotoxins isolated from *Bothrops* snake venoms on multilamellar liposomes: relationship to phospholipase A_2, anticoagulant and myotoxic activities. Biochim Biophys Acta 1070: 455–460.

55. Rufini S, Cesaroni P, Desideri A, Farias R, Gubenšek F, et al., (1992) Calcium ion-independent membrane leakage induced by phospholipase-like myotoxins. Biochemistry 31: 12424–12430.

56. Cintra-Francischinelli M, Caccin P, Chiavegato A, Pizzo P, Carmignoto G, et al., (2010) *Bothrops* snake myotoxins induce a large efflux of ATP and potassium with spreading of cell damage and pain. Proc Natl Acad Sci USA 107: 14140–14145.

57. Bustillo S, Gay CC, García Denegri ME, Ponce-Soto LA, Bal de Kier Joffe E, et al., (2012) Synergism between baltergin metalloproteinase and Ba SPII RP4 PLA_2 from *Bothrops alternatus* venom on skeletal muscle (C2C12) cells. Toxicon 59, 338–343.

58. Caccin P, Pellegatti P, Fernández J, Vono M, Cintra-Francischinelli M, et al. (2013) Why myotoxin-containing snake venoms possess powerful nucleotidases? Biochem Biophys Res Comm 430, 1289–1293.

3

Site-Specific Chemoenzymatic Labeling of Aerolysin Enables the Identification of New Aerolysin Receptors

Irene Wuethrich⁹, Janneke G. C. Peeters⁹, Annet E. M. Blom, Christopher S. Theile, Zeyang Li, Eric Spooner, Hidde L. Ploegh*, Carla P. Guimaraes

Whitehead Institute for Biomedical Research, Department of Biology, Massachusetts Institute of Technology, Cambridge, Massachusetts, United States of America

Abstract

Aerolysin is a secreted bacterial toxin that perforates the plasma membrane of a target cell with lethal consequences. Previously explored native and epitope-tagged forms of the toxin do not allow site-specific modification of the mature toxin with a probe of choice. We explore sortase-mediated transpeptidation reactions (sortagging) to install fluorophores and biotin at three distinct sites in aerolysin, without impairing binding of the toxin to the cell membrane and with minimal impact on toxicity. Using a version of aerolysin labeled with different fluorophores at two distinct sites we followed the fate of the C-terminal peptide independently from the N-terminal part of the toxin, and show its loss in the course of intoxication. Making use of the biotinylated version of aerolysin, we identify mesothelin, urokinase plasminogen activator surface receptor (uPAR, CD87), glypican-1, and CD59 glycoprotein as aerolysin receptors, all predicted or known to be modified with a glycosylphosphatidylinositol anchor. The sortase-mediated reactions reported here can be readily extended to other pore forming proteins.

Editor: Ludger Johannes, Institut Curie, France

Funding: Funding provided by R01 AI087879, http://grants.nih.gov/grants/funding/r01.htm. The funders had no role in study design, data collection and analysis, decision to publish, or preparation of the manuscript.

Competing Interests: The authors have declared that no competing interests exist.

* Email: ploegh@wi.mit.edu

⁹ These authors contributed equally to this work.

Introduction

Pore-forming toxins (PFTs) comprise the largest category of bacterial virulence factors [1]. One of the better studied examples is aerolysin secreted by *Aeromonas hydrophila* [2]. Aerolysin forms a homo-heptameric pore that spans the plasma membrane of the target cell [3] [4], leading to depletion of small ions [5] [6] [7], rapid loss of ATP, and ultimately cell death [8].

Aerolysin is secreted as an inactive monomeric precursor, proaerolysin, comprising a 43-residue C-terminal peptide (CP) [9] (Fig. 1*A*). The CP has chaperone features and appears to be required in the course of synthesis to properly fold proaerolysin into its soluble form. It not only prevents aggregation but also impedes premature pore formation by controlling the onset of heptamerization [10]. Proaerolysin is known to bind to N-glycosylated glycosylphosphatidylinositol (GPI)-anchored proteins at the target cell surface [11] [12]. Not only is the glycan important for binding but also the polypeptide to which it is attached [13].

Maturation of proaerolysin to aerolysin involves proteolytic cleavage in a flexible loop that precedes the C-terminal peptide. Furin is thought to play a major role in this process, but other proteases at the plasma membrane may participate as well [14] [15]. Following cleavage, monomers oligomerize to form a prepore complex on the cell surface [16], a step that requires release of the C-terminal peptide [17]. Removal of the C-terminal peptide induces the transition from prepore to the pore complex. The aerolysin heptamer undergoes a drastic concerted conforma-

tional change of the extramembranous region, accompanied by a vertical collapse of the complex, which ultimately leads to the insertion of a water-filled transmembrane beta-barrel into the lipid bilayer [17]. The CP is not part of the functional pore, as inferred from tryptophan fluorescence and energy transfer measurements [18]. Its fate after separation from the heptamer is unknown.

Insights into the mechanism of aerolysin intoxication have been obtained without the possibility of labeling discrete domains of the toxin at will. Being able to do so might allow a more detailed examination of the role and fate of each of the specific domains. It is still unclear which domains of aerolysin bind to the proteinaceous moieties of its receptors. Chemical labeling of exposed Lys or Cys residues usually results in a heterogeneous population of labeled proteins, making it impossible to accurately assess the identity of the molecular species responsible for activity. To overcome this technical challenge, we explore sortase-based site-specific chemoenzymatic labeling [19–21]. This allows us to investigate the fate of individual N- and C-terminal domains, while preserving toxin activity. Attachment of a single fluorophore at the very C-terminus of the C-terminal peptide makes it possible to directly visualize this chaperone's departure during aerolysin intoxication. Attachment of a single biotin group at the N-terminus of aerolysin enables us to identify novel cell surface receptors.

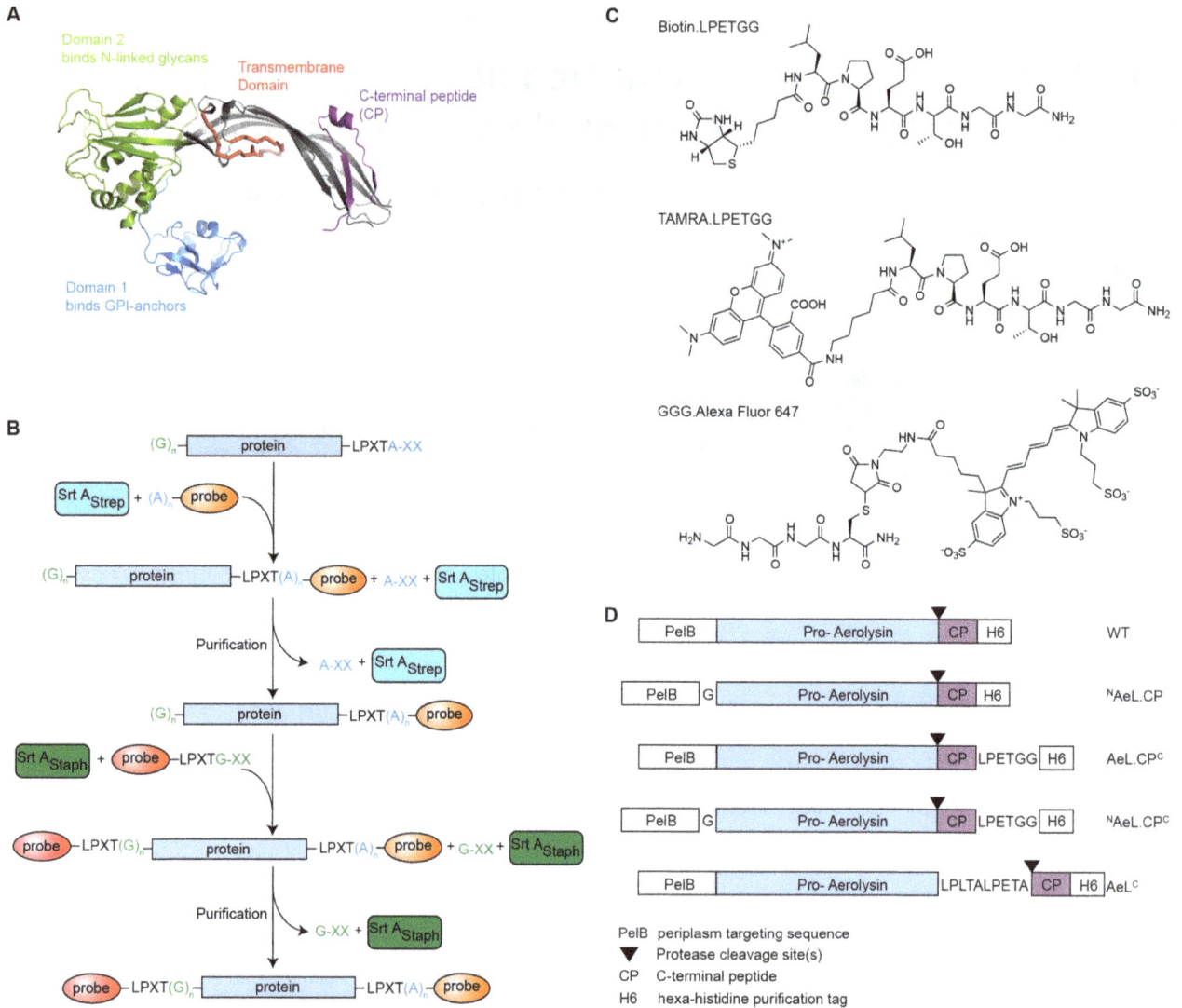

Figure 1. Strategies for site-specific labeling of proaerolysin. A Structure of the proaerolysin monomer (PDB: 1PRE). Proaerolysin consists of several different domains, two of which are responsible for receptor binding (domains 1 and 2), one containsing the trans-membrane domain, and the C-terminal peptide (CP), which functions as a chaperone and dissociates from the rest of the complex upon heptamer association and pore formation. **B** Sortase reaction mechanism. C-terminal sortagging: sortase cleaves after threonine in the context of its recognition motif resulting in the formation of a new covalent bond with the N-terminus of an added oligoglycine or oligoalanine nucleophile coupled to a label of choice. N-terminal sortagging: the N-terminal glycine of proaerolysin is recognized as a nucleophile by sortase and conjugated to an LPXTG/A probe bearing a label. **C** Structures of probes used in this study. Not depicted is AAA.Alexa Fluor 647, which is similar to GGG.Alexa Fluor 647, but with alanine replacing glycine. PelB: periplasm targeting sequence, cleaved off by the producer bacteria upon export of proaerolysin to the periplasm. H6: hexahistidine handle for affinity purification. Protease cleavage sites are recognized by target cell surface proteases such as furin. CP: C-terminal peptide, serves as a chaperone for proaerolysin. Upon its loss, proaerolysin is converted to mature aerolysin (AeL). **D** Scheme for wild type (WT) and sortaggable versions of proaerolysin with their designations. The LPXTG/A pentapeptides are sortase recognition motifs.

Materials and Methods

Antibodies, cell lines, constructs

Antibodies against CD59 (sc-28805) and mesothelin (sc-50427) were purchased from Santa Cruz Biotechnology. HRP-coupled secondary anti-rabbit antibody was from BD Biosciences. HeLa cells were purchased from American Type Culture Collection and cultured in Dulbecco's Modified Eagle Medium (DMEM) supplemented with 10% Fetal Bovine Serum (FBS). KBM7 cells were a kind gift from the T. R. Brummelkamp lab, and were described previously [22]. KBM7 cells were maintained in Iscove's Modified Dulbecco's Medium (IMDM) supplemented with 10%

FBS. The wild type proaerolysin construct [23] was a generous gift from F. G. van der Goot. Sortaggable variants were cloned by site-directed mutagenesis using the QuikChange kit (Agilent Technologies) following the manufacturer's instructions and using the following primers: NAeL.CP (introduction of a single glycine at N-terminus),

forward: 5'-AGCCGGCGATGGCCGGTATGGCAGAGC-CCGTC-3',

reverse: 5'-GACGGGCTCTGCCATACCGGCCATCGCC-GGCT-3'; AeL.CPC (introduction of LPETGG at C-terminus), forward: 5′-GCGTGACCCCTGCTGCCAATCAACTAC-CAGAGACCGGTGGACTCGAGCACCACCACCACCACC-ACTGAGATCC-3′,

reverse: 5′-GGATCTCAGTGGTGGTGGTGGTGGTGCT-CGAGTCCACCGGTCTCTGGTAGTTGATTGGCGCAGG-GGTCACGC-3′. ^{N}AeL.CP^C, was built using the forward primer 5′-AGCCGGCGATGGCCGGTATGGCAGAGCCCGTC-3′,

and the reverse primer 3′-GGATCTCAGTGGTGGTGG-TGGTGGTGCTCGAGTCCACCGGTCTCTGGTAGTTGA-TTGGCAGCAGGGGTCACGC-5′ with a PCR on WT proaer-olysin template using the Expand High Fidelity PCR system (Roche Diagnostics). AeL.^{C} (introduction of LPLTALPETA motive upstream of the C-terminal peptide) was done in a two-step-manner using QuikChange, according to the manufacturer's instructions:

5′-AGATCGGTGCTCCCCTCCCGCTCACTGCTGACA-GCAAGGGTG-3′,

3′-CACCTTGCTGTCAGCAGTGAGCGGGAGGGGAGC-ACCGATCT-5′;

5′-TCCCCTCCCGCTCACTGCTCTCCCGGAGACTGC-TGACAGCAAGGTGCGTCG-3′,

3′-CGACGCACCTTGCTGTCAGCAGTCTCCGGGAGA-GCAGTGAGCGGGAGGGGA-5′.

Expression and purification proaerolysin

Overnight cultures of *E. coli* BL21 (DE3) pLysS (Promega) transformed with the various aerolysin constructs and grown at 30°C were diluted 1:50 with LB broth supplemented with 200 µg/mL ampicillin plus 35 µg/mL chloramphenicol, and incubated at 37°C, shaking at 220 rpm, to an optical density of 0.5–0.6 at 600 nm. Expression of proaerolysin was induced with 1 mM isopropyl-beta-D-1-thiogalactopyranoside (IPTG) (Sigma), and the temperature was lowered to 26°C. After 4–5 hours, cells were harvested and centrifuged at 6000×g, 4°C for 20 min. Subsequent steps were carried out at 4°C. Cell pellets were resuspended in 10 ml lysis buffer per 1 L expression culture: 50 mM Tris-HCl pH 7.5, 300 mM NaCl, 0.5 mg/ml polymixin B (Sigma) supplemented with complete protease cocktail inhibitors (Roche) and 50 µg/ml phenylmethylsulfonyl fluoride (PMSF) (Sigma). The suspension was agitated for 45 minutes at 4°C and centrifuged at 6000×g for 30 min at 4°C. The supernatant was incubated at 4°C with 0.25 ml bed volume NiNTA agarose (Qiagen) per 1 L culture, overnight, with gentle rotation. The resin was washed with 20 column volumes of 50 mM Tris-HCl pH 7.5, 300 mM NaCl, 10 mM imidazole. The protein was eluted with 5 column volumes 50 mM Tris-HCl pH 7.5, 300 mM NaCl, 150 mM imidazole. The fractions were subjected to buffer exchange to 50 mM Tris-HCl pH 7.5, 300 mM NaCl, using a PD-10 desalting column (GE Healthcare). 10% (v/v) glycerol was added to the protein preparations, aliquots were snap-frozen, and stored at −80°C. Protein concentration was determined by Bradford assay (Bio-Rad Laboratories).

Toxicity assay

0.5×10^5 KBM7 WT cells were incubated for 1 h at 37°C with different concentrations of each of the aerolysin variants (as indicated in the figures) in a total volume of 100 µL. Cells were washed twice with cold PBS and resuspended in PBS containing 1 µg/mL propidium iodide and analyzed by flow cytometry. The percentage of PI negative controls was set to 100%, and the 50% lethal dosis (LC50) calculated in R. 0.001 was added to all concentration values to avoid taking a log2 of 0.

Flow cytometry

Data acquisition was performed on a FACS Calibur HTS (BD Biosciences) using the CellQuest Pro (BD Biosciences) software. Data were analyzed with FlowJo (Tree Star Inc.).

Sortase expression, purification, immobilization. Sortase expression, purification, immobilization

Sortase A (SortA) from *Staphylococcus aureus* (SrtA$_{Staph}$) and SortA from *Streptococcus pyogenes* (SrtA$_{Strep}$) were expressed and purified as described previously [21] [20]. Additionally we used a heptamutant form of Sortase A from *S. aureus* (SrtA$_{staph7M}$), which combined previously described mutations to give Ca^{2+} independence and increased activity [24] [25]. SrtA was immobilized on cyanogen bromide activated sepharose beads (Sigma) in a ratio of 1 g dry beads per 30 mg SrtA$_{Staph}$ or 40 mg SrtA$_{Staph7M}$. The beads were swelled in 50 mL of 1 mM HCl for five washes of five minutes each at 4°C. After extensive washing with ice-cold water the sortase was coupled to the beads in 100 mM NaHCO$_3$ and 500 mM NaCl for 2 hrs at 25°C or O.N. at 4°C (make sure the storage buffer of the SortA is exchanged as Tris will react with the beads). Finally, the coupled beads were washed and stored as a 50% bead slurry in 50 mM Tris (pH 7.4) and 150 mM NaCl at 4°C. All washes/filtrations were done in a plastic capped fritted column and the buffers were removed between steps by vacuum filtration. For long-term storage more than one week add 20% glycerol and store aliquots at −20°C.

Synthesis of sortase probes and sortase labeling

GGG.TAMRA, AAA.AF647, TAMRA.LPETGG and Bio-tin.LPETGG were synthesized as described in [20] [21]. Soluble sortase labeling reactions with SrtA$_{strep}$ and SrtA$_{staph}$ were performed as described [19] [20] [21] [26]. The SrtA$_{staph7M}$ has increased activity and reactions took place at 4°C and with 20% of sortase in relation to proaerolysin. Additionally, Ca^{2+} is no longer needed in the coupling buffer. Sortase immobilized to cyanogen bromide beads was filtered from the reaction solution. Otherwise reaction conditions are the same as the soluble sortase.

Fluorescence image scan

Fluorescence scans were obtained using a variable mode imager (Typhoon 9200; GE Healthcare).

SDS PAGE, Coomassie staining, and Immunoblot

SDS-PAGE was performed as described [27]. Gels were stained with Coomassie Brilliant Blue R250 (Thermo Scientific) according to the manufacturer's instructions. Proteins were blotted onto polyvinylidene difluoride (PVDF) membranes and probed with the appropriate antibodies, followed by chemoluminescence detection using Western Lightning ECL detection kit (Perkin Elmer Life Sciences) and exposure to XAR-5 films (Kodak).

Fluorescence microscopy

HeLa cells grown on coverslips were washed with ice-cold DMEM media and incubated on ice for 30 minutes with the appropriate concentrations of labeled or unlabeled aerolysin (as indicated in the figures). Cells were washed 3 times with ice-cold PBS, fixed with 4% paraformaldehyde in PBS for 20 minutes at room temperature to prevent activity of plasma membrane-associated proteases that cleave off the C-terminal peptide, washed with PBS, incubated for 1 minute in PBS containing 1 µg/mL Hoechst stain, and mounted with glycerol on coverslips. Alternatively, cells were shifted to 37°C after Hoechst staining. All images were collected on a PerkinElmer Ultraview Multispectral Spinning

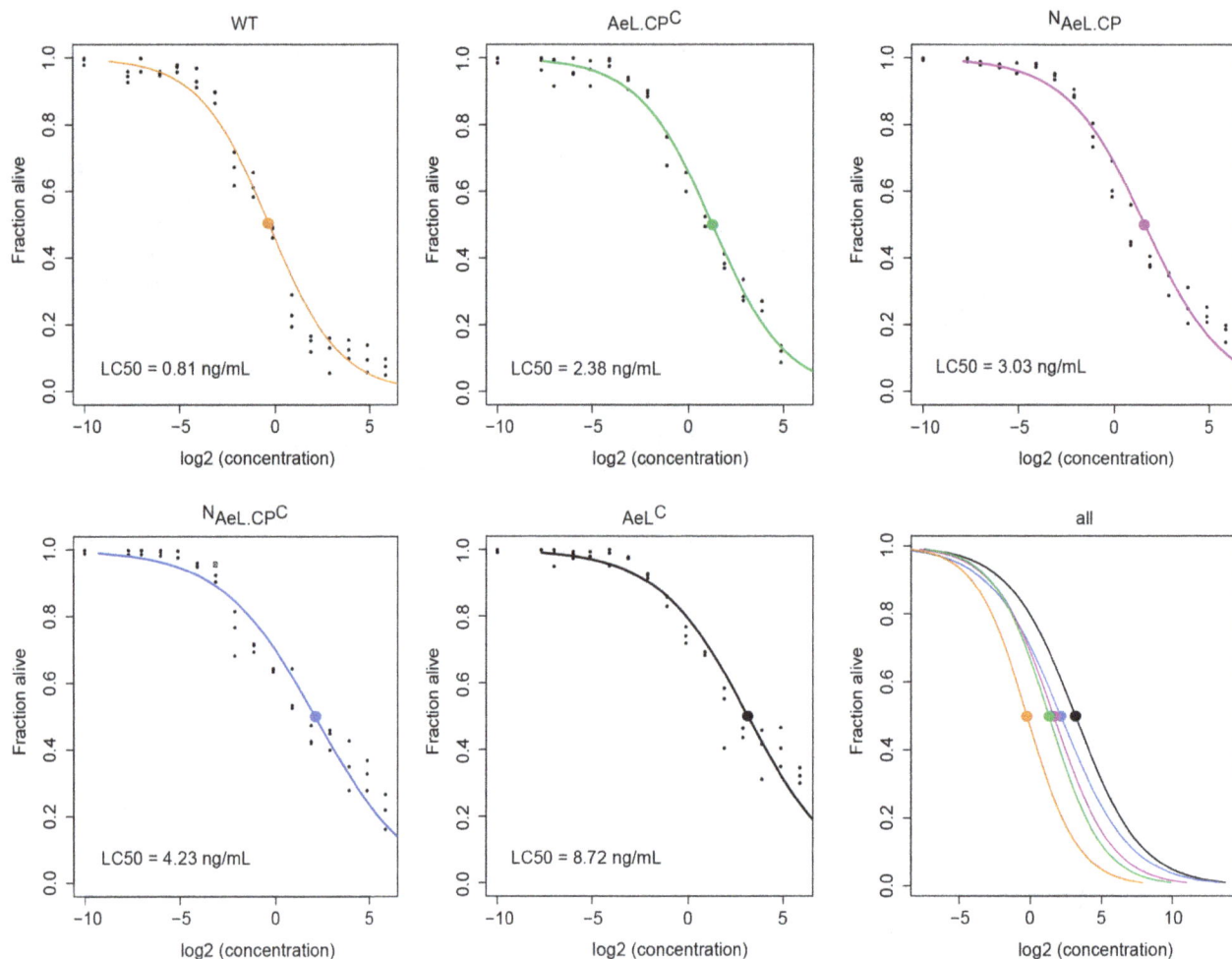

Figure 2. Impact of aerolysin modification on toxic activity. Aerolysin variants were titrated on KBM7 cells. 0.5×10^5 cells per sample were incubated with toxin for 1 hour at 37°C in a total volume of 100 μL, stained with propidium iodide (PI), and the PI negative percentage determined by flow cytometry. The concentration range for the aerolysin variants ranged from 60 ng/mL to 4 pg/μL. Every condition was tested in triplicate. The percentage of PI negative controls was set to 100%, and the 50% lethal dose (LC50) calculated in R. 0.001 was added to all concentration values to avoid taking a log2 of 0.

Disk Confocal Microscope equipped with a Yokogawa CSU-22 spinning disk confocal on a Zeiss Axiovert 200 motorized inverted microscope with Chroma 488/568/647 and 458/515/647 triple dichroic mirrors and Prior emission filter wheel, Perkin Elmer laser launch with 100 mW argon gas laser (488 nm, 514 nm), 100 mW krypton gas laser (568 nm), and 405 nm, 440 nm and 640 nm solid state lasers with AOTF for laser line selection/attenuation and fiber-optic delivery system, a Zeiss 1.4 NA oil immersion 63x objective lens and a Prior piezo-electric objective focusing device for maintenance of focus. Images were acquired with a Hamamatsu ORCA ER cooled CCD camera controlled with Volocity software. Confocal images were collected using an exposure time of 500 ms and 1×1 binning. For time-lapse microscopy, laser power was set to 77% for the 100 mW krypton gas laser (568 nm), and to 100% for the 640 nm 40 mW solid-state laser. Number of frames: 1 per image. Acquisition frequency: 1 frame per 25 seconds. Brightness was adjusted on displayed images (identically for compared image sets) using Fiji software.

Immunoprecipitation

~ 10^7 HeLa cells per condition were incubated with 120 μg [Biotin]AeL.CP or WT aerolysin for 30 min at 4°C, washed, scraped, and lysed in buffer containing 0.5% (v/v) NP40, 10 mM Tris-HCl pH 7.4, 150 mM NaCl, 5 mM $MgCl_2$, supplemented with complete protease cocktail inhibitors (Roche) and 50 μg/ml phenylmethylsulfonyl fluoride (PMSF) (Sigma). Immunoprecipitations were performed for 3 h at 4°C with rotation using 20 μL neutravidin-sepharose beads (Thermo Scientific) per sample. Samples were eluted by boiling in reducing sample buffer and subjected to SDS-PAGE, followed by immunoblotting or mass spectrometry.

Mass spectrometry

Bands were excised, reduced, alkylated and digested with trypsin at 37C overnight. The resulting peptides were extracted, concentrated and injected onto a Dionex RSLCnano HPLC equipped with a self-packed Jupiter 3 μm C18 analytical column (0.075 mm by 10 cm, Phenomenex). Peptides were eluted using standard reverse-phase gradients. The effluent from the column

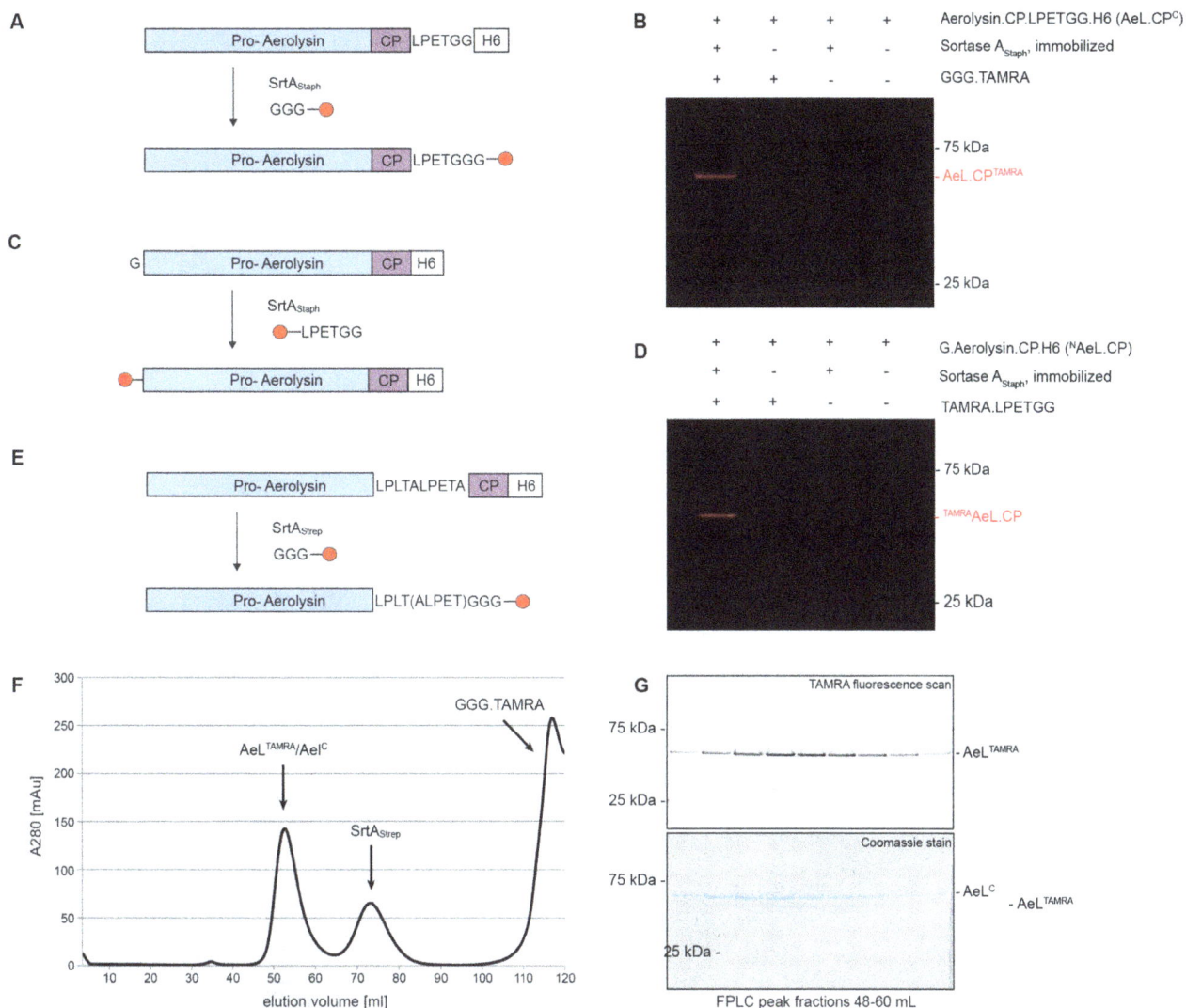

Figure 3. Installation of a single label on proaerolysin. The fluorophore carboxytetramethylrhodamine (TAMRA) was installed at the N-terminus of aerolysin (^{N}AeL.CP), at the C-terminus of aerolysin upstream of the CP (AeL^C) and at the C-terminus of the C-terminal peptide (AeL.CP^C) with sortase. **A, C, E** Schematic representation of the sortagging reactions using of ^{N}AeL.CP, AeL.CP^C, AeL^C respectively. **B, D** Sortagging of ^{N}AeL.CP and AeL.CP^C respectively, with respective control conditions, resolved by SDS PAGE and imaged with a fluorescence scanner. Product is visible by fluorescent signal. SrtA$_{Strep}$ and SrtA$_{Staph}$ recognize and cleave LPXTA and LPXTG motives, respectively. **F** Purification of labeled AeL^{TAMRA}, gel filtration. The first peak in the A280 elution profile corresponds to aerolysin, the second to sortase, and the third to free nucleophile. **G** Analysis of the first peak of the gel filtration elution profile with SDS PAGE followed by fluorescence image scan and Coomassie stain. A fraction of Ael^C is not converted to fluorescent product.

was analyzed using a Thermo Orbitrap Elite mass spectrometer (nanospray configuration) operated in a data dependent manner. The resulting fragmentation spectra were correlated against the known database using SEQUEST. Scaffold Q+S (Proteome Software) was used to provide consensus reports for the identified proteins.

Results

Strategies for site-specific labeling of proaerolysin

Sortases A (SrtA) recognize a pentapeptide motif specific to an individual bacterial enzyme, e.g., LPXTG for SrtA from *Staphylococcus aureus* (SrtA$_{Staph}$) and LPXTA for SrtA from *Streptococcus pyogenes* (SrtA$_{Strep}$) (where X is any aminoacid). SrtA cleaves the peptide bond between the threonine and glycine or

alanine, respectively, yielding a thioacyl intermediate, which is then resolved by a nucleophilic attack of the N-terminus of an oligoglycine- or oligoalanine-containing nucleophile (Fig. 1*B*). This results in the formation of a new peptide bond [28] [26]. Because SrtA$_{Staph}$ and SrtA$_{Strep}$ enzymes are orthogonal to one another it is possible to introduce two distinct labels into one and the same protein or virus [29] [30] [31].

Hexa-histidine tags have been genetically installed at the C-terminus of proaerolysin [23]. However, site-specific fluorescent labeling of the C-terminus of mature aerolysin has not previously been attempted, an essential requirement for live-cell imaging. Using sortases we installed biotin and fluorophore probes onto different domains of proaerolysin (Fig. 1*C*). Labels were placed at: the N-terminus of proaerolysin (^{N}AeL.CP), the C-terminus of the C-terminal peptide (AeL.CP^C), the C-terminus of aerolysin

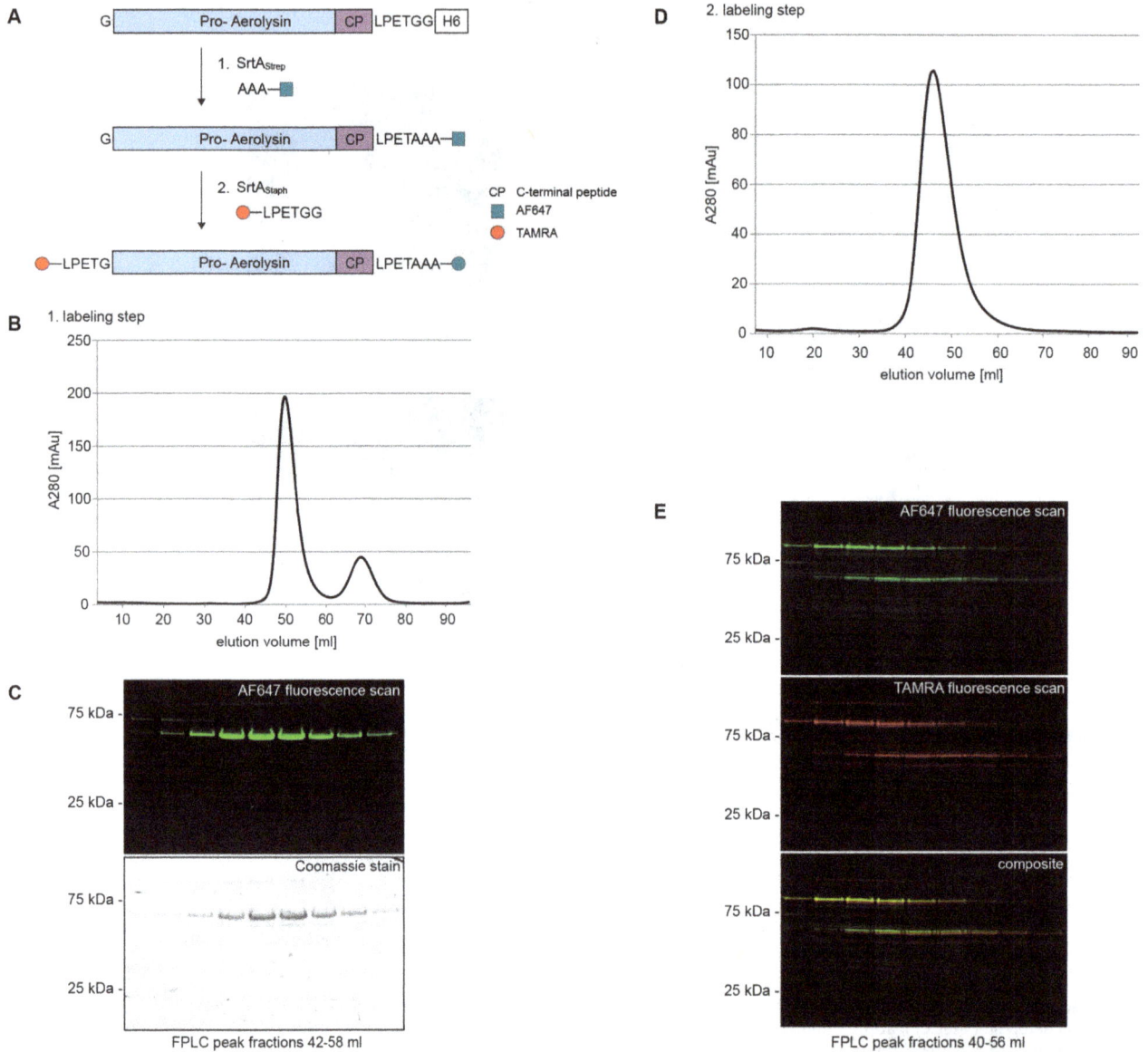

Figure 4. Double-labeling of proaerolysin. Double-labeling was achieved with a two-step approach. **A** Schematic representation of the dual labeling strategy of proaerolysin. **B** We used SrtA$_{Strep}$ to install an oligoalanine coupled to the fluorophore AF647 at the C-terminus of proaerolysin, followed by a gel filtration purification step. **C** Elution profiles were analyzed by SDS-PAGE, fluorescence scan and coomassie stain. **D** The reaction product was subjected to the second round of sortagging with SrtA$_{Staph7M}$ and LPETG-coupled TAMRA fluorophore for N-terminal labeling. SrtA$_{Staph}$ does not recognize or cleave LPXTA, hence the C-terminal label remains intact. A single peak is observed on the elution profile as immobilized sortase was used for the reaction and removed prior to gel filtration. **E** Elution profiles were analyzed by SDS-PAGE followed by fluorescence scan.

preceeding the chaperone (AeL^C), as well as creating a double-label variant (^{N}AeL.CP^C). The different sortaggable proaerolysin versions are schematically diagrammed in Fig. 1D.

Aerolysin activity

The different versions of sortaggable aerolysin were titrated on KBM7 cells. Toxin concentrations ranging from 60 ng/mL to 4 pg/mL were assayed in triplicate. The assay was performed for all aerolysin versions and concentrations in a single experiment on aliquots of the same batch of cells. Cells (3.5×10^5 per sample) were intoxicated for 1 hour at 37°C, washed, stained with propidium iodide and analyzed by flow cytometry. The percentage of live cells was determined and the median lethal concentration (LC50)

calculated (Fig. 2). Compared to wild type (WT) aerolysin, all of the modified versions showed a slight decrease in toxicity. The difference was greatest for AeL^C, which was ~10 fold less toxic than the WT. Modifying the N terminus with a single glycine impaired toxicity ~3 fold. This was comparable to the loss of activity observed for the C-terminal modified version. Modification of both the N and C terminus of proaerolysin reduced toxic activity further and revealed the toxicity of ^{N}proAeL^C to be intermediate between the WT and AeL^C.

Installation of a single label on proaerolysin

Proaerolysin was labeled at either its N- or C-terminus with a peptide coupled to carboxy-tetramethylrhodamine (TAMRA)

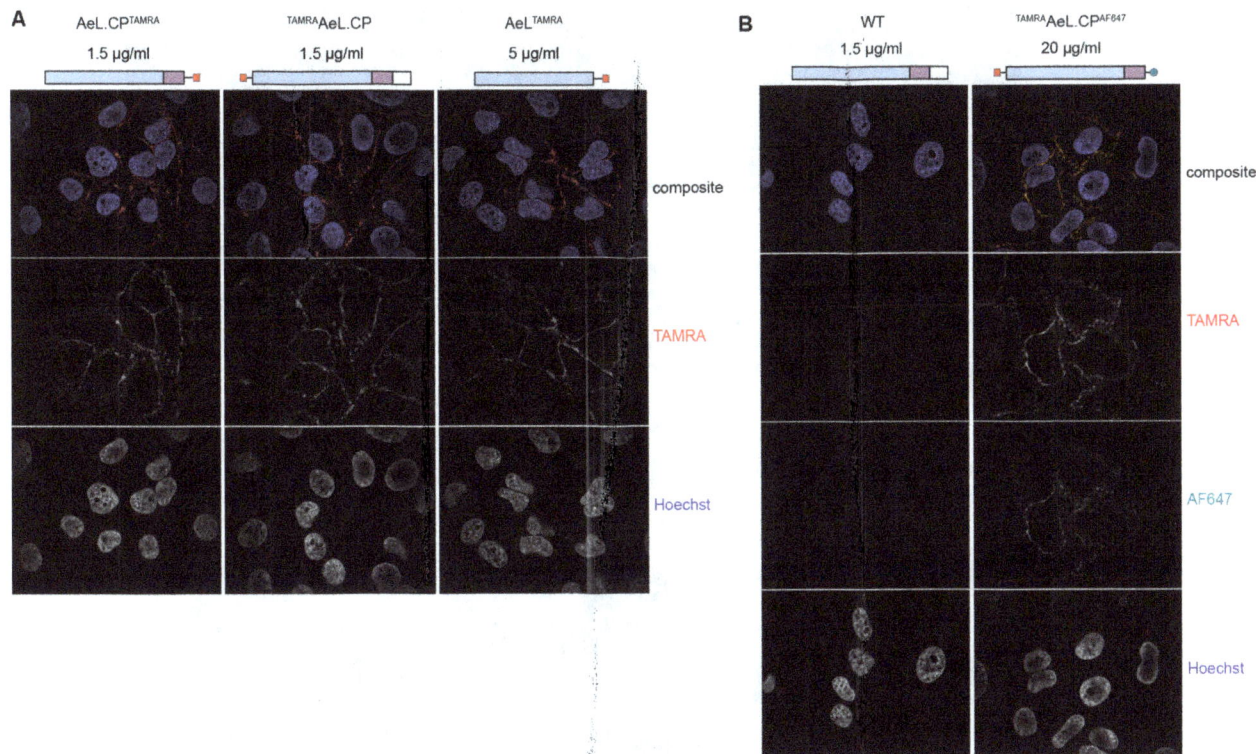

Figure 5. Aerolysin imaging. Aerolysin variants, fluorescently labeled, bind to the cell surface of HeLa cells. Images were acquired by confocal fluorescence microscopy. **A** Single labeled aerolysin versions. For comparable signal intensity, different aerolysin concentrations were required as indicated. **B** Double-labeled aerolysin and unlabeled aerolysin control.

[Figs. 3A and 3C]. Fluorescent product was observed only when all the components of the labeling reaction mixture were co-mixed. No background labeling detected (Fig. 3B and 3D). The labeling efficiency was near-quantitative, as previously demonstrated for cholera toxin [32] and various other proteins [30] [33]. N-terminally labeled proaerolysin (^{Tamra}AeL.CP) migrated slightly faster on SDS-PAGE than the C-terminally labeled AeL.CP^{TAMRA}.

To label AeL^C, we introduced a tandem sortase recognition site, LPLTALPETA, upstream of the protease cleavage site(s) that precede(s) the C-terminal peptide (Fig. 3E). We empirically determined that installation of a single sortase recognition motif, either LPLTA or LPETG, was insufficient to yield a good substrate for sortase and failed to yield a labeled product (data not shown).

Sortagged product was purified by fast protein liquid chromatography (FPLC) to separate the product from free dye-conjugated nucleophile and sortase (Fig. 3F). The fractions of the elution profile containing aerolysin were resolved by reducing SDS-PAGE and analyzed by fluorescence scan followed by coomassie staining. For this construct, labeling was incomplete (yield <50%) (Fig. 3G). Prolonged incubation times, different reaction temperatures and increasing the concentration of nucleophile did not further improve the extent of labeling (data not shown).

Double-labeling of proaerolysin

Labeling with two different probes was achieved by combining sortases with different specificities, SrtA$_{Staph}$ and SrtA$_{Strep}$, such that the product of the first reaction was not recognized as a substrate for the second (Fig. 4A). In the first step, the C-terminus of ^{N}AeL.CP^C was reacted with AAA.Alexa Fluor 647 by SrtA$_{Strep}$

with near-complete labeling efficiency. The product was purified by FPLC and used as a substrate for the second labeling reaction (Fig. 4B). The elution peak containing ^{N}AeL.CP^{AF647} also contained a minor fraction of higher and lower molecular weight species (Fig. 4C), the identity of which is not known.

TAMRA.LPETGG was appended to the N-terminus of ^{N}AeL.CP^{AF647} in a second labeling step. We used immobilized SrtA$_{Staph7M}$ to simplify sortase removal. Free nucleophile was removed by size exclusion chromatography (Fig. 4D). Labeling was monitored by SDS-PAGE, followed by fluorescence imaging (Fig. 4E). Two prominent polypeptides were visible in both channels (AF647: peudo color green; TAMRA: pseudo color red), one around 50 kDa, and a second around 100 kDa. In addition, a third polypeptide with an apparent molecular weight of 150 kDa was detected in the TAMRA channel but not in the AF647 channel. Image overlay showed co-localization of the 50 and 100 kDa species, most probably oligomers that lost the CP.

Aerolysin imaging. Next we checked whether the different labeled proaerolysin versions would still bind to cells. Cell preparation, incubation, and the subsequent washing steps prior to fixation were done at 4°C to prevent activity of cell surface proteases that would otherwise activate proaerolysin. Confocal fluorescence microscopy revealed a rim-staining pattern for single-labeled proaerolysin (Fig. 5A). To acquire images with the same image acquisition settings (laser intensity, exposure time, gain), 3.3 times more (5 µg/mL) AeL^{TAMRA} had to be added to cells compared to both ^{TAMRA}AeL.CP and AeL.CP^{TAMRA} (1.5 µg/mL). 20 µg/mL double-labeled ^{TAMRA}AeL.CP^{AF647} was required for an adequate signal to noise ratio (Fig. 5B). Both fluorophores were visible as rim staining, and co-localized at the plasma membrane. Shifting the intoxicated cells to 37°C for 10 minutes

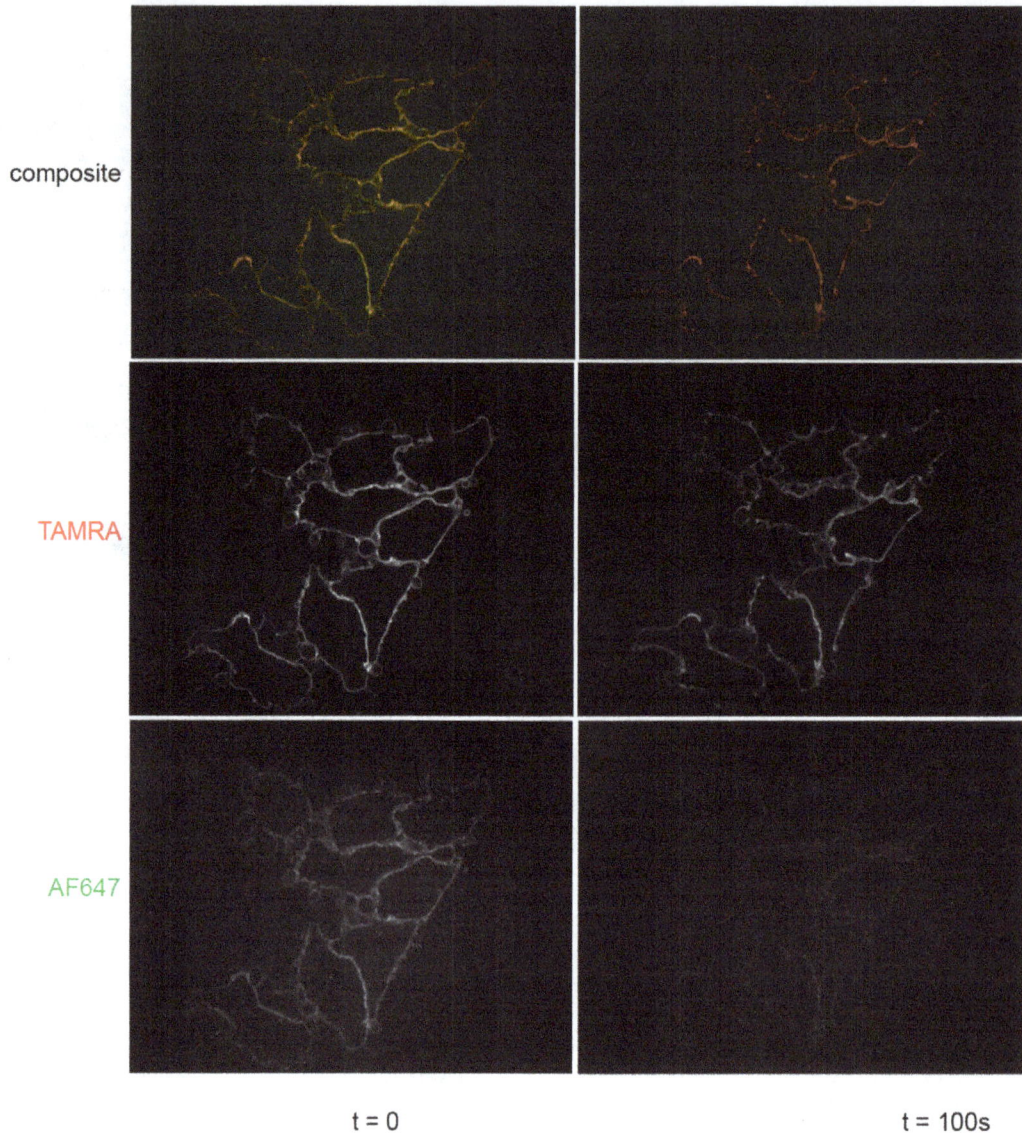

Figure 6. Dissociation of the C-terminal chaperone in the course of intoxication. HeLa cells were incubated with ^{TAMRA}AeL.CP^{AF647} for 30 minutes at 4°C, washed, and the temperature shifted to 37°C. Images were acquired by confocal microscopy.

prior to imaging resulted in cell detachment, indicative of intoxication (data not shown).

Dissociation of the C-terminal chaperone in the course of intoxication. We used the double-labeled version of aerolysin to monitor the fate of the C-terminal chaperone during aerolysin intoxication. HeLa cells were incubated with ^{TAMRA}AeL.CP^{AF647} for 30 minutes on ice, washed, and then shifted to 37°C. Confocal microscopy showed an initial overlapping surface staining pattern for both fluorophores. The intensity of the AF647 signal decreased over time to almost background level in ~120 seconds, whereas the signal for TAMRA suffered loss of intensity to a much smaller extent and remained well above background (Fig. 6). This is indicative of separation of the two labels, and hence consistent with loss of the C-terminal peptide.

Identification of new aerolysin receptors. Aerolysin was sort°gged with biotin at its N-terminus (Fig. 7A) and incubated with HeLa cells at 4°C. Upon cell lysis, using a mild detergent, biotinylated aerolysin and its bound materials were recovered with

neutravidin beads. The eluted proteins were separated on a reducing SDS-PAGE gel, and analyzed by mass spectrometry. Five GPI-anchored proteins were identified: mesothelin, urokinase plasminogen activator surface receptor (uPAR, CD87), glypican-1, complement decay accelerating factor (CD55), and CD59 glycoprotein; each represented by multiple exclusive unique peptide coverage (Fig. 7B). Interaction was confirmed for mesothelin and CD59 by immunoblot in an independent experiment (Fig. 7C).

Discussion

Aerolysin is the first example of a pore-forming toxin to which a site-specific, chemoenzymatic labeling strategy has been applied. Sortagging allows maximal versatility in the choice of functionalities to be installed [28] [33]. Sortase accepts protein substrates in their native tertiary or quaternary structure. This eliminates two common problems of genetic fusion proteins: aggregation and

A

IP: neutravidin beads
IB: anti-biotin

C

IP: neutravidin beads
IB: anti-mesothelin

IP: neutravidin beads
IB: anti-CD59

B Aerolysin interactors, Mass Spectrometry Hits

MSLN_HUMAN UniProt Q13421 Mesothelin 12 exclusive unique peptides
MALPTARPLLGSCGTPALGSLLFLLFSLGWVQPSRTLAGETGQEAAPLDGVLANPPNISSLSPRQLLGFPCAEVSGLSTERVRELAVALAQKNVKLSTEQLRCLAHRLSEPPEDLDALPLDLLLFLNPDAFSGPQACTRFFSRITKANVDLLPRGAPERQRLLPAALACWGVRGSLLSEADVRALGGLACDLPGRFVAESAEVLLPRLVSCPGPLDQDQQEAARAALQGGGPPYGPPSTWSVSTMDALRGLLPVLGQPIIRSIPQGIVAAWRQRSSRDPSWRQPERTILRPRFRREVEKTACPSGKKAREIDESLIFYKKWELEACVDAALLATQMDRVNAIPFTYEQLDVLKHKLDELYPQGYPESVIQHLGYLFLKMSPEDIRKWNVTSLETLKALLEVNKGHEMSPQAPRRPLPQVATLIDRFVKGRGQLDKDTLDTLTAFYPGYLCSLSPEELSSVPPSSIWAVRPQDLDTCDPRQLDVLYPKARLAFQNMNGSEYFVKIQSFLGGAPTEDLKALSQQNVSMDLATFMKLRTDAVLPLTVAEVQKLLGPHVEGLKAEERHRPVRDWILRQRQDDLDTLGLGLQGGIPNGYLVLDLSMQEALSGTPCLLGPGPVLTVLALLLASTLA

UPAR_HUMAN UniProt Q03405 Urokinase plasminogen activator surface receptor (CD87) 6 exclusive unique peptides
MGHPPLLPLLLLLHTCVPASWGLRCMQCKTNGDCRVEECALGQDLCRTTIVRLWEEGEELELVEKSCTHSEKTNRTLSYRTGLKITSLTEVVCGLDLCNQGNSGRAVTYSRSRYLECISCGSSDMSCERGRHQSLQCRSPEEQCLDVVTHWIQEGEEGRPKDDRHLRGCGYLPGCPGSNGFHNNDTFHFLKCCNTTKCNEGPILELENLPQNGRQCYSCKGNSTHGCSSEETFLIDCRGPMNQCLVATGTHEPKNQSYMVRGCATASMCQHAHLGDAFSMNHIDVSCCTKSGCNHPDLDVQYRSGAAPQPGPAHLSLTITLLMTARLWGGTLLWT

GPC1_HUMAN UniProt P35052 Glypican-1 14 exclusive unique peptides
MELRARGWWLLCAAAALVACARGDPASKSRSCGEVRQIYGAKGFSLSDVPQAEISGEHLRICPQGYTCCTSEMEENLANRSHAELETALRDSSRVLQAMLATQLRSFDDHFQHLLNDSERTLQATFPGAFGELYTQNARAFRDLYSELRLYYRGANLHLEETLAEFWARLLERLFKQLHPQLLLPDDYLDCLGKQAEALRPFGEAPRELRLRATRAFVAARSFVQGLGVASDVVRKVAQVPLGPECSRAVMKLVYCAHCLGVPGARPCPDYCRNVLKGCLANQADLDAEWRNLLDSMVLITDKFWGTSGVESVIGSVHTWLAEAINALQDNRDTLTAKVIQGCGNPKVNPQGPGPEEKRRRGKLAPRERPPSGTLEKLVSEAKAQLRDVQDFWISLPGTLCSEKMALSTASDDRCWNGMARGRYLPEVMGDGLANQINNPEVEVDITKPDMTIRQQIMQLKIMTNRLRSAYNGNDVDFQDASDDGSGSGSGDGCLDDLCSRKVSRKSSSSRTPLTHALPGLSEQEGQKTSAASCPQPPTFLLPLLLFLALTVARPRWR

DAF_HUMAN UniProt P08174 Complement decay-accelerating factor (CD55) 7 exclusive unique peptides
MTVARPSVPAALPLLGELPRLLLLVLLCLPAVVWGDCGLPPDVPNAQPALEGRTSFPEDTVITYKCEESFVKIPGEKDSVICLKGSQWSDIEEFCNRSCEVPTRLNSASLKQPYITQNYFPVGTVVEYECRPGYRREPSLSPKLTCLQNLKWSTAVEFCKKKSCPNPGEIRNGGQIDVPGGILFGATISFSCNTGYKLFGSTSSFCLISGSSVQWSDPLPECREIYCPAPPQIDNGIIQGERDHYGYRQSVTYACNKGFTMIGEHSIYCTVNNDEGEWSGPPPECRGKSLTSKVPPTVQKPTTVNVPTTEVSPTSQKTTTKTTTPNAQATRSTPVSRTTKHFHETTPNKGSGTTSGTTRLLSGHTCFTLTGLLGTLVTMGLLT

CD59_HUMAN UniProt P13987 CD59 glycoprotein 2 exclusive unique peptides
MGIQGGSVLFGLLLVLAVFCHSGHSLQCYNCPNPTADCKTAVNCSSDFDACLITKAGLQVYNKCWKFEHCNFNDVTTRLRENELTYYCCKKDLCNFNEQLENGGTSLSEKTVLLLVTPFLAAAWSLHP

signal peptide (removed from mature form)
MS coverage
Lipidation (GPI anchor)
removed from mature form

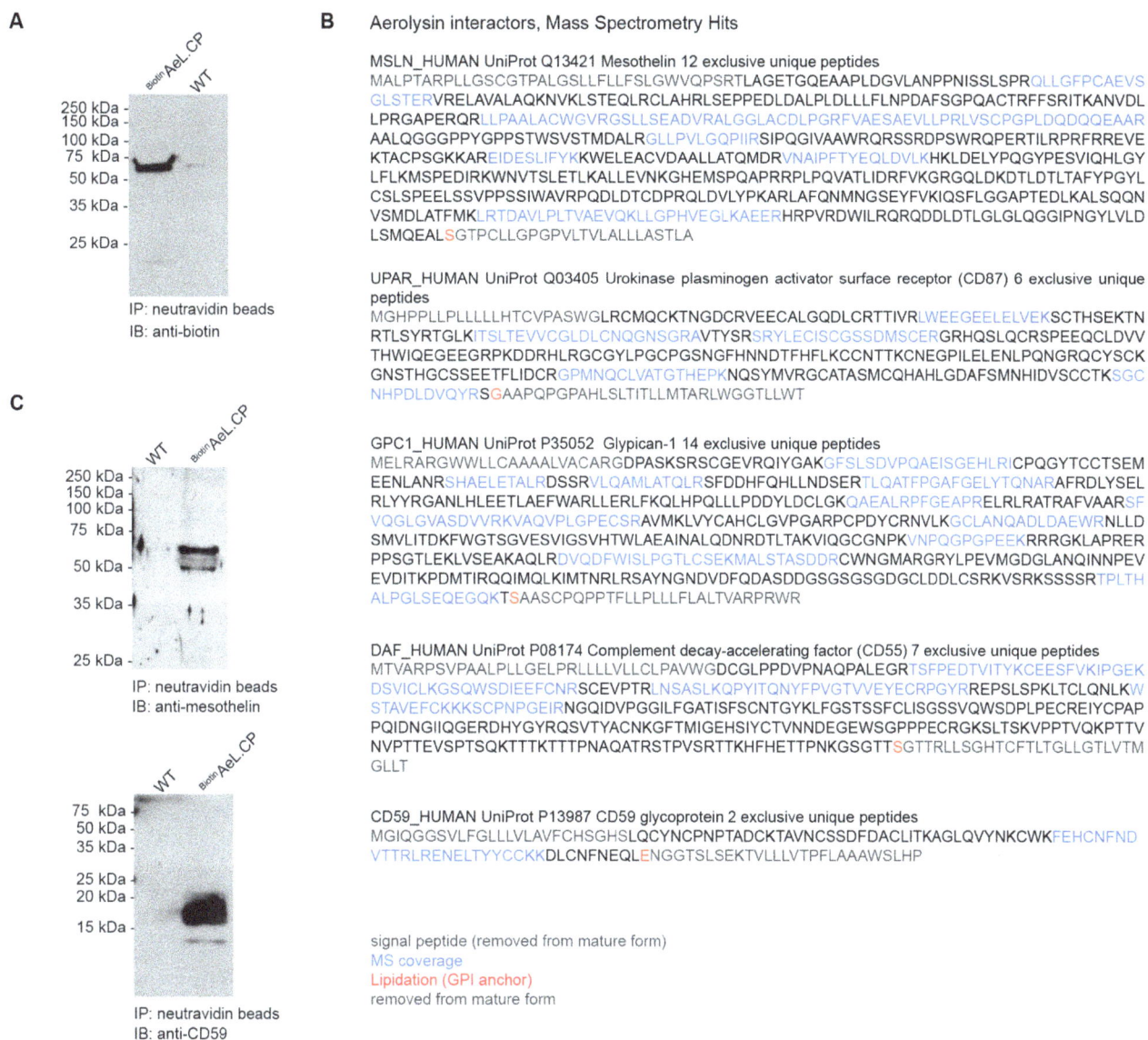

Figure 7. Identification of new aerolysin receptors. BiotinAeL.CP was used to identify new GPI-anchored proteins that bind Aerolysin. **A** Biotin.LPETG was attached to the N-terminus of proaerolysin via sortagging. The purified reaction product was analyzed by immunoblot. **B** HeLa cells were incubated with BiotinAeL.CP for 3 hours at 4°C and subsequently lysed with 0.5% NP-40. After pull-down with neutravidin beads, proteins were eluted, analyzed by SDS-PAGE, and subjected to mass spectrometry. Five GPI-anchored proteins were identified. UniProt accession codes are indicated. Peptides identified by mass spectrometry, lipidated amino acids, signal peptides, as well as peptides cleaved off from the pro-proteins are highlighted. **C** Binding of BiotinAeL.CP to mesothelin and to CD59 was verified by immunoblot.

non-functional folding. Aerolysin tolerates only subtle modifications [34]. A dramatic conformational change must take place for the soluble aerolysin monomer to form the homo-heptameric pore upon binding to a suitable receptor [17]; a point mutation can lock the protein into a particular conformation [35] and/or impede oligomerization [9], preventing toxicity. This leaves only three sites readily amenable to site-specific alteration: the very N-terminus, the very C-terminus, and the slightly more variable sequence that flanks the protease cleavage site(s) preceding the C-terminal peptide [36]. While it is true that addition of a few residues, a single glycine at the N-terminus of aerolysin, or the LPXTG/A motif diminishes toxicity (anywhere from a factor of 3 up to a factor of 10, Fig. 2), we have shown that enzymatic modification of any of these three aerolysin sites nonetheless yields

a functional product fully capable of intoxication. It is not immediately obvious from the aerolysin crystal structure whether the N-terminus is critically engaged in receptor binding or pore-formation [37]. Genetic appendage of an affinity tag at the C-terminus of the C-terminal peptide for purification purposes is standard, but its effect on toxicity has not been systematically investigated. As observed in this study, internal modification of aerolysin has the most detrimental effect. The anomalous mobility on SDS-PAGE of TAMRAproAeL compared to proAeLTAMRA (calculated molecular weights: 55.5 kDa for TAMRAproAeL and 54.8 kDa for AeL.CPTAMRA) we attribute to the relative positioning of the fluorophores, and the incomplete denaturation and/or differences in SDS binding. Alternatively TAMRAAeL.CP may have lost its C-terminal peptide, which has a molecular weight of approximately 3.7 kDa. However, unless proteases were present in the sortagging reaction, or aerolysin could somehow activate autocatalytically, this we consider less likely. AeL.CP^{TAMRA} was clearly not affected in this manner, or it would have lost its fluorescence.

We show that modification of mature aerolysin not only at its N-terminus and C-terminal end of the CP (in the context of the holotoxin), but also at the newly generated C-terminus after cleavage of the CP is readily achievable using sortase. After the CP is cleaved off by the sortase reaction, it remains associated with non-receptor-bound aerolysin and continues to exert its function as a chaperone. By inhibiting aggregation and premature pore-formation, it maintains the molecule's toxic potential [10].

Introduction of five additional amino acids in addition to the sortase recognition site was necessary to achieve successful sortase-mediated modification. Placing the LPXTG/A pentapeptide in a flexible loop generally increases flexibility of the protein backbone and thus accessibility, which in certain cases is required for proper sortase action [28] [32]. We did not determine which of the two motifs within this tandem sequence was recognized and used by sortase. The fact that modification of this site by addition of amino acids only modestly affects toxicity suggests that the new C-terminus has no critical function in the mature pore. Still, even though the five amino acid extension rendered the site accessible to sortase, the sortagging reaction could not be driven to completion. Presumably there is residual steric hindrance that interferes with accessibility for sortase.

Site-specific N- and C-terminal labeling of a single polypeptide using sortases of different specificity has been demonstrated in earlier work [29]. Applying the same strategy on aerolysin, obtained data are entirely consistent with double labeling. SrtA$_{Strep}$ not only accepts oligoalanine, but also oligoglycine as a nucleophile, albeit with different kinetics [29] [38]. The N-terminal glycine of ^{N}AeL.CP^{label} acts as a nucleophile, and can resolve the substrate-sortase thioacyl intermediate. This may result in concatenation of a fraction of aerolysin monomers, and would explain the detection of the 100 kDa and 150 kDa protein bands in the double-labeling reactions. These molecular weights are compatible with dimer and trimer formation, respectively. Dimers of aerolysin appear to contribute to the protein's stability and have been detected in solution [39] [40] [41]. Dissociation in the presence of SDS is dependent on detergent concentration. Van der Goot et al. reported that "the dimer begins to come apart at 0.0125% SDS and is nearly completely dissociated by 0.025% detergent" [39]. The SDS concentration in our system is 0.1% (w/v), which should be sufficient to achieve denaturation. However, we know of several examples where non-covalent oligomers might be formed in the presence of SDS or resist to denaturing conditions, for example, the Cholera toxin B subunit [21]. How the enzymatic modification of aerolysin affects these properties is not known.

Installation of fluorescent tags does not compromise the ability of aerolysin to bind to its receptors. The different toxin amounts required to achieve equivalent binding reflect the differences in LC50 observed for the unlabeled, sequence-modified aerolysin variants. Moreover, the immediate detachment of the adherent HeLa cells shortly after temperature shift is a clear indication of the toxicity of the aerolysin variants. In the case of AeL^{TAMRA},

where the unlabeled fraction constitutes the majority after reaction, it is not possible to infer toxicity of the labeled fraction, although the unlabeled, altered sequence of the input aerolysin preparation used for labeling is of course toxic.

With the double labeled ^{TAMRA}AeL.CP^{AF647} construct in hand, we could not only confirm the toxicity of the labeled fraction itself, but also visualize the loss of aerolyin's C-terminal peptide in the course of intoxication by microscopy. We thus confirm the previous findings of van der Goot et al that the chaperone is not part of the functional pore and separates from the active toxin [18].

A further application of sortagged aerolysin is the identification of new GPI-anchored human cell surface proteins that serve as receptors for the toxin. Previously, it was known that aerolysin binds to a subset of N-glycanated GPI-anchored proteins [11] [12] [42], where not only the GPI anchor, but also the receptor polypeptide moiety plays a role [13]. Plasma membrane micro-domains act as a concentration platform for such GPI-anchored proteins [43]. The earliest identified receptor was Thy-1 from mouse lymphocytes [44]. Others are an unidentified 80 kD protein on baby hamster kidney cells [6], an unidentified 47 kD receptor on rat erythrocytes [45], the variant surface glycoprotein (VSG) of *Trypanosoma brucei* over-expressed in mammalian cells, *Leishmania major* CD63, but only when expressed in Chinese hamster ovary cells [11], and murine contactin [46]. In addition, aerolysin binds to human complement decay accelerating factor (CD55) [47]. In our assay we were able to detect CD55, attesting to the power of our approach, along with mesothelin, urokinase plasminogen activator surface receptor (uPAR, CD87), glypican-1, and CD59 glycoprotein, a novel set of molecularly identified GPI-anchored proteins not previously associated with aerolysin binding. Of note, CD59 was specifically excluded as an aerolysin receptor in previous work [13]. We speculate that the reason for this observed difference might be of a technical nature. The fact that we identify CD59 with two different analysis methods, immunoblot and mass spectrometry, makes us confident that CD59 is a true interaction partner of aerolysin.

Sortagging converts aerolysin into a versatile and valuable tool to study the 'GPI-ome' as a means of further characterizing lipid rafts where most GPI-anchored proteins are clustered [48], The sortagging strategy described here should be applicable also to other members of the bacterial pore-forming toxin family and may facilitate further biophysical studies on membrane interactions and pore formation.

Acknowledgments

We are grateful to Gisou van der Goot for the plasmid encoding proaerolysin; Thijn Brummelkamp for KBM7 cells; Wendy Salmon for assistance with fluorescence microscopy; George Bell for statistics; Lenka Kundrat for help with figures; and all the Ploegh laboratory members for helpful discussions and suggestions.

Author Contributions

Conceived and designed the experiments: IW JGCP CPG. Performed the experiments: IW JGCP AEMB. Analyzed the data: IW JGCP AEMB HLP CPG. Contributed reagents/materials/analysis tools: IW JGCP AEMB CST ZL ES. Contributed to the writing of the manuscript: IW HLP CPG.

References

1. Alouf JE (2005) The Comprehensive Sourcebook of Bacterial Protein Toxins. Third Edition. Academic Press. ISBN: 978-0-12-088445-2.
2. Bernheimer AW, Avigad LS (1974) Partial characterization of aerolysin, a lytic exotoxin from Aeromonas hydrophila. Infection and Immunity 9: 1016–1021.
3. Wilmsen HU, Leonard KR, Tichelaar W, Buckley JT, Pattus F (1992) The aerolysin membrane channel is formed by heptamerization of the monomer. EMBO J 11: 2457–2463.

4. Moniatte M, van der Goot FG, Buckley JT, Pattus F, van Dorsselaer A (1996) Characterisation of the heptameric pore-forming complex of the Aeromonas toxin aerolysin using MALDI-TOF mass spectrometry. FEBS Lett 384: 269–272.

5. Wilmsen HU, Pattus F, Buckley JT (1990) Aerolysin, a hemolysin from Aeromonas hydrophila, forms voltage-gated channels in planar lipid bilayers. J Membr Biol 115: 71–81.

6. Abrami L, Fivaz M, Glauser PE, Parton RG, van der Goot FG (1998) A pore-forming toxin interacts with a GPI-anchored protein and causes vacuolation of the endoplasmic reticulum. The Journal of Cell Biology 140: 525–540.

7. Krause KH, Fivaz M, Monod A, van der Goot FG (1998) Aerolysin induces G-protein activation and Ca2+ release from intracellular stores in human granulocytes. J Biol Chem 273: 18122–18129.

8. Fennessey CM, Ivie SE, McClain MS (2012) Coenzyme depletion by members of the aerolysin family of pore-forming toxins leads to diminished ATP levels and cell death. Mol Biosyst 8: 2097–2105.

9. Pernot L, Schiltz M, van der Goot FG (2010) Preliminary crystallographic analysis of two oligomerization-deficient mutants of the aerolysin toxin, H132D and H132N, in their proteolyzed forms. Acta Crystallogr Sect F Struct Biol Cryst Commun 66: 1626–1630.

10. Iacovache I, Degiacomi MT, Pernot L, Ho S, Schiltz M, et al. (2011) Dual chaperone role of the C-terminal propeptide in folding and oligomerization of the pore-forming toxin aerolysin. PLoS Pathog 7: e1002135.

11. Diep DB, Nelson KL, Raja SM, Pleshak EN, Buckley JT (1998) Glycosylphos-phatidylinositol anchors are binding determinants for the channel-forming toxin aerolysin. J Biol Chem 273: 2355–2360.

12. Hong Y, Ohishi K, Inoue N, Kang JY, Shime H, et al. (2002) Requirement of N-glycan on GPI-anchored proteins for efficient binding of aerolysin but not Clostridium septicum alpha-toxin. EMBO J 21: 5047–5056.

13. Abrami L, Velluz M-C, Hong Y, Ohishi K, Mehlert A, et al. (2002) The glycan core of GPI-anchored proteins modulates aerolysin binding but is not sufficient: the polypeptide moiety is required for the toxin-receptor interaction. FEBS Lett 512: 249–254.

14. Howard SP, Buckley JT (1985) Activation of the hole-forming toxin aerolysin by extracellular processing. J Bacteriol 163: 336–340.

15. Abrami L, Fivaz M, Decroly E, Seidah NG, Jean F, et al. (1998) The pore-forming toxin proaerolysin is activated by furin. J Biol Chem 273: 32656–32661.

16. van der Goot FG, Pattus F, Wong KR, Buckley JT (1993) Oligomerization of the channel-forming aerolysin precedes insertion into lipid bilayers. Biochemistry. 32(10): 2636–42.

17. Degiacomi MT, Iacovache I, Pernot L, Chami M, Kudryashev M, et al. (2013) Molecular assembly of the aerolysin pore reveals a swirling membrane-insertion mechanism. Nat Chem Biol. 9(10): 623–9.

18. van der Goot FG, Hardie KR, Parker MW, Buckley JT (1994) The C-terminal peptide produced upon proteolytic activation of the cytolytic toxin aerolysin is not involved in channel formation. J Biol Chem 269: 30496–30501.

19. Popp MW, Antos JM, Ploegh HL (2009) Site-specific protein labeling via sortase-mediated transpeptidation. Curr Protoc Protein Sci Chapter 15: Unit15.3.

20. Guimaraes CP, Witte MD, Theile CS, Bozkurt G, Kundrat L, et al. (2013) Site-specific C-terminal and internal loop labeling of proteins using sortase-mediated reactions. Nat Protoc 8: 1787–1799.

21. Theile CS, Witte MD, Blom AEM, Kundrat L, Ploegh HL, et al. (2013) Site-specific N-terminal labeling of proteins using sortase-mediated reactions. Nat Protoc 8: 1800–1807.

22. Carette JE, Guimaraes CP, Varadarajan M, Park AS, Wuethrich I, et al. (2009) Haploid genetic screens in human cells identify host factors used by pathogens. Science 326: 1231–1235.

23. Iacovache I, Paumard P, Scheib H, Lesieur C, Sakai N, et al. (2006) A rivet model for channel formation by aerolysin-like pore-forming toxins. EMBO J 25: 457–466.

24. Chen I, Dorr BM, Liu DR (2011) A general strategy for the evolution of bond-forming enzymes using yeast display. Proceedings of the National Academy of Sciences 108: 11399–11404.

25. Hirakawa H, Ishikawa S, Nagamune T (2012) Design of Ca2+-independent Staphylococcus aureus sortase A mutants. Biotechnol Bioeng 109: 2955–2961.

26. Popp MW, Antos JM, Grotenbreg GM, Spooner E, Ploegh HL (2007) Sortagging: a versatile method for protein labeling. Nat Chem Biol 3: 707–708.

27. Laemmli UK (1970) Cleavage of structural proteins during the assembly of the head of bacteriophage T4. Nature 227: 680–685.

28. Popp MW, Ploegh HL (2011) Making and breaking peptide bonds: protein engineering using sortase. Angew Chem Int Ed Engl 50: 5024–5032.

29. Antos JM, Chew, Guimaraes CP, Yoder NC, Grotenbreg GM, et al. (2009) Site-specific N- and C-terminal labeling of a single polypeptide using sortases of different specificity. J Am Chem Soc 131: 10800–10801.

30. Hess GT, Cragnolini JJ, Popp MW, Allen MA, Dougan SK, et al. (2012) M13 bacteriophage display framework that allows sortase-mediated modification of surface-accessible phage proteins. Bioconjug Chem 23: 1478–1487.

31. Hess GT, Guimaraes CP, Spooner E, Ploegh HL, Belcher AM (2013) Orthogonal labeling of M13 minor capsid proteins with DNA to self-assemble end-to-end multiphage structures. ACS Synth Biol 2: 490–496.

32. Guimaraes CP, Carette JE, Varadarajan M, Antos J, Popp MW, et al. (2011) Identification of host cell factors required for intoxication through use of modified cholera toxin. The Journal of Cell Biology 195: 751–764.

33. Witte MD, Theile CS, Wu T, Guimaraes CP, Blom AEM, et al. (2013) Production of unnaturally linked chimeric proteins using a combination of sortase-catalyzed transpeptidation and click chemistry. Nat Protoc 8: 1808–1819.

34. Diep DB, Lawrence TS, Ausió J, Howard SP, Buckley JT (1998) Secretion and properties of the large and small lobes of the channel-forming toxin aerolysin. Mol Microbiol 30: 341–352.

35. Tsitrin Y, Morton CJ, el-Bez C, Paumard P, Velluz M-C, et al. (2002) Conversion of a transmembrane to a water-soluble protein complex by a single point mutation. Nat Struct Biol 9: 729–733.

36. van der Goot FG, Lakey J, Pattus F, Kay CM, Sorokine O, et al. (1992) Spectroscopic study of the activation and oligomerization of the channel-forming toxin aerolysin: identification of the site of proteolytic activation. Biochemistry 31: 8566–8570.

37. Tucker AD, Parker MW, Tsernoglou D, Buckley JT (1990) Crystallization of a proform of aerolysin, a hole-forming toxin from Aeromonas hydrophila. J Mol Biol 212: 561–562.

38. Race PR, Bentley ML, Melvin JA, Crow A, Hughes RK, et al. (2009) Crystal structure of Streptococcus pyogenes sortase A: implications for sortase mechanism. J Biol Chem 284: 6924–6933.

39. van der Goot FG, Ausió J, Wong KR, Pattus F, Buckley JT (1993) Dimerization stabilizes the pore-forming toxin aerolysin in solution. J Biol Chem 268: 18272–18279.

40. Fivaz M, Velluz MC, van der Goot FG (1999) Dimer dissociation of the pore-forming toxin aerolysin precedes receptor binding. J Biol Chem 274: 37705–37708.

41. Barry R, Moore S, Alonso A, Ausió J, Buckley JT (2001) The channel-forming protein proaerolysin remains a dimer at low concentrations in solution. J Biol Chem 276: 551–554.

42. Howard SP, Buckley JT (1982) Membrane glycoprotein receptor and hole-forming properties of a cytolytic protein toxin. Biochemistry 21: 1662–1667.

43. Abrami L, van der Goot FG (1999) Plasma membrane microdomains act as concentration platforms to facilitate intoxication by aerolysin. The Journal of Cell Biology 147: 175–184.

44. Nelson KL, Raja SM, Buckley JT (1997) The glycosylphosphatidylinositol-anchored surface glycoprotein Thy-1 is a receptor for the channel-forming toxin aerolysin. J Biol Chem 272: 12170–12174.

45. Cowell S, Aschauer W, Gruber HJ, Nelson KL, Buckley JT (1997) The erythrocyte receptor for the channel-forming toxin aerolysin is a novel glycosylphosphatidylinositol-anchored protein - Cowell −2003 - Molecular Microbiology - Wiley Online Library. Mol Microbiol 25: 343–350.

46. MacKenzie CR, Hirama T, Buckley JT (1999) Analysis of receptor binding by the channel-forming toxin aerolysin using surface plasmon resonance. J Biol Chem 274: 22604–22609.

47. Andrew AJ, Kao S, Strebel K (2011) C-terminal Hydrophobic Region in Human Bone Marrow Stromal Cell Antigen 2 (BST-2)/Tetherin Protein Functions as Second Transmembrane Motif. Journal of Biological Chemistry 286: 39967–39981.

48. Simons K, Sampaio JL (2011) Membrane Organization and Lipid Rafts. Cold Spring Harb Perspect Biol. 3(10): a004697 doi: 10.1101/cshperspect.a004697.

A New Ochratoxin A Biodegradation Strategy Using *Cupriavidus basilensis* Őr16 Strain

Szilamér Ferenczi[1*⍟], **Mátyás Cserháti**[2⍟], **Csilla Krifaton**[2], **Sándor Szoboszlay**[2], **József Kukolya**[3], **Zsuzsanna Szőke**[4], **Balázs Kőszegi**[4], **Mihály Albert**[5], **Teréz Barna**[6], **Miklós Mézes**[7], **Krisztina J. Kovács**[1], **Balázs Kriszt**[2]

1 Institute of Experimental Medicine, Laboratory of Molecular Neuroendocrinology, Budapest, Hungary, 2 Szent István University, Department of Environmental Protection and Safety, Gödöllő, Hungary, 3 Central Environmental and Food Science Research Institute, Department of Microbiology, Budapest, Hungary, 4 Soft Flow Hungary R&D Ltd., Pécs, Hungary, 5 CEVA Phylaxia Ltd, Budapest, Hungary, 6 University of Debrecen, Department of Genetics and Applied Microbiology, Debrecen, Hungary, 7 Szent István University, Department of Nutrition, Gödöllő, Hungary

Abstract

Ochratoxin-A (OTA) is a mycotoxin with possibly carcinogenic and nephrotoxic effects in humans and animals. OTA is often found as a contaminant in agricultural commodities. The aim of the present work was to evaluate OTA-degrading and detoxifying potential of *Cupriavidus basilensis* ŐR16 strain. *In vivo* administration of OTA in CD1 male mice (1 or 10 mg/kg body weight for 72 hours or 0.5 mg/kg body weight for 21 days) resulted in significant elevation of OTA levels in the blood, histopathological alterations- and transcriptional changes in OTA-dependent genes (*annexinA2, clusterin, sulphotransferase* and *gadd45* and *gadd153*) in the renal cortex. These OTA-induced changes were not seen in animals that have been treated with culture supernatants in which OTA was incubated with *Cupriavidus basilensis* ŐR16 strain for 5 days. HPLC and ELISA methods identified ochratoxin α as the major metabolite of OTA in *Cupriavidus basilensis* ŐR16 cultures, which is not toxic *in vivo*. This study has demonstrated that *Cupriavidus basilensis* ŐR16 efficiently degrade OTA without producing toxic adventitious metabolites.

Editor: Gayle E. Woloschak, Northwestern University Feinberg School of Medicine, United States of America

Funding: This study was supported by the TÁMOP-4.2.1.B-11/2/KMR-2011-0003, KTIA-AIK_12-1-2013-0017, Research Centre of Excellence-17586-4/2013/TUDPOL, TÁMOP 4.2.1/B-09/1/KONV-2010–0007 and the work was supported by grants from Hungarian Research Fund OTKA 109622 to K.J.K.; 109744 to Sz.F., and Research Centre of Excellence - 8526-5/2014/TUDPOL. The funders had no role in study design, data collection and analysis, decision to publish, or preparation of the manuscript.

Competing Interests: The authors (Mihály A, Szőke Zs and Kőszegi B) are employed by a commercial company (CEVA Phylaxia Ltd and Soft Flow Hungary R&D Ltd.).

* Email: ferenczi@koki.hu

⍟ These authors contributed equally to this work.

Introduction

Ochratoxin-A (OTA) is a hazardous mycotoxin produced by number of *Aspergillus* and *Penicillium* species [1]. Mycotoxins are extracellular secreted secondary metabolites of moulds that are harmful or toxic to animals and humans [2]. The chemical structure of OTA molecule (*N*-{[(3*R*)-5-chloro-8-hydroxy-3-methyl-1-oxo-3,4-dihydro-1*H*-isochromen-7-yl]carbonyl}-L-phenylalanine) includes a β-phenylalanine-dihydroisocoumarine derivative, which is very stable at high temperature and resistant to hydrolysis, hence processing of raw materials in feed and food industry does not eliminate the OTA and the toxin remains intact in the end-products. The OTA is often found as a contaminant in cereal grains or other crops and plant products such as red wine, coffee beans, peanuts, cocoa beans, and different spices [3-5]. Dried Distillers Grains with Solubles (DDGS) remaining after bioethanol production from maize is a valuable protein source for animal nutrition, but high mycotoxin content of DDGS limits its application [6]. On the other hand, the mycotoxin is also capable to accumulate in several animal-derived food products (meat, egg, blood and milk products) [7].

Chronic OTA exposure is the major causative chemical of mycotoxin-induced porcine nephropathy [8,9] and Balkan endemic nephropathy (BEN) in humans [10-13]. The OTA-induced nephropathy is characterized by degeneration of epithelial cells in the renal proximal tubules, glomerulus degeneration in renal cortex area and interstitial fibrosis resulting in polyuria and various changes in hematological and biochemical parameters [14]. On the other hand, chemical structure of OTA shows similarity to the amino acid phenylalanine, thus the toxin is able to interrupt the protein synthesis [15,16]. Influence of OTA as a causal chemical substance of different types of cancer such as renal adenocarcinoma and liver tumor have been described in laboratory rodents and in humans, as well [17,18]. OTA affects the expression of several genes related to cell damage, apoptosis, cellular stress, such as Growth arrest and DNA-damage-inducible proteins (*gadd45* and *gadd153*), *annexins, sulfotransferase* and *clusterin* [19].

Several strategies can be used to reduce OTA levels in animal feed and human food. The most important are preventive methods since they avoid the contamination of commodities in the first place. However, fully implemented Hazard Analysis and

Critical Control Points (HACCP) schemes are rare, and when the individual measures fail or are not in place, OTA remains in feed and food products. Decontamination or detoxification procedures can be used to remove or to reduce OTA levels. Remediation processes are often used to eliminate, reduce or avoid the toxic effects of OTA. The widely used physical adsorbents have some disadvantages including limited efficiency, high cost and nonspecific binding of some important nutrients, such as vitamins or minerals and therapeutic agents. Biological methods have been considered as an alternative to physical and chemical treatments. The biodegradation is the most promising approach to control mycotoxins and these methods are important postharvest strategies to protect the animal and consumer health.

Several enzymes may be involved in the microbiological degradation of OTA. However, little information is available and very few have been purified and characterized. The first reported protease able to hydrolyze OTA was carboxypeptidase A (CPA) (EC 3.4.17.1) from bovine pancreas [20].

Previously more than fifteen species of bacteria [21] have been shown to degrade OTA – but not yet any *Cupriavidus* species – and many species of fungi have also been reported. However, vast majority of this biodegradation by microorganisms cannot be regarded as detoxification since the toxicity after the biotransformation was not elucidated. To develop a bacterial strain to efficient biodegradation of OTA, selection of the most active and environmentally safe microbes is required. The aim of the present work was to evaluate the OTA-degrading and detoxifying potential of a *Cupriavidus basilensis* strain, which mycotoxin-degrading ability was presumable based on its genome project [22].

Traditional chemical analysis and immunochemical methods are unable to detect the toxic effect of all potential degradation products; therefore it is important to monitor toxicity *in vivo*. Moreover, the European Food Safety Authority reported that contamination of animal feed by mycotoxins may be reduced by mycotoxin-detoxifying agents but the additive effects of the resulting metabolite(s)/degradation products(s) must also be monitored in appropriate toxicological studies. Thus, development of *in vivo* studies is essential to investigate biodegradation and detoxification efficiency directly on the renal cortical area, the most sensitive organ for OTA in animals and humans, as well. For this purpose the application of a rodent based *in vivo* toxicological experiment can be the most suitable approach, in which two markers are analysed: alterations in the kidney and spleen weight and changes in the expression of OTA-affected genes in the kidney tissue [19]. This method in combination with analytical and immunochemical techniques was applied to analyse OTA and residuals toxicity after biodegradation.

Materials and Methods

2.1 Reagents

Ochratoxin-A (OTA) (Fermentek, Israel), methyl- methanesulfonate (MMS) (Sigma-Aldrich Co., USA), OTalpha standard (Biopure, cat. number: BRM S02053, lot. number: L12503A), dimethyl-sulfoxid - DMSO (Sigma-Aldrich Co., USA), Tris-(hydroximethyl)- aminomethane, Tris (Sigma_Aldrich, USA), modified Luria-Bertani (LB) medium (1 g triptone, 0,5 g yeast extract, 0,9 g NaCl in 1000 ml distilled water) were used.

2.2 Bacterial strain and culture conditions in the biodegradation test

The strain *Cupriavidus basilensis* ŐR16, was isolated from a Hungarian pristine soil sample. It was identified by molecular taxonomy as *C. basilensis* and deposited in the National Collection of Agricultural and Industrial Microorganisms (NCAIM BO2487). Cells were streaked on LB agar plates and incubated at 28°C for 72 h. Single colonies were inoculated into 50 ml liquid LB medium and incubated at 170 rpm at 28°C for 72 h. The optical density of the cultures was adjusted to 0.6 ($OD_{600} = 0.6$) and 50 ml was added to 1350 ml sterile modified LB medium to which OTA (28 mg OTA was dissolved in the 1400 ml modified LB medium) had been added reaching a 20 mg/l final concentration. A no inoculated control with 20 mg/l OTA content and a control culture without OTA was applied. Control culture was essential since in toxicity testing animals are presumably sensitive to metabolic by-products of the *C. basilensis* ŐR16 strain. Samples were incubated (170 rpm, 28°C) for 5 days. One-millilitre samples from the flasks were removed at the 1st, 2nd, 3rd, 5th day, centrifuged at 25,000 × g at 4°C for 20 min and both supernatant and pellet were stored at −20°C until further use. At the 5th day (end-point) of the experiment the entire pellet material was removed (25,000 × g at 4°C for 20 min) and the supernatant was concentrated by a factor of 100 on an Edwards Micromodulyo lyophilisator and the lyophilised supernatant was used in the animal experiments. Remaining OTA concentrations in the supernatant were analyzed by High Performance Liquid Chromatography (Wessling Hungary Ltd., Hungary) and the supernatant and pellet were analysed by ELISA (Soft Flow Ltd., Hungary).

2.3 Analysis of samples for remaining toxin concentration

2.3.1 Enzyme-linked immunosorbent assay (ELISA). The OTA toxin concentrations at the zero point in the supernatant and also in the pellet on the 1st, 2nd, 3rd and 5th day of the degradation experiment were determined by TOXI-WATCH ELISA kit (Cat#301051, Soft Flow Hungary R& D Ltd., Hungary) according to the manufacturer's specifications. Assay range: (0.1375 ng/ml–44 ng/ml, limit of detection: 0.130 ng/ml). 0.1M PBS buffer with 3% sodium-hydrogen-carbonate $NaHCO_3$, (4:1 v/v%) was used for sample dilution, while standards contain the same solution (PBS/3% $NaHCO_3$ 4:1 ratio).

The 201052-5G9 (Soft Flow Hungary Ltd., Hungary) monoclonal antibody specifically binds to the mycotoxin OTA. The immunogen used to generate the hybridoma 5G9 was OTA-BSA conjugate. The 201052-5G9 antibody cross-reacts with ochratox-in-B (9.3%). Measurements were carried out in triplicate and the measurements were performed on Thermo Scientific Multiskan EX photometric microplate absorbance reader.

2.3.2 High-performance liquid chromatography (HPLC). HPLC analyses were carried out by Wessling Hungary Ltd., an accredited laboratory, using a HPLC series 1100 from Agilent Technologies, USA.

The supernatant collected at the beginning and on the 1st, 2nd, 3rd, 5th day of the degradation experiment, was analyzed for OTA and its derivative OT-α. The bacterial pellet was suspended in 1 ml methanol and centrifuged (3,000 × g for 10 min at <10°C), then the supernatant was analysed for OTA. Results for degradation potential were corrected with the pellet analysis.

Protocols for the immuno-affinity column cleaning, derivatization, LC separation and fluorescence detection of the compounds were carried out according to European Standard (EN) and International Organization for Standardization (ISO) (EN ISO 15141-1:2000 standard) for OTA. For the determination of OTα, the column, eluent composition and detection parameters were modified (see in Supplementary Materials, Table S1). HPLC measurements were carried out in triplicates.

2.4 Animals

Adult, 7–9 week old, male CD1 mice (from the colony breed at the Institute of Experimental Medicine, Budapest) were used. Animals had free access to rodent food and water and were maintained under controlled conditions (temperature, $21 \pm 1°C$; humidity, 65%; light-dark cycle, 12-h light/12-h dark, lights on at 07:00). All procedures were conducted in accordance with the guidelines set by the European Communities Council Directive (86/609 EEC) and the protocol was approved by the Institutional Animal Care and Use Committee of the Institute of Experimental Medicine, Budapest Hungary (permit number: PEI/001/35-4/ 2013).

2.5 Measuring of the blood OTA concentrations by ELISA

Extraction of OTA was carried out from 50 µl plasma sample with 100 µl chloroform (Sigma-Aldrich Co., USA) and 10µl 0.1 M H_3PO_4. The mixture was vortexed and incubated on Bio RS-24 vertical rotator (Biosan) rotating 25 rpm for 20 min then vortexed again and centrifuged for 10 min at $10000 \times g$. The lower phase was transferred to a microcentrifuge tube, vortexed with 100 µl 3% (w/v) $NaHCO_3$ solution, and incubated on the vertical rotator (25 rpm, 10 min). The phases were let to split and the upper phase was used for further measurements.

The OTA concentration of the extract was measured by Toxi-Watch OTA ELISA Kit (Cat#301051, Soft Flow Hungary Ltd., Hungary). Measurements were performed on a Thermo Scientific Multiskan EX photometric microplate absorbance reader. Measurements were carried out in triplicate. The recovery was 77.6 ± 5.42 % as was measured with 20 ng/ml OTA spiked blood plasma samples.

2.6 Animal treatment

Male CD1 mice were housed and treated according to OECD guideline for the testing of chemicals No. 407 with full access to food and drinking water. Body weight, food and water consumption was recorded daily. OTA was dissolved in DMSO and a stock solution in 100 mg/ml OTA concentration was prepared, stored at 4°C. Thereafter this master solution was diluted into sterile drinking water containing 10 mM Tris (pH 8) to reach the required experimental OTA dose. OTA and vehicle solutions were administered daily via oral gavage (200µl/animal) in the morning hours.

For testing OTA, three different dosage groups (n = 7-10/ group) were formed. For acute tests 1 mg/kg bw and 10 mg/kg bw sacrificed after 72 h; for chronic test 0.5 mg/kg bw, sacrificed after 21 day. Sterile drinking water supplemented with 10 mM Tris and equal concentration of DMSO with high dose OTA group in acute experiment and equal concentration of DMSO with chronic experiment were applied as control. As genotoxic control, MMS was used in 100 mg/kg bw dose for the 72 h experiment and 40 mg/kg bw dose for the 21 day experiment [23].

For testing OTA detoxification by *C. basilensis* Őr16, samples and controls originated from the degradation experiment were applied (section 2.2). The lyophilized supernatant from the biodegradation experiment with *C. basilensis* Őr16 strain was dissolved in 11.2 ml sterile tap water containing Tris and DMSO following the same procedures that used in high OTA content preparation (10 mg/kg bw). The theoretical OTA concentration of this solution is 2.5 mg/ml, calculated by initial OTA quantity (28 mg OTA). This stock solution was used for the treatment of high OTA deg group (group treated with theoretical 10 mg/kg body weight Ochratoxin A). Forty µl from this solution was added to each 10g body weight (0.1 mg theoretical OTA quantity).

Following dilutions were made from this stock solution for the lower OTA deg groups treatment (group treated with 1 mg/kg body weight and 0.5 mg/kg bw Ochratoxin A) by using sterile tap water containing 10 mM Tris (pH 8) and balanced DMSO. Doses were calculated from the animal weights and administered via oral gavages.

The animal treatment with intact Ochratoxin A and the biodegradation experiment were carried out from same OTA batch. Animals were decapitated, trunk blood collected on ice, spleen and kidney were removed and their weights were measured. Kidney was cut longitudinally resulting in half kidneys. One half was fixed in 10% buffered formalin solution for histological examination. From the other half of the kidney, the cortex and medulla were separated and frozen immediately in dry ice and stored at −80°C to prevent RNA degradation.

2.7 Quantitative Real-Time PCR

Frozen kidney cortex tissue samples were homogenized by IKA Ultra Turrax in TRI Reagent Solution (Ambion, USA) and total RNA was isolated with QIAGEN RNeasy Mini Kit (Qiagen, USA) according the manufacturer's instruction. To eliminate genomic DNA contamination DNase I treatment were used and 100 µl Rnase-free DNase I (1 unit DNase) (Thermo Scientific, USA) solution was added. Sample quality control and the quantitative analysis were carried out by NanoDrop (Thermo Scientific, USA). Amplification was not detected in the RT-minus controls. The cDNA synthesis was performed with the High Capacity cDNA Reverse Transcription Kit (Applied Biosystems, USA). Primers for the comparative Ct experiments were designed by Primer Express 3.0 Program. The primers (Microsynth, Balgach) were used in the Real-Time PCR reaction with Fast EvaGreen qPCR Master Mix (Biotium, USA) on ABI StepOne-Plus instrument was listed in Table S2.

List of the genes: peptidylprolyl isomerase A (*ppia*, NM_008907), annexin A2 (*anxa2*, NM_007585), clusterin (*clu*, NM_013492), DNA-damage inducible transcript 3 (*gadd153*, NM_007837), growth arrest and DNA-damage-inducible 45 alpha (*gadd45a*, NM_007836) and sulfotransferase (*sult1c2*, NM_026935).

The gene expression was analyzed by ABI Step One 2.1 program. The amplicon was tested by Melt Curve Analysis on ABI Step OnePlus Instrument. Experiments were normalized to *ppia* (peptidylprolyl isomerase A) expression [24].

2. 8 Histology

Formalin fixed kidney samples were processed and embedded in paraffin using the standard protocol. Sections of 4 µm were stained with haematoxylin and eosin. Slides were analysed by an expert veterinary pathologist in a blinded manner.

2.9 Statistical analysis

Data are expressed as means $\pm$ SD. The data were first subjected to a Kolmogorov-Smirnov normality test. Data passing this test, were analyzed by One way ANOVA followed by the Tukey's *post hoc* test. Data showed non-Gaussian distribution, the Kruskal-Wallis test was used. Statistical analysis was performed using GraphPad PRISM version 6 software (GraphPad Software, USA). $P \leq 0.05$ was considered significant.

Results

3.1 Ochratoxin-A biodegradation by *Cupriavidus basilensis* ŐR16

The biodegradation ability of *Cupriavidus basilensis* ŐR16 strain to detoxify OTA was monitored by different analytical approaches. The HPLC and ELISA results are summarised in Fig. 1, where samples originating from the OTA degradation experiments (1st, 2nd, 3rd, 5th day) are indicated as a function of time. OTA concentration in the no inoculated control remained 20 mg/l during the incubation (5 days) measured by HPLC and ELISA. In the bacterial pellet ELISA detected lower than 0.004% residual OTA of the original concentration (20 mg/l). The first day of incubation *Cupriavidus basilensis* ŐR16 cells degraded 0.15% of the initial OTA content, but this OTA content reduced by the 5th day below 0.004%, thus OTA elimination from the matrix was attributed to metabolic activity. OTA content in the supernatants reduced continuously during the 5-day incubation and the OTA was completely degraded (94% decrease measured by ELISA, 100% decrease by HPLC). Based on the HPLC results OTA was metabolized to OTα, since OTα content increased in parallel by OTA decrease.

3.2 Water, food consumption and body weight change of mice

Food and water consumption did not change significantly during acute or chronic OTA administration with the supernatant samples from biodegradation study. Body weight of the treated animals in either experiment also did not alter significantly.

3.3 Blood OTA content in acute and chronic toxicities

Low levels of OTA were detected in the blood of vehicle or MMS-treated control animals (5.30± 3.9 and 3.20±4.9 ng/ml respectively). Acute mycotoxin treatment significantly elevated OTA concentration in the blood OTA 1 (269.73 ± 60.6 ng/ml OTA in blood plasma, p = 0.0055), and OTA 10 (1969.28 ±654.6 ng/ml OTA in blood plasma, p = 0.0023) groups. However, significantly lower levels of OTA were detected in plasma samples of mice treated with 10 mg/kg bw biodegraded OTA products in acute tests (101.18±11.4 ng/ml OTA,

p = 0.0236) (Fig. 2A). Chronic (21 days) OTA treatment (0.5 mg/kg bw) resulted in 231.35± 50.23 ng/ml OTA level in the blood (p = 0.0001), however that elevation of OTA levels were not seen in animals treated with the same dose of biodegraded OTA (Fig. 2B). The batches of high quality animal feed were also tested by SFH laboratory (Soft Flow Hungary Ltd., Hungary), and traces of OTA were detected (3.05±0.12 µg/kg feed).

3.4 Effect of OTA on the spleen and kidney weight

Spleen and kidney are sensitive indicators of OTA toxicity. The acute OTA administration did not influence significantly the kidney wet weight, but the spleen wet weights normalized to body weight decreased significantly in both MMS and OTA treated groups (p = 0.0096, p = 0.0109 and p = 0,0393) (Fig. S1B in Supplementary Materials). On the other hand chronic OTA administration decreased significantly the kidney wet weight normalized to body weight only in the OTA treated group (p = 0.0059) (Fig. S1C in Supplementary Materials). The spleen wet weight normalized to body weight did not show statistically significant differences between the MMS and OTA treated groups (Fig. S1D in Supplementary Materials). The bacterial residuals did not showed toxic effects on the spleen and the kidney in both experiments as showed by their wet weight normalized to body weight.

3.5 Histopathological analysis of renal cortex tissue

Animals treated with OTA (1 mg/kg bw or 10 mg/kg bw) for 72 h showed clear degenerative lesions mainly located in the inner part of the cortex. Sporadic cell necrosis of the tubular epithelium with cell detachment to the tubular lumen was detectable. Multifocal tubular necrosis also occurred. Dispersed apoptotic bodies, cell size reduction and condensed chromatin in nucleus were observed at high OTA dosed groups and in the chronically treated animals. Beyond degenerative changes tubular cell regeneration has been detected in the chronic OTA treated group. Mice treated with biodegraded OTA and their residuals did not exhibit remarkable histopathological changes. The *Cupriavidus basilensis* Őr16 alone showed similar histology to vehicle group (Fig. 3).

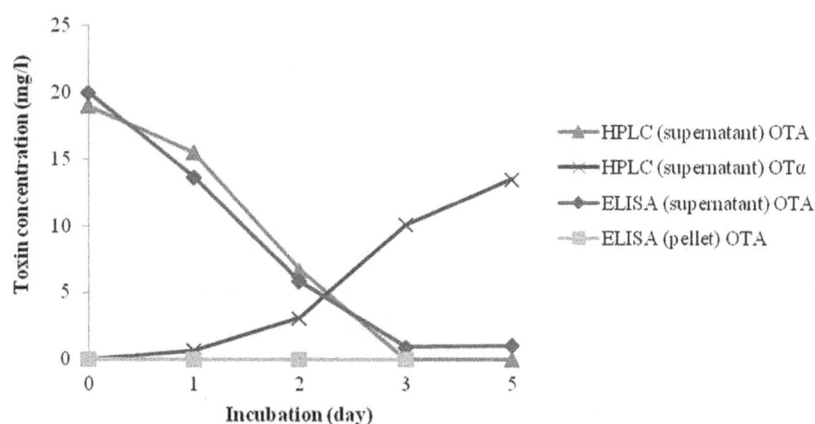

Figure 1. Ochratoxin-A biodegradation by *Cupriavidus basilensis* ŐR16 during 5 day incubation. Continuous decrease of the OTA concentration is detected in the supernatant and pellet, while OTα concentration is increasing. Abbreviations: HPLC (supernatant OTA) – OTA concentration in the supernatant originated from the degradation experiment measured by HPLC, HPLC (supernatant OTα) – OTα concentration in the supernatant originated from the degradation experiment measured by HPLC, ELISA (supernatant) OTA – OTA concentration in the supernatant originated from the degradation experiment measured by ELISA, ELISA (pellet) OTA – OTA concentration in the pellet originated from the degradation experiment measured by ELISA. Measurements were carried out in triplicate, SD>3%.

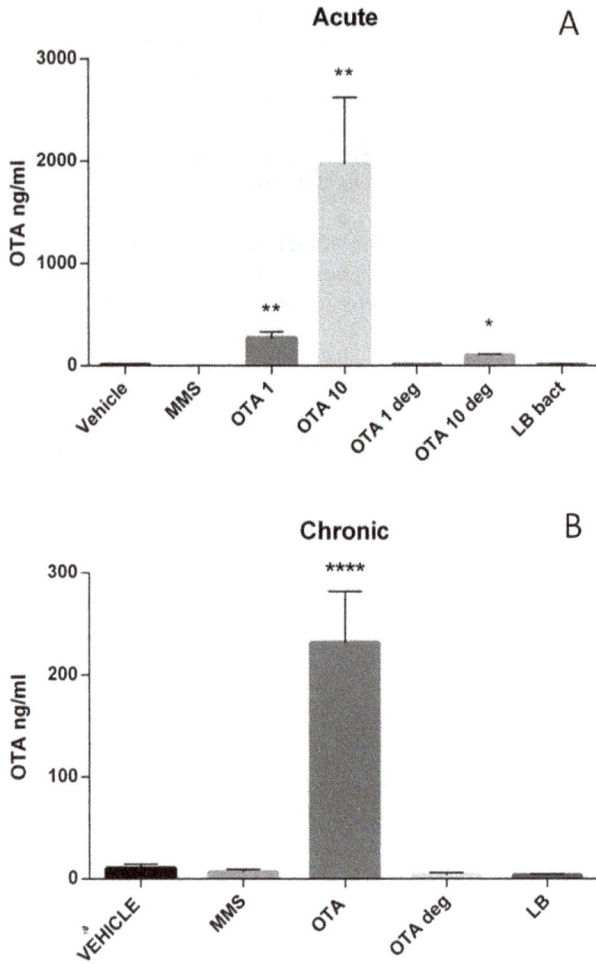

Figure 2. OTA concentration in the plasma (ng/ml) analyzed by ELISA after 72 hours of treatment (A). OTA 1 and OTA 10 groups show elevated OTA concentrations in blood plasma. The OTA 10 deg group shows increased OTA content. Abbreviations: MMS- Group treated with methyl methanesulfonate, OTA 1 and OTA 10- Groups treated with 1 and 10 mg/kg body weight Ochratoxin A, OTA 1 deg and OTA 10 deg- Groups treated with 1 and 10 mg/kg body weight Ochratoxin A + *Cupriavidus basilensis* ŐR16 in modified Luria- Bertani medium, LB bact- *Cupriavidus basilensis* ŐR16 in modified Luria- Bertani medium (Kruskal-Wallis test was used). OTA concentrations in the plasma (ng/ml) analyzed by ELISA after 21 days of treatment (B). The OTA 0.5 group shows elevated OTA blood concentrations. Abbreviations: MMS – Group treated with methyl methanesulfonate, OTA 0.5 – Group treated with 0.5 mg/kg body weight Ochratoxin A, OTA 0.5 deg – Group treated with 0.5 mg/kg body weight Ochratoxin A + *Cupriavidus basilensis* ŐR16 in modified Luria- Bertani medium, LB bact – *Cupriavidus basilensis* ŐR16 in modified Luria- Bertani medium. (One way ANOVA followed by the Tukey's *post hoc* test were used) Data are presented as mean ± SD (n = 7–10, **p<0.01)

3.6 Effect of acute OTA and OTA biodegradation residuals on the expression of various marker genes in the kidney

The high dose OTA and the MMS treatment significantly increased *gadd 45* (p = 0.00014) and *gadd 153* (p = 0.0112) mRNA levels (Fig. 4 A and B). The *Cupriavidus basilensis* ŐR16-metabolized OTA residuals did not influence mRNA levels of marker genes. LB with the bacterial strain did not change the expressions of genotoxic marker genes. The acute OTA admin-

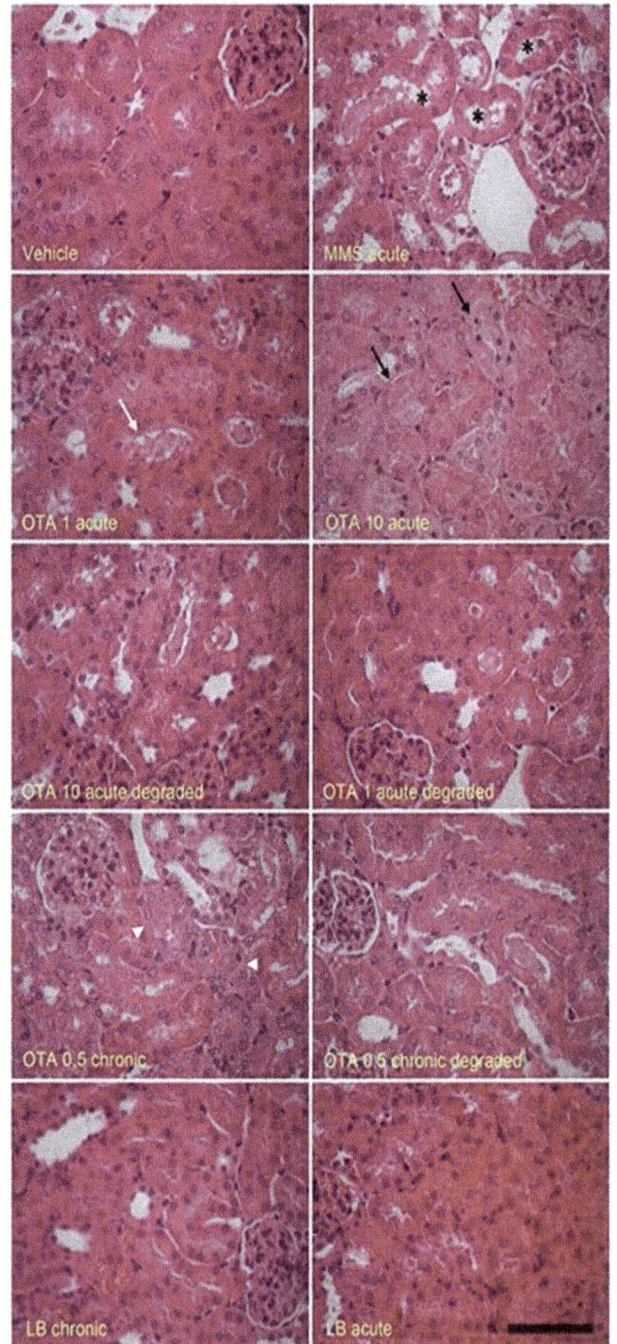

Figure 3. Histology of the kidneys following OTA and degraded OTA administrations. Photomicrographs showing hematoxylin-eosine stained kidney sections. Abbreviations: MMS- –methyl methanesulfonate treated animals, OTA 1 and OTA 10 – Groups treated with 1 and 10 mg/kg body weight Ochratoxin A, OTA 1 deg and OTA 10 deg – Groups treated with 1 and 10 mg/kg body weight Ochratoxin A + *Cupriavidus basilensis* ŐR16 in modified Luria-Bertani medium, OTA 0.5 – Group treated with 0.5 mg/kg body weight Ochratoxin A, OTA 0.5 deg – Group treated with 0.5 mg/kg body weight Ochratoxin A + *Cupriavidus basilensis* ŐR16 in modified Luria-Bertani medium, LB bact – *Cupriavidus basilensis* ŐR16 in modified Luria- Bertani medium. Symbols: asterisk- dilated tubules with detached necrotic epithelial cells, white arrow- detached necrotic epithelial cells, black arrow-necrotic tubular cells, white arrowhead- tubular cell regeneration. Scale bar: 100 μm.

istration with high dosage significantly elevated the *annexin2* mRNA expression (p = 0.0101). The end products of the OTA biodegradation did not change the *annexin2* mRNA expression in the kidney cortex samples (Fig. 5A). Elevated expression level of *clusterin* was observed in the high dose OTA treated group (p = 0.000141), however metabolites of the biodegraded OTA did not influence the *clusterin* mRNA levels (Fig. 5B). Animals treated with high OTA dosage showed significant decrease in the *sult1c2* mRNA levels (p = 0.000129). The biodegraded OTA did not influence the *sult1c2* mRNA expression in the renal cortex (Fig. 6).

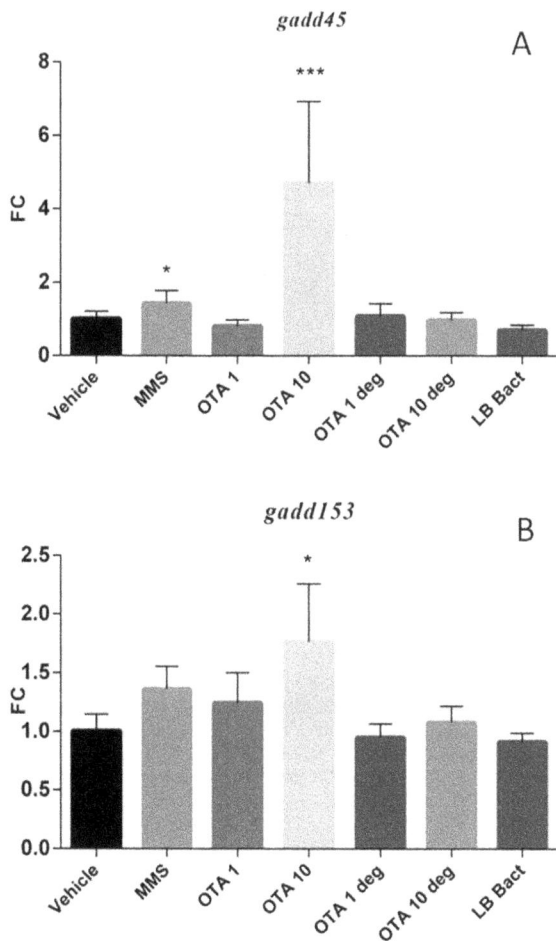

Figure 4. Effect of acute (72 hours) OTA treatment on *gadd45* mRNA expression (A). MMS and OTA 10 elevated the *gadd45* mRNA level. The metabolised OTA by *Cupriavidus basilensis* ŐR16 (OTA 1 deg and OTA 10 deg groups) not influenced the mRNA level (One way ANOVA followed by the Tukey's *post hoc* test were used). Effect of acute (72 hours) OTA treatment on *gadd153* mRNA expression (B). OTA 10 elevated the *gadd153* mRNA level. The metabolised OTA by *Cupriavidus basilensis* ŐR16 (OTA 1 deg and OTA 10 deg groups) not influenced the mRNA level. (Kruskal-Wallis test was used) Abbreviations: MMS – Group treated with methyl methanesulfonate, OTA 1 and OTA 10 – Groups treated with 1 and 10 mg/kg body weight Ochratoxin A, OTA 1 deg and OTA 10 deg – Groups treated with 1 and 10 mg/kg body weight Ochratoxin A + *Cupriavidus basilensis* ŐR16 in modified Luria-Bertani medium, LB bact- *Cupriavidus basilensis* ŐR16 in modified Luria-Bertani medium. Data are presented as mean ± SD (n = 7–10, * p<0.05, ***p< 0.001)

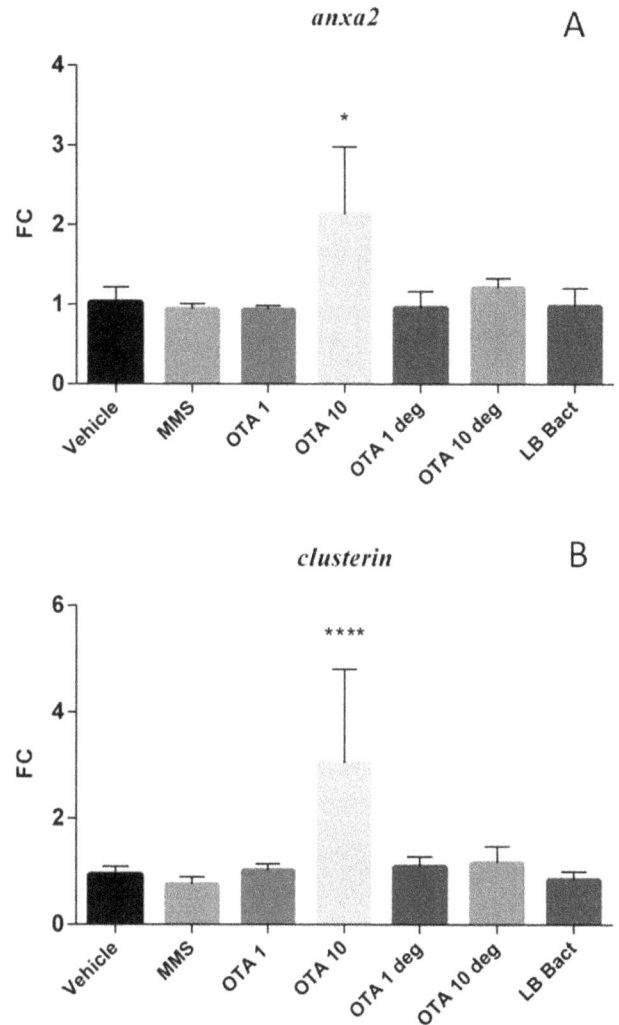

Figure 5. Effect of acute (72 hours) OTA treatment on *annexin2* mRNA expression (A). OTA 10 elevated the *annexin2* mRNA level. The metabolised OTA by *Cupriavidus basilensis* ŐR16 (OTA 1 deg and OTA 10 deg groups) did not influence the mRNA level (Kruskal-Wallis test was used). Effect of acute (72 hours) OTA treatment on *clusterin* mRNA expression (B). OTA 10 elevated the *clusterin* mRNA level. The metabolised OTA by *Cupriavidus basilensis* ŐR16 (OTA 1 deg and OTA 10 deg groups) did not influence the mRNA level. (One way ANOVA followed by the Tukey's *post hoc* test were used) Abbreviations: MMS – Group treated with methyl methanesulfonate, OTA 1 and OTA 10 – Groups treated with 1 and 10 mg/kg body weight Ochratoxin A, OTA 1 deg and OTA 10 deg- Groups treated with 1 and 10 mg/kg body weight Ochratoxin A + *Cupriavidus basilensis* ŐR16 in modified Luria-Bertani medium, LB bact – *Cupriavidus basilensis* ŐR16 in modified Luria-Bertani medium. Data are presented as mean ± SD (n = 7–10, ** p<0.01, *** p<0.001).

3.7 Effect of chronic OTA and OTA biodegradation residuals on the expression of marker genes in the kidney

The chronic low dose OTA exposure significantly induced *gadd45* (p = 0.0001) and *gadd153* (p = 0.0141) mRNA levels in the kidney. MMS and OTA degradation products did not affect the mRNA levels of the genotoxic markers (Fig. 7A and 7B). The *annexin2* expression was increased in OTA treated animals (p = 0.000177) (Fig. 8A). On the other hand *clusterin* mRNA

sulfotransferase

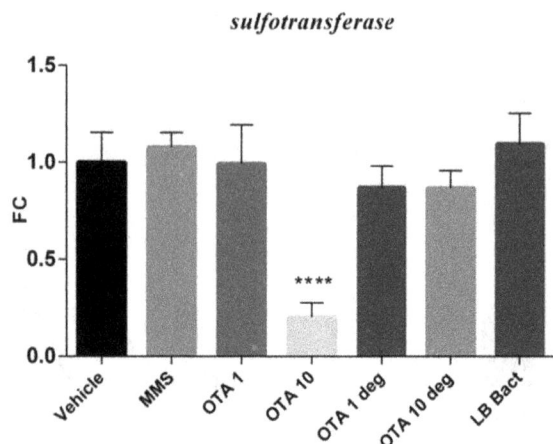

Figure 6. Effect of acute (72 hours) OTA treatment on *sult1c2* **mRNA expression.** OTA 10 elevated the *sult1c2* mRNA level alone. The metabolised OTA by *Cupriavidus basilensis* ŐR16 (OTA 1 deg and OTA 10 deg groups) not influenced the mRNA level. (One way ANOVA followed by the Tukey's *post hoc* test were used) Abbreviations: MMS-Group treated with methyl methanesulfonate, OTA 1 and OTA 10-Groups treated with 1 and 10 mg/kg body weight Ochratoxin A, OTA 1 deg and OTA 10 deg- Groups treated with 1 and 10 mg/kg body weight Ochratoxin A + *Cupriavidus basilensis* ŐR16 in modified Luria- Bertani medium, LB bact- *Cupriavidus basilensis* ŐR16 in modified Luria- Bertani medium. Data are presented as mean ± SD (n = 7–10, **** p<0.0001)

expression was up-regulated in the MMS (non significant) and OTA 0.5 (p = 0.0002) groups. The degraded OTA remnants did not affect *clusterin* expression (Fig. 8B). In contrast, the *sult1c2* mRNA expression was decreased significantly (p = 0.0005) in the renal cortex during the OTA administration in the chronic experiment; while the biodegraded OTA did not show effect on the *annexin2* and *sult1c2* mRNA expressions in the kidney (Fig. 8A and Fig. 9).

Discussion

Several studies on OTA degrading, adsorbing and detoxifying agents have been published recently. Certain *Lactobacillus* species have moderate OTA degradation capacity however, the toxicity of the metabolites remains unclear [25]. Moreover, *Bacillus licheniformis* degraded 92.5% of OTA at 37°C and OTα, as degradation product, was detected [26]; while *Brevibacterium spp*. strains showed 100% degradation of OTA [27]. Furthermore an OTA degrading enzyme was identified in *Aspergillus niger*, which is capable to metabolize the OTA to phenylalanine and OTα [28]. Some *Trichosporon* species have the ability to cleave OTA selectively into phenylalanine and OTα but then the presumed nephrotoxic effect of other alternative metabolites were not investigated at gene expression level [29]. *Trichosporon mycotox-inivorans* was classified as a novel species due to ability to detoxify OTA [30]. This yeast, when introduced to the diet of broiler chickens completely abolished OTA effects on the immune system [31]. However, a recent study was raising doubts over the safety of *T. mycotoxinivorans* as it was associated with cystic fibrosis and the death of a patient with histological documented *Trichosporon* pneumonia [32].

In our experiment the OTA-degrading potential of *C. basilensis* ŐR16 and acute/chronic toxicity of the degraded products were analysed. The OTA was degraded efficiently by the 5th day of biodegradation. Moreover, metabolised form of OTA was also

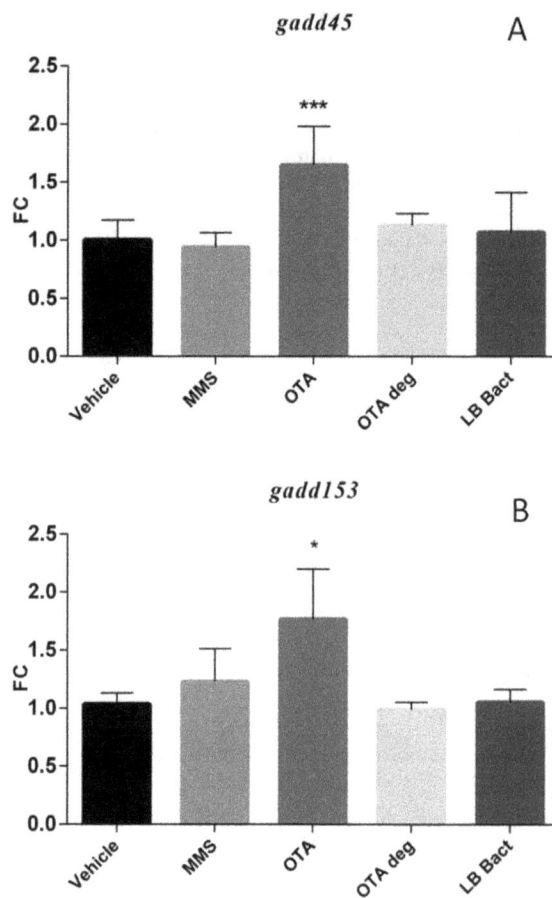

gadd45 A

gadd153 B

Figure 7. Effect of chronic (21 days) OTA treatment on *gadd45* **mRNA expression (A).** The OTA 0.5 mg/kg bw chronic administration elevated the *gadd45* mRNA level. The metabolised OTA by *Cupriavidus basilensis* ŐR16 (OTA 0.5 deg group) not influenced the mRNA levels (One way ANOVA followed by the Tukey's *post hoc* test were used). Effect of chronic (21 days) OTA treatment on *gadd153* mRNA expression (**B**). The OTA 0.5 mg/kg bw chronic administration elevated the *gadd153* mRNA level. The metabolised OTA by *Cupriavidus basilensis* ŐR16 (OTA 0.5 deg group) did not influence the mRNA level (Kruskal-Wallis test was used). Abbreviations: MMS – Group treated with methyl methanesulfonate, OTA 0.5 – Group treated with 0.5 mg/kg body weight Ochratoxin A, OTA 0.5 deg – Group treated with 0.5 mg/kg body weight Ochratoxin A + *Cupriavidus basilensis* ŐR16 in modified Luria-Bertani medium, LB bact – *Cupriavidus basilensis* ŐR16 in modified Luria-Bertani medium. Data are presented as mean ± SD (n = 7–9, *p< 0.05***p<0.001)

measured. Two pathways may be involved in OTA microbiolog-ical degradation. First, OTA can be biodegraded through the hydrolysis of the amide bond that links the L-β-phenylalanine molecule to the OTα moiety. Since OTα and L-β-phenylalanine are virtually non-toxic, this mechanism can be considered to be a detoxification pathway. Second, a more hypothetical process involves OTA being degraded via the hydrolysis of the lactone ring [33]. In this case, the final degradation product is an opened lactones form of OTA, which has similar toxicity than OTA when administered to rats [34,35]. In the present study OTα was detected by HPLC, and also the time-curve detected increasing OT-α concentration parallel with the OTA-decrease. Based on this phenomenon cleavage of the amide bond that links the L-β-phenylalanine molecule to the OTα moiety is hypothesized

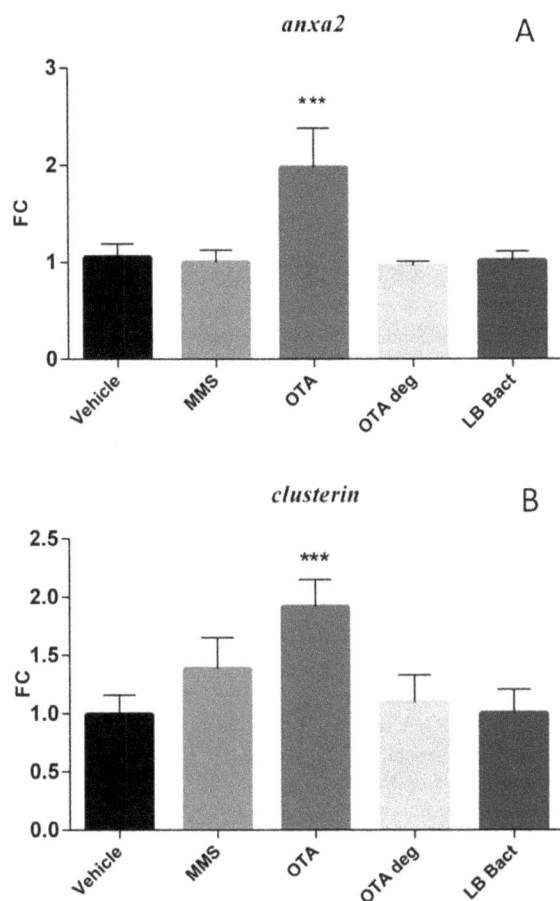

Figure 8. Effect of chronic (21 days) OTA treatment on *annexin2* mRNA expression (A). The OTA 0.5 mg/kg bw chronic administration elevated the *annexin2* mRNA level. The metabolised OTA by *Cupriavidus basilensis* ŐR16 (OTA 0.5 deg group) did not influence the mRNA level. (One way ANOVA followed by the Tukey's *post hoc* test were used) Effect of chronic (21 days) OTA treatment on *clusterin* mRNA expression (**B**). The MMS and OTA 0.5 mg/kg bw chronic administration elevated the *clusterin* mRNA level. The metabolised OTA by *Cupriavidus basilensis* ŐR16 (OTA 0.5 deg group) did not influence the mRNA level. (One way ANOVA followed by the Tukey's *post hoc* test were used) Abbreviations: MMS – Group treated with methyl methanesulfonate, OTA 0.5 – Group treated with 0.5 mg/kg body weight Ochratoxin A, OTA 0.5 deg – Group treated with 0.5 mg/kg body weight Ochratoxin A + *Cupriavidus basilensis* ŐR16 in modified Luria-Bertani medium, LB bact – *Cupriavidus basilensis* ŐR16 in modified Luria- Bertani medium. Data are presented as mean ± SD (n = 7–9, *** p<0.001)

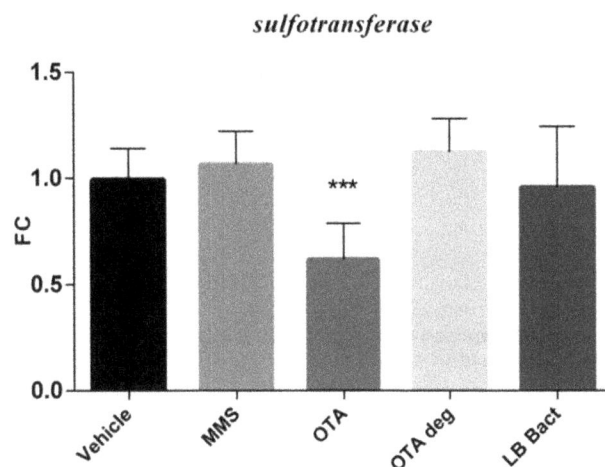

Figure 9. Effect of chronic (21 days) OTA treatment on *sult1c2* mRNA expression. The OTA 0.5 mg/kg bw chronic administration elevated the *sult1c2* mRNA level. The metabolised OTA by *Cupriavidus basilensis* ŐR16 (OTA 0.5 deg group) did not influence the mRNA level. (One way ANOVA followed by the Tukey's *post hoc* test were used) Abbreviations: MMS – Group treated with methyl methanesulfonate, OTA 0.5 – Group treated with 0.5 mg/kg body weight Ochratoxin A, OTA 0.5 deg- Group treated with 0.5 mg/kg body weight Ochratoxin A + *Cupriavidus basilensis* ŐR16 in modified Luria-Bertani medium, LB bact- *Cupriavidus basilensis* ŐR16 in modified Luria-Bertani medium. Data are presented as mean ± SD (n = 6–9, **p<0.01)

(Fig. 10). This observation was confirmed by *in vivo* toxicological tests.

The major metabolite of the bacterial OTA degradation is the OTα, which is a non-toxic metabolite of the OTA but then formations of other toxic residuals are possible [36,37]. Chemical analysis and immunochemical methods are less sensitive to detect all potential harmful degradation products, therefore it is important to monitor for toxicity by *in vivo* methods.

After oral administration of various doses of OTA in acute and chronic experiments, significant elevation of the OTA concentrations were found in plasma. Even in control animals OTA levels above the detection limit were found, which could be attributed to natural contamination, as it was reported previously [38–40]. OTA concentration in the plasma showed positive correlation with the administered mycotoxin doses. On the other hand elevated OTA concentration was detected in the blood samples after acute exposure with high doses of biodegraded OTA metabolites; however, this OTA concentration was only 5.1 % compared to the OTA level detected in the OTA 10 group (Fig. 2A). Presumably the residual non degraded OTA was accumulated in the blood. This result was confirmed by ELISA tests which detected 94% biodegradation efficiency of the *Cupriavidus basilensis* ŐR16 (Fig. 1).

The long-term OTA exposure during the chronic mycotoxin treatment significantly decreased the kidney weight but then the acute treatment with the detoxified metabolites of OTA did not affect it, which alteration is the most toxins sensitive. These observations were established by previous reports in which chronic OTA exposure induced nephropathy in animals and humans, as well [8,12,13]. The OTA degradation by *Cupriavidus basilensis* ŐR16 completely abolished these effects. This phenomenon was confirmed by histopathology analysis. The high dose of acute and the lower dose of chronic OTA treatment induced toxicities related malformations in renal cortex tissue (Fig. 3). These results were also detected in previous studies of Lühe and co-workers in acute experiments and also in chronic experiments on rodent models by Rached and colleagues [19,41]. In the present work, neither the *Cupriavidus basilensis* ŐR16 with modified LB, nor the degraded OTA residuals formed pathological disorders.

The spleen, the other mycotoxin sensitive organ, was examined with different OTA dosages in acute and chronic experiments. The spleen weight was significantly decreased after acute OTA and MMS exposure, but the chronic OTA and MMS treatments did not decrease the spleen weight significantly. The rapid OTA accumulation in the blood after high dosage treatment could explain the suppression of immune system and the lymphoid organ weight loss. Similar observations were published in case of broiler chickens after chronic OTA administration [42,43]. Moreover, by analysing blood samples and lymphoid organs of humans and

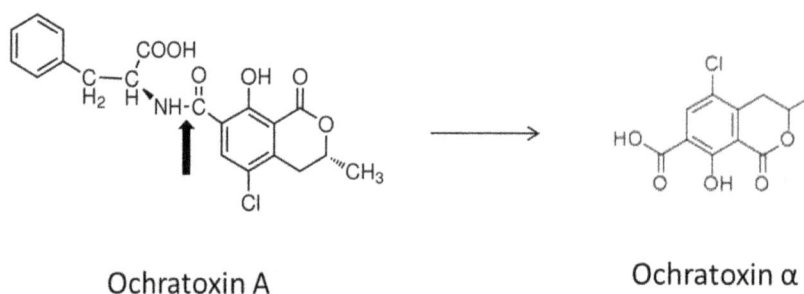

Figure 10. Proposed cleavage of Ochratoxin A by *Cupriavidus basilensis* **ŐR16.** The amide bond hydrolysis (up arrow) resulting Ochratoxin α as a major degradation product.

other mammalians, altered immune functions were also detected [44]. Histopathological examinations were demonstrated that the immunotoxic effect and histological malformation regarding the degraded OTA residuals and the *Cupriavidus basilensis* ŐR16 strain was not detected at histopathological level. Our bacterial OTA degradation strategy is an effective detoxification process by toxicological and physiological point of view.

Previous molecular genetic analysis demonstrated that the OTA influences the expression of genotoxic, apoptotic, detoxification and inflammation related genes in a dose dependent manner. This study revealed 254 genes which expression changed by at least two-fold after acute (3 day) OTA exposure (1 and 10 mg/kg bw). Eighty-nine genes were up regulated and 165 were down regulated. In the present work dose and time dependent Discriminator Genes were selected [19]. These genes are useful markers in the renal cortex for monitoring possible toxic effects of the end products after biodegradation. The selected, robust up- or down-regulated marker genes along with the adjusted experimental circumstances encompass the complete toxic action of OTA and the applied indicators are sensitive for many of the possible toxicities of the bio-converted OTA residuals. The expressions of OTA induced marker genes were detected by quantitative-real-time-PCR measurement; since one of the major effects of OTA is the DNA damaging action [45]. The *gadd 45* and *gadd 153* genes serves as markers to demonstrate the genotoxic effect and DNA damage induction of OTA, besides these genes are monitoring the biodegradation of OTA. By the degradation of OTA, the toxicity is eliminating which results unaltered *gadd 45* and *gadd 153* mRNA levels. MMS treated animals served as positive control, because MMS is a well-studied genotoxic chemical that induces alterations in *gadd 45* and *gadd 153* mRNA expressions [46]. While OTA up-regulated the expression of *gadd 45* and *gadd 153* in a dose dependent manner, the metabolised OTA by *Cupriavidus basilensis* ŐR16 completely eliminated this up-regulation in both experiments. Furthermore, the OTA is involved in renal tumour formation. The *clusterin* and *annexin2* play important role in the apoptotic processes and in the renal tumour formation [47]. Previous studies have demonstrated *annexin 2* (*anxa2*) up-regulation by acute OTA treatment in the renal cortex of rats, which resulted similar mRNA expression level that was described in our acute experiment in mice [19]. *Annexin2* is a cofactor for DNA polymerase alpha subunit that plays an important role in the DNA repair and in the development of different cancers [48]. Furthermore *annexin2* is a substrate for an oncogene associated kinase [49]. Elevated level of *annexin2* was described in the kidney carcinoma formation in rat [50]. The OTA biodegradation by *Cupriavidus basilensis* ŐR16 strain abolished the up-regulation of both marker genes in both acute

and chronic treatments, indicating that the biodegradation was a detoxification as well.

Sulfotransferase 1c2 serves as a marker for the cellular and detoxification processes, which has been identified as an OTA-induced gene in acute (72 hours) mycotoxin treatment [19]. *Sulfotransferase* takes part in xenobiotic detoxification, carcinogen activation, prodrug processing, and cellular signalling pathways [51]. Our work demonstrated that *sulfotransferase 1c2* expression decreased after acute and chronic OTA exposure. OTA biodegradation by *Cupriavidus basilensis* ŐR16 strain abolished the *sulfotransferase* mRNA down-regulation in both experiments.

Based on our present results, the major metabolite of OTA biodegradation by *Cupriavidus basilensis* ŐR16 is Ochratoxin α. This metabolite is not toxic *in vitro* and here we found that biodegradation product does not display nephrotoxic effects *in vivo*. In summary, by application of *Cupriavidus basilensis* ŐR16, OTA is degraded efficiently without bioactive intermediates and by-products; therefore *Cupriavidus basilensis* ŐR16 is worth further study for possible use for the decontamination of raw materials, to reduce OTA concentration.

Supporting Information

Figure S1 The acute OTA administration did not influence significantly the kidney normalized weight (**A**). (Kruskal-Wallis test was used). The acute OTA administration significantly decreased the spleen normalized weights of animals in the MMS, OTA 1 and OTA 10 groups (**B**). (Kruskal-Wallis test was used). Abbreviations: MMS – Group treated with methyl methanesulfonate, OTA 1 and OTA 10 – Groups treated with 1 and 10 mg/body weight kg Ochratoxin A, OTA 1 deg and OTA 10 deg- Groups treated with 1 and 10 mg/body weight kg Ochratoxin A + *Cupriavidus basilensis* ŐR16 in modified Luria-Bertani medium, LB bact - *Cupriavidus basilensis* ŐR16 in modified Luria-Bertani medium. Data are presented as mean ± SD (n = 7-10, *p<0.05,**p<0.01,). The chronic OTA administration significantly decreased the kidney normalized weight of animals in the OTA 0.5 groups (**C**). (One way ANOVA followed by the Tukey's *post hoc* test were used). The chronic OTA administration decreased the spleen normalized weight of animals in the MMS and OTA 0.5 groups (**D**). The alterations were not significant. (Kruskal-Wallis test was used). Abbreviations: MMS – Group treated with methyl methanesulfonate, OTA 0.5 – Group treated with 0.5 mg/body weight kg Ochratoxin A, OTA 0.5 deg – Group treated with 0.5 mg/body weight kg Ochratoxin A + *Cupriavidus basilensis* ŐR16 in modified Luria-Bertani medium, LB bact – *Cupriavidus basilensis* ŐR16 in modified Luria- Bertani medium. Data are presented as mean ± SD (n = 7-10, **p<0.01).

Table S1   Detailed information about analytical methods for ochratoxin-A, and its derivative ochratoxin-α.

Table S2   The nucleotide sequence of the oligonucleotid primers.

Acknowledgments

We thank the excellent technical assistance to Julianna Benkő and Máté Sipos. We thank the critical reading of the manuscript to Frank Mandy.

Author Contributions

Conceived and designed the experiments: SF MM B. Kriszt SS. Performed the experiments: SF MC CK ZS MA B. Kőszegi. Analyzed the data: SF CK JK ZS MA. Contributed reagents/materials/analysis tools: TB MC. Wrote the paper: SF CK ZS MM B. Kriszt KJK.

References

1. van der Merwe KJ, Steyn PS, Fourie L, Scott DB, Theron JJ (1965) Ochratoxin A, a toxic metabolite produced by Aspergillus ochraceus Wilh. Nature 205: 1112–1113.
2. Walker R (2002) Risk assessment of ochratoxin: current views of the European Scientific Committee on Food, the JECFA and the Codex Committee on Food Additives and Contaminants. Adv Exp Med Biol 504: 249–255.
3. Raters M, Matissek R (2005) Study on distribution of mycotoxins in cocoa beans. Mycotoxin Res 21: 182–186.
4. Zimmerli B, Dick R (1995) Determination of ochratoxin A at the ppt level in human blood, serum, milk and some foodstuffs by high-performance liquid chromatography with enhanced fluorescence detection and immunoaffinity column cleanup: methodology and Swiss data. J Chromatogr B Biomed Appl 666: 85–99.
5. Vega FE, Posada F, Peterson SW, Gianfagna TJ, Chaves F (2006) Penicillium species endophytic in coffee plants and ochratoxin A production. Mycologia 98: 31–42.
6. Rodrigues I, Naehrer K (2012) A three-year survey on the worldwide occurrence of mycotoxins in feedstuffs and feed. Toxins (Basel) 4: 663–675.
7. Duarte SC, Lino CM, Pena A (2012) Food safety implications of ochratoxin A in animal-derived food products. Vet J 192: 286–292.
8. Krogh P, Hald B, Pedersen EJ (1973) Occurrence of ochratoxin A and citrinin in cereals associated with mycotoxic porcine nephropathy. Acta Pathol Microbiol Scand B Microbiol Immunol 81: 689–695.
9. Krogh P (1977) Ochratoxin A residues in tissues of slaughter pigs with nephropathy. Nord Vet Med 29: 402–405.
10. Elling F, Krogh P (1977) Fungal toxins and Balkan (endemic) nephropathy. Lancet 1: 1213.
11. Krogh P, Hald B, Plestina R, Ceovic S (1977) Balkan (endemic) nephropathy and foodborn ochratoxin A: preliminary results of a survey of foodstuffs. Acta Pathol Microbiol Scand B 85: 238–240.
12. Hald B (1991) Ochratoxin A in human blood in European countries. IARC Sci Publ: 159–164.
13. Stoev SD (1998) The role of ochratoxin A as a possible cause of Balkan endemic nephropathy and its risk evaluation. Vet Hum Toxicol 40: 352–360.
14. Stoev SD, Vitanov S, Anguelov G, Petkova-Bocharova T, Creppy EE (2001) Experimental mycotoxic nephropathy in pigs provoked by a diet containing ochratoxin A and penicillic acid. Vet Res Commun 25: 205–223.
15. Dirheimer G, Creppy EE (1991) Mechanism of action of ochratoxin A. IARC Sci Publ: 171–186.
16. Heller K, Roschenthaler (1978) Inhibition of protein synthesis in Streptococcus faecalis by ochratoxin A. Can J Microbiol.24: 467–472.
17. Castegnaro M, Pfohl-Leszkowicz A, Bartsch H, Tillmann T, Mohr U (2005) Re: Comments on paper by Son et al. Toxicol Lett 156: 315; author reply 317.
18. Clark HA, Snedeker SM (2006) Ochratoxin a: its cancer risk and potential for exposure. J Toxicol Environ Health B Crit Rev 9: 265–296.
19. Luhe A, Hildebrand H, Bach U, Dingermann T, Ahr HJ (2003) A new approach to studying ochratoxin A (OTA)-induced nephrotoxicity: expression profiling in vivo and in vitro employing cDNA microarrays. Toxicol Sci 73: 315–328.
20. Pitout MJ (1969) The hydrolysis of ochratoxin A by some proteolytic enzymes. Biochem Pharmacol 18: 485–491.
21. Abrunhosa L, Paterson RR, Venancio A (2010) Biodegradation of ochratoxin a for food and feed decontamination. Toxins (Basel) 2: 1078–1099.
22. Cserhati M, Kriszt B, Szoboszlay S, Toth A, Szabo I, et al. (2012) De novo genome project of Cupriavidus basilensis OR16. J Bacteriol 194: 2109–2110.
23. Zeljezic D, Domijan AM, Peraica M (2006) DNA damage by ochratoxin A in rat kidney assessed by the alkaline comet assay. Braz J Med Biol Res 39: 1563–1568.
24. Cui X, Zhou J, Qiu J, Johnson MR, Mrug M (2009) Validation of endogenous internal real-time PCR controls in renal tissues. Am J Nephrol 30: 413–417.
25. Piotrowska M, Zakowska Z (2005) The elimination of ochratoxin A by lactic acid bacteria strains. Pol J Microbiol 54: 279–286.
26. Petchkongkaew A, Taillandier P, Gasaluck P, Lebrihi A (2008) Isolation of Bacillus spp. from Thai fermented soybean (Thua-nao): screening for aflatoxin B1 and ochratoxin A detoxification. J Appl Microbiol 104: 1495–1502.
27. Rodriguez H, Reveron I, Doria F, Costantini A, De Las Rivas B, et al. (2011) Degradation of ochratoxin a by Brevibacterium species. J Agric Food Chem 59: 10755–10760.
28. Stander MA, Bornscheuer UT, Henke E, Steyn PS (2000) Screening of commercial hydrolases for the degradation of ochratoxin A. J Agric Food Chem48: 5736–5739.
29. Schatzmayr G, Heidler D, Fuchs E, Nitsch S, Mohnl M, et al. (2003) Investigation of different yeast strains for the detoxification of ochratoxin A. Mycotoxin Res19: 124–128.
30. Molnar O, Schatzmayr G, Fuchs E, Prillinger H (2004) Trichosporon mycotoxinivorans sp. nov., a new yeast species useful in biological detoxification of various mycotoxins. Syst Appl Microbiol 27: 661–671.
31. Politis I, Fegeros K, Nitsch S, Schatzmayr G, Kantas D (2005) Use of Trichosporon mycotoxinivorans to suppress the effects of ochratoxicosis on the immune system of broiler chicks. Br Poult Sci 46: 58–65.
32. Hickey PW, Sutton DA, Fothergill AW, Rinaldi MG, Wickes BL, et al. (2009) Trichosporon mycotoxinivorans, a novel respiratory pathogen in patients with cystic fibrosis. J Clin Microbiol 47: 3091–3097.
33. Karlovsky P (1999) Biological detoxification of fungal toxins and its use in plant breeding, feed and food production. Nat Toxins 7: 1–23.
34. Xiao H, Madhyastha S, Marquardt RR, Li S, Vodela JK, et al. (1996) Toxicity of ochratoxin A, its opened lactone form and several of its analogs: structure-activity relationships. Toxicol Appl Pharmacol 137: 182–192.
35. Li S, Marquardt RR, Frohlich AA, Vitti TG, Crow G (1997) Pharmacokinetics of ochratoxin A and its metabolites in rats. Toxicol Appl Pharmacol 145: 82–90.
36. Creppy EE, Stormer FC, Roschenthaler R, Dirheimer G (1983) Effects of two metabolites of ochratoxin A, (4R)-4-hydroxyochratoxin A and ochratoxin alpha, on immune response in mice. Infect Immun 39: 1015–1018.
37. Bruinink A, Rasonyi T, Sidler C (1998) Differences in neurotoxic effects of ochratoxin A, ochracin and ochratoxin-alpha in vitro. Nat Toxins 6: 173–177.
38. Aoudia N, Tangni EK, Larondelle Y (2008) Distribution of ochratoxin A in plasma and tissues of rats fed a naturally contaminated diet amended with micronized wheat fibres: effectiveness of mycotoxin sequestering activity. Food Chem Toxicol 46: 871–878.
39. Mantle PG (2008) Interpretation of the pharmacokinetics of ochratoxin A in blood plasma of rats, during and after acute or chronic ingestion. Food Chem Toxicol 46: 1808–1816.
40. Arbillaga L, Vettorazzi A, Gil AG, van Delft JH, Garcia-Jalon JA, et al. (2008) Gene expression changes induced by ochratoxin A in renal and hepatic tissues of male F344 rat after oral repeated administration. Toxicol Appl Pharmacol 230: 197–207.
41. Rached E, Hoffmann D, Blumbach K, Weber K, Dekant W, et al. (2008) Evaluation of putative biomarkers of nephrotoxicity after exposure to ochratoxin a in vivo and in vitro. Toxicol Sci 103: 371–381.
42. Singh GS, Chauhan HV, Jha GJ, Singh KK (1990) Immunosuppression due to chronic ochratoxicosis in broiler chicks. J Comp Pathol 103: 399–410.
43. Hassan ZU, Khan MZ, Saleemi MK, Khan A, Javed I, et al. (2012) Immunological responses of male White Leghorn chicks kept on ochratoxin A (OTA)-contaminated feed. J Immunotoxicol 9: 56–63.
44. Al-Anati L, Petzinger E (2006) Immunotoxic activity of ochratoxin A. J Vet Pharmacol Ther 29: 79–90.
45. Obrecht-Pflumio S, Dirheimer G (2000) In vitro DNA and dGMP adducts formation caused by ochratoxin A. Chem Biol Interact 127: 29–44.
46. Beard SE, Capaldi SR, Gee P (1996) Stress responses to DNA damaging agents in the human colon carcinoma cell line, RKO. Mutat Res 371: 1–13.
47. Miyake H, Hara S, Arakawa S, Kamidono S, Hara I (2002) Over expression of clusterin is an independent prognostic factor for nonpapillary renal cell carcinoma. J Urol 167: 703–706.
48. Kumble KD, Hirota M, Pour PM, Vishwanatha JK (1992) Enhanced levels of annexins in pancreatic carcinoma cells of Syrian hamsters and their intrapancreatic allografts. Cancer Res 52: 163–167.
49. Skouteris GG, Schroder CH (1996) The hepatocyte growth factor receptor kinase-mediated phosphorylation of lipocortin-1 transduces the proliferating signal of the hepatocyte growth factor. J Biol Chem 271: 27266–27273.
50. Tanaka T, Kondo S, Iwasa Y, Hiai H, Toyokuni S (2000) Expression of stress-response and cell proliferation genes in renal cell carcinoma induced by oxidative stress. Am J Pathol 156: 2149–2157.
51. Runge-Morris MA (1997) Regulation of expression of the rodent cytosolic sulfotransferases. FASEB J 11: 109–117.

5

Discovery and Characterization of a Potent and Selective Inhibitor of *Aedes aegypti* Inward Rectifier Potassium Channels

Rene Raphemot[1,2], Matthew F. Rouhier[3], Daniel R. Swale[1], Emily Days[4], C. David Weaver[2,4], Kimberly M. Lovell[2,6], Leah C. Konkel[2,6], Darren W. Engers[2,6], Sean F. Bollinger[2,6], Corey Hopkins[2,5,6], Peter M. Piermarini[3]*, Jerod S. Denton[1,2,4,5]*

1 Department of Anesthesiology, Vanderbilt University Medical Center, Nashville, TN, United States of America, 2 Department of Pharmacology, Vanderbilt University School of Medicine, Nashville, TN, United States of America, 3 Department of Entomology, Ohio Agricultural Research and Development Center, The Ohio State University, Wooster, OH, United States of America, 4 Institute of Chemical Biology, Vanderbilt University School of Medicine, Nashville, TN, United States of America, 5 Institute for Global Health, Vanderbilt University, Nashville, TN, United States of America, 6 Department of Chemistry, Vanderbilt University School of Medicine, Nashville TN, United States of America

Abstract

Vector-borne diseases such as dengue fever and malaria, which are transmitted by infected female mosquitoes, affect nearly half of the world's population. The emergence of insecticide-resistant mosquito populations is reducing the effectiveness of conventional insecticides and threatening current vector control strategies, which has created an urgent need to identify new molecular targets against which novel classes of insecticides can be developed. We previously demonstrated that small molecule inhibitors of mammalian Kir channels represent promising chemicals for new mosquitocide development. In this study, high-throughput screening of approximately 30,000 chemically diverse small-molecules was employed to discover potent and selective inhibitors of *Aedes aegypti* Kir1 (*Ae*Kir1) channels heterologously expressed in HEK293 cells. Of 283 confirmed screening 'hits', the small-molecule inhibitor VU625 was selected for lead optimization and in vivo studies based on its potency and selectivity toward *Ae*Kir1, and tractability for medicinal chemistry. In patch clamp electrophysiology experiments of HEK293 cells, VU625 inhibits *Ae*Kir1 with an IC_{50} value of 96.8 nM, making VU625 the most potent inhibitor of *Ae*Kir1 described to date. Furthermore, electrophysiology experiments in *Xenopus* oocytes revealed that VU625 is a weak inhibitor of *Ae*Kir2B. Surprisingly, injection of VU625 failed to elicit significant effects on mosquito behavior, urine excretion, or survival. However, when co-injected with probenecid, VU625 inhibited the excretory capacity of mosquitoes and was toxic, suggesting that the compound is a substrate of organic anion and/or ATP-binding cassette (ABC) transporters. The dose-toxicity relationship of VU625 (when co-injected with probenecid) is biphasic, which is consistent with the molecule inhibiting both *Ae*Kir1 and *Ae*Kir2B with different potencies. This study demonstrates proof-of-concept that potent and highly selective inhibitors of mosquito Kir channels can be developed using conventional drug discovery approaches. Furthermore, it reinforces the notion that the physical and chemical properties that determine a compound's bioavailability in vivo will be critical in determining the efficacy of Kir channel inhibitors as insecticides.

Editor: Joseph Clifton Dickens, United States Department of Agriculture, Beltsville Agricultural Research Center, United States of America

Funding: This work was funded by a grant from the Foundation for the National Institutes of Health through the Vector-Based Transmission of Control: Discovery Research (VCTR) program of the Grand Challenges in Global Health initiative. This work was also supported in part by a grant from the National Institute of Diabetes and Digestive and Kidney Diseases (1R01DK082884; JSD). The funders had no role in study design, data collection and analysis, decision to publish, or preparation of the manuscript.

Competing Interests: The authors have declared that no competing interests exist.

* Email: piermarini.1@osu.edu (PMP); jerod.s.denton@vanderbilt.edu (JSD)

Introduction

Mosquitoes are vectors of protozoan, filarial nematode, and viral pathogens that cause numerous human diseases, including malaria, lymphatic filariasis, and dengue fever. These diseases impose an enormous burden on global health and profoundly impair socioeconomic advancement in developing countries [1]. The overuse of a limited number of insecticides has led to the emergence of insecticide-resistant populations of mosquitoes, which is hampering the effectiveness of vector control efforts [2,3,4]. Consequently, there is a need to identify new molecular targets against which insecticides can be developed and deployed.

An emerging body of evidence from our group supports the idea that inward rectifier potassium (Kir) channels represent viable targets for insecticide development [5,6,7]. Kir channels are tetrameric proteins that conduct K^+ ions across the cell membrane and thereby generate an ionic current that underlies various cellular functions. Dipteran insects possess three major Kir channel subtypes, denoted Kir1, Kir2 and Kir3. In *Drosophila melanogaster*, there are three genes that encode Kir channels

(*Dr*Kir1, *Dr*Kir2, *Dr*Kir3), which play important roles in osmoregulation, immunity, and development [8,9,10,11]. In *Aedes aegypti*, there are five Kir channel genes (*AeKir1, AeKir2A, AeKir2B, AeKir2B'* and *AeKir3*), which are expressed in various body segments and tissues such as the carcass (thorax and abdomen), head, Malpighian tubules, midgut, and hindgut [6,12]. We showed previously in vitro that the *A. aegypti* Kir1 (*Ae*Kir1) channel mediates strong inward rectifying K^+ currents that are blocked by barium and the small molecule inhibitors, VU573 and VU590 [7,12,13]. Moreover, a hemolymph injection of either VU573 or VU590 inhibits the excretion of urine by adult female mosquitoes, leads to abdominal bloating, and incapacitates mosquitoes within 24 h [5].

Taken together, the above studies indicate that Kir channels represent promising molecular targets for insecticides that have a novel mechanism of action by disrupting the renal-dependent regulation of extracellular fluid homeostasis (i.e., renal failure). However, in mammals, Kir channels regulate the electrical excitability of neurons and cardiac cells, hormone secretion, and transport of K^+ ions across epithelial tissues of the kidney and gut [14]. Missense mutations that perturb the activity of Kir channels cause human diseases of the heart, nervous system, pancreas, and kidney [15,16,17]. Thus, efforts aimed at developing insecticides to target Kir channels must verify that lead compounds do not perturb the functions of mammalian Kir channels.

As such, the above 'tool' compounds VU573 and VU590 allowed us to establish proof-of-concept, but are not suitable for insecticide development, in part, because they inhibit mammalian Kir channels with greater potency than *Ae*Kir1 [18,19]. Here, we aim to discover new chemical probes of *Ae*Kir1 channels that exhibit improved potency and selectivity compared to the tool compounds by optimizing and validating an existing fluorescent thallium (Tl^+) flux-based assay of *Ae*Kir1 function [5] for high-throughput screening (HTS) of small molecule libraries. Screening approximately 30,000 small molecules from the chemical library of the Vanderbilt Institute of Chemical Biology (VICB) resulted in the identification of 283 compounds with activity against *Ae*Kir1 channels. We focus on the in vitro and in vivo activity of one of these compounds, N-(3-methoxyphenyl)-2-methyl-1-propylin-doline-5-sulfonamide (VU625), which exhibits nanomolar affinity and is highly selective for *Ae*Kir1 over mammalian Kir channels.

Materials and Methods

Tl^+ flux assays

Tl^+ flux assays were performed essentially as described previously [13,18,19]. Briefly, stably transfected T-Rex-HEK-293 cells expressing *Ae*Kir1 channels were cultured overnight in 384-well plates (20,000 cells/20 µL/well black-walled, clear-bottomed BD PureCoat amine-coated plates (BD, Bedford, MA) with a plating media containing DMEM, 10% dialyzed FBS and 1 µg/mL tetracycline. The next day, the cell culture medium was replaced with a dye-loading solution containing assay buffer (Hanks Balanced Salt Solution with 20 mM HEPES, pH 7.3), 0.01% (*w/v*) Pluronic F-127 (Life Technologies, Carlsbad, CA), and 1.2 µM of the thallium-sensitive dye Thallos-AM (TEFlabs, Austin, TX). Following 1 hr incubation at room temperature, the dye-loading solution was washed from the plates and replaced with 20 µL/well of assay buffer.

The plates were transferred to a Hamamatsu Functional Drug Screening System 6000 (FDSS6000; Hamamatsu, Hamamatsu (or Bridgewater, NJ), Japan) where 20 µL/well of test compounds in assay buffer (as prepared below) were added and allowed to incubate with the cells for 20 min. After the incubation period, a baseline recording was collected at 1 Hz for 10 s (excitation 470 ± 20 nm, emission 540 ± 30 nm) followed by a Tl^+ stimulus buffer addition (10 µL/well) and data collection for an additional 4 min. The Tl^+ stimulus buffer contains in (mM) 125 $NaHCO_3$, 1.8 $CaSO_4$, 1 $MgSO_4$, 5 glucose, 12 Tl_2SO_4, 10 HEPES, pH 7.4. For Tl^+ flux assays on the mammalian channels Kir2.x, Kir4.1 and Kir6.2/SUR1 expressing cells, the Tl^+ stimulus buffer contained 1.8 mM Tl_2SO_4. Also, Tl^+ flux assays on Kir3.1/3.2/mGlu8 expressing cell, required addition of an EC_{80} concentration of glutamate (Sigma-Aldrich, St. Louis, MO) with the Tl^+ stimulus buffer [19].

The test compounds were transferred to daughter polypropyl-ene 384-well plates (Greiner Bio-One, Monroe, NC) using an Echo555 liquid handler (Labcyte, Sunnyvale, CA), and then diluted into assay buffer to generate a 2X stock in 0.6% DMSO (0.3% final). For Tl^+ flux assays on Kir6.2/SUR1 expressing cells, test compounds were diluted in assay buffer containing diazoxide (250 µM final) to induce channel activation [20]. Concentration-response curves (CRCs) were generated by screening compounds at 3-fold dilution series in 4-point (1 µM–30 µM) or 11-point (1 nM–30 µM) CRCs.

Tl^+ flux data were analyzed as previously described [19,21,22] using a combination of Excel (Microsoft Corp, Redmond, WA) with XLfit add-in (IDBS, Guildford, Surrey, UK) and OriginPro (OriginLab, Northampton, MA) software. Raw data were opened in Excel and each data point in a given trace was divided by the first data point from that trace (static ratio) followed by subtraction of data points from control traces generated in the presence of vehicle controls. The slope of the fluorescence increase beginning 5 s after Tl^+ addition and ending 15 s after Tl^+ addition was calculated.

Compound synthesis

2,2,2-trifluoro-1-(2-methylindolin-1-yl)ethan-1-one. The reagents and conditions are illustrated in Figure S1. To a round bottom flask equipped with a magnetic stir bar, 2-methylindoline (4.8 mL, 37 mmol, 1 eq.) and pyridine (46 mL) were added. The reaction mixture was cooled to 0°C and trifluoroacetic anhydride (6.3 mL, 44 mmol, 1.2 eq.) was added dropwise. The reaction mixture was allowed to warm to room temperature and was stirred an additional 2 hours. The reaction was quenched with water (50 mL) and diluted with DCM (100 mL). The organic layer was separated and washed subsequently with water (50 ml) and brine (50 mL), dried over Na_2SO_4, and concentrated under reduced pressure. The crude material (8.33g, 98%) was used without purification. LCMS: $R_T = 0.785$ min, $[M+H]^+ = 229.6$; >98%.

2-methyl-1-(2,2,2-trifluoroacetyl)indoline-5-sulfonyl chloride: Chlorosulfonic acid (22 mL, 330 mmol, 9 equiv.) was added to a 100 mL round bottom flask equipped with a reflux condensor, and cooled to 0°C. To this, 2,2,2-trifluoro-1-(2-methylindolin-1-yl)ethan-1-one, (8.5 g, 37 mmol, 1 eq.) was added dropwise. The reaction mixture was removed from the ice bath. The vial was heated to 40°C for 1 hour. The reaction was subsequently cooled to room temperature and PCl_5 (7.7 g, 37 mmol, 1 equiv.) was added slowly. After gas evolution ceased, the reaction mixture was heated to 80°C for 1 hour. The reaction mixture was cooled to room temperature and then placed in an ice bath. Water was added very slowly to the reaction mixture. Subsequently, DCM was added and the reaction was filtered through a phase separator. The organic layer was concentrated under reduced pressure and used without subsequent purification (6.46 g, 53%).

N-(3-methoxyphenyl)**-2-methylindoline-5-sulfonamide**: 2-methyl-1-(2,2,2-trifluoroacetyl)indoline-5-sulfonyl chloride (2.5 g,

7.6 mmol, 1 eq.) was diluted with DCM (10 mL). 3-methoxyaniline (1.71 mL, 15.2 mmol, 2 eq.) followed by N,N-Diisopropylethylamine (5.3 mL, 31 mmol, 4 eq.) was added to the reaction. Reaction progress was monitored by LCMS. Once the reaction was deemed complete, it was diluted with DCM (40 mL) and washed with water (2x, 50 mL) and brine (50 mL). The organic layer was dried over Na_2SO_4 and concentrated under reduced pressure. Purification by flash chromatography (0%–100% EtOAc in Hexanes) afforded the desired product (2.66 g, 85%). LCMS: $R_T = 0.800$ min., $[M+H]^+ = 414.7$; >98% @ 220 and @ 254 nm. The trifluoroacetate was removed by stirring in a 1:1:1 mixture of MeOH, THF, and 10% NaOH affording the title compound (782 mg, 38%). LCMS: $R_T = 0.665$ min., $[M+H]^+ = 318.8$; >98% @ 220 and @ 254 nm.

N-(3-methoxyphenyl)-2-methyl-1-propionylindoline-5-sulfonamide (VU0077625): N-(3-methoxyphenyl)-2-methylindoline-5-sulfonamide (11 mg, 0.035 mmol, 1 eq.) was diluted with DCM (0.3 mL). To this reaction, pyridine was added (0.011 mL, 0.14 mmol, 4 eq.) followed by propionyl chloride (0.003 mL, 0.05 mmol, 1.5 eq.). Reaction progress was monitored by LCMS. Once the reaction was deemed complete it was concentrated under forced air and heat and was subsequently purified on preparative HPLC (3 mg, 26%). ^{1}H NMR (400.1 MHz, $CDCl_3$) δ ppm): 8.17 (bs, 1 H); 7.67 (dd, $J = 1.69$, 8.72 Hz, 1 H); 7.58 (s, 1 H); 7.16 (t, $J = 8.25$ Hz, 1 H); 6.69–6.57 (m, 4 H); 4.58 (bs, 1 H); 3.74 (s, 3 H); 3.38–3.32 (m, 1 H); 2.66–2.47 (m, 4 H); 1.29–1.22 (m, 5 H). HRMS (TOF, ES^+) $C_{19}H_{23}N_2O_4S$ $[M+H]^+$ calc'd for 375.1379, found 375.1381.

Patch clamp electrophysiology

T-REx-HEK293-AeKir1 cells were voltage clamped in the whole-cell configuration of the patch clamp technique after overnight induction with tetracycline (1 µg/ml) essentially as described earlier [5]. Briefly, patch electrodes were pulled from silanized 1.5 mm outer diameter borosilicate microhematocrit tubes using a Narishige PC-10 two-stage puller. Electrode resistance ranged from 3.5 to 5.5 MΩ when filled with the following intracellular solution (in mM): 135 KCl, 2 $MgCl_2$, 1 EGTA, 10 HEPES free acid, 2 Na_2ATP (Roche, Indianapolis, IN), pH 7.3, 275 mOsm. The standard bath solution contained (in mM): 135 NaCl, 5 KCl, 2 $CaCl_2$, 1 $MgCl_2$, 5 glucose, 10 HEPES free acid, pH 7.4, 290 mOsm. Whole-cell currents were recorded under voltage-clamp conditions using an Axopatch 200B amplifier (Molecular Devices, Sunnyvale, CA). Electrical connections to the amplifier were made using Ag/AgCl wires and 3 M KCl/agar bridges. Electrophysiological data were collected at 5 kHz and filtered at 1 kHz. Data acquisition and analysis were performed using pClamp 9.2 software (Axon Instruments). All recordings were made at room temperature (20–23°C).

Heterologous expression of AeKir1 and AeKir2B in Xenopus oocytes

AeKir1 and AeKir2B channels were expressed heterologously in *Xenopus laevis* oocytes as described previously [6]. In brief, defolliculated *Xenopus* oocytes (purchased from Ecocyte Bioscience, Austin, TX) were injected with 10 ng (0.35 ng/nL) of either AeKir1 or AeKir2B cRNA and cultured for 3–7 days in OR3 media at 18°C. Oocytes injected with 28 nl of nuclease-free H_2O served as controls.

Electrophysiology of Xenopus oocytes

All electrophysiological experiments on *Xenopus* oocytes were performed at room temperature. The compositions of the solutions used in these experiments are shown in Table 1. When present,

VU625 was dissolved in solution *III* or solution *V* to a final concentration of 0.1, 1, 5, 15, or 50 µM (0.05% DMSO). All solutions were delivered by gravity to a RC-3Z oocyte chamber (Warner Instruments, Hamden, CT) via polyethylene tubing at a flow rate of ~2 ml/min. Solution changes were made with a Rheodyne Teflon 8-way Rotary valve (Model 5012, Rheodyne, Rohnert Park, CA).

Electrophysiological recordings from oocytes were conducted as described previously [6] In brief, each oocyte was transferred to the holding chamber under superfusion with solution *I* and impaled with two conventional-glass microelectrodes backfilled with 3 M KCl (resistances of 0.5–1.5 MΩ) to measure membrane potential (V_m) and whole-cell membrane current (I_m), respectively. Current-voltage (I–V) relationships of oocytes were acquired as described previously [6]. In brief, the oocytes were subjected to a voltage-stepping protocol consisting of 20 mV steps from −140 mV to +40 mV (100 ms each). After the conclusion of the voltage-stepping protocol, the clamp was turned off and a new solution was superfused through the chamber for ~90 s before acquiring another I–V relationship. All V_m and I_m values were recorded by a Digidata 1440A Data Acquisition System (Molecular Devices) and the Clampex module of pCLAMP. The I–V plots were generated using the Clampfit module of pCLAMP.

To evaluate the inhibition of AeKir1 and AeKir2B activity by VU625, we focused on the maximal inward currents elicited by the voltage-stepping protocol, which occur at a voltage of −140 mV. For AeKir1 oocytes, the background, inward currents in solution *II* (i.e., 0.5 mM K^+) were subtracted from those in 1) solution *III* (i.e., 10 mM K^+) to calculate the total inward current for an oocyte before exposure to VU625 (I_A), and 2) solution *III* with VU625 to calculate the inward current after exposure to the small molecule (I_B). The percent inhibition of the inward current was calculated by subtracting I_B from I_A and then dividing by I_A. For AeKir2B oocytes, a similar protocol was followed and similar calculations were made, except solution *IV* replaced solution *II* and solution *V* replaced solution *III*.

Mosquito colony

The *Aedes aegypti* mosquito colony used in the present study is identical to that described previously [6]. As before, only adult female mosquitoes 3–10 days post emergence were utilized for experiments.

Mosquito toxicology experiments

Adult female mosquitoes for injection were anesthetized on ice and impaled through the metapleuron using a pulled-glass capillary attached to a nanoliter injector (Nanoject II, Drummond Scientific Company, Broomall, PA). Each mosquito received a single hemolymph injection of 69 nL of solution. The injection solution consisted of a potassium-rich phosphate buffered saline (K^+-PBS), 15% DMSO, 1% β-cyclodextrin, 0.1% Solutol, and a concentration of VU625 to deliver the doses indicated. In experiments where probenecid was used, water-soluble probenecid (Biotium, Hayward CA) was included in the injection solution at 50 mM, thereby providing a dose of 3.4 nmol per mosquito.

The K^+-PBS solution consisted of the following in mM: 92.2 NaCl, 47.5 KCl, 10 Na_2HPO_4, and 2 KH_2PO_4 (pH 7.5). A total of 10 mosquitoes were injected for a given treatment or dose, and then were placed into small cages within a rearing chamber (28°C, 80% relative humidity, 12:12 light:dark) and allowed free access to a solution of 10% sucrose. The mosquitoes were observed at 24 hr after injection. For each treatment, 3–7 replicates of 10 mosquitoes each were performed.

Table 1. Compositions (in mM) of solutions used in *Xenopus* oocyte electrophysiology.

Solution #	I	II	III	IV	V
NaCl	96	88.5	88.5	73.5	73.5
NMDG-Cl	0	9.5	0	24.5	0
KCl	2	0.5	10	0.5	25
MgCl$_2$	1.0	1.0	1.0	1.0	1.0
CaCl$_2$	1.8	1.8	1.8	1.8	1.8
HEPES	5	5	5	5	5

The pH of all solutions was adjusted to 7.5 with NMDG-OH.
The osmolality of each solution was verified to be 190 mOsm kg^{-1} H$_2$O ($\pm$5 mOsm kg^{-1} H$_2$O) by vapor pressure osmometry.
NMDG = N-methyl-D-glucamine.

Mosquito excretion experiments

The excretory capacity of mosquitoes was measured as described [6]. In brief, after anesthetizing mosquitoes on ice, their hemolymph was injected as described above with 900 nL of a K$^+$-PBS vehicle containing 1.15% DMSO, 0.077% β-cyclodextrin, and 0.008% Solutol, or the vehicle containing VU625 (0.77 mM) to deliver a dose of 690 pmol of VU625 per mosquito. In experiments where probenecid was used, the vehicle was supplemented with water-soluble probenecid (3.08 mM) to deliver a dose of 3.4 nmol of probenecid per mosquito. After injection, the mosquitoes were placed immediately in a graduated, packed-cell volume tube (MidSci, St. Louis, MO; 5 mosquitoes per tube) and held at 28°C. The volume of urine excreted at 60 min post injection was measured as described previously [6], and all mosquitoes were confirmed to be alive at the end of 60 min period. For each treatment, 6–18 independent trials of 5 mosquitoes per treatment were performed.

Statistical analyses

Tl+ flux assay. The Z′ value was calculated as described earlier [21], using the following formula:

$$Z' = 1 - \left(3SD_p + 3SD_n\right)/|Mean_p + Mean_n|$$

where SD is standard deviation, p and n are vehicle control and compound inhibited flux values respectively.

To compare the effect of DMSO on *Ae*Kir1-mediated Tl$^+$ flux, a one-way ANOVA was performed with a Tukey's multiple comparison test. Prism software (GraphPad Software) was used to generate CRC from Tl$^+$ flux. Half-inhibition concentration (IC$_{50}$) values were calculated from fits using a four parameter logistic equation.

Mosquito toxicology and urine excretion. Prism (GraphPad Software) was used to generate a dose-response curve for the toxicity of VU625; the doses (x-axis) were first log transformed and then the mortality data was normalized using Prism, where the smallest value and largest values in a data set equal '0%' and '100%', respectively. The data were then fitted using a 'biphasic' algorithm (<100 constraint) to calculate potencies (ED$_{25}$ and ED$_{75}$ values). To compare 1) the toxic effects among the vehicle, probenecid, VU625, and VU625 + probenecid treatments, and 2) the excretory capacity among the vehicle, probenecid, VU625, and VU625 + probenecid treatments, one-way ANOVAs were performed with Newman-Keuls posttests.

Results

Discovery of novel *Ae*Kir1 inhibitors via HTS

In an effort to discover mosquito-specific inhibitors of *Ae*Kir1, we optimized a Tl$^+$ flux assay for HTS of large libraries of chemically diverse small molecules. The assay utilizes a monoclonal T-REx-HEK293 cell line that expresses *Ae*Kir1 from a tetracycline-inducible promoter [5]. The fluorescent dye, Thallos, is used to report the inward flux of Tl$^+$ through the *Ae*Kir1 channel pore in a population of cells plated in individual wells of a 384-well plate. As shown in Figure 1A, overnight induction of *Ae*Kir1 expression with tetracycline leads to a robust Tl$^+$ flux compared to control cells that were not treated with tetracycline. This assay enables more than 300 compounds to be tested simultaneously in a single plate, and thousands of compounds to be tested daily, for effects on *Ae*Kir1 activity.

The assay was validated for HTS by meeting a series of performance benchmarks. First, the assay was tested for its tolerance to the small-molecule vehicle DMSO at concentrations up to 10% v/v. As shown in Fig. 1B, the Tl$^+$-flux mediated by *Ae*Kir1 is unaffected by DMSO concentrations up to 1.3% v/v as compared to the 0% DMSO control (one-way ANOVA, P < 0.0001). Next, the assay was tested for uniformity and reproducibility of HTS performance. As shown in Fig. 1C, the average Z′ statistic for these experiments was 0.69±0.05 (Z′≥0.5 is suitable for HTS), indicating that the assay is robust and will enable modulators of *Ae*Kir1 to be identified in HTS with a low false-positive rate.

Approximately 30,000 compounds from the VICB library were screened at a nominal concentration of 10 μM for inhibition of *Ae*Kir1. From this primary screen and following confirmation testing in tetracycline-induced and uninduced T-REx-HEK293-*Ae*Kir1 cells (see Methods), 283 authentic channel-dependent modulators were selected for further study. Because our ultimate goal is to develop Kir channel inhibitors that are active against mosquitoes and not humans, these 'hits' were subsequently tested for dose-dependent activity against a panel of mammalian Kir channels, which included Kir1.1, Kir2.1, Kir2.2, Kir2.3, Kir3.1/3.2, Kir4.1, Kir7.1(M125R), and Kir6.2/SUR1 [18,19,21]. Four-point concentration response curves (CRCs) were generated for the 283 compounds, resulting in 17 inhibitors with 11 unique chemical scaffolds that exhibited dose-dependent inhibition of *Ae*Kir1 with IC$_{50}$ values below 5 μM and little to no activity (IC$_{50}$≥30 μM) against mammalian Kir channels (data not shown). These compounds were subsequently purchased from commercial vendors, freshly dissolved in DMSO, and assayed in 11-point CRCs against *Ae*Kir1 via the Tl$^+$-flux assay.

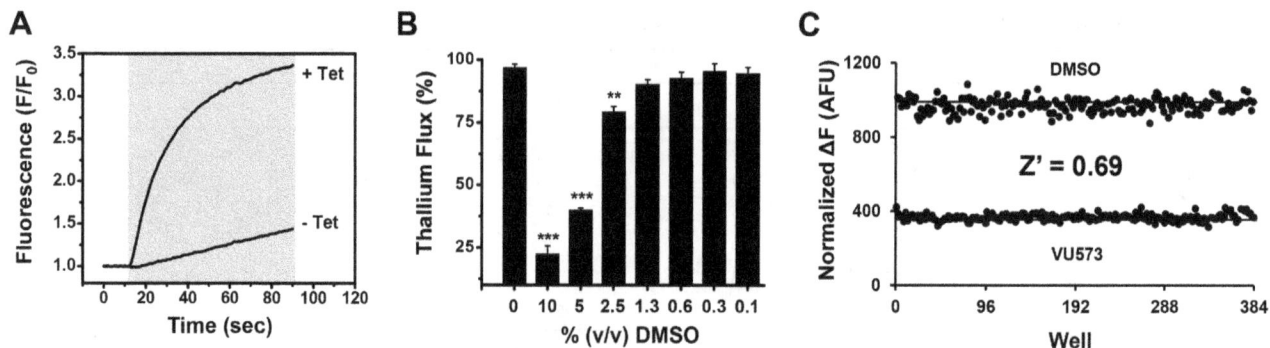

Figure 1. Tl$^+$ flux assay of AeKir1 channel activity for high-throughput screening. (A) Representative Tl$^+$-induced changes in Thallos fluorescence in T-Rex-HEK293-AeKir1 cells cultured overnight with (+Tet) or without (-Tet) tetracycline. The shaded box indicates the cell exposure to Tl$^+$. (B) DMSO concentrations up to 1.3% v/v DMSO have no effect on Tl$^+$ flux through AeKir1. Data are means ±SEM ($n = 3$). One-way ANOVA P< 0.0001, and asterisks (**, ***) indicate P<0.01 or P<0.001 respectively, when compared to 0% DMSO (Tukey's test). (C) Representative checkerboard analysis using 100 μM VU573 or 0.1% v/v DMSO as the vehicle control. The mean peak fluorescence amplitude of each sample population is indicated with a solid line and alternating samples for DMSO (top) and VU573 (bottom) are graphed as individual points. The mean ±SD Z' calculated over 6 plates on 3 separate days was 0.69±0.05.

VU625 is a potent and preferential inhibitor of AeKir1 vs. mammalian Kir and AeKir2B channels

From the aforementioned Tl$^+$ flux assays, one compound—N-(3-methoxyphenyl)-2-methyl-1-propionylindoline-5-sulfonamide, termed VU625—was found to inhibit AeKir1 in 11-point CRCs with an IC$_{50}$ of 0.32 μM (95% CI: 0.25–0.39 μM) and a Hill coefficient value of 0.98 (95% CI: 0.8–1.2) (Fig. 2A–C). VU625 also had no significant effects on the mammalian Kir channels assayed via Tl$^+$ flux with the exception of G-protein coupled Kir channels comprised of Kir3.1/3.2 subunits (IC$_{50}$ = 8.6 μM; Table S1). Furthermore, in radioligand displacement assays against 68 mammalian GPCR's, ion channels, and transporters, 10 μM VU625 was active (defined as >50% ligand displacement) against only three targets: adenosine A1 receptor (76% displacement), melatonin MT1 receptor (56% displacement) and 5-HT$_{2B}$ receptor (69% displacement) (Table S2).

To further confirm the activity of VU625 obtained from Tl$^+$-flux assays, we used patch-clamp electrophysiology to assay the inhibition of AeKir1 expressed in T-REx-HEK293 cells. In whole-cell patch clamp recordings, VU625 inhibited AeKir1 channel

activity with an IC$_{50}$ of 96.8 nM (95% CI: 75.4–124.2 nM) and a Hill coefficient value of 1.02 (95% CI: 0.8–1.3) (Fig. 3A, B).

In a previous paper, we demonstrated that other small molecule inhibitors of AeKir1 (i.e., VU573 and VU590) can have different pharmacological effects on AeKir2B [6]. Thus, we sought to determine the effects of VU625 on AeKir2B channel activity, utilizing Xenopus oocytes heterologously expressing AeKir2B. AeKir1 expressing oocytes served as positive controls. Figure 3C shows that VU625 inhibits AeKir1- and AeKir2B-mediated K$^+$ currents with IC$_{50}$ values of 3.8 μM (95% CI: 2.3–6.3 μM) and 45.1 μM (95% CI: 31.7–64.2 μM), respectively. Thus, VU625 inhibits both AeKir1 and AeKir2B channels, albeit with greater affinity for AeKir1. It should be noted that the reduction in VU625 potency observed in Xenopus oocytes compared to HEK cells is typical for a small-molecule inhibitor of Kir channels and has been observed for structurally diverse compounds and Kir channels [5,6,19,23].

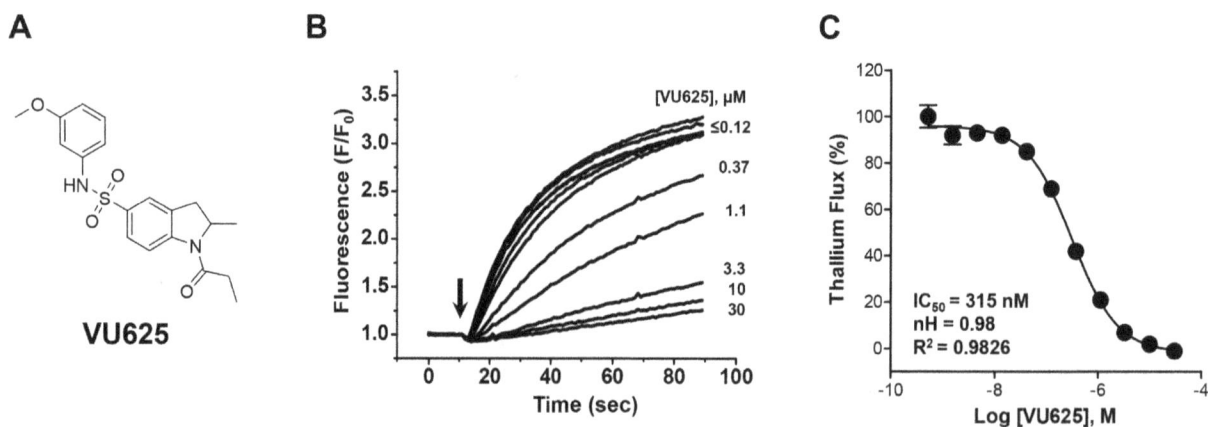

Figure 2. VU625 is a potent inhibitor of AeKir1 in Tl$^+$ flux assays. (A) Chemical structure of VU625. (B) Dose-dependent inhibition of the AeKir1-mediated Tl$^+$ flux by VU625 with concentrations ranging from ≤0.12 to 30 μM. The arrow indicates when Tl$^+$ was added to the extracellular bath. (C) Concentration-response curves of VU625 derived from Tl$^+$ flux assays. The IC$_{50}$ and Hill-coefficient (nH) values are 315 nM (95% CI: 254.4–390.2 nM) and 0.98 respectively. Data are mean ±SEM. $n = 4$ independent experiments performed in triplicate.

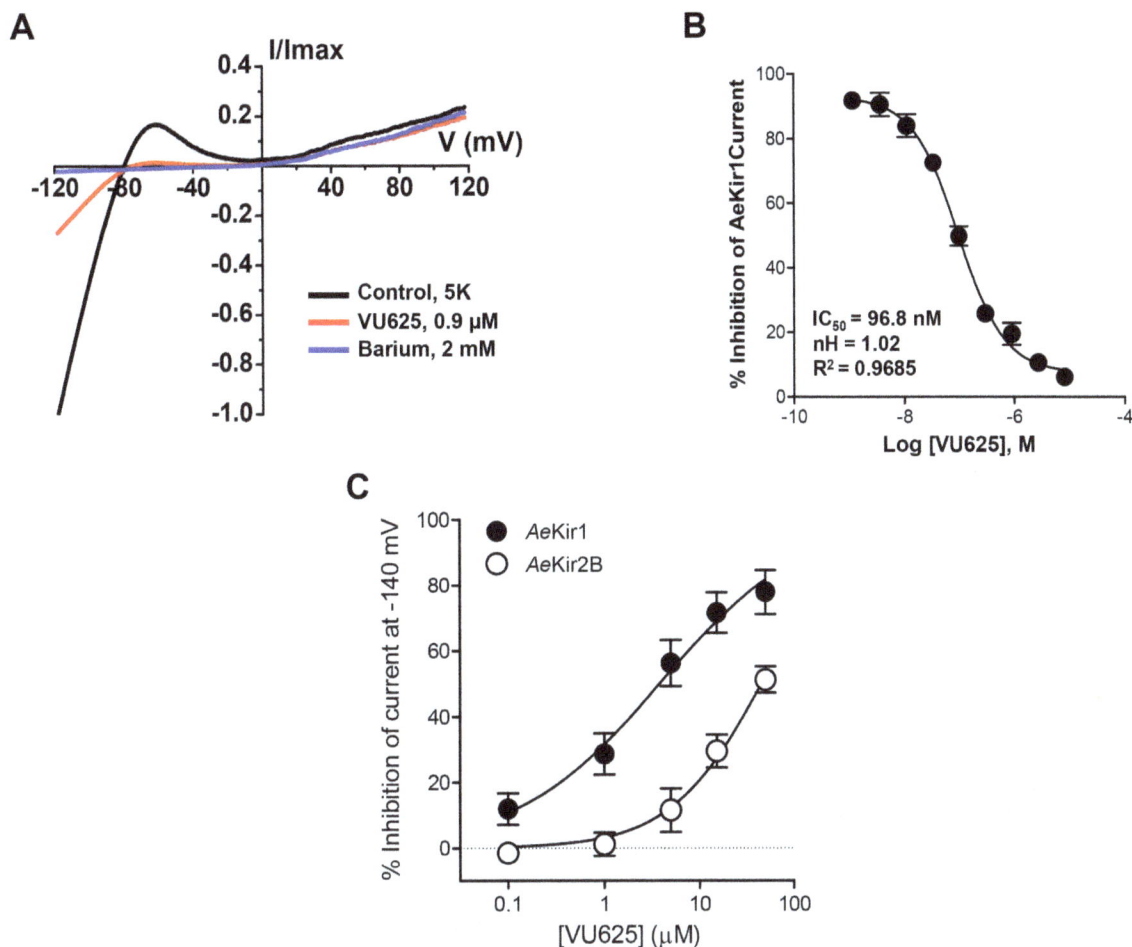

Figure 3. VU625 is a potent and preferential inhibitor of AeKir1 over AeKir2B in whole-cell electrophysiology. (A) Normalized AeKir1 current-voltage relationships obtained from heterologous expression in T-Rex-HEK293 cells, illustrating VU625-dependent inhibition before (control) and after addition of 0.9 µM VU625. Residual AeKir1 currents were inhibited with 2 mM barium. Cells were voltage clamped at −75 mV and ramped between −120 mV and +60 mV. (B) Concentration-response curve of VU625 derived from patch clamp experiments ($n = 4$–6). The IC_{50} of VU625 is 96.8 nM (95% CI: 75.4–124.2 nM). (C) Concentration-response curves of current inhibition mediated by heterologous expression in Xenopus oocytes of AeKir1 (filled circles) and AeKir2B (open circles) channels after bath application of VU625. $n = 4$–5 oocytes per concentration. The calculated IC_{50} values of VU625 for AeKir1 and AeKir2B current inhibition are 3.8 µM (95% CI: 2.3–6.3 µM) and 45.1 µM (95% CI: 31.7–64.2 µM), respectively.

Chemical lead optimization and structure-activity relationships

Because of its potency, clean ancillary pharmacology and chemical tractability (Figures 2–3, Tables S1–S2), VU625 was selected for lead optimization (**3a**, Table 2). We partitioned the compound into three areas for structure-activity relationship (SAR) exploration denoted as the sulfonamide, central core, and southern amide portions (Fig. 4A). The first generation libraries held the sulfonamide and the central core sections constant and diversified the southern amide portion (Table 2). The synthetic scheme (Fig. 4B) for this portion was straightforward and started with protection of the amine with trifluoroacetamide (TFAA, pyridine) followed by sulfonyl chloride formation ($ClSO_3$, PCl_5). Next, the sulfonamide was formed, the protecting group was removed, and either the amide or sulfonamide was formed (see Methods for details). Little tolerance for steric bulk was seen in this portion of the molecule. That is, the trifluoroacetamide (VU0477197, **3b**, Table 2) retained potency (0.58 µM), however, larger aromatic amides were much less active (**3c–g**, Table 2). The same trend was observed for the sulfonamide compounds, with smaller sulfonamides retaining nanomolar activity (VU0477691, **3k**, 0.76 µM; VU0477692, **3l**, 0.82 µM) and the larger aromatic group leading to less activity (**3h**, Table 2).

Next, we evaluated the left-hand sulfonamide portion of the molecule, however, all efforts to change the 3-methoxyaryl moiety led to significant reductions in potency (see Table S3). Finally, we explored the central core with the intent of establishing the minimal pharmacophore needed for activity against AeKir1. To this end, the indoline core was replaced with simple aryl, heteroaryl or biaryl groups which all led to compounds with much reduced activity (>10-fold loss of potency). However, an interesting SAR was seen with very closely related 6,6- or 6,5-indole or dihydroquinolinone-like structures (**4a–f**, Table 3). The simple N-methyl indole (VU0481807, **4a**, 0.55 µM, Table 3) retained most of the activity as VU625 and addition of a 2-methyl (VU0486620, **4b**, 0.97 µM, Table 3) led to a further minor reduction in activity. Expanding the ring system and addition of a lactam (**4c–e**, Table 3) was not productive. Lastly, removal of the methyl group in the indoline system of VU625, led to a ~3-fold loss of potency (VU0483404, **4f**, 1.15 µM, Table 3).

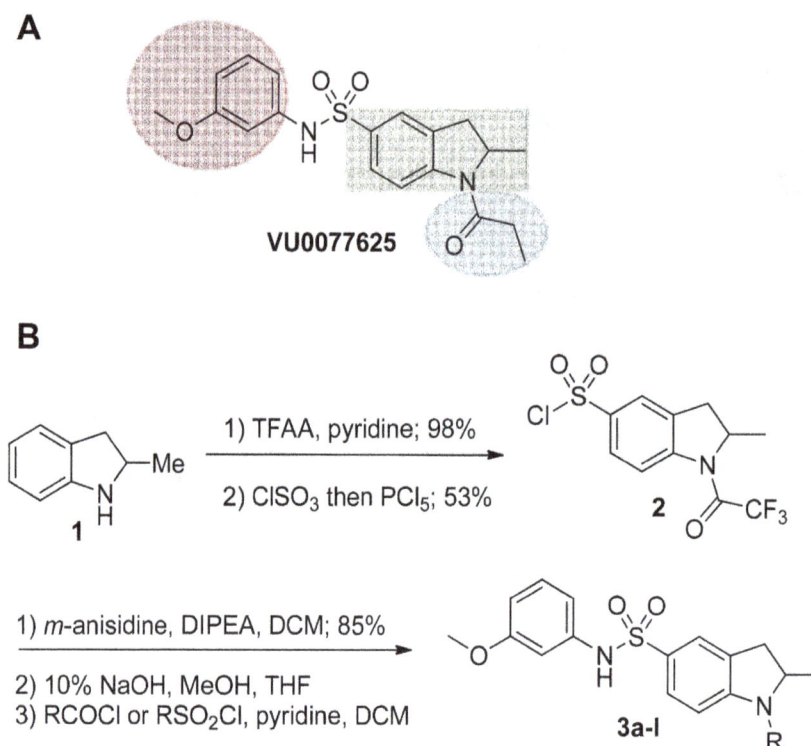

Figure 4. Design and chemical lead optimization strategy for VU625. (A) Modular approach to assess three areas of diversification of VU625: sulfonamide (red shading), central core (green shading), and southern amide (blue shading) portions. (B) General synthetic approach to access VU625 and analogs around the amide and sulfonamide portions.

Figure 5 summarizes the SAR observed for the VU625 scaffold. The left-hand sulfonamide portion offered the least amount of SAR traction as only the 3-methoxyphenyl (and weaker 2-methoxyphenyl) sulfonamide provided activity. Replacement with an amide, or substituting the 3-methoxyphenyl for other aryl groups all led to less potent compounds. Replacement of the proponamide in the southern fraction was tolerated as long as the substituent was small and aliphatic. Sulfonamides could be exchanged, although there was an observed ~2-3-fold loss of activity. Lastly, the central core was also important for potency. Only very similar compounds such as indole and des-methyl indoline were tolerated.

VU625-induced toxicity is increased by probenecid

Injection of the *Ae*Kir1 channel inhibitors VU573 or VU590 into the hemolymph of adult female *A. aegypti* mosquitoes leads to their incapacitation and/or death within 24 h [5,6]. Surprisingly, injection of a high dose (i.e. 690 pmol per mosquito) of VU625, which is a more potent inhibitor of *Ae*Kir1 than VU573 and VU590, into the hemolymph of mosquitoes had no significant effects on mosquito behavior or survival within 24 h (Fig. 6). Thus, we hypothesized that the lack of in vivo effects could be due to poor bioavailability of VU625 as a result of metabolic detoxification and/or excretion by the mosquito.

We therefore tested whether probenecid, which is a broad-spectrum inhibitor of organic anion transporters (OATs) and ATP-binding cassette (ABC) transporters [24,25,26], would improve the efficacy of VU625. Interestingly, both probenecid and VU625 have a sulfonamide moiety in their chemical structure (Fig. S2). As shown in Fig. 6, the injection of probenecid (3.4 nmol per mosquito) along with VU625 (690 pmol per mosquito)

significantly increases the toxicity of VU625 within 24 h compared to injection of VU625 or probenecid alone. The abdomens of these mosquitoes were not severely bloated and obvious sub-lethal effects (e.g., loss of flight) were not apparent.

We next sought to characterize the dose-response relationship of VU625 in mosquitoes when co-injected with a constant dose of probenecid (3.4 nmol per mosquito). As shown in Fig. 7, co-injection of VU625 with probenecid induces mortality in mosquitoes within 24 h in a biphasic manner with 25% and 75% efficacious doses (ED_{25} and ED_{75}) of 9.96 pmol and 502 pmol, respectively. This biphasic dose-response relationship suggests the inhibition of at least two distinct molecular targets for which VU625 has different affinities, which is consistent with the inhibition of both *Ae*Kir1 and *Ae*Kir2B channels by VU625 (Fig. 3C).

VU625-induced reduction of urine excretion is enhanced by probenecid

We showed previously that pharmacological inhibition of *Ae*Kir1 with the small molecule inhibitors VU573 and VU590 leads to a decrease in the excretory capacity of *A. aegypti* mosquitoes after loading their hemolymph with 900 nl of a PBS vehicle [5] [6]. Therefore, we sought to similarly determine the effects of VU625 on mosquito excretory capacity. As shown in Fig. 8, mosquitoes injected with the PBS vehicle excreted 644 ± 24.18 nL of urine within the next hour. Consistent with the toxicity studies, we found that adding VU625 (0.77 mM) to the vehicle, which delivers 690 pmol of VU625 per mosquito, did not significantly decrease the excretory capacity (583.3 ± 29.52 nL/ female) compared to the vehicle controls (Fig. 8). Interestingly, adding probenecid (50 mM) to the vehicle, which delivers

Table 2. Structure-activity relationships and lead optimization summary of VU0077625 scaffold.

Cmpd	R	VU#	IC$_{50}$±SEM (μM)
3a		VU0077625	0.36±0.02
3b		VU0477197	0.58±0.04
3c		VU0477684	5.20±0.40
3d		VU0477693	4.41±1.11
3e		VU0477694	3.87±1.97
3f		VU0477688	>30
3g		VU0477685	4.40±0.50
3h		VU0477686	3.29±0.89
3i		VU0477687	2.09±0.49
3j		VU0477690	2.82±0.48
3k		VU0477691	0.76±0.00
3l		VU0477692	0.82±0.48

IC$_{50}$ values were derived from 11-point CRCs on AeKir1 in Tl$^+$ flux experiments performed in triplicate on two separate days.

3.4 nmol of probenecid per mosquito, causes a small but significant reduction in excretory capacity to 467.8±33.53 nL/female, suggesting a potential role of probenecid-sensitive transporters in urine excretion. However, adding both VU625 (0.77 mM) and probenecid (50 mM) to the vehicle significantly decreases the excretory capacity the furthest to 236.7±24.53 nL/female.

Discussion

Here, we report the discovery of VU625, the first sub-micromolar inhibitor of a mosquito Kir channel. VU625 is one of 283 confirmed AeKir1 inhibitors identified in a HTS of approximately 30,000 compounds from the VICB library. It was chosen for lead optimization based on its potency (IC$_{50}$ = 96.8 nM), greater than 80-fold selectivity for the AeKir1 channel over 8 mammalian Kir channels, and clean ancillary pharmacology among a panel of 68 critical mammalian off-targets comprised of voltage-gated ion channels, ion transporters, and receptors (i.e., neurotransmitter, peptide, and G-protein coupled). VU625 is the most potent and selective mosquito Kir channel inhibitor reported to date.

This study provides proof-of-concept that conventional drug discovery approaches can be employed successfully to identify small-molecule tools for probing the physiology of insect Kir channels and potential lead compounds for insecticide development. A similar approach has been used recently in insecticide discovery efforts targeting mosquito G-protein coupled receptors [27].

VU625 exhibits inhibitory activity against both AeKir1 and AeKir2B, albeit with greater affinity for AeKir1. To date, we have reported the activity of two other small-molecule inhibitors of mosquito Kir channels that exhibit differential pharmacology. VU590 is a selective inhibitor of AeKir1 over AeKir2B, whereas VU573 inhibits AeKir1 and activates AeKir2B [6]. Thus, VU625 potentially represents a broad-spectrum, small-molecule blocker of mosquito Kir channels, pending the characterization of its effects on the other mosquito Kir channels (AeKir2A, AeKir2B' and AeKir3 channels), which to date have not yet been expressed functionally in a heterologous system ([12]; Denton and Piermarini, personal observations). Once the distinguishing pharmacological properties of each of these Kir channel inhibitors are fully characterized, they can potentially be employed to determine the relative contributions of Kir channel subtypes in the physiology of various mosquito tissues. This would provide an important

Table 3. Structure-activity relationships and lead optimization summary for the central core portion of VU0077625 scaffold.

Cmpd	R	VU#	IC$_{50}$±SEM (μM)
4a		VU0481807	0.55±0.08
4b		VU0486620	0.97±0.10
4c		VU0481811	>30
4d		VU0483082	>30
4e		VU0483402	>30
4f		VU0483404	1.15±0.05

IC$_{50}$ values were derived from 11-point CRCs on AeKir1 in Tl$^+$ flux experiments performed in triplicate on two separate days.

chemical tool set to validate and complement studies of mosquito Kir channels that employ functional genetic approaches (e.g., RNA interference).

Given the superior in vitro potency of VU625 compared to the AeKir1 inhibitors VU573 [5] and VU590 [6], we expected VU625 to elicit superior in vivo toxicity. Thus, we were surprised when high doses of VU625 elicited no observable effects on mosquito survival or excretory capacity when injected directly into the hemolymph. Since mosquitoes have evolved robust protective mechanisms for detoxifying and excreting xenobiotics that would harm them otherwise [28,29], we investigated whether the molecule may be detoxified and/or excreted.

Preliminary experiments with PBO did not improve the efficacy of VU625, suggesting that detoxification of the compound by cytochrome P450s is unlikely to contribute to its poor in vivo efficacy. The co-injection of VU625 with probenecid rescued not only its toxicity, but also its effects on excretory capacity, which suggests that VU625 is likely a substrate of OATs and/or ABC transporters in the mosquitoes and may be rendered ineffective in

vivo through excretion. The potent toxicity of VU625 when co-injected with probenecid may be due to the ability of VU625 to inhibit at least two Kir channels, some of which are expressed in the central and peripheral nervous systems, such as Kir1 and Kir2B' [8,12,30,31], and/or a synergistic effect of probenecid that maintains high circulating concentrations of VU625 by preventing its renal excretion. Indeed, it is conceivable that the sulfonamide moiety in the structures of VU625 and probenecid causes them to be substrates for OATs and/or ABC transporters. Overall, these findings highlight efficient xenobiotic transport mechanisms in mosquitoes that render a nanomolar inhibitor of AeKir1 (VU625) ineffective in vivo, even when introduced directly to the hemolymph. The tissues that contribute to the excretion of VU625 remain to be determined, but presumably involve the Malpighian tubules and/or gut [32,33].

Lastly, the medicinal chemistry efforts put forth in the present study may be a valuable first step in determining which structural moieties are important for the excretion of VU625 by xenobiotic transporters and/or its in vivo activity in mosquitoes. Future

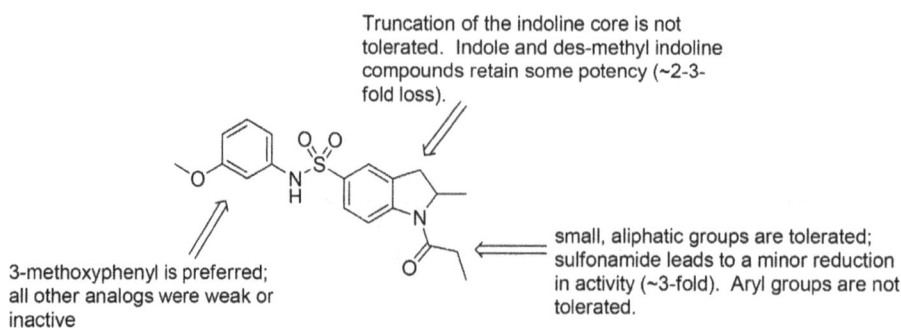

Truncation of the indoline core is not tolerated. Indole and des-methyl indoline compounds retain some potency (~2-3-fold loss).

3-methoxyphenyl is preferred; all other analogs were weak or inactive

small, aliphatic groups are tolerated; sulfonamide leads to a minor reduction in activity (~3-fold). Aryl groups are not tolerated.

Figure 5. Summary of structure-activity relationship (SAR). Summary of observed SAR of over 100 analogs synthesized exploring all three regions of VU625.

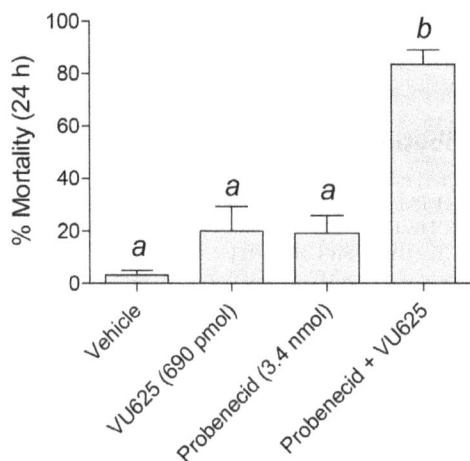

Figure 6. Effects of probenecid and VU625 on survival of adult female mosquitoes (*A. aegypti*). Percent mortality of mosquitoes at 24 h post-injection. Each mosquito was injected with 69 nl of the vehicle containing VU625 (10 mM), probenecid (50 mM), or both, to deliver the desired doses: 690 pmol of VU625, 3.4 nmol probenecid. $n = 6–7$ trials of 10 mosquitoes each per treatment. Lower-case letters indicate statistical categorization of the means as determined by a one-way ANOVA with a Newman-Keuls post-test ($P < 0.05$).

studies should assess the in vivo efficacy and probenecid-mediated clearance of the VU625 analog series we generated to determine if any of these compounds exhibit potent toxicity in mosquitoes without probenecid.

Perspectives

Here, we show a direct relationship between in vitro pharmacology and in vivo toxicity of VU625, which is consistent with our previous studies [5,6] suggesting that Kir channel inhibitors are promising chemicals for insecticide development. To date, none of

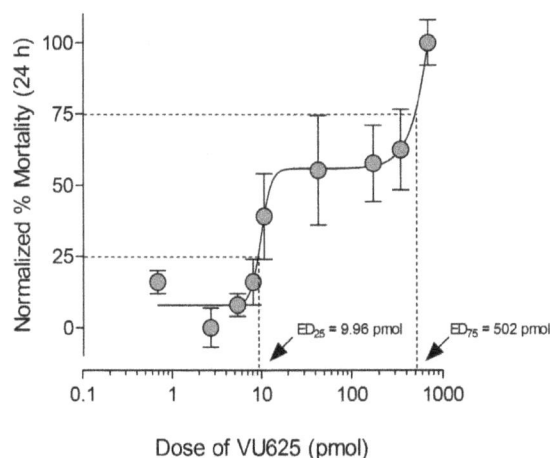

Figure 7. The dose-response curve of the toxic effects of VU625 on adult female mosquitoes (*A. aegypti*) is biphasic. Normalized percent mortality of mosquitoes at 24 h post-injection. Each mosquito was injected with 69 nL of the vehicle containing probenecid (50 mM) and an appropriate concentration of VU625 to deliver the doses of VU625 indicated and 3.4 nmol of probenecid. The ED_{25} and ED_{75} were determined by fitting a non-linear biphasic curve to the data. $n = 3–4$ trials of 10 mosquitoes each per dose.

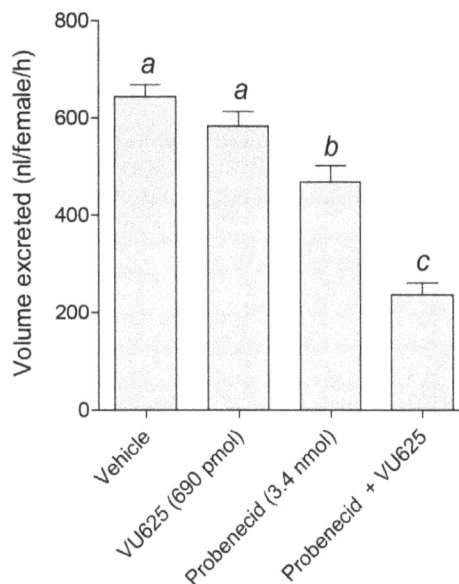

Figure 8. Effects of probenecid and VU625 on the in vivo excretory capacity of adult female mosquitoes (*A. aegypti*). Amount of urine excreted by mosquitoes 1 h after injection with 900 nL of the vehicle (K^+-PBS_{50} containing 1.8% DMSO, 0.077% β-cyclodextrin, and 0.008% Solutol), or the vehicle containing VU625 (0.77 mM), probenecid (3.85 mM), or both, to deliver the desired doses: 690 pmol of VU625, 3.4 nmol probenecid. Values are means $\pm$SEM; $n = 6–18$ trials of 5 mosquitoes per treatment. Lower-case letters indicate statistical categorization of the means as determined by a one-way ANOVA with a Newman-Keuls posttest ($P < 0.05$).

the Kir channel inhibitors we have reported (i.e. VU573, VU590, VU625) exhibit toxicity when applied to the cuticle (Piermarini, unpublished observations), which is a waxy, lipophilic structure that creates a physical barrier to insecticide permeation into the hemocoel of mosquitoes. This lack of topical activity severely limits the potential use of the present Kir channel inhibitors as active compounds for incorporation into insecticide-treated bed nets and indoor-residual sprays. The efficacy of common insecticides, such as permethrin, is dependent in part on their lipophilic nature [34,35]. Thus, future chemistry efforts will focus on lipophilic inhibitors of Kir channels. Furthermore, prioritizing initial HTS 'hits' according to their hydrophobicity may facilitate the discovery of more suitable small-molecules compounds for insecticide development.

Supporting Information

Figure S1 Reagents and conditions: (A) TFAA, pyridine, 0°C; (B) ClSO₃H, 40°C, 1 h; PCl₅, rt; (C) 3-methoxyaniline, DIEA, rt; MeOH:10% NaOH (1:1:1); (D) pyridine, CH₂Cl₂, ClCOCH₂CH₃.

Figure S2 VU625 and probenecid share a sulfonamide moiety. The sulfonamide moiety contained in the chemical structure of VU625 and probenecid is shaded in blue.

Table S1 Selectivity of VU625 against human Kir channels assessed in Tl⁺ flux assays. $n = 2$ independent experiments in triplicate.

Table S2 Summary of results obtained from the activity of the VU625 compound in radioligand binding assays. The significant results are highlighted in grey.

Table S3 SAR around the left-hand sulfonamide. IC_{50} values were derived from 11-point CRCs on AeKir1 in Tl^+ flux experiments performed in triplicate on two separate days.

References

1. WHO (2013) World Malaria Report WHO; World Health Organization.
2. Ranson H, N'Guessan R, Lines J, Moiroux N, Nkuni Z, et al. (2011) Pyrethroid resistance in African anopheline mosquitoes: what are the implications for malaria control? Trends Parasitol 27: 91–98.
3. Asidi A, N'Guessan R, Akogbeto M, Curtis C, Rowland M (2012) Loss of household protection from use of insecticide-treated nets against pyrethroid-resistant mosquitoes, benin. Emerg Infect Dis 18: 1101–1106.
4. Maharaj R (2011) Global trends in insecticide resistance and impact on disease vector control measures. Open Access Insect Physiology: 27.
5. Raphemot R, Rouhier MF, Hopkins CR, Gogliotti RD, Lovell KM, et al. (2013) Eliciting renal failure in mosquitoes with a small-molecule inhibitor of inward-rectifying potassium channels. PLoS One 8: e64905.
6. Rouhier MF, Raphemot R, Denton JS, Piermarini PM (2014) Pharmacological Validation of an Inward-Rectifier Potassium (Kir) Channel as an Insecticide Target in the Yellow Fever Mosquito *Aedes aegypti*. PLoS One 9:e100700.
7. Raphemot R, Estevez-Lao TY, Rouhier MF, Piermarini PM, Denton JS, et al. (2014) Molecular and functional characterization of Anopheles gambiae inward rectifier potassium (Kir1) channels: A novel role in egg production. Insect Biochem Mol Biol 51: 10–19.
8. Döring F, Wischmeyer E, Kühnlein RP, Jäckle H, Karschin A (2002) Inwardly Rectifying K (Kir) Channels in *Drosophila*. J Biol Chem 277: 25554–25561.
9. Evans JM, Allan AK, Davies SA, Dow JA (2005) Sulphonylurea sensitivity and enriched expression implicate inward rectifier K^+ channels in *Drosophila* melanogaster renal function. J Exp Biol 208: 3771–3783.
10. Eleftherianos I, Won S, Chtarbanova S, Squiban B, Ocorr K, et al. (2011) ATP-sensitive potassium channel (K_{ATP})–dependent regulation of cardiotropic viral infections. Proc Natl Acad Sci 108: 12024–12029.
11. Dahal GR, Rawson J, Gassaway B, Kwok B, Tong Y, et al. (2012) An inwardly rectifying K^+ channel is required for patterning. Development 139: 3653–3664.
12. Piermarini PM, Rouhier MF, Schepel M, Kosse C, Beyenbach KW (2013) Cloning and functional characterization of inward-rectifying potassium (Kir) channels from Malpighian tubules of the mosquito *Aedes aegypti*. Insect Biochem Mol Biol 43: 75–90.
13. Raphemot R, Kadakia RJ, Olsen ML, Banerjee S, Days E, et al. (2013) Development and validation of fluorescence-based and automated patch clamp-based functional assays for the inward rectifier potassium channel kir4.1. Assay Drug Dev Technol 11: 532–543.
14. Hibino H, Inanobe A, Furutani K, Murakami S, Findlay I, et al. (2010) Inwardly Rectifying Potassium Channels: Their Structure, Function, and Physiological Roles. Physiol Rev 90: 291–366.
15. Denton JS, Pao AC, Maduke M (2013) Novel diuretic targets. Am J Physiol Renal Physiol 305: F931–942.
16. Pattnaik BR, Asuma MP, Spott R, Pillers DA (2012) Genetic defects in the hotspot of inwardly rectifying K^+ (Kir) channels and their metabolic consequences: a review. Mol Genet Metab 105: 64–72.
17. Denton JS, Jacobson DA (2012) Channeling dysglycemia: ion-channel variations perturbing glucose homeostasis. Trends Endocrinol Metab 23: 41–48.
18. Lewis LM, Bhave G, Chauder BA, Banerjee S, Lornsen KA, et al. (2009) High-throughput screening reveals a small-molecule inhibitor of the renal outer medullary potassium channel and Kir7.1. Mol Pharmacol 76: 1094–1103.
19. Raphemot R, Lonergan DF, Nguyen TT, Utley T, Lewis LM, et al. (2011) Discovery, characterization, and structure-activity relationships of an inhibitor of inward rectifier potassium (Kir) channels with preference for Kir2.3, Kir3.x, and Kir7.1. Front Pharmacol 2: 75.
20. Raphemot R, Swale DR, Dadi PK, Jacobson DA, Cooper P, et al. (2014) Direct Activation of beta-cell K_{ATP} Channels with a Novel Xanthine Derivative.Mol Pharmacol. 85: 858–65.
21. Raphemot R, Weaver CD, Denton JS (2013) High-throughput screening for small-molecule modulators of inward rectifier potassium channels. J Vis Exp. 71: 4209.
22. Niswender CM, Johnson KA, Luo Q, Ayala JE, Kim C, et al. (2008) A novel assay of Gi/o-linked G protein-coupled receptor coupling to potassium channels provides new insights into the pharmacology of the group III metabotropic glutamate receptors. Mol Pharmacol 73: 1213–1224.
23. Bhave G, Chauder BA, Liu W, Dawson ES, Kadakia R, et al. (2011) Development of a selective small-molecule inhibitor of Kir1.1, the renal outer medullary potassium channel. Mol Pharmacol 79: 42–50.
24. Feller N, Broxterman HJ, Währer DC, Pinedo HM (1995) ATP-dependent efflux of calcein by the multidrug resistance protein (MRP): no inhibition by intracellular glutathione depletion. FEBS Lett 368: 385–388.
25. Jaehde U, Sörgel F, Reiter A, Sigl G, Naber KG, et al. (1995) Effect of probenecid on the distribution and elimination of ciprofloxacin in humans. Clin Pharmacol Ther 58: 532–541.
26. Hill G, Cihlar T, Oo C, Ho ES, Prior K, et al. (2002) The anti-influenza drug oseltamivir exhibits low potential to induce pharmacokinetic drug interactions via renal secretion-correlation of in vivo and in vitro studies. Drug Metab Dispos 30: 13–19.
27. Meyer JM, Ejendal KF, Avramova LV, Garland-Kuntz EE, Giraldo-Calderon GI, et al. (2012) A "genome-to-lead" approach for insecticide discovery: pharmacological characterization and screening of *Aedes aegypti* D_1-like dopamine receptors. PLoS Negl Trop Dis 6: e1478.
28. Li X, Schuler MA, Berenbaum MR (2007) Molecular mechanisms of metabolic resistance to synthetic and natural xenobiotics. Annu Rev Entomol 52: 231–253.
29. Dermauw W, Van Leeuwen T (2014) The ABC gene family in arthropods: Comparative genomics and role in insecticide transport and resistance. Insect Biochem Mol Biol 45C: 89–110.
30. Baker DA, Nolan T, Fischer B, Pinder A, Crisanti A, et al. (2011) A comprehensive gene expression atlas of sex- and tissue-specificity in the malaria vector, *Anopheles gambiae*. BMC Genomics 12: 296.
31. Rouhier MF, Piermarini PM (2014) Identification of life-stage and tissue-specific splice variants of an inward rectifying potassium (Kir) channel in the yellow fever mosquito *Aedes aegypti*. Insect Biochem Mol Biol 48C: 91–99.
32. O'Donnell MJ (2009) Too much of a good thing: how insects cope with excess ions or toxins in the diet. J Exp Biol 212: 363–372.
33. O'Donnell MJ (2008) Insect Excretory Mechanisms. In: Simpson SJ, editor.Advances in Insect Physiology.London: Academic Press. pp.1–122.
34. Tice CM (2001) Selecting the right compounds for screening- does Lipinski's Rule of 5 for pharmaceuticals apply to agrochemicals? Pest Manag Sci 57: 3–16.
35. Akamatsu M (2011) Importance of physicochemical properties for the design of new pesticides. J Agric Food Chem 59: 2909–2917.

Acknowledgments

The authors thank Nuris Acosta (The Ohio State University), and the Vanderbilt High-Throughput Screening Center for technical assistance.

Author Contributions

Conceived and designed the experiments: RR MFR DRS ED CDW KML LCK DWE SFB CH PMP JSD. Performed the experiments: RR MFR DRS ED KML LCK DWE SFB PMP. Analyzed the data: RR MFR DRS ED CDW KML LCK DWE SFB CH PMP JSD. Contributed reagents/materials/analysis tools: CDW KML LCK DWE SFB. Wrote the paper: RR MFR DRS CDW CH PMP JSD.

6

Genome-Wide Association Analysis of Tolerance to Methylmercury Toxicity in *Drosophila* Implicates Myogenic and Neuromuscular Developmental Pathways

Sara L. Montgomery[1], Daria Vorojeikina[1], Wen Huang[2], Trudy F. C. Mackay[2], Robert R. H. Anholt[2], Matthew D. Rand[1]*

1 Department of Environmental Medicine, University of Rochester School of Medicine and Dentistry, Rochester, New York, United States of America, 2 Department of Biological Sciences, Genetics Program, and W. M. Keck Center for Behavioral Biology, North Carolina State University, Raleigh, North Carolina, United States of America

Abstract

Methylmercury (MeHg) is a persistent environmental toxin present in seafood that can compromise the developing nervous system in humans. The effects of MeHg toxicity varies among individuals, despite similar levels of exposure, indicating that genetic differences contribute to MeHg susceptibility. To examine how genetic variation impacts MeHg tolerance, we assessed developmental tolerance to MeHg using the sequenced, inbred lines of the *Drosophila melanogaster* Genetic Reference Panel (DGRP). We found significant genetic variation in the effects of MeHg on development, measured by eclosion rate, giving a broad sense heritability of 0.86. To investigate the influence of dietary factors, we measured MeHg toxicity with caffeine supplementation in the DGRP lines. We found that caffeine counteracts the deleterious effects of MeHg in the majority of lines, and there is significant genetic variance in the magnitude of this effect, with a broad sense heritability of 0.80. We performed genome-wide association (GWA) analysis for both traits, and identified candidate genes that fall into several gene ontology categories, with enrichment for genes involved in muscle and neuromuscular development. Overexpression of glutamate-cysteine ligase, a MeHg protective enzyme, in a muscle-specific manner leads to a robust rescue of eclosion of flies reared on MeHg food. Conversely, mutations in *kirre*, a pivotal myogenic gene identified in our GWA analyses, modulate tolerance to MeHg during development in accordance with *kirre* expression levels. Finally, we observe disruptions of indirect flight muscle morphogenesis in MeHg-exposed pupae. Since the pathways for muscle development are evolutionarily conserved, it is likely that the effects of MeHg observed in *Drosophila* can be generalized across phyla, implicating muscle as an additional hitherto unrecognized target for MeHg toxicity. Furthermore, our observations that caffeine can ameliorate the toxic effects of MeHg show that nutritional factors and dietary manipulations may offer protection against the deleterious effects of MeHg exposure.

Editor: Dennis C. Ko, Duke University, United States of America

Funding: Funding by P30 ES001247, T32 ES07026 (http://www.niehs.nih.gov/) National Institute of Environmental Sciences (MDR, SLM), GM045146, R21 ES021719, (http://www.nigms.nih.gov/) National Institute of General Medical Sciences (RRHA, TFCM), and NCSU Initiative for Biological Complexity, North Carolina State University (WH). The funders had no role in study design, data collection and analysis, decision to publish, or preparation of the manuscript.

Competing Interests: The authors have declared that no competing interests exist.

* Email: matthew_rand@urmc.rochester.edu

Introduction

Methylmercury (MeHg) is a potent environmental neurotoxin that presents a risk to human health. MeHg exposures occur predominantly through dietary intake of fish species that harbor elevated levels of the organometal. Historic accidental MeHg poisonings in Minamata, Japan (1950's) and Iraq (1970's) demonstrated that the neurotoxic effects of MeHg result primarily from fetal exposures [1,2]. In congenital Minamata disease, MeHg-exposed pregnant women with little to no neurological signs give birth to children with a range of severe clinical manifestations akin to cerebral palsy, including mental retardation, ataxia and motor deficits, growth retardation, speech and auditory deficits [3]. Clinical cases of Minamata disease, and limited samples of human fetal brain histopathology associated with them, have consolidated the notion that the developing nervous system is a target tissue for MeHg toxicity [4–6].

Large-scale epidemiologic studies that have investigated outcomes of prenatal MeHg exposure through seafood diets have yielded incongruent results with respect to neurological deficits [7,8]. Subsequent studies have explored genetic predisposition and nutritional modifiers as factors that confer tolerance or susceptibility to MeHg among populations and in individuals [9–11]. In addition to neurotoxicity, recent population studies have identified MeHg effects on cardiovascular factors (e.g., heart rate variability and blood pressure) [12,13] and the immune system [14,15]. While less well studied, there is evidence that overall fetal and infant growth rates are inversely related to prenatal MeHg exposure [16,17]. Given the prevailing focus on neural-specific mechanisms, the extent to which other developing organ systems are affected by MeHg during development has not been fully explored.

MeHg distributes rapidly and ubiquitously in living tissues and demonstrates an exceptionally high affinity for biological thiols, including glutathione (GSH) and protein thiols [18,19]. As a result, the potential molecular and cellular pathways perturbed by MeHg during development are numerous. Thus, natural variation in phenotypic outcomes of MeHg exposure (e.g. tolerance or susceptibility) is the consequence of MeHg interaction with multiple gene products. However, few studies investigating MeHg mechanisms have focused on genetic variation as the underlying framework for variation in MeHg susceptibility. Conducting genome-wide association (GWA) analyses for MeHg susceptibility is challenging in human populations as both the extent of early developmental exposure and its postnatal manifestations are difficult to quantify, and environmental exposure in human populations cannot be controlled precisely. Thus, genome-wide studies on the genetic underpinnings of variation in MeHg exposure are best performed in a model system, where exposure conditions, environmental growth conditions and genetic back-ground can be controlled and effects of MeHg exposure precisely quantified. Fundamental insights based on evolutionarily con-served biological processes can then be extrapolated to human populations.

Drosophila melanogaster presents an excellent genetic model system for quantitative genetic analyses of complex traits, and has resulted in the identification of genetic networks that underlie several stress responses, such as starvation resistance, chill coma recovery, startle behavior, oxidative stress sensitivity, and exposure to alcohol [20–23]. The recent establishment of the *Drosophila melanogaster* Genetic Reference Panel (DGRP), consisting of 205 wild-derived inbred fly strains with fully sequenced genomes, enables GWA studies in a population where all genetic variants are known [24,25]. Linkage disequilibrium decays rapidly within *Drosophila* [24] and the limited population structure in the DGRP can be corrected for by taking into account segregating inversions and genomic relatedness [25]. In addition, the Drosophila model allows for rapid assessment of candidate genes through functional analyses of mutants.

Here, we have used the DGRP lines to perform a GWA analysis for variation in tolerance/susceptibility to MeHg toxicity during development. We measured the development of flies exposed to MeHg during larval and pupal stages by scoring eclosion (adult hatching) as a phenotypic endpoint. In addition, we examined development on MeHg food supplemented with caffeine, a previously identified dietary modifier of MeHg toxicity in fly development [26]. We find significant genetic variation in tolerance to MeHg as well as in modulation of MeHg toxicity by caffeine. Gene network and gene ontology analyses reveal, among others, an enrichment of genes related to development of muscle and the neuromuscular junction. We present a character-ization of pupal MeHg phenotypes and functional analyses in mutant and transgenic flies that confirm a role for muscle development as a target for MeHg toxicity.

Materials and Methods

Drosophila Stocks

The following lines were obtained from the Bloomington *Drosophila* Stock Center (Indiana University): $Mi\{MIC\}kirre^{MI07148}$, (#41549), $Mi\{MIC\}kirre^{MI00678}$ (#41463) and $P\{EP\}$-$kirre^{G1566}$ (#32593), Mef2-RFP (#26882), y^1w^{67c23} (#6599), w^{1118}(#5905), Mef2-Gal4 (#27390), and the entire *Drosophila melanogaster* Genetic Reference Panel (DGRP). The DGRP is a set of fully sequenced inbred lines generated by 20 generations of full-sib mating of progeny of wild-caught females from the Raleigh, NC population [24]. UAS-GCLc5 and UAS-GCLc 6 were kindly provided by Dr. William C. Orr, Southern Methodist University, Dallas TX [60]. All stocks were maintained at 25°C with 60% humidity and reared on cornmeal-molasses-agar culture medium.

MeHg tolerance assays

Eclosion on MeHg food was assayed as previously described [27,61]. Briefly, 30–50 first instar larvae (mixed sexes) were seeded on MeHg-containing media (0–15 µM). Assays for each treatment condition were performed on n = 150–300 larvae in three vials with 50 larvae each. On day 13 after larvae seeding, the number of eclosed adult flies were counted and expressed as percent of larvae applied to the food. To assess overall developmental tolerance on MeHg media, an eclosion index was calculated by normalizing the mean eclosion rate for each MeHg concentration to the eclosion on 0 µM MeHg for each strain. An overall eclosion index was then generated by summing the normalized percent eclosion values obtained on the 5, 10, and 15 µM MeHg treatments for each strain. For example, if a strain exhibits 95% eclosion on 5 µM MeHg, 50% eclosion on 10 µM MeHg and 5% eclosion on 15 µM MeHg, the eclosion index would be 95+50+5 = 150. Some DGRP strains demonstrated less than 60% eclosion on 0 µM MeHg (9 lines total), exhibiting poor baseline eclosion behavior. These lines were omitted from the analyses, for a total of 167 DGRP lines.

Parallel assays assessing the modulating effects of caffeine on eclosion rates were also determined on 0 µM and 10 µM MeHg with and without 2 mM caffeine (LKT Laboratories; St. Paul MN). This concentration of caffeine was previously characterized as a sub-toxic and tolerance-promoting dose in two wild-type *Drosophila* strains [26]. Eclosion values were normalized to the 0 µM MeHg condition for each strain. A caffeine difference index was determined for each line by subtracting the normalized eclosion rate on 10 µM MeHg alone from that on 10 µM MeHg+ 2 mM caffeine. Lines exhibiting 0% eclosion on 10 µM MeHg and 10 µM+2 mM caffeine were omitted from GWA analysis, leaving 139 lines for GWA analysis.

Quantitative genetic analyses

We performed a mixed effects model analysis of variance (ANOVA) using the model $Y = \mu + D + L + D \times L + \varepsilon$ to partition phenotypic variation, where Y is the response variable, μ is the overall mean, D is the fixed effect for dose, and L and $D \times L$ are the random effects for line and dose by line interaction. Significance of the effects was tested using type III F tests implemented in SAS Proc Mixed (SAS Institute). Broad sense heritability was calculated as $H^2 = \frac{\sigma_L^2 + \sigma_{DXL}^2}{\sigma_L^2 + \sigma_{DXL}^2 + \sigma_\varepsilon^2}$. For the effect of caffeine, because there was only a single dose of MeHg, a simpler model was fitted as $Y = \mu + L + \varepsilon$, and $H^2 = \frac{\sigma_L^2}{\sigma_L^2 + \sigma_\varepsilon^2}$.

Genome-wide association analysis

We performed genome-wide association analysis on line means of the phenotype using the DGRP analysis portal (http://dgrp2. gnets.ncsu.edu; [24,25]). Briefly, the hatching index or caffeine index was used to fit a mixed model for each variant in the form of $Y = \mu + M + g + \varepsilon$, where Y is the line means adjusted for *Wolbachia* infection and five major inversion polymorphisms (*In(2L)t, In(2R)NS, In(3R)Y, In(3R)P, In(3R)Mo*) in the DGRP, μ is

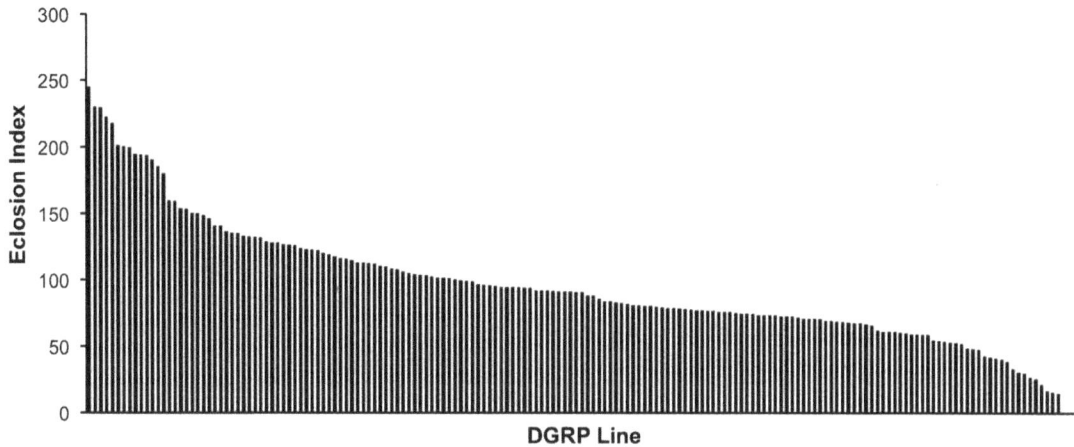

Figure 1. Genetic variation in MeHg tolerance during development. 176 DGRP lines were assayed in triplicate for eclosion on media containing 0, 5, 10 and 15 μM MeHg. A cumulative index (Eclosion Index) was generated by summing the percent eclosion on 5, 10 and 15 μM MeHg food for each strain (see methods). The histogram represents a rank ordering of the eclosion index for each of the DGRP lines.

the overall population mean, M is the effect of DNA variant being tested, and g is a polygenic component with covariance between lines determined by their genomic relationship [25]. For Wolbachia infection adjustment we fit a linear model with the infection status and major inversion genotypes as covariates and the raw phenotypes as the response variable. Residuals from this linear model were used as inputs for GWAS. We performed 2,180,555 tests for association for the MeHg treatment alone, restricting the analyses to variants for which at least 6 lines contain the minor allele (for a minor allele frequency, MAF, >3.6%). We performed 2,357,353 tests for association for the MeHg+caffeine treatment, restricting the analysis to variants for which at least 4 lines contained the minor allele (MAF>2.9%).

GeneMANIA network analysis

Polymorphism-based single marker analysis for MeHg and MeHg+caffeine was used to identify top candidate genes found to be associated with developmental tolerance to MeHg. Candidate genes were uploaded to the GeneMANIA prediction server (www.genemania.org), a web interface to identify networks of gene functions associated with a query list of genes [39]. Functional networks were derived using automatic query-dependent gene weighting and biological function-based gene ontology (GO) weighting to identify interactions based on co-expression, co-localization, genetic, and physical interactions of query and non-query genes related to biological integration networks. Outputs from GeneMANIA were constructed in tabular form and in graphical form using a Cytoscape plugin v3.1.0 (Cytoscape). Functional enrichment is based on the GO categories and is reported as Q-values of a false discovery rate (FDR) using a corrected hypergeometric test for enrichment. Coverage ratios for

the number of annotated genes in the displayed network versus the number of genes with that annotation in the genome are also reported. Q-values are derived using the Benjamini-Hochberg procedure. Categories are displayed up to a Q-value cutoff of 0.1.

Muscle phenotype characterization

Mef2>RFP L1 larvae were seeded onto 0, 10, and 15 μM MeHg media and monitored until pupae formation at 25°C. Stage 6–12 pupae were selected based on established developmental landmarks such as the appearance of green in Malpighian tubules, body color, eye color, bristles development and wing color [62]. Pupae were dissected from their case and positioned on a Superfrost microscope slide (VWR International; Radnor, PA) for fluorescent reporter imaging of the indirect flight muscles (IFMs) within the thorax. Phosphate-buffered saline (PBS) was added drop-wise to each dissected pupae to avoid desiccation. Fluorescent microscopy was performed with a Leitz Orthoplan 2 microscope (Leica Microsystems; Buffalo Grove, IL) equipped with a SPOT Insight QE 4.2 Camera (SPOT Imaging Solutions; Sterling Heights, MI) and imaging software using a 4× objective. Images were assembled in Microsoft PowerPoint.

Functional validation of candidate genes

Functional validation of candidate genes related to muscle development was performed with eclosion assays using *kir-re*[MI07148], *kirre*[MI00678] and *kirre*[G1566] mutants (Bloomington *Drosophila* Stock Center, Indiana University). Eclosion on MeHg food (0–15 μM) was assayed for the *kirre* mutants and the corresponding y^1w^{67c23} control strain. Experiments overexpressing *UAS-GCLc5* and *UAS-GCLc6* were conducted by using the

Table 1. ANOVA table for MeHg tolerance.

Source of Variation	Df	MS (Type III)	F	P value	σ^2 (SE)
Line	172	0.0909	12.42	<0.0001	0.0299 (0.0035)
Error	346	0.0073			0.0073 (0.0006)

Phenotype = hatching rate for each replicate at 5, 10, 15 μM MeHg normalized to the line means of hatching rate at 0 μM MeHg. Residuals are weighted by the square of number of flies assayed.

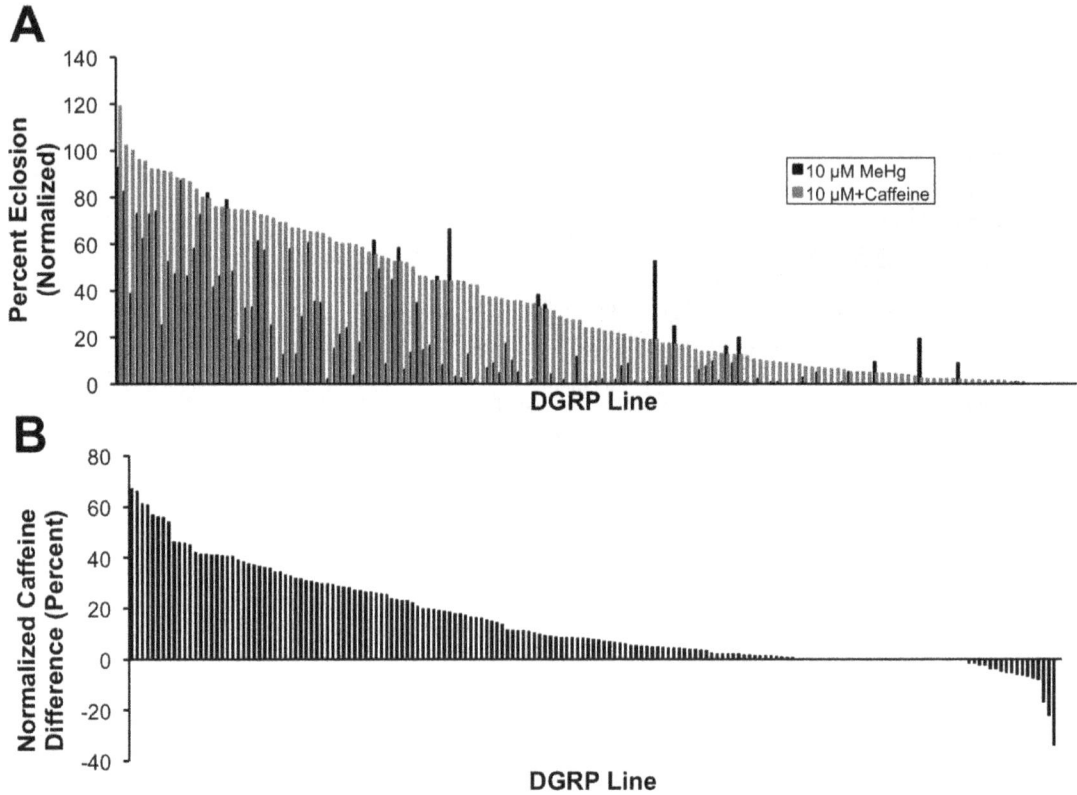

Figure 2. Caffeine effect on MeHg tolerance exhibits genetic variation. (A) Eclosion rates of DGRP lines were determined on 0 μM and 10 μM MeHg food with and without addition of 2 mM caffeine. The histogram is a rank ordered expression of eclosion rates on the MeHg+caffeine condition (gray bars) paired with the respective line on MeHg alone (black bars). (B) A caffeine difference index was determined for each DGRP line by subtracting the normalized eclosion rate on 10 μM MeHg from that on 10 μM MeHg+2 mM caffeine. Positive values indicate a beneficial effect of caffeine and negative values indicate a detrimental effect of caffeine relative to 10 μM MeHg alone. Lines showing 0% eclosion on both MeHg alone and MeHg+caffeine were omitted from the analyses leaving 139 lines for GWA analyses.

muscle-specific *Mef2-Gal4* driver. Female *Mef2-GAL4* flies were bred with male *UAS-GCLc5*, *UAS-GCLc6* or *w*[1118] control flies, and progeny assayed for eclosion on MeHg media (0–25 μM). Rates of eclosion for indicated strains at each MeHg concentration are expressed in proportions (% eclosion). Assays were performed to achieve n = 150 larvae. Statistical consideration of differences between experimental and control fly strains are therefore comparisons of proportion values and not of continuous values. Since error determinations in proportion values become restricted at the edges (*i.e.* near 100%), an analysis of variance (ANOVA) was not used. Statistical analyses of eclosion assays were therefore done using a pairwise 2-tailed z-test, treating each MeHg concentration categorically. *p*-values of less than 0.01 were considered significant.

Gene expression

GCLc and *kirre* gene expression was measured by quantitative real-time PCR (qRT-PCR) of RNA extracts isolated from first instar larvae or staged pupae. For the indicated genotypes, RNA was extracted by pooling 15–20 larvae or 20–25 pupae. The tissue was homogenized and RNA extracted with Trizol (Invitrogen; Grand Island, NY). qRT-PCR quantification was performed on a Bio-Rad CFZ Connect Real-Time PCR Detection System using CFX Manager software. cDNA synthesis and reverse transcription was performed in a Bio-Rad iScript SYBR Green one-step

Table 2. ANOVA table for caffeine effect.

Source of Variation	Df	MS (Type III)	F	P value	σ² (SE)
Dose	2	66.4455	10788	<0.0001	Fixed
Line	172	0.1983	32.21	<0.0001	0.0155 (0.0027)
Dose × Line	344	0.0711	11.55	<0.0001	0.0231 (0.0019)
Error	3	0.0062			0.0062 (0.0003)

Phenotype = (hatching rate for each replicate at 10 μM MeHg + Caffeine normalized to the line means of hatching rate at 0 μM MeHg) – (line means of hatching rate at 10 μM MeHg normalized to the line means of hatching rate at 0 μM MeHg). Residuals are weighted by the square of number of flies assayed.

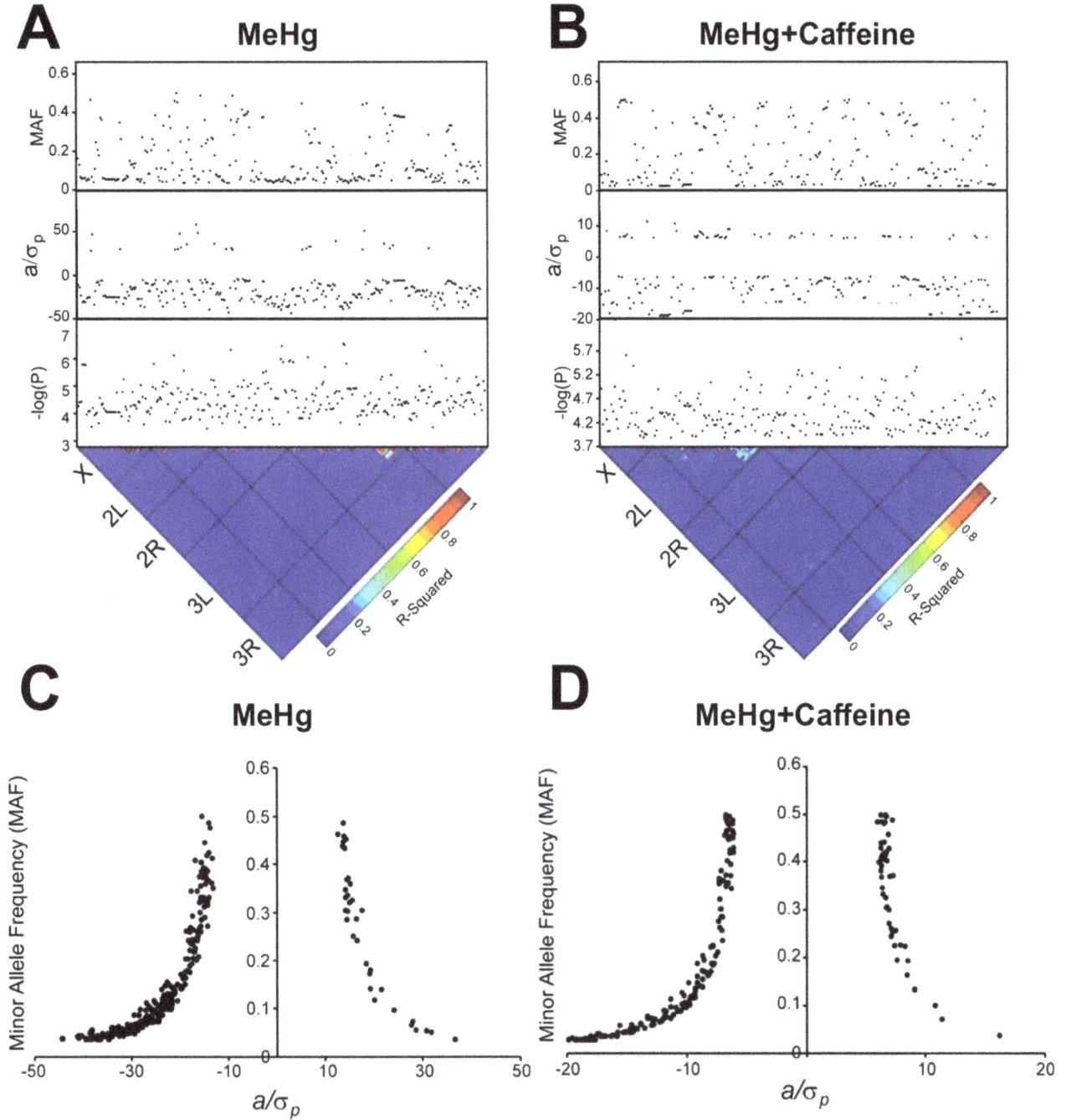

Figure 3. Genome-wide association analysis of eclosion on MeHg with and without caffeine supplementation. Single marker analyses using ANOVA of 2,180,555 (MeHg alone) and 2,357,353 (MeHg+caffeine) polymorphic alleles across 167 (MeHg alone) and 139 (MeHg+caffeine) DGRP lines, respectively, resolved (A) 350 and (B) 239 polymorphic markers ($p<10^{-4}$, MAF>3%). Depicted is a heat map for linkage disequilibrium (LD) based on r^2 values where the black bars represent the five major *Drosophila* chromosome arms. Red indicates high LD, while blue indicates low LD. The black dots represent polymorphic marker associations for eclosion on MeHg or MeHg+caffeine. p values ($\log_{10}(p)$), effect size (a/σ_P), and the minor allele frequency (MAF) are shown. (C,D) MAF *vs.* effect size. All 350 (C) or 239 (D) polymorphic markers associated with phenotypic variation for eclosion on MeHg or MeHg+caffeine, respectively, are depicted. a/σ_P indicates effect size ([mean of major allele class – mean of minor allele class]/2), where negative a/σ_P indicates the minor allele is associated with increased MeHg tolerance with respect to eclosion.

reaction (Bio-Rad; Hercules, CA). Twenty-five μL reactions containing 40 ng RNA template, iScript SYBR Green reaction mix (2x), iScript reverse transcriptase for one-step RT-PCR, and forward and reverse primers (10 μM final concentration) were used. The *Drosophila Rp49* gene was used for normalization of expression. Gene expression levels were determined by the comparative C_T method [63]. The following primers were used; *Rp49*: 5′-AGTATCTGATGCCCAACATCG-3′ and 5′-TTCC-GACCAGGTTACAAGAAC-3′, *GCLc*: 5′-ATGACGAGGAG-AATGAGCTG-3′, and 5′-CCATGGACTGCAAAATAGCTG-

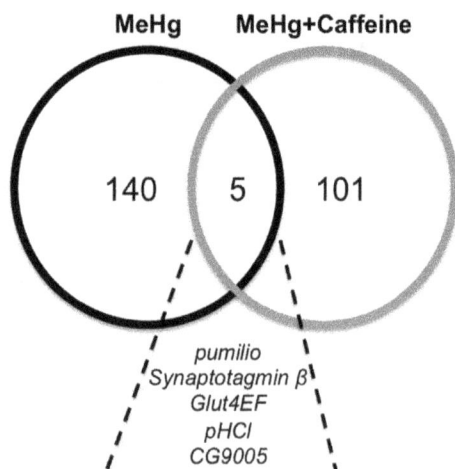

Figure 4. Overlap of genes identified by common polymorphic markers for variance in MeHg and MeHg+caffeine treatments. Candidate genes were identified from one or more associated polymorphisms in GWA analyses. A total of 145 and 106 genes were identified for MeHg and MeHg+caffeine, respectively. In common between the two treatments are 5 genes: *pumilio*, *Synaptotagmin* β, *Glut4EF*, *pHCl*, and *CG9005*.

3′, *kirre*: 5′-TGGACTGGCCATTAATCTTACC-3′ and 5′-AA-CGATCGCCACCGAAAT-3′.

Results

Quantitative genetic analysis of natural variation in tolerance to MeHg during development

To characterize natural genetic variation in tolerance and susceptibility to MeHg during development, we examined 176 DGRP lines in an eclosion assay on four concentrations ([MeHg] = 0, 5, 10, 15 µM, Table S3) of MeHg-containing food. We found substantial phenotypic variation in susceptibility to MeHg as measured by an eclosion index (see Materials and Methods for definition) across the DGRP lines, ranging from 0 to 244.6 (Fig.1). ANOVA for variation in MeHg tolerance across the four concentrations of MeHg showed significant variation for Line and the Dose × Line interaction term (Table 1). The broad sense heritability (H^2) was 0.86, indicating a strong genetic component to variation in MeHg tolerance, which provides a basis for GWA analysis (Table 1). To explore dietary modulation of MeHg toxicity, we examined the effects of caffeine co-administration (Fig. 2A, B, Table S3), which has previously been shown to attenuate MeHg developmental toxicity in a limited set of fly lines [26,27]. Addition of 2 mM caffeine to 10 µM MeHg supplemented food resulted in increased MeHg tolerance in the majority of the lines (Figure 2A, B), with only 12 lines exhibiting decreased MeHg tolerance with caffeine supplementation (Fig 2B). The variation in the modulating effect of caffeine can be seen clearly by subtraction of the eclosion rate on MeHg alone from that on MeHg+caffeine (Figure 2B). The modulating effect of caffeine on MeHg exposure varies significantly across the lines with $H^2 = 0.80$ (Table 2).

Polymorphic markers associated with MeHg tolerance

We performed single marker GWA analyses to identify polymorphic markers (single nucleotide polymorphisms (SNPs), insertions and deletions) associated with MeHg tolerance and the

modulatory effect of caffeine on MeHg toxicity. Line means for both traits were approximately normally distributed (Fig. S1); therefore, we did not transform the data. Quantile-quantile plots show a clear enrichment of variants with p-values $<10^{-4}$ for MeHg tolerance, but no evidence for enrichment for the modulatory effect of caffeine (Fig. S2). In the MeHg tolerance GWA, one SNP (in *pHCl*) nearly met a Bonferroni-adjusted significance level, and 14 SNPs (in *pHCl*, *eco*, *CG44245 CG33981* and *CG15221*) had false discovery rates (FDR) of FDR <0.2 (Table S1).

In *Drosophila*, we can use GWA analysis as an exploratory hypothesis-generating tool, and test hypotheses more rigorously in secondary screens using mutations or targeting RNAI for candidate genes implicated by the GWA analysis. Therefore, we used a lenient reporting threshold of $p<10^{-4}$ for both GWA analyses (Tables S1, S2). We identified 350 polymorphisms in or near 145 genes associated with variation in eclosion rates on MeHg food (Fig. 3A) and 239 polymorphisms in or near 106 genes (Fig. 3B) associated with the modulatory effect of caffeine on MeHg treatment. Most polymorphisms associated with the two analyses had MAF <0.15, and, as expected, we found inverse relationships of effect size and allele frequency (Figs. 3C, 3D). Rarer alleles were associated with greater tolerance to MeHg and modulation of the effect by caffeine with respect to larva-adult viability for a majority of the polymorphisms (Figs. 3C, 3D), suggesting these alleles have other deleterious effects on fitness. There was little linkage disequilibrium between the most significant polymorphisms (Figs. 3A, 3B).

Candidate genes associated with MeHg tolerance

We found five genes in common between the two GWA analyses for exposure to MeHg in the presence or absence of caffeine: *pumilio* (*pum*, *CG9755*), *Synaptotagmin* β (*Sytβ*, *CG42333*), *Glut4EF* (*CG34360*), *pHCl* (*CG44099*) and *CG9005* (Fig. 4). *pum* is an Armadillo repeat RNA binding protein involved in repression of translation and has two human homologs, PUM1 and PUM2. *pum* has functional implications in cellular and developmental processes including embryonic patterning, synaptic transmission, dendrite morphogenesis, pole cell migration, and learning and memory [28,29]. *Sytβ* is one of seven Synaptotagmin family members in *Drosophila* with predicted function in synaptic vesicle exocytosis [30]. *Sytβ* localizes to the developing CNS as well as to specific motor neuron termini [31]. *Glut4EF* is a zinc finger transcription factor and homolog of the human glucose transporter (GLUT4) enhancer factor [32]. In flies, *Glut4EF* influences wing positioning with mutants giving a stretched out wing phenotype [32]. Mammalian Glut4EF is important for glucose uptake in muscles and associates with the MEF2A transcription factor [33]. *pHCl* encodes a gamma-aminobutyric acid A receptor, a ligand gated chloride channel that is expressed in the embryonic nervous system [34]. *CG9005* encodes a protein of unknown function that has two human homologs, Hsap/KIAA1370 and Hsap/FAM214B. RNAi knockdown of *CG9005* in flies has effects on development of the notum [35]. Therefore, four of the five overlapping genes share functions in the domain of neuromuscular function and neural development, suggesting that these biological processes are likely associated with MeHg tolerance during development.

A particularly noteworthy gene identified by GWA with MeHg alone is the metal transcription factor (*MTF-1*) gene, which was represented with six SNPs (Table S1). *MTF-1* is a conserved transcriptional regulator and the primary responder to heavy metal toxicity insult [36]. While better known for conferring resistance to divalent metal ions and inorganic mercury [37], *MTF-1* regulates expression of metallothionein proteins and is

Table 3. GeneMANIA network analyses reveals both overlapping and unique biological functions among GWA genes from MeHg alone and MeHg+caffeine.

MeHg alone				MeHg + Caffeine			
Function	FDR	Network	Genome	Function	FDR	Network	Genome
muscle organ development	1.73E-11	24	247	*transmembrane receptor protein tyrosine kinase signaling*	3.40E-05	12	129
muscle structure development	1.73E-11	26	294	*enzyme linked receptor protein tyrosine kinase signaling pathway*	1.26E-04	13	187
muscle cell differentiation	3.38E-10	20	184	**muscle organ development**	3.04E-04	14	247
striated muscle cell differentiation	7.56E-09	18	170	**muscle structure development**	3.04E-04	15	294
muscle tissue development	7.58E-08	16	151	regulation of cell differentiation	9.79E-04	14	283
striated muscle tissue development	7.58E-08	16	150	tissue morphogenesis	1.05E-03	14	289
skeletal muscle organ development	7.58E-08	17	173	protein phosphorylation	1.53E-03	13	258
visceral muscle development	1.83E-07	7	14	epithelium development	3.80E-03	13	286
skeletal muscle tissue development	2.34E-07	15	141	adult behavior	3.80E-03	9	126
urogenital system development	1.00E-06	11	71	genital disc development	4.04E-03	6	44
renal system development	1.00E-06	11	71	response to organic substance	4.98E-03	12	261
cell migration	1.25E-06	17	217	embryonic morphogenesis	4.98E-03	11	213
cell motility	2.31E-06	17	227	regulation of nervous system development	4.98E-03	10	176
localization of cell	3.63E-06	17	235	**skeletal muscle organ development**	4.98E-03	10	173
regulation of muscle tissue development	4.45E-06	10	65	regulation of cell development	4.98E-03	11	217
regulation of striated muscle tissue development	4.45E-06	10	65	**neuromuscular junction development**	5.23E-03	8	106
regulation of muscle organ development	8.81E-06	10	70	**skeletal muscle fiber development**	5.64E-03	8	108
tube development	2.30E-05	13	149	morphogenesis of an epithelium	5.64E-03	12	269
tissue migration	3.42E-05	8	44	**muscle cell differentiation**	5.76E-03	10	184
transmembrane receptor protein tyrosine kinase sig.	3.51E-05	12	129	**muscle tissue development**	6.63E-03	9	151
enzyme linked receptor protein signaling pathway	4.00E-05	14	187	**striated muscle tissue development**	6.63E-03	9	150
cell-cell adhesion	7.98E-05	10	90	synapse organization	6.63E-03	9	149
striated muscle cell development	9.81E-05	12	144	hindgut morphogenesis	6.63E-03	6	55
renal filtration cell differentiation	9.81E-05	5	12	**muscle fiber development**	6.80E-03	8	116

GeneMANIA derived biological network integration results from MeHg and MeHg+caffeine GWA genes. Overlapping networks with muscle related function (bold text)and receptor signaling/tyrosine kinase function (italicized bold text) are indicated. Also shown are False discovery rate (FDR) and coverage indicated by the number of the genes in the 'Network' with a given function relative to all the genes in the 'Genome' identified with that function.

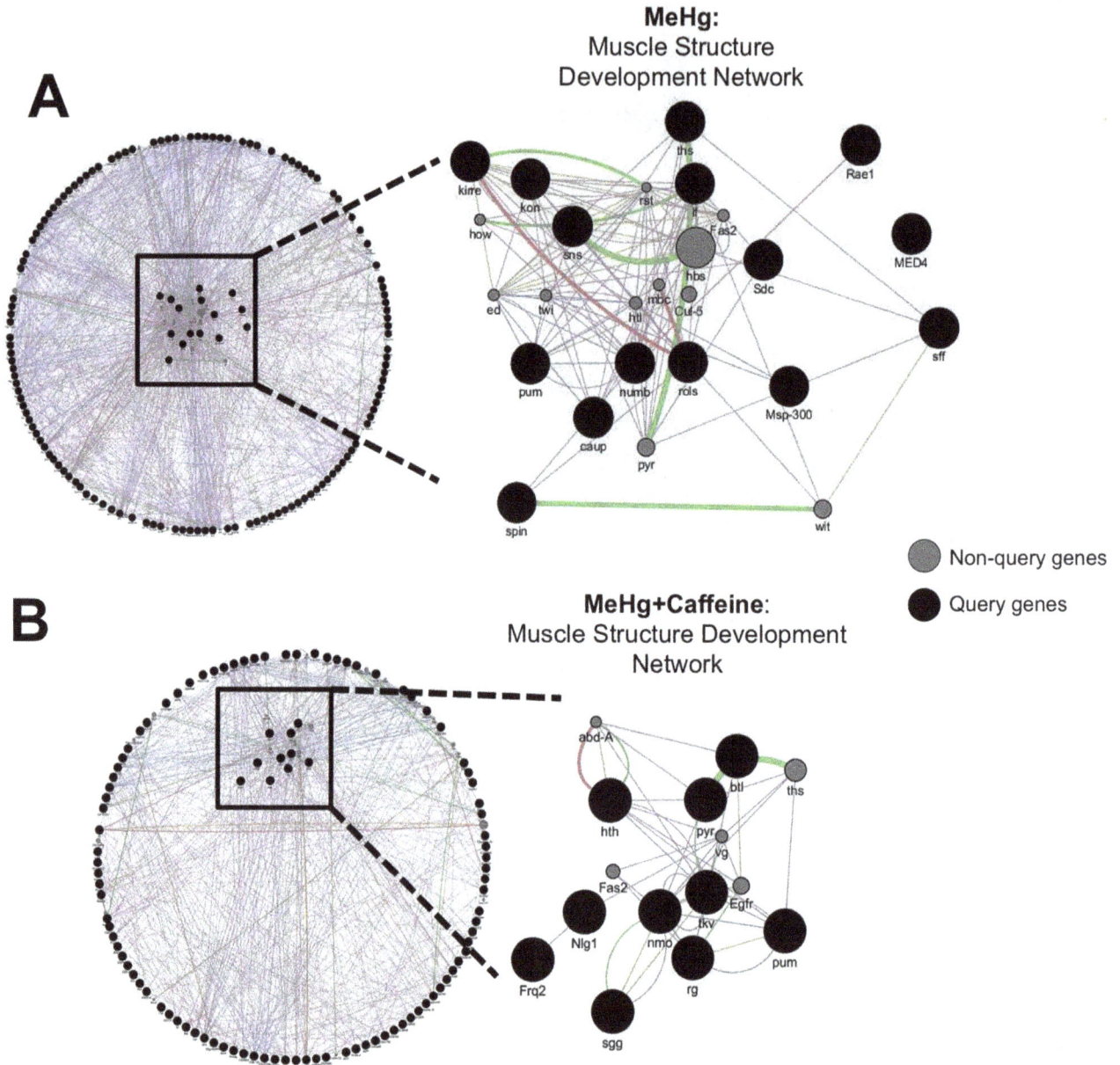

Figure 5. A shared functional network among non-overlapping genes identified in GWA of MeHg alone and MeHg+caffeine treatments. Network maps generated by GeneMANIA illustrate an example of a shared network for muscle structure development of genes identified in the GWA for MeHg alone (A) and MeHg+caffeine (B). Interactions are identified at the level of co-expression (purple lines), co-localization (blue lines), genetic interactions (green lines) and physical interactions (red lines). Query genes from the GWA analyses are represented by black circles and non-query genes (computationally recruited to complete network associations) are indicated by gray circles. The cluster of genes comprising the network is sorted to the inside of the circle, while the remaining query genes, not associated with the network, remain on the periphery.

effective in moderating oxidative stress [38]. MTF-1 responds robustly to inorganic mercury in *Drosophila*; however, its function in MeHg tolerance in flies remains to be investigated.

Functional gene networks related to MeHg tolerance

To assess to what extent genes associated with variation in MeHg tolerance can be assembled into genetic networks that represent biological pathways, we used the GeneMANIA [39] algorithm. The results from such analyses generate hypotheses regarding biological processes associated with phenotypic variation that can subsequently be tested by disrupting hub genes though

mutational analyses or targeted RNAi. Although only five candidate genes overlapped between the MeHg alone versus MeHg+caffeine treatments, we found substantial enrichment for genes associated with a number of muscle development functions for MeHg treatment both with and without caffeine and an additional overlap for the functional category of receptor protein kinase signaling (Table 3). One of the resulting GeneMANIA functional categories is assigned the "muscle structure development" network term and is shown schematically in Figure 5A and B for MeHg alone and MeHg+caffeine, respectively. Genes on the query list that are enriched for the "muscle structure develop-

Table 4. MeHg: Muscle structure development network query genes.

Gene Name	Fly Base ID	No. SNPs	Gene Function	Protein Function	CG #	Human Homolog
If	FBgn0001250	11	Axon guidance, muscle attachment, myofibril assembly	integrin alpha chain	CG9623	-
kirre	FBgn0028369	1	Myoblast fusion	immunoglobulin	CG3653	Kirrel/NEPH1
Sff	FBgn0036544	1	NMJ development	Protein serine/threonine kinase	CG6114	-
Rae1	FBgn0034646	1	Negative regulation of synaptic growth at NMJ	WD40 repeat	CG9862	RAE1
Rols	FBgn0041096	1	Myoblast fusion	zinc finger, ankyrin repeat	CG32096	-
Kon	FBgn0032683	1	Muscle attachment, muscle organ development, neurogenesis	laminin G domain, concanavalin A-like lectin	CG10275	CSPG4
pum	FBgn0003165	1	Regulation of synaptic growth at NMJ, synaptic transmission, dendrite morphogenesis, pole cell migration	RNA binding protein	CG9755	PUM1/PUM2
Msp-300	FBgn0261836	1	Skeletal muscle development, flight, locomotion	actin-binding, actinin-type, spectrin repeat	CG42768	
caup	FBgn0015919	1	Muscle cell fate commitment	Tale/IRO homebox family	CG10605	IRX3
spin	FBgn0086676	1	Regulation of synaptic growth at NMJ, locomotion, nervous system remodeling, glial migration	unknown	CG8428	SPNS1/2/3
ths	FBgn0033652	1	Myoblast migration, heart development	FGF receptor binding, growth factor	CG12443	-
sns	FBgn0024189	1	Myoblast fusion, nephrocyte diaphragm assembly	immunoglobulin	CG33141	NPHS1
Sdc	FBgn0010415	1	Regulation of synaptic growth at NMJ, motor neuron axon guidance	heparin sulfate proteoglycan, cytoskeletal binding	CG10497	-
numb	FBgn0002973	3	Muscle cell fate specification, neurogenesis	Notch binding	CG3779	NUMB/NUMBL
MED4	FBgn0035754	1	Muscle organ development	RNA Pol II cofactor activity	CG8609	MED4

Genes identified in the GWA for MeHg that constitute the "Muscle Structure Development" network are listed. The human homologs listed were identified in Flybase.

ment" category under analysis are listed in Tables 4 and 5. Five core genes in the network derived from the GWA analysis of the effects of MeHg alone act in muscle cell fusion and muscle attachment and development: *inflated* (*if*, *CG9623*), *kin of irre* (*kirre*, a.k.a. *dumbfounded* (*duf*) *CG3653*), *sticks and stones* (*sns*, *CG331441*), *kon-tiki* (*kon*, *CG10275*) and *rolling pebbles* (*rols*, *CG32096*) (Fig. 5A and Table 4). Also of note are five genes that play a role in neuromuscular junction development and integrity; *sugar free frosting* (*sff*, *CG6114*), *rae1* (*CG9862*), *pum* (*CG9755*), *spinster* (*spin*, *CG8428*) and *Syndecan* (*Sdc*, *CG10497*) (Fig. 5A and Table 4). Nine of these 15 genes have human homologs (Table 4). Among the 10 genes in the "muscle structure development" network with MeHg+caffeine treatments eight have human homologs (Table 5). It is of interest that eight of these 10 genes are transcriptionally responsive to caffeine (Table 5).

In summary, although the genes identified largely differ between the GWA analysis of effects of MeHg alone and MeHg+caffeine, the top GWA genes in both cases were functionally enriched for playing roles in muscle and neuromuscular junction development. This suggests that genes affecting muscle development contribute to the mechanisms of tolerance to MeHg toxicity during development.

Functional assessment of sensitivity of muscle development to MeHg toxicity

To functionally assay developing muscle tissue as a sensitive MeHg target, we examined flies that carry a gene known to affect MeHg tolerance expressed under the muscle specific enhancer *myocyte enhancing factor 2* (*Mef2*) [40]. We induced expression of glutamate-cysteine ligase (GCL), the highly conserved, rate-limiting enzyme for the synthesis of glutathione (GSH). GSH is a small molecule thiol compound present in all cells and is a first line of defense to MeHg toxicity, forming a conjugate that enhances MeHg excretion [41]. Elevated expression of GCL gives resistance to MeHg toxicity [42]. Using the *Gal4>UAS* system, we over-expressed the catalytic subunit of GCL (GCLc) using two independent lines carrying the *UAS-GCLc* construct (*GCLc5*, *GCLc6*) with the *Mef2-Gal4* driver (Fig. 6B). GCLc expression in muscle shows a robust enhancement of tolerance to MeHg in the eclosion assay (Fig. 6A), consistent with the notion that protection of muscle development is critical to overall development of the fly and completion of eclosion under MeHg toxicity stress.

We further examined flies carrying mutations in *kirre*, one of the core myogenic candidate genes identified in our GWA study. The *kirre*^{G1566} mutation is a viable mutant of *kirre* carrying a *P*-element insert in exon 10 (Fig. 7A). The *kirre*^{MI07148} and *kirre*^{MI00678} mutations carry a *Minos* element insert in an intronic

Table 5. MeHg+caffeine: Muscle structure development network query genes.

Gene Name	Fly Base ID	No. SNPs	Gene Function	Protein Function	CG #	Human Homolog	Caff induced
Hth	FBgn0001235	3	Somatic muscle development, peripheral nervous system development, neuron differentiation	DNA binding protein	CG17117	MEIS1/2/3	low
Nmo	FBgn0011817	1	Positive regulation of synaptic growth at NMJ, eye and wing development	Protein kinase	CG7892	NLK	Y
pum	FBgn0003165	1	Regulation of synaptic growth at NMJ, synaptic transmission, dendrite morphogenesis, Pole cell migration	RNA binding protein	CG9755	PUM1/PUM2	Y
Tkv	FBgn0003716	1	Positive regulation of synaptic growth at NMJ, neuromuscular synaptic transmission, TGF-β signaling pathway	TGF beta receptor/Serine-threonine kinase	CG14026	BMPR1/ACVR1	Y
Pyr	FBgn0033649	1	Myoblast migration, cardioblast differentiation	FGF receptor binding, growth factor	CG13194	-	Y
Sgg	FBgn0003371	1	Negative regulation of synaptic growth at NMJ, circadian clock, epithelial cell morphogenesis	Serine threonine kinase	CG2621	GSK3A/B	Y
Nlg1	FBgn0051146	1	NMJ development, synaptic growth at NMJ	Carboxyesterase	CG31146	-	N
Frq2	FBgn0083228	1	NMJ development, synaptic transmission, regulation of neurotransmitter secretion	Ca++ binding guanylate cyclase activator	CG5744	KCNIP/NCALD	low
btl	FBgn0005592	1	Negative regulation of axon extension, tracheal outgrowth/open tracheal system	Tyrosine Kinase	CG32134	FGFR1/2/3/5, RET	N
rg	FBgn0266098	1	Neuromuscular junction development, mushroom body development, short-term memory, compound eye	Protein kinase binding	CG44835	LRBA, NBEA	low

Genes identified in the GWA for MeHg+caffeine that constitute the "Muscle Structure Development" network are listed. The human homologs listed were identified in Flybase. In addition, response to caffeine for each gene was adapted from the modENCODE treatment expression data in the Flybase record for each gene.

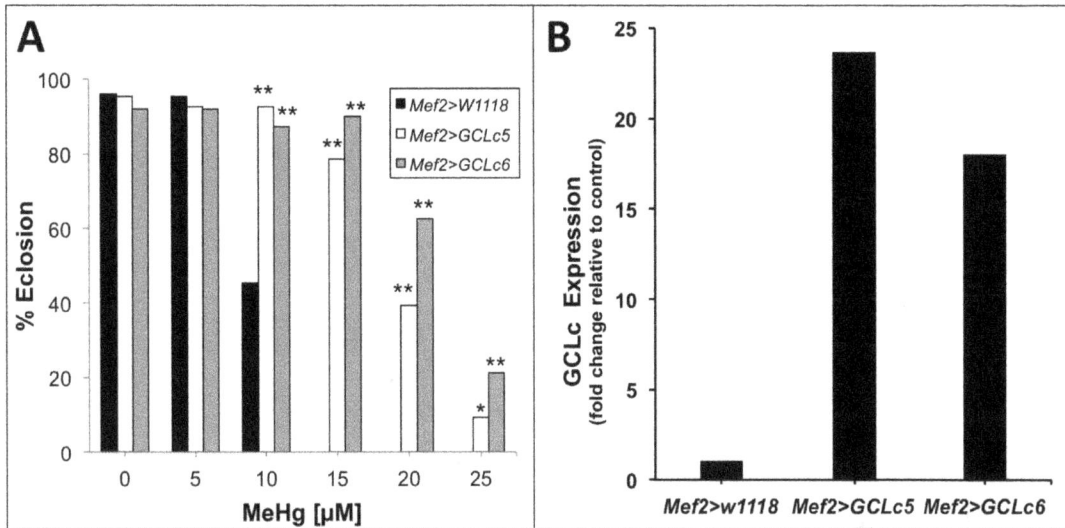

Figure 6. Muscle-specific expression of glutamate-cysteine ligase (GCL) rescues eclosion on MeHg. (A) Eclosion assays comparing flies expressing the catalytic subunit of GCL in two independent *UAS* responder lines (*GCLc5* and *GCLc6*) using the muscle-specific *Mef2-GAL4* driver (Mef2) with control flies (*Mef2>w^1118*). Statistical analyses by *z*- test, n = 150 flies/bar. * *p* <0.001 and **p<0.0001 relative to *Mef2>w^1118*. (B) Expression of *GCLc* mRNA in P12 pupae thoracic RNA extracts (pooled sample of n = 20 pupae) measured via qRT-PCR.

region of four of the seven transcripts (Fig. 7A). Analysis by qRT-PCR demonstrates that transcript levels are substantially reduced in the *kirre*^MI07148 mutant and essentially absent in the *kirre*^G1566 mutant (Fig. 7C), consistent with the predicted effect on transcripts encompassing the respective insertions. A moderate but significant reduction in MeHg tolerance is seen with both the *kirre*^MI07148 and *kirre*^G1566 mutants, specifically with exposure to 10 µM MeHg (Fig. 7B). Consistent with the corresponding expression levels, the *kirre*^G1566 mutant showed the lowest MeHg tolerance with the *kirre*^MI07148 mutant giving an intermediate tolerance relative to the *yw* control line at 10 µM exposures (Fig. 7B). Unexpectedly, the *kirre*^MI00678 mutant shows a significant increase in MeHg tolerance at the 5, 10 and 15 µM exposures (Fig. 7B), and concomitantly, *kirre mRNA* levels are seen to be elevated relative to the y^1w^{67c23} control line (Fig. 7C). These findings are consistent with the notion that modulation in the levels of *kirre* expression affects sensitivity of muscle development to MeHg.

Identification of an indirect flight muscle phenotype in MeHg-exposed pupae

With MeHg exposure, eclosion commonly fails in late pupal stages resulting in the accumulation of dark pupae, particularly at 10–15 µM MeHg. Based on our GWA results we examined various stages of MeHg-exposed pupae for potential muscle phenotypes using a line of flies that expresses red fluorescent protein (RFP) constitutively in muscles (*Mef2>RFP*). *Mef2>RFP* larvae were exposed to various concentrations of MeHg and collected at various pupal stage endpoints. Fluorescent imaging of these pupae reveals the prominent pattern of the indirect flight muscle groups, notably the dorsal longitudinal muscles (DLMs) at their attachment sites under the notum. We observe an overall disruption of DLM morphogenesis with MeHg treatments, despite an apparent normal development of ectodermal structures as well as the specialized organs of the bristles and eyes (Fig. 8A, B). Following MeHg exposure, early pupae (P6) show a reduction in size of the DLM fiber bundles and an apparent displacement of forming DVM muscles (Fig. 8A, C upper panels, open arrows). At later stages (P12), in addition to reduced fiber size, a "ball" of

RFP-positive tissue is seen indicative of a failure of DLM myofiber maturation, elongation and attachment to tendon cells on the notum epithelium (Fig. 8B, C lower panels).

Discussion

Natural variation in tolerance to MeHg toxicity

We sought to elaborate a fuller spectrum of the molecular networks and the tissue targets that influence MeHg toxicity outcomes through an unbiased query of polymorphisms across the entire genome of a diverse panel of developing animals. We find that variation in MeHg tolerance is under significant genetic control. Furthermore, we demonstrate that variation in response to a dietary modifier of MeHg toxicity, caffeine, is also genetically variable. This latter finding adds an additional level of complexity to interpreting outcomes of MeHg exposure, namely, that dietary factors may influence MeHg toxicity, but their efficacy, in itself, is subject to genetic pre-disposition. Nonetheless, for more than two thirds of the fly lines assayed, a beneficial effect of caffeine on MeHg toxicity was observed. Translating this finding to mammalian models and to humans has the potential to identify a means of moderating MeHg exposure effects through the diet.

GWA identifies an association of MeHg tolerance with genes and networks in muscle development

We used a lenient statistical threshold of $p<10^{-4}$ for identification of candidate genes associated with phenotypic variation. This threshold does not reach genome-wide significance based on Bonferroni multiple testing correction or permutation, but nonetheless serves as a hypothesis generating mechanism which identifies the top polymorphisms in a population where all polymorphisms are known. Candidate genes identified at this nominal threshold can be further verified through the use of mutants or by asking to what extent candidate genes are members of a network with a probability that is significantly higher than expected by chance.

The top candidate genes from our GWA analyses of MeHg tolerance were enriched for functions in muscle development.

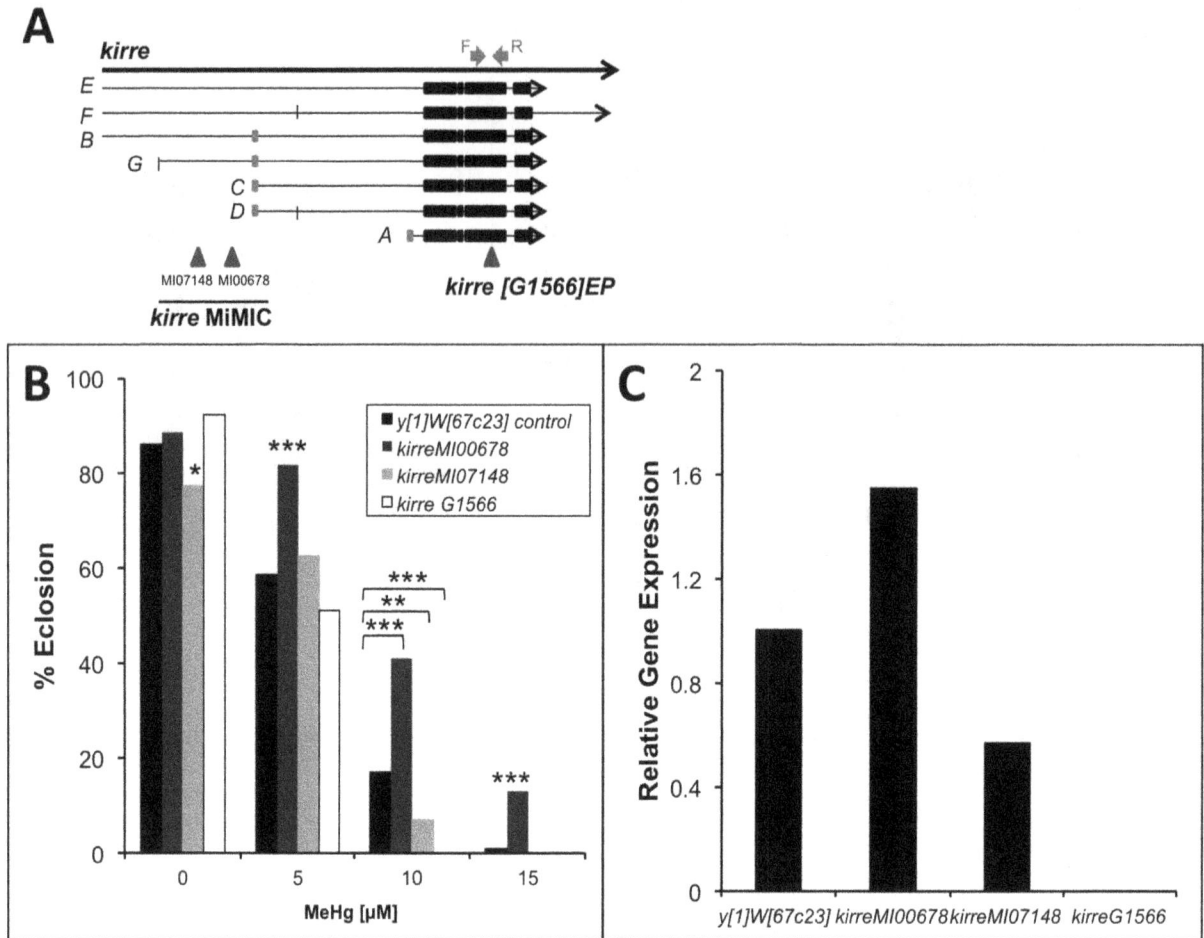

Figure 7. Altered MeHg tolerance in *kirre* mutant flies. (A) Schematic representation of mutant lines targeting *kirre*. *kirre*[M107148] is located at X: 2921499 targeting *kirre* transcripts E, F, B and G. *kirre*[MI00678] is located at X: 2952881 targeting E, F, B and G transcripts. *kirre*[G1566] is located at X: 3025507 in Exon 10 targeting all 7 splice variants of *kirre*. Gray arrows depict the location of the forward and reverse primers used for qRT-PCR analysis. (B) Eclosion assays of *kirre* mutant lines (MiMIC and EP) compared to y^1w^{67c23} control line. Statistical analyses done by z- test. $N = 300$ flies/bar. * $p < 0.01$, ** $p < 0.001$ and *** $p < 0.0001$ relative to y^1w^{67c23}. (C) Expression of *kirre* mRNA in P12 pupae thoracic RNA extracts (pooled sample of n = 20 pupae) measured via qRT-PCR.

kirre(duf), *sns*, *if*, *kon* and *rols* are central players in myoblast fusion, myotube elongation and attachment and myofibrillogenesis in both embryonic and adult muscle development in flies [43]. Adult indirect flight muscles (IFMs) are an excellent model to study muscle development [43]. IFMs are comprised of dorsal longitudinal muscles (DLMs) and dorso-ventral muscles (DVMs), which act antagonistically. DLMs form through a process whereby persistent larval oblique muscles serve as templates for the recruitment and fusion of myoblasts that migrate from the notal region of the imaginal wing disc [44]. Myoblast homing and fusion to growing myotubes is mediated by *kirre* and *sns*, these being Ig-domain proteins and cognate ligand partners that mediate cell adhesion and the formation of multinucleate syncytial cells [45]. In this process, *kirre* interacts directly with *rols*, a scaffolding protein, to facilitate myoblast fusion [46]. Subsequent splitting of the growing myotube occurs to generate three and then six distinct fiber bundles in each hemithorax. Concurrently the bundles elongate with the tips eventually anchoring to tendon cell attachment sites, a process that requires *kon* [43] [47]. The fact that polymorphisms in these five core pathway genes are among the top associations with variation in MeHg tolerance strongly supports the hypothesis that muscle development is a MeHg target.

MeHg appears to disrupt myotube growth, fiber bundle splitting and, apparently, anchoring at the myotendinous junction in DLMs at the pupal stage (Fig. 8), a phenotype entirely consistent with disruption of the function of one or more genes listed above. Furthermore, *kirre* mutants that reduce expression levels demonstrated enhanced susceptibility to MeHg toxicity (Fig. 7). This effect was moderate and likely due to a redundant function for *kirre* and *roughest* (*rst*) [48]. Nonetheless, a *kirre* mutant causing increased expression results in a corresponding increase in MeHg tolerance (Fig. 7) reinforcing the notion that *kirre* can moderate MeHg toxic effects. A concerted role for muscle development in MeHg toxicity is strongly supported by our finding that pan-muscular expression of the MeHg protective enzyme, GCLc, gives a robust rescue of the MeHg effect on eclosion. How MeHg interacts with myogenic genes and/or their products remains to be characterized. A potential role of these genes is consistent with the notion that failure to eclose, a behavior that requires concerted contractions of newly formed adult muscles, results from MeHg disrupting the integrity of forming muscles.

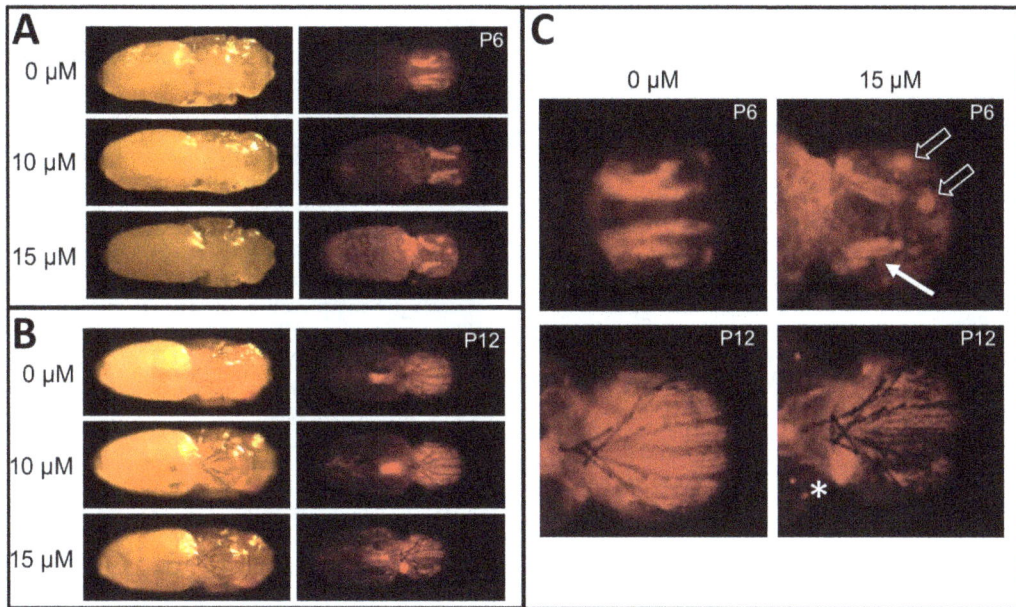

Figure 8. MeHg disruption of DLM muscle development. (A, B) *Mef2>RFP* pupae reared on indicated concentration of MeHg to stage P6 (A) or P12 (B) and imaged by bright light and red fluorescence to reveal DLM morphology. (C) Close-up image of selected panel from A and B. The solid arrow indicates reduced DLM bundle size and defects in DLM bundle splitting with MeHg. Open arrows indicate displacement of attachment sites of DVM bundles. Asterisks (*) indicates failure of extension and anchoring of the DLM resulting in myofibers coalesced in a ball. The development of eyes and bristles appear unaffected by MeHg treatment.

Genes with a function in formation of the neuromuscular junction (NMJ) were also enriched in our network analyses, notably, *sff*, *pum*, *spin*, *Sdc*, *nmo*, *tkv*, *sgg*, *nlg1* and *frq2*. NMJ-related genes are more highly represented in the MeHg+caffeine treatment. Six of the seven genes with NMJ function have human homologs and, intriguingly, are induced by caffeine as indicted by modENCODE treatment data in the FlyBase entry for each gene. Overall, these findings support the notion that clinical motor deficits may stem from effects of MeHg at the level of the motor unit. NMJ establishment and maintenance relies upon coordinated expression of factors that mediate targeting of the growing axon and connecting nerve terminals with muscle fibers, which are subsequently reinforced through a mechanism reliant upon vesicular trafficking [49]. It is therefore plausible that MeHg tolerance could arise from a favorable expression profile of the above genes that is influenced by natural polymorphic variation and can be modulated by caffeine. The effects of MeHg on the electrophysiological function of mature NMJ is well characterized [50], however, the extent to which MeHg alters NMJ formation in development is not clear.

Our findings present a paradigm shift in the hypothesis that the developing nervous system is preferentially targeted and exceptionally sensitive to MeHg. Myogenesis and neurogenesis share several conserved molecular pathways, and furthermore, the development of motor systems is intrinsically reliant on coordinated signals between developing muscle cells and neurons. It is not surprising that myogenesis could be an equally sensitive target for MeHg and that neurological deficits in animal models and humans observed thus far could include a yet unappreciated neuromuscular component.

We have previously characterized a MeHg-specific activation of the Notch receptor target gene *Enhancer of split mDelta* (*E(spl)mδ*) in *Drosophila* cells and embryos [51]. *E(spl)mδ* is unexpectedly expressed in embryonic muscle precursors as well as in differentiated larval muscles at late embryonic stages [51]. Furthermore, MeHg exposure during embryo development, as well as ectopic *E(spl)mδ* expression in muscle precursors, results in disrupted muscle patterning and concomitant defects in motor neuron outgrowth and branching [51,52]. While it remains to be seen if *E(spl)mδ* functions similarly in developing muscles at pupal stages, a recent study has identified a central role for Notch signals in maintaining migrating myoblast in a fusion incompetent state until encountering their myotube destination during IFM development [48]. Together, these data reinforce the notion that MeHg targets developing muscle in *Drosophila*, and further highlight the potential role for Notch signals, in addition to the gene candidates identified here, to mediate detrimental MeHg effects.

Multiple functions of candidate genes in development and MeHg toxicity

Several of the genes identified here have pleiotropic functions in development. Importantly, a number of genes have central functions in neurogenesis, neuronal differentiation and axon outgrowth, for example, *numb*, *if*, *kon*, *spin* and *Sdc*. While several steps in muscle development rely on autonomous signaling mechanisms and muscle-specific cues, in certain contexts a neural scaffold is required for appropriate muscle development [53]. Notably, denervation of the individual IFM fibers during early pupal stages affect subsequent myoblast proliferation contributing to reduced muscle bundle size in the DLM and DVM [53]. Thus, the phenotypes seen here may reflect an underlying MeHg-sensitive neural mechanism that remains to be characterized.

Alternatively, natural variation in MeHg tolerance may stem from effects on development of organs critical for dealing with toxic insult and excretion. *kirre* and *sns* are fundamental for morphogenesis of the Garland cell nephrocyte, a major site of waste removal and filtration of insect hemolymph [45,54]. *kirre/sns* function analogously to their vertebrate orthologs Neph1 and

Nephrin, which direct morphogenesis of the slit diaphragm of the podocyte in the mammalian glomerulus of the kidney [55,56]. In addition, *rols* functions in the normal morphogenesis of the Malpighian tubule, the renal organ of the fly [57]. Therefore, *kirre, sns* and *rols* may also influence MeHg tolerance by supporting development of essential excretory organs in addition to directing proper myogenesis during development.

Caffeine as a modulator of MeHg toxicity

We found that caffeine modulates MeHg toxicity, and in most cases shows an enhancement of tolerance to MeHg. Interestingly, caffeine has a positive impact on neurodegenerative disease, such as Parkinson's disease [58]. However, in some cases caffeine shows a negative effect on development with MeHg. There is a strong genetic component to the natural variation of the MeHg modulating effect of caffeine in flies, which parallels reports of genetic variation in caffeine effects in humans [59]. These findings emphasize the need to approach the issue of MeHg tolerance and susceptibility with a greater understanding of the role of individual genetic background, as well as dietary behaviors, particularly in investigations of fish-eating human population studies where MeHg exposures are most common.

Summary

We have identified muscle development as a prominent target for MeHg by associating genetic variation in the DGRP with MeHg toxicity. This finding expands the window of inquiry into mechanisms of MeHg toxicity. Candidate genes identified here set the stage for translational studies in vertebrates, and possibly in human populations, to assess to what extent muscle morphogenesis is compromised by this ubiquitous environmental toxin.

Supporting Information

Figure S1   Q-Q plots for eclosion train exhibited under MeHg alone and MeHg+caffeine treatments.

Figure S2   Q-Q plots for P-values under MeHg alone and MeHg+caffeine treatments.

Table S1   Genome Wide Association results for MeHg alone. Minor and major allele identities and counts are indicated for each polymorphism (SNP = single nucleotide polymorphism; INS = insertion; DEL = deletion; MNP = multiple nucleotide polymorphism). P-values and false discovery rates (FDR) are also indicated (See Materials and Methods). Gene identifications include the Flybase gene ID number (FB ID), gene name and location of the polymorphism.

Table S2   Genome Wide Association results for MeHg + Caffeine. (See legend for Table S2.)

Table S3   Eclosion assay raw data. Results of individual trials for eclosion assays are presented for each RAL line on food containing MeHg (concentration in μM) and Caffeine (2 mM) indicated in the column header. Results are expressed in percent (%) eclosion for 50 L1 larvae assayed in each trial (except for a few trials were 30 L1 larvae were assayed, indicated by italics).

Author Contributions

Conceived and designed the experiments: MDR SLM DV. Performed the experiments: SLM DV. Analyzed the data: SLM WH. Contributed reagents/materials/analysis tools: MDR RRHA TFCM. Wrote the paper: MDR SLM RRHA WH TFCM. Software development for analyses: WH.

References

1. Harada M (1995) Minamata disease: methylmercury poisoning in Japan caused by environmental pollution. Crit Rev Toxicol 25: 1–24.
2. Amin-Zaki L, Elhassani S, Majeed MA, Clarkson TW, Doherty RA, et al. (1974) Intra-uterine methylmercury poisoning in Iraq. Pediatrics 54: 587–595.
3. Harada M (1978) Congenital Minamata disease: intrauterine methylmercury poisoning. Teratology 18: 285–288.
4. Sabbagh K (1977) ECT and the media. Br Med J 2: 1215.
5. Choi BH, Lapham LW, Amin-Zaki L, Saleem T (1978) Abnormal neuronal migration, deranged cerebral cortical organization, and diffuse white matter astrocytosis of human fetal brain: a major effect of methylmercury poisoning in utero. J Neuropathol Exp Neurol 37: 719–733.
6. Al-saleem T (1976) Levels of mercury and pathological changes in patients with organomercury poisoning. Bull World Health Organ 53 Suppl: 99–104.
7. Debes F, Budtz-Jorgensen E, Weihe P, White RF, Grandjean P (2006) Impact of prenatal methylmercury exposure on neurobehavioral function at age 14 years. Neurotoxicol Teratol 28: 536–547.
8. Myers GJ, Davidson PW, Shamlaye CF, Axtell CD, Cernichiari E, et al. (1997) Effects of prenatal methylmercury exposure from a high fish diet on developmental milestones in the Seychelles Child Development Study. Neurotoxicology 18: 819–829.
9. Llop S, Engstrom K, Ballester F, Franforte E, Alhamdow A, et al. (2014) Polymorphisms in ABC transporter bgenes and concentrations of mercury in newborns - evidence from two Mediterranean birth cohorts. PLoS One 9: e97172.
10. Julvez J, Smith GD, Golding J, Ring S, Pourcain BS, et al. (2013) Prenatal methylmercury exposure and genetic predisposition to cognitive deficit at age 8 years. Epidemiology 24: 643–650.
11. Myers GJ, Davidson PW, Strain JJ (2007) Nutrient and methyl mercury exposure from consuming fish. J Nutr 137: 2805–2808.
12. Valera B, Dewailly E, Poirier P (2013) Association between methylmercury and cardiovascular risk factors in a native population of Quebec (Canada): a retrospective evaluation. Environ Res 120: 102–108.
13. Goodrich JM, Wang Y, Gillespie B, Werner R, Franzblau A, et al. (2013) Methylmercury and elemental mercury differentially associate with blood pressure among dental professionals. Int J Hyg Environ Health 216: 195–201.
14. Passos CJ, Mergler D (2008) Human mercury exposure and adverse health effects in the Amazon: a review. Cad Saude Publica 24 Suppl 4: s503–520.
15. Nyland JF, Fillion M, Barbosa F, Jr., Shirley DL, Chine C, et al. (2011) Biomarkers of methylmercury exposure immunotoxicity among fish consumers in Amazonian Brazil. Environ Health Perspect 119: 1733–1738.
16. Lee BE, Hong YC, Park H, Ha M, Koo BS, et al. (2010) Interaction between GSTM1/GSTT1 polymorphism and blood mercury on birth weight. Environ Health Perspect 118: 437–443.
17. Ramon R, Ballester F, Aguinagalde X, Amurrio A, Vioque J, et al. (2009) Fish consumption during pregnancy, prenatal mercury exposure, and anthropometric measures at birth in a prospective mother-infant cohort study in Spain. Am J Clin Nutr 90: 1047–1055.
18. Hughes WL (1957) A physicochemical rationale for the biological activity of mercury and its compounds. Ann N Y Acad Sci 65: 454–460.
19. Rabenstein DL, Evans CA (1978) The mobility of methylmercury in biological systems. Bioinorg Chem 8: 107–101, 104.
20. Morgan TJ, Mackay TFC (2006) Quantitative trait loci for thermotolerance phenotypes in Drosophila melanogaster. Heredity (Edinb) 96: 232–242.
21. Jordan KW, Craver KL, Magwire MM, Cubilla CE, Mackay TFC, et al. (2012) Genome-wide association for sensitivity to chronic oxidative stress in Drosophila melanogaster. PLoS One 7: e38722.
22. Weber AL, Khan GF, Magwire MM, Tabor CL, Mackay TFC, et al. (2012) Genome-wide association analysis of oxidative stress resistance in Drosophila melanogaster. PLoS One 7: e34745.
23. Morozova TV, Mackay TFC, Anholt RRH (2011) Transcriptional networks for alcohol sensitivity in Drosophila melanogaster. Genetics 187: 1193–1205.
24. Mackay TFC, Richards S, Stone EA, Barbadilla A, Ayroles JF, et al. (2012) The Drosophila melanogaster Genetic Reference Panel. Nature 482: 173–178.
25. Huang W, Massouras A, Inoue Y, Peiffer J, Ramia M, et al. (2014) Natural variation in genome architecture among 205 Drosophila melanogaster Genetic Reference Panel lines. Genome Res. 24: 1193–1208.
26. Rand MD, Lowe JA, Mahapatra CT (2012) Drosophila CYP6g1 and its human homolog CYP3A4 confer tolerance to methylmercury during development. Toxicology 300: 75–82.

27. Rand MD, Montgomery SL, Prince L, Vorojeikina D (2014) Developmental toxicity assays using the Drosophila model. Curr Protoc Toxicol 59: 1 12 11–11 12 20.

28. Baines RA (2005) Neuronal homeostasis through translational control. Mol Neurobiol 32: 113–121.

29. Dubnau J, Chiang AS, Grady L, Barditch J, Gossweiler S, et al. (2003) The staufen/pumilio pathway is involved in Drosophila long-term memory. Curr Biol 13: 286–296.

30. Littleton JT, Bai J, Vyas B, Desai R, Baltus AE, et al. (2001) synaptotagmin mutants reveal essential functions for the C2B domain in Ca2+-triggered fusion and recycling of synaptic vesicles in vivo. J Neurosci 21: 1421–1433.

31. Adolfsen B, Saraswati S, Yoshihara M, Littleton JT (2004) Synaptotagmins are trafficked to distinct subcellular domains including the postsynaptic compartment. J Cell Biol 166: 249–260.

32. Yazdani U, Huang Z, Terman JR (2008) The glucose transporter (GLUT4) enhancer factor is required for normal wing positioning in Drosophila. Genetics 178: 919–929.

33. Knight JB, Eyster CA, Griesel BA, Olson AL (2003) Regulation of the human GLUT4 gene promoter: interaction between a transcriptional activator and myocyte enhancer factor 2A. Proc Natl Acad Sci U S A 100: 14725–14730.

34. Schnizler K, Saeger B, Pfeffer C, Gerbaulet A, Ebbinghaus-Kintscher U, et al. (2005) A novel chloride channel in Drosophila melanogaster is inhibited by protons. J Biol Chem 280: 16254–16262.

35. Mummery-Widmer JL, Yamazaki M, Stoeger T, Novatchkova M, Bhalerao S, et al. (2009) Genome-wide analysis of Notch signalling in Drosophila by transgenic RNAi. Nature 458: 987–992.

36. Balamurugan K, Egli D, Selvaraj A, Zhang B, Georgiev O, et al. (2004) Metal-responsive transcription factor (MTF-1) and heavy metal stress response in Drosophila and mammalian cells: a functional comparison. Biol Chem 385: 597–603.

37. Egli D, Selvaraj A, Yepiskoposyan H, Zhang B, Hafen E, et al. (2003) Knockout of 'metal-responsive transcription factor' MTF-1 in Drosophila by homologous recombination reveals its central role in heavy metal homeostasis. EMBO J 22: 100–108.

38. Bahadorani S, Mukai S, Egli D, Hilliker AJ (2010) Overexpression of metal-responsive transcription factor (MTF-1) in Drosophila melanogaster ameliorates life-span reductions associated with oxidative stress and metal toxicity. Neurobiol Aging 31: 1215–1226.

39. Warde-Farley D, Donaldson SL, Comes O, Zuberi K, Badrawi R, et al. (2010) The GeneMANIA prediction server: biological network integration for gene prioritization and predicting gene function. Nucleic Acids Res 38: W214–220.

40. Olson EN, Perry M, Schulz RA (1995) Regulation of muscle differentiation by the MEF2 family of MADS box transcription factors. Dev Biol 172: 2–14.

41. Dutczak WJ, Ballatori N (1994) Transport of the glutathione-methylmercury complex across liver canalicular membranes on reduced glutathione carriers. J Biol Chem 269: 9746–9751.

42. Toyama T, Shinkai Y, Yasutake A, Uchida K, Yamamoto M, et al. (2011) Isothiocyanates reduce mercury accumulation via an Nrf2-dependent mechanism during exposure of mice to methylmercury. Environ Health Perspect 119: 1117–1122.

43. Weitkunat M, Schnorrer F (2014) A guide to study Drosophila muscle biology. Methods.

44. Fernandes JJ, Keshishian H (1996) Patterning the dorsal longitudinal flight muscles (DLM) of Drosophila: insights from the ablation of larval scaffolds. Development 122: 3755–3763.

45. Kesper DA, Stute C, Buttgereit D, Kreisköther N, Vishnu S, et al. (2007) Myoblast fusion in Drosophila melanogaster is mediated through a fusion-restricted myogenic-adhesive structure (FuRMAS). Dev Dyn 236: 404–415.

46. Bulchand S, Menon SD, George SE, Chia W (2010) The intracellular domain of Dumbfounded affects myoblast fusion efficiency and interacts with Rolling pebbles and Loner. PLoS One 5: e9374.

47. Devenport D, Bunch TA, Bloor JW, Brower DL, Brown NH (2007) Mutations in the Drosophila alphaPS2 integrin subunit uncover new features of adhesion site assembly. Dev Biol 308: 294–308.

48. Gildor B, Schejter ED, Shilo BZ (2012) Bidirectional Notch activation represses fusion competence in swarming adult Drosophila myoblasts. Development 139: 4040–4050.

49. Menon KP, Carrillo RA, Zinn K (2013) Development and plasticity of the Drosophila larval neuromuscular junction. Wiley Interdiscip Rev Dev Biol 2: 647–670.

50. Levesque PC, Atchison WD (1988) Effect of alteration of nerve terminal Ca2+ regulation on increased spontaneous quantal release of acetylcholine by methyl mercury. Toxicol Appl Pharmacol 94: 55–65.

51. Engel GL, Rand MD (2014) The Notch target E(spl)mdelta is a muscle-specific gene involved in methylmercury toxicity in motor neuron development. Neurotoxicol Teratol 43C: 11–18.

52. Engel GL, Delwig A, Rand MD (2012) The effects of methylmercury on Notch signaling during embryonic neural development in Drosophila melanogaster. Toxicol In Vitro 26: 485–492.

53. Fernandes JJ, Keshishian H (2005) Motoneurons regulate myoblast proliferation and patterning in Drosophila. Dev Biol 277: 493–505.

54. Zhuang S, Shao H, Guo F, Trimble R, Pearce E, et al. (2009) Sns and Kirre, the Drosophila orthologs of Nephrin and Neph1, direct adhesion, fusion and formation of a slit diaphragm-like structure in insect nephrocytes. Development 136: 2335–2344.

55. Srinivas BP, Woo J, Leong WY, Roy S (2007) A conserved molecular pathway mediates myoblast fusion in insects and vertebrates. Nat Genet 39: 781–786.

56. Sohn RL, Huang P, Kawahara G, Mitchell M, Guyon J, et al. (2009) A role for nephrin, a renal protein, in vertebrate skeletal muscle cell fusion. Proc Natl Acad Sci U S A 106: 9274–9279.

57. Putz M, Kesper DA, Buttgereit D, Renkawitz-Pohl R (2005) In Drosophila melanogaster, the rolling pebbles isoform 6 (Rols6) is essential for proper Malpighian tubule morphology. Mech Dev 122: 1206–1217.

58. Prediger RD (2010) Effects of caffeine in Parkinson's disease: from neuroprotection to the management of motor and non-motor symptoms. J Alzheimers Dis 20 Suppl 1: S205–220.

59. Yang A, Palmer AA, de Wit H (2010) Genetics of caffeine consumption and responses to caffeine. Psychopharmacology (Berl) 211: 245–257.

60. Orr WC, Radyuk SN, Prabhudesai L, Toroser D, Benes JJ, et al. (2005) Overexpression of glutamate-cysteine ligase extends life span in Drosophila melanogaster. J Biol Chem 280: 37331–37338.

61. Mahapatra CT, Bond J, Rand DM, Rand MD (2010) Identification of methylmercury tolerance gene candidates in Drosophila. Toxicol Sci 116: 225–238.

62. Bainbridge SP, Bownes M (1981) Staging the metamorphosis of Drosophila melanogaster. J Embryol Exp Morphol 66: 57–80.

63. Livak KJ, Schmittgen TD (2001) Analysis of relative gene expression data using real-time quantitative PCR and the 2(-Delta Delta C(T)) Method. Methods 25: 402–408.

7

Mercury and Selenium in Stranded Indo-Pacific Humpback Dolphins and Implications for Their Trophic Transfer in Food Chains

Duan Gui[1], Ri-Qing Yu[2], Yong Sun[1], Laiguo Chen[3], Qin Tu[1], Hui Mo[4], Yuping Wu[1]*

1 Guangdong Provincial Key Laboratory of Marine Resources and Coastal Engineering, School of Marine Sciences, Sun Yat-Sen University, Guangzhou, China, **2** Department of Biology, University of Texas at Tyler, Tyler, Texas, United States of America, **3** Urban Environment and Ecology Research Center, South China Institute of Environmental Sciences (SCIES), Ministry of Environmental Protection, Guangzhou, China, **4** South China Botanical Garden, Chinese Academy of Sciences, Guangzhou, China

Abstract

As top predators in the Pearl River Estuary (PRE) of China, Indo-Pacific humpback dolphins (*Sousa chinensis*) are bioindicators for examining regional trends of environmental contaminants in the PRE. We examined samples from stranded *S. chinensis* in the PRE, collected since 2004, to study the distribution and fate of total mercury (THg), methylmercury (MeHg) and selenium (Se) in the major tissues, in individuals at different ages and their prey fishes from the PRE. This study also investigated the potential protective effects of Se against the toxicities of accumulated THg. Dolphin livers contained the highest concentrations of THg (32.34 ± 58.98 µg g^{-1} dw) and Se (15.16 ± 3.66 µg g^{-1} dw), which were significantly different from those found in kidneys and muscles, whereas the highest residue of MeHg (1.02 ± 1.11 µg g^{-1} dw) was found in dolphin muscles. Concentrations of both THg and MeHg in the liver, kidney and muscle of dolphins showed a significantly positive correlation with age. The biomagnification factors (BMFs) of inorganic mercury (Hg$_{inorg}$) in dolphin livers (350×) and MeHg in muscles (18.7×) through the prey fishes were the highest among all three dolphin tissues, whereas the BMFs of Se were much lower in all dolphin tissues. The lower proportion of MeHg in THg and higher Se/THg ratios in tissues were demonstrated. Our studies suggested that *S. chinensis* might have the potential to detoxify Hg via the demethylation of MeHg and the formation of tiemannite (HgSe) in the liver and kidney. The lower threshold of hepatic THg concentrations for the equimolar accumulation of Se and Hg in *S. chinensis* suggests that this species has a greater sensitivity to THg concentrations than is found in striped dolphins and Dall's porpoises.

Editor: Dwayne Elias, Oak Ridge National Laboratory, United States of America

Funding: This research was supported by the National Natural Science Foundation of China (Grant no. 41276147); a Science and Research Project of the Marine Non-profit Industry (Grant no. 201105011-5); the Ocean Park Conservation Foundation, Hong Kong; the National Key Technology R & D Program (Grant no. 2011BAG07B05-3); and the Sousa chinensis Conservation Action Project from the Administrator of Ocean and Fisheries of Guangdong Province, China. The funders had no role in study design, data collection and analysis, decision to publish, or preparation of the manuscript.

Competing Interests: The authors have declared that no competing interests exist.

* Email: exwyp@mail.sysu.edu.cn

Introduction

Mercury (Hg) in its inorganic form is a ubiquitous pollutant that is globally distributed by atmospheric transportation. Less toxic Hg(II) in environments can easily be converted into the highly toxic methylmercury (MeHg), primarily by sulfate- and iron-reducing bacteria and methanogens [1–7] through the putative Hg methylation genes *hgc*A and *hgc*B via the acetyl CoA pathway [5]. MeHg is a strong neurotoxic substance; once it is bioavailable in aquatic ecosystems, it can be bioaccumulated and biomagnified quickly through aquatic food webs, which creates a health threat to humans and aquatic mammals such as dolphins [3].

The estuary of the Pearl River, which is the third longest river in China, is a traditional nursery for fisheries and provides an ideal habitat for Indo-Pacific humpback dolphins (*Sousa chinensis*). The Pearl River Estuary (PRE) region contains a group of cities that include Guangzhou, Shenzhen and Hong Kong, forming one of the largest local and global economic hubs in southern China. Rapid industrial development and urbanization in recent decades have undermined the habitats of local fish and dolphins in the estuary. *S. chinensis* is considered one of the most endangered species (the National Key Species for Protection, Grade 1) in China. The Chinese government has delimitated the PRE as a national nature reserve for *S. chinensis*. Recent studies have indicated a decreasing trend of total mercury (THg) concentration in sediments with distance away from the PRE and toward the South China Sea [8] and showed an accelerated input of THg in sediment cores in recent decades [9]. These results suggest that THg contamination in this region has been strongly correlated with industrial development. Contamination by Hg(II) and MeHg was also observed in surface water in the tributary (e.g., Dong River) of the Pearl River Delta. However, THg and MeHg contamination in Indo-Pacific humpback dolphins and the interaction between THg toxicity and Se accumulation in their bodies have not been systematically studied in this ecosystem [10,11].

In aquatic ecosystems, dolphins are top predators that have long lifespans, which increases their potential to accumulate Hg(II) and MeHg [12]. MeHg is easily accumulated in the livers of cetaceans, likely as a result of the ability of the liver to store and biotransform toxic contaminants [13]. The accumulation of Hg(II) and MeHg might cause detrimental effects on the reproduction system, immune responses, central nervous system and organs such as the liver and kidneys [14,15].

Previous studies have reported that selenium (Se) can mitigate the toxicity of MeHg in the liver of cetaceans by forming a highly insoluble Se–Hg compound after demethylating MeHg [16,17]. The presence of the nontoxic Se–Hg compound was confirmed in the cytoplasm of hepatic cells in *Stenella coeruleoalba*, and an equimolar ratio between Se and THg was reported in liver tissue with a high THg concentration [18,19]. This phenomenon likely explains the ability of cetaceans to tolerate high THg concentrations without directly observable adverse effects and exhibit a low MeHg residue in the brain tissue. Se is a micronutrient that plays an important role in enzymes (e.g., glutathione peroxidase) in the maintenance of normal organ functions. Adverse biological effects occur when there is a deficiency of bioavailable Se, and an Hg-induced Se deficiency can lead to MeHg or THg toxicity [20]. The present investigation examined samples from dolphins stranded in the PRE, which have been collected since 2004, to study the distribution and fate of toxic pollutants (THg, MeHg and Se) in the major organs, in individuals at different ages and in their prey fishes from the PRE. The aims of the study were also to investigate the potential protective effects of Se against the toxicities of accumulated THg, and to provide evidence for the conservation of this endangered species.

Materials and Methods

Ethics Statement

This study on the Indo-Pacific humpback dolphins was approved by the Ministry of Agriculture of Chinese government under permit number 2003-54. The protocol was specifically verified by the Administration of Ocean and Fisheries of Guangdong Province, China under permit number 1999-583. No issue on ethics was concerned in this study.

Samples and chemical analysis

The tissue samples of *S. chinensis* were collected from dead and stranded animals along the PRE of the South China Sea from 2004 to 2012 (**Fig. 1**). Before performing the necropsies, the biological parameters were measured and tooth specimens were acquired to determine the age of specific individuals according to the method described by Jefferson [21] and Myrck et al. [22]. According to the report from Jefferson et al. [23], male dolphins inhabiting the PRE reach sexual maturity at 12–14 years, whereas females generally reach maturity at 9–10 years. Accordingly, the specimen assigned ID numbers from 21 to 28 in the present study were considered adults, and those with assigned numbers 1 to 20 were considered juveniles (**Table S1**). The liver, kidney and muscle tissue samples were placed in clean and acid-washed plastic bags and stored at $-20°C$ immediately after collection. Information based on previous studies [21,24] indicated that the Indo-Pacific humpback dolphins have specific preferences for prey fishes. Based on that, 13 species of fish were collected from the PRE. Whole-body fish samples were smashed for metal analysis. All samples (dolphin and fish) were kept frozen until processing.

Samples were processed and prepared by a method similar to that of previous studies [25], in which portions of the different tissue samples were freeze-dried (Freeze-drying system, Labconco, Kansas City, Missouri, USA) for 48 h at $40–133×10^{-3}$ mBar and $-49°C$. The dried samples were then ground with an automatic agate mortar (Retsch, Germany) for 10 min. The concentration of THg in the dried tissue samples was measured without pretreatment or digestion by using the Hydra-C Automated Direct Hg Analyzer (Teledyne Instruments, Leeman Labs, USA). All specimens were analyzed in batches that included a procedural blank and standard reference material DORM-3 (National Research Council of Canada, Canada). The procedural blank and the reference material were treated and measured in the same way as the tissue samples. To analyze the MeHg concentration, tissue samples were digested in a KOH–methanol solution at $65°C$ for 4 h. The extractants were subjected to aqueous ethylation, separation by gas chromatography and detection by cold vapor atomic fluorescence spectrometry (CVAFS) (TEKRAN Model 2700 with an automated MERX purge and trap system, Brooks Rand Labs, USA) modified from USEPA method 1630 [26].

The digestion and preparation of dried tissue samples for Se analysis followed the methods described by Hung et al. [10]. Approximately 0.2 g of tissue samples was weighed in Teflon digestion tubes and soaked overnight in a mixture of 2 ml of double-distilled deionized water (3-D water) and 5 ml of 70% nitric acid (Merck, Germany). The digestion tubes were then sealed, placed in a microwave oven (Xin Tuo, model XT-9912, China) and subjected to a pressure increase of 65 psi for 15 m. After cooling, 2 ml H_2O_2 was added to the sample solution. The pressure was then increased to 65 psi for 15 m. The resulting digests were cooled and filtered through disposable syringe filter discs (0.45 μm pores, 25 mm diameter, with a mixed cellulose-ester filtering material, Jing Teng, China) equipped with 50-ml plastic syringes. The filtrates were transferred to 25-ml volumetric flasks and diluted with 3-D water. The samples were kept in acid-washed PVC tubes at $4°C$ prior to trace element analysis. The concentration of Se was measured by an inductively coupled plasma mass spectrometer (ICP-MS) (Agilent 7700, USA) with the procedural blank and reference TORT-2 included with every batch of tissue samples.

Quality assurance/quality control (QA/QC)

The precision and accuracy of the analytical methods were determined and monitored using the certified material TORT-2 (lobster hepatopancreas) and DORM-3 (fish protein) from the National Research Council of Canada. The recovery rates for THg, MeHg and Se were approximately 95.3%, 94.9% and 94.3%, respectively.

Statistical analysis

Statistical analyses were performed using SPSS (Statistical Package for the Social Sciences) software (StatSoft, ver. 22, USA), and the level of statistical significance was defined as $p < 0.05$. Grubbs' test was used to identify outliers, which were removed before further calculations. The Kolmogorov–Smirnoff test was used to assess the normality of the data distribution; if the data were not in normality, all the data were log_{10}-transformed to improve normality prior to analysis to best fit the underlying assumptions of the analysis of variance. The correlation between measured parameters was assessed by coefficient of determination (R^2). Differences in the concentrations of MeHg, THg and Se were analyzed among the groups (adult males, adult females, juvenile males and juvenile females) by using one-way ANOVA followed by Tukey's post-hoc tests. The contaminant concentrations of the

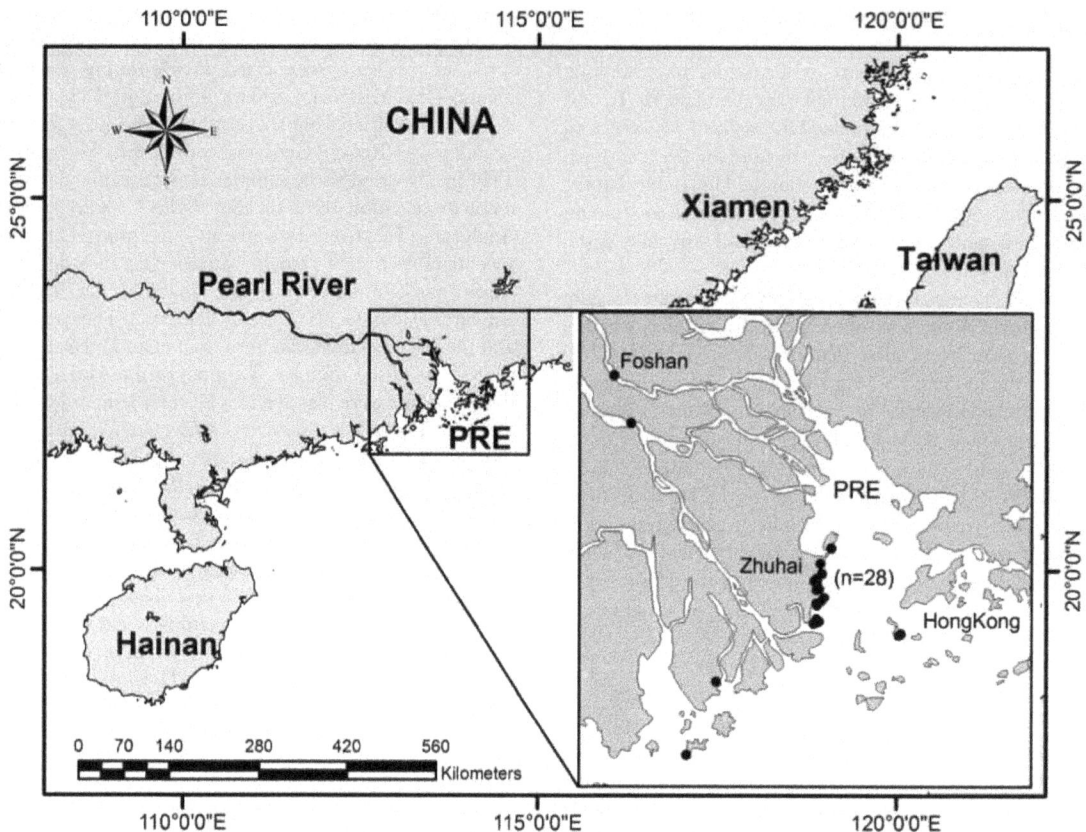

Figure 1. Sampling sites in the Pearl River Estuary (PRE) where the stranded Indo-Pacific humpback dolphins (n = 28) were collected from 2004 to 2012.

stranded dolphins that exhibited a large dispersion were analyzed by non-parametric tests.

Results

The total Hg, Se and MeHg concentrations and their related ratios were determined in the tissue samples from the liver (n = 28), kidney (n = 22) and muscle (n = 15) of Indo-Pacific humpback dolphins (**Table 1**). The mean concentrations of THg, Se and MeHg in 13 fish species from the PRE were summarized in **Table 2**. The average THg concentration in the prey fish species was 0.146 µg g^{-1} dw, with a range from 0.062 to 0.303 µg g^{-1} dw, and the average Se concentration was 2.23 µg g^{-1} dw, with a range from 1.93 to 3.34 µg g^{-1} dw. No significant differences in concentrations were found for the different fish species except the predatory species *Arius sinensis* and *Pampus argenteus*, which showed high THg concentrations. The potential biomagnification factor of inorganic mercury (Hg$_{inorg}$) in the dolphin tissue from the prey fishes was the highest in the liver tissue (350-fold) and the lowest in the muscle tissue (4.78-fold) (**Table 2**). For MeHg, dolphin muscle tissue had the highest biomagnification factor (18.7-fold), followed by liver tissue (14.3-fold) and kidney tissue (9.6-fold). Overall, Se in dolphin tissues showed the lowest potential for biomagnification of the three contaminants. For all dolphin individuals, muscle represents around 30% of total body mass, while other tissues (e. g., liver and kidney) contribute much less to the total body weight (<5%).

The highest mean concentration of THg was found in dolphin liver tissue (32.3±59.0 µg g^{-1} dw), whereas a lower concentration

was found in the kidneys (4.52±5.53 µg g^{-1} dw), with the smallest residue level shown in the muscle tissue (1.45±1.62 µg g^{-1} dw). The difference in THg accumulation among the three tissues was significant ($p<0.05$) (**Table 1**). Conversely, a significant difference in MeHg accumulation among different tissues was not found. Dolphin muscle tissue contained the highest MeHg concentration (1.02±1.11 µg g^{-1} dw), followed by liver (0.79±0.61 µg g^{-1} dw) and kidney (0.53±0.49 µg g^{-1} dw). Se concentrations displayed a similar profile as THg, with the highest mean value found in the liver tissue (15.2±19.4 µg sg^{-1} dw), followed by kidney (7.57±3.47 µg g^{-1} dw) and muscle tissue (1.89±1.69 µg g^{-1} dw).

The log$_{10}$-transformed concentrations of both THg and MeHg in the liver, kidney and muscle tissue of dolphins showed a significantly positive correlation with the log$_{10}$-transformed values of age (**Fig. 2A, B**). However, the slopes between tissue MeHg with age were much lower than those between THg and age for the three tissues. The MeHg/THg ratio in the livers and kidneys significantly decreased with age, while the MeHg/THg ratio in the muscles showed no trend with age (**Fig. 2C**). The mean percentage of MeHg/THg in the liver, kidney and muscle tissue was 18±15, 29±22 and 77±23, respectively (**Table 1**), indicating that the MeHg concentrations in the liver and kidney tissue represented 30% or less of the THg, which was generally lower than the MeHg/THg fraction that appeared in the prey fish (ranging from 18% to 83%, with an average of 42%, **Table 2**). The dolphin muscle tissue showed the highest MeHg/THg ratio. Se accumulation in the liver and kidney tissue significantly increased with age, whereas the concentration of Se in muscle tissue was not obviously affected by age (**Fig. 2D**).

Table 1. The mean concentrations and standard deviations (SD), in µg g^{-1} dry weight, of total mercury (THg), selenium (Se) and methyl mercury (MeHg); the molar ratio (%) of Se to THg; and the percentage (%) of MeHg/THg in liver, kidney and muscle tissue of Indo-Pacific humpback dolphins from the Pearl River Estuary (PRE), China.

		Liver (n=28)					Kidney (n=22)					Muscle (n=15)				
		THg	Se	MeHg	Se:THg	MeHg:THg	THg	Se	MeHg	Se:THg	MeHg:THg	THg	Se	MeHg	Se:THg	MeHg:THg
JM (n=13)	Mean	4.24	5.63	0.49	8.51	25	1.27	5.67	0.26	37.7	43.4	0.58	1.52	0.48	10.6	78.7
	SD	5.12	3.54	0.35	5.90	14.5	1.65	2.86	0.21	27.8	22.2	0.40	0.42	0.36	6.67	12.9
JF (n=7)	Mean	2.27	5.09	0.47	7.14	23.4	1.73	6.95	0.36	15.46	27.5	1.29	2.78	0.43	7.82	66.9
	SD	1.36	1.20	0.15	2.59	6.66	1.14	1.83	0.16	8.6	11.9	1.91	2.67	0.34	2.64	32.3
	p values	n.s.	n.s.	n.s.	n.s.	n.s.	n.s.	n.s.	n.s.	n.s.	n.s.	n.s.	n.s.	n.s.	n.s.	n.s.
AM (n=3)	Mean	84.3	35.6	1.56	1.07	1.88	8.21	10.3	0.98	3.13	11	2.27	1.61	2.03	0.90	89.4
	SD	8.19	6.93	0.44	0.14	0.64	1.19	2.68	0.35	0.35	3.39	0	0	0	0	0
AF (n=5)	Mean	116	41.8	1.56	0.99	1.89	13.4	11.1	1.06	2.29	7.42	3.18	1.43	2.72	0.79	85.6
	SD	81.8	24.9	0.46	0.11	0.91	5.16	2.45	0.60	0.47	2.18	1.05	0.24	0.94	0.21	6.47
	p values	n.s.	n.s.	n.s.	n.s.	n.s.	n.s.	n.s.	n.s.	n.s.	n.s.	n.s.	n.s.	n.s.	n.s.	n.s.
M (n=16)	Mean	3.19	5.63	0.60	9.08	20.7	2.87	6.73	0.43	29.7	36.1	0.82	1.53	0.70	9.01	80.4
	SD	3.76	3.54	0.44	5.76	15.9	3.32	3.42	0.39	28.4	23.7	0.70	0.39	0.64	7.07	12.5
F (n=12)	Mean	31.6	20.4	0.93	4.92	14.4	6.90	8.79	0.67	9.61	18.6	2	2.2	1.29	4.81	73.9
	SD	50.3	24.2	0.62	3.90	11.8	6.77	2.96	0.54	9.17	13.4	1.88	2.13	1.28	4.01	27.4
	p values	n.s.	0.016	n.s.	n.s.	n.s.	n.s.	n.s.	n.s.	n.s.	n.s.	n.s.	n.s.	n.s.	n.s.	n.s.
All (n=28)	Mean	32.3	15.2	0.79	6.03	18.5	4.52	7.57	0.53	21.5	29.0	1.45	1.89	1.02	6.75	76.9
	SD	59.0	19.4	0.61	5.40	15.3	5.53	3.47	0.49	25.3	22.5	1.62	1.69	1.11	6.26	23.3

JM: juvenile male (<12 years); JF: juvenile female (<9 years); AM: adult male (>12 years); AF: adult female (>9 years).
n.s.: not significant.

Table 2. The mean concentrations and standard deviations (SD), in $\mu g\ g^{-1}$ dry weight, of total mercury (THg), inorganic mercury (Hg$_{inorg}$), methylmercury (MeHg), selenium (Se), and the percentage (%) of MeHg/THg in the prey fishes (whole body) for Indo-Pacific humpback dolphins and their average biomagnification factors (BMFs) in the dolphin tissues collected from the Pearl River Estuary (PRE), China.

Species	Family	Sample number	THg		Hg$_{inorg}$		MeHg		Se		MeHg/THg
			Mean	SD	Mean	SD	Mean	SD	Mean	SD	Mean
Johnius belengerii	Sciaenidae	3	0.146	0.075	0.100	0.079	0.046	0.01	2.51	0.41	25
Collichthys lucidus	Sciaenidae	4	0.134	0.106	0.073	0.082	0.060	0.026	2.61	0.47	45
Clupanodon thrissa	Clupeidae	2	0.182	0.129	0.147	0.127	0.036	0.002	1.87	0.58	20
Coilia mystus	Engraulidae	5	0.158	0.152	0.121	0.144	0.037	0.008	1.99	0.43	23
Pampus argenteus	Stromateidae	3	0.221	0.111	0.189	0.119	0.032	0.008	2.22	0.22	15
Harpadon nehereus	Synodontidae	2	0.079	0.024	0.030	0.016	0.048	0.009	2.06	0.63	61
Cynoglossus bilineatus	Cynoglossidae	3	0.077	0.024	0.039	0.015	0.038	0.015	2.21	0.33	50
Sillago sihama	Sillaginidae	3	0.166	0.036	0.029	0.017	0.137	0.044	1.99	0.27	83
Arius sinensis	Ariidae	2	0.303	0.007	0.247	0.006	0.056	0.001	1.93	0.08	19
Selaroides leptolepis	Carangidae	2	0.118	0.065	0.079	0.058	0.039	0.007	1.99	0.40	33
Mugil cephalus	Mugilidae	2	0.062	0.002	0.033	0.005	0.030	0.003	1.94	0.32	48
Odontamblyopus rubicundus	Taenioididae	2	0.161	0.027	0.053	0.002	0.107	0.028	3.34	0.35	67
Odontamblyopus lacepedii	Taenioididae	3	0.077	0.000	0.033	0.009	0.044	0.009	2.39	0.53	57
Mean biomagnification factor	Dolphin liver				350		14.3		6.8		
Mean biomagnification factor	Dolphin kidney				44.3		9.6		3.4		
Mean biomagnification factor	Dolphin muscle				4.78		18.7		0.8		

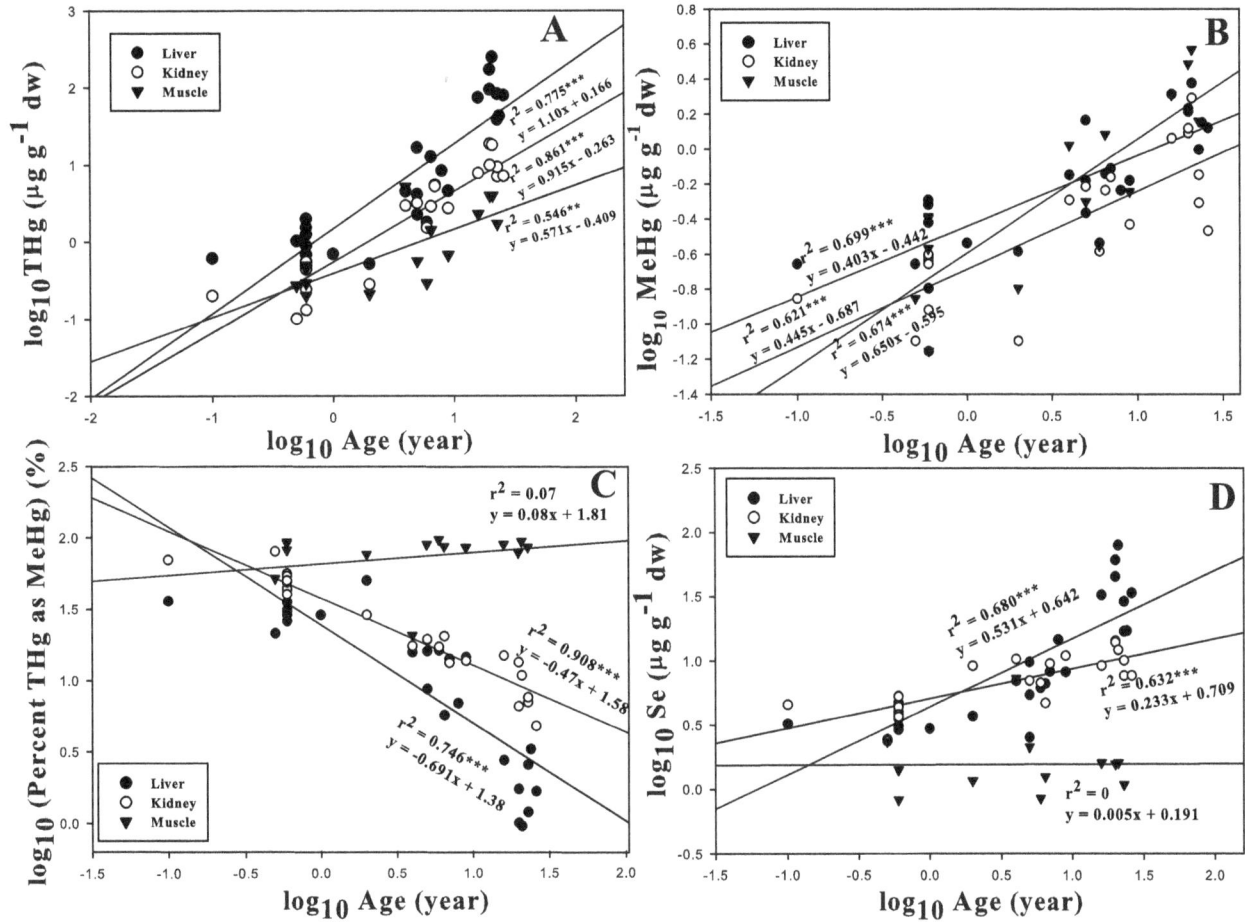

Figure 2. Relationships of dolphin age with the concentrations of THg, MeHg, Se and MeHg/THg ratio in the liver, kidney and muscle tissue, respectively, in the Indo-Pacific humpback dolphins stranded in the Pearl River Estuary (PRE) region.

The mean molar ratio of Se to THg was highest in the kidney tissue (21.5 ± 25.3) and the lowest in the liver (6.04 ± 5.40), with a medium ratio observed in the muscle tissue (6.75 ± 6.26) (**Table 1**). The molar ratios of Se/THg in the livers and kidneys of the juveniles were eight-fold higher than in the adult livers and 14-fold higher than in the adult kidneys, respectively. A significant positive correlation was found between the concentrations of Se and THg in both the livers and kidneys (**Fig. 3A, B**). The $\log_{10}$ Se/THg molar ratios showed strongly negative regressions with the $\log_{10}$ MeHg levels in the livers ($p<0.05$) and kidneys ($p<0.05$) (**Fig. 3C, D**). A significantly positive relationship between THg and MeHg was observed in the livers, with an inflection range of 8.4–16.9 µg g^{-1} dw of THg (**Fig. 4**).

No significant differences were found in the THg and MeHg concentrations in the liver and muscle tissues between males and females. Only the mean Se concentrations in the liver tissue were significantly different between males and females ($p<0.05$) (**Table 1**).

Discussion

Compared with the kidneys and muscles, extremely high concentrations of THg were found in the livers of *S. chinensis* (32.3 ± 59.0 µg g^{-1} dw), although the upper limits of the THg concentrations in the livers were lower than those found in dolphins from the waters of Hong Kong (906 µg g^{-1} dw) [27].

This phenomenon may be related to the detoxification function of marine mammal livers in terms of storage and biotransformation. The tolerance limit of THg in mammalian hepatic tissues appears to be within the range of 100 to 400 µg g^{-1} wet weight (ww) [28]. The THg concentrations shown in **Table 1** are below this range; however, a dolphin analyzed in our laboratory was found with a liver THg concentration of 1374 µg g^{-1} dw. Albeit not as high as the results from Japan (1600 µg g^{-1} dw) [29] and the Mediterranean (13150 µg g^{-1} dw) [30], the THg concentrations detected in the liver samples of *S. chinensis* in the PRE were high enough to cause damage to the internal organs of the contaminated individuals.

The accumulation of MeHg tended to increase with age (**Fig. 2**) but at a lower rate than that of THg. No obvious trend existed between the MeHg/THg ratio (%) and age in the muscle samples, whereas the liver and kidney samples showed a decreasing trend of MeHg with age, which could be ascribed to a slow demethylation process that occurs in livers and kidneys but not in muscles [29,31]. Among the three tissue types, muscle tissue accumulated the highest MeHg concentrations, which is consistent with the hypothesis that lack of demethylation mechanisms occur in muscles [32]. Based on studies of several small mammals [33], the lethal level of MeHg in brain tissue was proposed to be in the range of 12–30 µg g^{-1} ww (equivalent to 60–150 µg g^{-1} dw). However, the highest MeHg concentration in the brain tissue

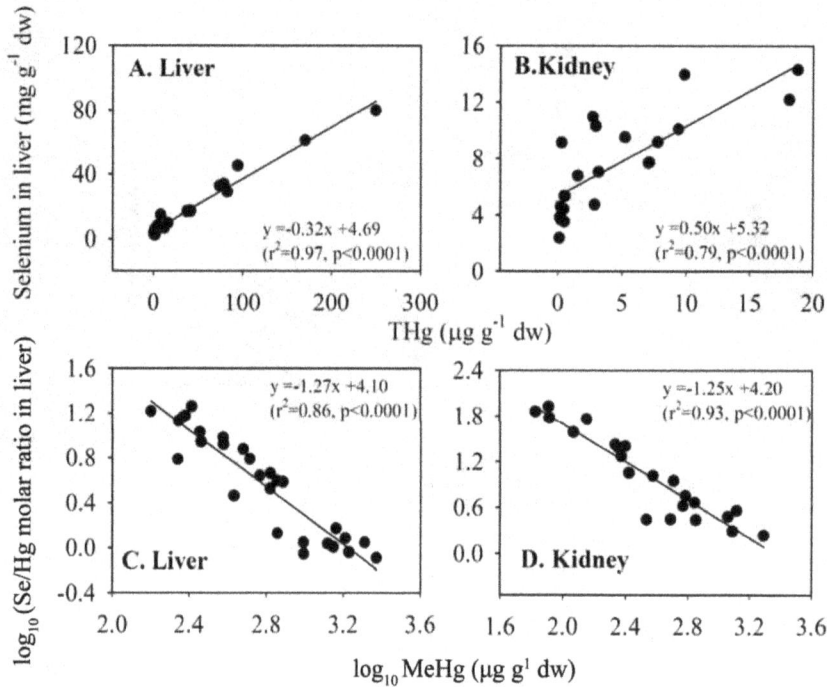

Figure 3. Regression analysis of Se with THg, and of $\log_{10}$ (Se/Hg) with $\log_{10}$ MeHg in the liver and kidney of Indo-Pacific humpback dolphins (n = 28) stranded in the Pearl River Estuary (PRE) region.

(0.41 µg g^{-1}) from our previous study (unpublished data) was significantly lower than the lethal level.

The relationships between age and THg concentration in livers and kidneys of different species of marine mammal have been extensively examined [12,30,34], and indicate that the hepatic and renal THg concentrations increase with age. This correlation implies a higher capability for the bioaccumulation of toxic elements than for their elimination throughout these animals' life span. In addition, as the size of the prey and the quantities of food tends to increase in proportion with the growth of the dolphins, the trophic transfer of the toxic metals may also progressively increase

[35]. In the present study, the THg concentration increased with age in the livers, kidneys and muscles (**Fig. 2**).

Because of the difficulties in tracking down the prey fish species of dolphins in natural habitats to analyze their tissue contaminant residues, the trophic transfer of THg, MeHg and Se from prey fish to dolphin has scarcely been studied, even though dolphins are considered one of the top predators in the ocean. Through a comparison of the mean concentrations of THg, MeHg and Se from the prey fish to dolphin tissues, our studies outline the first direct evidence of the biomagnification processes of contaminants in this cetacean (**Table 2**). For Hg$_{inorg}$, the average concentrations

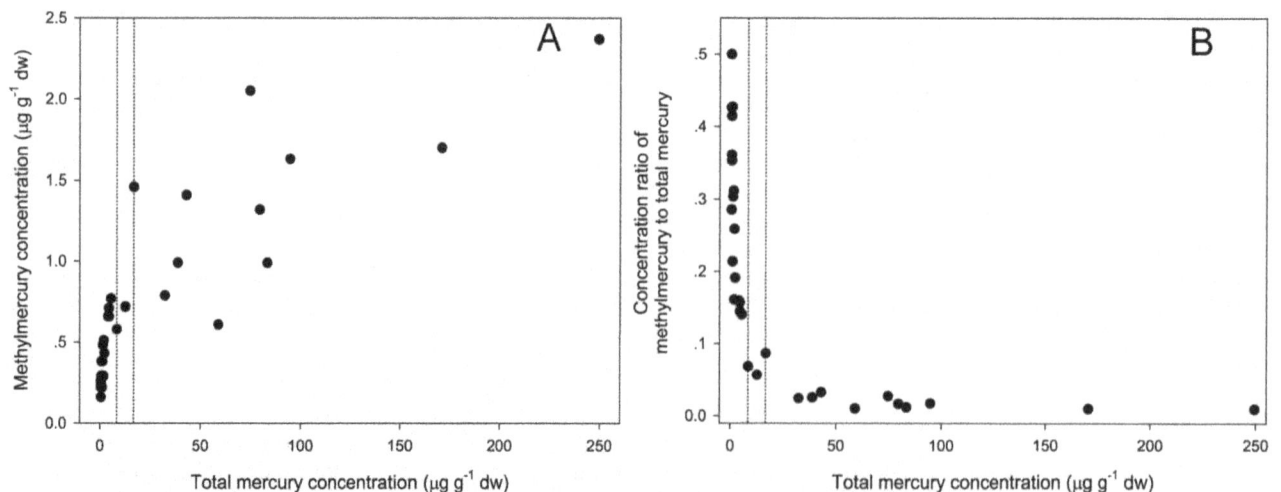

Figure 4. MeHg concentration (µg g^{-1} dw) (A) and concentration ratio of MeHg to THg (B) against THg concentration (µg g^{-1} dw) in the liver samples of the stranded Indo-Pacific humpback dolphins in the Pearl River Estuary region (n = 28).

in the three dolphin tissues were 4.78- to 350-fold greater than the concentrations detected in their prey fish, suggesting that a significant biomagnification process could occur for Hg, especially in the liver. The present study also showed that concentrations of MeHg in the cetacean tissue were 9- to 18-fold higher than the concentrations in the prey fish because of the high assimilation and bioaccumulation capability of MeHg across trophic levels. Conversely, trophic transfer of Se was weak except in dolphin livers. The concentrations of Se in the dolphin muscle tissue were even lower than the concentrations found in the prey fish (BMF< 1), which is likely due to the lack of accumulation or rapid elimination of Se in this tissue. The comparison of THg, Se and MeHg between the dolphin organ tissues and prey fish indicated that THg and MeHg could significantly accumulate in dolphin organs. However, whether THg and MeHg can threaten the health of this cetacean is best determined by the molar ratio of Se/THg, which will be discussed below.

In the marine environment, the dominant portion of Hg in fish and squid is present in the form of MeHg [36]. However, the majority of Hg accumulated in the internal organs of cetaceans appears as inorganic Hg(II), especially in the liver, indicating that a demethylation of MeHg occurs in the liver [34,37]. The formation of the compound Se–Hg, resulting from the combination of a demethylation product (i.e., Hg(II)) and Se, appears to be the last step in the demethylation processes, leading to the fossilization of THg and Se in the form of an inert compound [17,19,38]. In the present study, the relationship between the $\log_{10}$ Se/THg value and $\log_{10}$ MeHg concentration in the livers and kidneys of Indo-Pacific humpback dolphins showed a significant negative correlation (**Fig. 3**). This finding strongly suggests that the Se–Hg compound was formed, causing the fraction of Se/THg in the form of the Se–Hg compound to decrease with respect to the increased MeHg levels [39]. The significant positive relationship between Se and THg and the significant negative correlation between the proportion of MeHg in THg and the THg concentration further confirms that detoxification processes act on MeHg in the livers and kidneys of the dolphins (**Fig. 3** and **Fig. S1**), similar to the results reported for other cetaceans [18,37].

The molar ratio of Se/THg can be considered an indicator of the extent of toxicity caused by Hg contamination because the toxic effects are alleviated after the formation of the Se–Hg compound, which is stable and has no relevant biological impact. Se can be combined with other elements to form various compounds. A molar ratio between Se and THg higher than 1 implies that Se is providing potential protection against Hg toxicity. However, a ratio below 1 suggests limited Se protection against Hg toxicity [40,41]. In the present study, the average molar ratios of Se to THg in the liver, kidney and muscle tissue were 6.03, 21.48 and 6.75, respectively, which are all significantly higher than 1. The high Se/THg ratios in tissues were due to the fact that juveniles comprised most of the analyzed samples and low THg concentrations were found in these samples. However, certain adults had molar ratios below 1 and were in danger of suffering Hg toxicity. According to Caurant et al. [38], young animals were still unable to demethylate MeHg efficiently, leading to higher mean percentages of MeHg/THg concentrations in juveniles than adults. We concluded that a molar ratio of Se/THg of 1 in the organs of adults can be used as an indicator of demethylation processes in the organs. The mean molar ratios of Se/THg in the liver samples of adult dolphins were approximately 1, whereas the mean value in the kidneys was 2.65. However, this

pattern does not preclude the possibility of the demethylation process occurring in the kidneys. Se, as the constituent of selenoprotein P and selenoenzymes, also plays an important role in maintaining the normal functions of the kidneys in addition to its detoxification function against Hg.

The relationship between THg and MeHg in dolphin livers may indirectly reveal how demethylation occurs. In this study (**Fig. 4**A), when the THg concentration was lower than 8.4 µg g^{-1} dw, the MeHg concentration increased significantly, indicating that no demethylation occurred when the body burden of THg was low. However, when the THg concentration increased from 8.4 µg g^{-1} dw to 16.9 µg g^{-1} dw, the increase of MeHg in the livers slowed down because the demethylation process was presumably occurring, although we lack the direct chemical and biochemical evidence to confirm this assumption. The concentration ratio of MeHg to THg was 1.86± 0.8% (Mean ± SD, n = 9) when the THg concentration exceeded 16.9 µg g^{-1} dw, whereas the concentration ratio was 27±11% (Mean ± SD, n = 16) when the THg concentration was below 8.4 µg g^{-1} dw (**Fig. 4**B). Therefore, it is assumed that the demethylation processes could be activated when the THg concentration reaches a threshold range (i.e. 8.4–16.9 µg g^{-1} dw). According to Palmisano et al. [42], mercury is generally stored as MeHg in the livers of dolphins initially, and after a threshold value (100 µg g^{-1} ww) is reached, demethylation takes place with the co-accumulation of Se/THg at a molar ratio of 1:1. In the livers of S. chinensis, Se was significantly related to THg ($R^2 = 0.9740$, $p<0.05$), and the molar ratios of Se/THg in most our samples were far higher than 1 (**Fig. S2**), suggesting that Se was involved in the detoxification process of MeHg.

The co-accumulation of Se/THg with a molar ratio of 1:1 in the livers of cetaceans after a threshold value is reached has been reported by several authors in striped dolphins and Dall's porpoises [42,43]. Together, these results indicated that exceeding the threshold value of THg was a necessarily initial step before triggering the demethylation processes. Compared with the threshold value of striped dolphins (100 µg g^{-1} ww) and Dall's porpoises (20–30 µg g^{-1} dw), a lower THg concentration was found in the present study for S. chinensis. These differences could be attributed to the metabolism and varying foraging habits among the cetacean species, which might also influence the accumulation of Hg and Se, as reflected in the Se/THg molar ratios [12,44]. The lower threshold of hepatic THg concentrations for the equimolar accumulation of Se and Hg in S. chinensis suggests that this species has a greater sensitivity to THg concentrations than is found in striped dolphins and Dall's porpoises.

Conclusions

This study is the first comprehensive investigation on the distribution and fate of THg, MeHg and Se in livers, kidneys and muscles of Indo-Pacific Humpback Dolphins collected for almost 10 years from the PRE of China, and in the prey fishes from the PRE. The results clearly showed that THg and Se were mainly accumulated in dolphin livers while the highest residue of MeHg was found in dolphin muscles. This study contains the first experimental evidence for the potential trophic transfer from the fish to Indo-Pacific Humpback dolphins, showing a high biomagnification factor of Hg_{inorg} in liver (350×) and MeHg in muscle (18.7×). Our studies suggest that the Indo-Pacific humpback dolphins may have the potential to detoxify Hg via the demethylation of MeHg and the formation of tiemannite (HgSe) in the liver and kidney.

Supporting Information

Figure S1 Relationship between log THg (μg g^{-1} dw) and percentage of MeHg/THg in the liver, kidney and muscle of *Sousa chinesis* stranded in the PRE.

Figure S2 (A) Individuals with molar ratio of Se/Hg higher than the threshold range (8.4–16.9 μg g^{-1} dw). (B) Individuals with molar ratio of Se/Hg lower than the threshold range (8.4–16.9 μg g^{-1} dw).

Table S1 Sampling information of *Sousa chinensis* stranded in the Pearl River Estuary.

Acknowledgments

We thank the Guangdong Pearl River Estuary Chinese White Dolphin National Nature Reserve for the logistic service; Mr. Wenzhi Lin, Mr. Xi Chen and Mr. Yinku Wang for collecting samples.

Author Contributions

Conceived and designed the experiments: YW. Performed the experiments: YS QT HM. Analyzed the data: DG RY YS. Contributed reagents/materials/analysis tools: RY DG. Contributed to the writing of the manuscript: DG YW RY YS. Supervised the research: YW RY LC. Revised the manuscript: DG YR YW.

References

1. Compeau G, Bartha R (1985) Sulfate-reducing bacteria: principal methylators of mercury in anoxic estuarine sediment. Appl Environ Microbiol 50: 498–502.
2. Fleming EJ, Mack EE, Green PG, Nelson DC (2006) Mercury methylation from unexpected sources: molybdate-inhibited freshwater sediments and an iron-reducing bacterium. Appl Environ Microbiol 72: 457–464.
3. Hong YS, Hunter S, Clayton LA, Rifkin E, Bouwer EJ (2012) Assessment of mercury and selenium concentrations in captive bottlenose dolphin's (*Tursiops truncatus*) diet fish, blood, and tissue. Sci Total Environ 414: 220–226.
4. Gilmour CC, Podar M, Bullock AL, Graham AM, Brown SD, et al. (2013) Mercury Methylation by Novel Microorganisms from New Environments. Environ Sci Technol 47: 11810–11820.
5. Parks JM, Johs A, Podar M, Bridou R, Hurt RA, et al. (2013) The genetic basis for bacterial mercury methylation. Science 339: 1332–1335.
6. Yu RQ, Flanders J, Mack EE, Turner R, Mirza MB, et al. (2012) Contribution of coexisting sulfate and iron reducing bacteria to methylmercury production in freshwater river sediments. Environ Sci Technol 46: 2684–2691.
7. Yu RQ, Reinfelder JR, Hines ME, Barkay T (2013) Mercury methylation by the methanogen Methanospirillum hungatei. Appl Environ Microbiol 79: 6325–6330.
8. Shi JB, Ip C, Zhang G, Jiang G, Li X (2010) Mercury profiles in sediments of the Pearl River Estuary and the surrounding coastal area of South China. Environ Pollut 158: 1974–1979.
9. Yu X, Li H, Pan K, Yan Y, Wang WX (2012) Mercury distribution, speciation and bioavailability in sediments from the Pearl River Estuary, Southern China. Mar Pollut Bull 64: 1699–1704.
10. Hung CL, So MK, Connell DW, Fung CN, Lam MH, et al. (2004) A preliminary risk assessment of trace elements accumulated in fish to the Indo-Pacific Humpback dolphin (*Sousa chinensis*) in the northwestern waters of Hong Kong. Chemosphere 56: 643–651.
11. Wu Y, Shi J, Zheng GJ, Li P, Liang B, et al. (2013) Evaluation of organochlorine contamination in Indo-Pacific humpback dolphins (*Sousa chinensis*) from the Pearl River Estuary, China. Sci Total Environ 444: 423–429.
12. Kunito T, Nakamura S, Ikemoto T, Anan Y, Kubota R, et al. (2004) Concentration and subcellular distribution of trace elements in liver of small cetaceans incidentally caught along the Brazilian coast. Mar Pollut Bull 49: 574–587.
13. Thompson DR (1990) Metal levels in marine vertebrates. CRC PRESS, BOCA RATON, FL(USA): 143–182.
14. Endo T, Hisamichi Y, Kimura O, Haraguchi K, Baker CS (2008) Contamination levels of mercury and cadmium in melon-headed whales (*Peponocephala electra*) from a mass stranding on the Japanese coast. Sci Total Environ 401: 73–80.
15. Dietz R, Riget F, Born E (2000) An assessment of selenium to mercury in Greenland marine animals. Sci Total Environ 245: 15–24.
16. Moreira I, Seixas T, Kehrig H, Fillmann G, Di Beneditto A, et al. (2009) Selenium and mercury (total and organic) in tissues of a coastal small cetacean, *Pontoporia blainvillei*. J Coast Res: 866–870.
17. Lailson-Brito J, Cruz R, Dorneles PR, Andrade L, Azevedo AdF, et al. (2012) Mercury-Selenium Relationships in Liver of Guiana Dolphin: The Possible Role of Kupffer Cells in the Detoxification Process by Tiemannite Formation. PLoS ONE 7: e42162.
18. Nakazawa E, Ikemoto T, Hokura A, Terada Y, Kunito T, et al. (2011) The presence of mercury selenide in various tissues of the striped dolphin: evidence from μ-XRF-XRD and XAFS analyses. Metallomics 3: 719–725.
19. Nigro M (1994) Mercury and selenium localization in macrophages of the striped dolphin, Stenella coeruleoalba. Journal of the Marine Biological Association of the United Kingdom Plymouth 74: 975–978.
20. Khan MAK, Wang F (2009) Mercury-selenium compounds and their toxicological significance: Toward a molecular understanding of the mercury-selenium antagonism. Environ Toxicol Chem 28: 1567–1577.
21. Jefferson TA (2000) Population biology of the Indo-Pacific hump-backed dolphin in Hong Kong waters. Wildlife monographs: 1–65.
22. Myrck AC Jr., Hohn AA, Sloan PA, Kimura M, Stanley DD (1983) Estimating age of spotted and spinner dolphins (*Stenella attenuata* and *Stenella longirostris*) from teeth.
23. Jefferson TA, Hung SK, Robertson KM, Archer FI (2012) Life history of the Indo-Pacific humpback dolphin in the Pearl River Estuary, southern China. Mar Mammal Sci 28: 84–104.
24. Barros NB, Jefferson TA, Parsons E (2004) Feeding habits of Indo-Pacific humpback dolphins (*Sousa chinensis*) stranded in Hong Kong. Aquat Mamm 30: 179–188.
25. Ruelas-Inzunza JR, Horvat M, Pérez-Cortés H, Páez-Osuna F (2003) Methylmercury and total mercury distribution in tissues of gray whales (*Eschrichtius robustus*) and spinner dolphins (*Stenella longirostris*) stranded along the lower Gulf of California, Mexico. Cienc Mar 29: 1–8.
26. U.S.EPA Method 1630 Methyl Mercury in Water by Distillation, Aqueous Ethylation, Purge and Trap, and Cold Vapor Atomic Fluorescence Spectrometry. US Environmental Protection Agency Office of Water Office of Science and Technology Engineering and Analysis Division (4303) 401 M Street SW Washington, DC 20460.
27. Parsons E (1998) Trace metal pollution in Hong Kong: Implications for the health of Hong Kong's Indo-Pacific hump-backed dolphins (*Sousa chinensis*). Science of the Total Environment 214: 175–184.
28. Wagemann R, Muir DCG (1984) Concentrations of heavy metals and organochlorines in marine mammals of northern waters: overview and evaluation. Western Region, Department of Fisheries and Oceans Canada.
29. Honda K, Tatsukawa R, Itano K, Miyazaki N, Fujiyama T (1983) Heavy metal concentrations in muscle, liver and kidney tissue of striped dolphin, *Stenella coeruleoalba*, and their variations with body length, weight, age and sex. Agric Biol Chem 47: 1219–1228.
30. Leonzio C, Focardi S, Fossi C (1992) Heavy metals and selenium in stranded dolphins of the Northern Tyrrhenian (NW Mediterranean). Sci Total Environ 119: 77–84.
31. Martoja R, Berry JP (1981) Identification of tiemannite as a probable product of demethylation of mercury by selenium in cetaceans. A complement to the scheme of the biological cycle of mercury [detoxification]. Vie Milieu.
32. Storelli M, Ceci E, Marcotrigiano G (1998) Comparison of total mercury, methylmercury, and selenium in muscle tissues and in the liver of *Stenella coeruleoalba* (Meyen) and *Caretta caretta* (Linnaeus). Bull Environ Contam Toxicol 61: 541–547.
33. Wren CD (1986) A review of metal accumulation and toxicity in wild mammals: I. Mercury. Environ Res 40: 210–244.
34. Meador J, Ernest D, Hohn A, Tilbury K, Gorzelany J, et al. (1999) Comparison of elements in bottlenose dolphins stranded on the beaches of Texas and Florida in the Gulf of Mexico over a one-year period. Arch Environ Contam Toxicol 36: 87–98.
35. André J, Ribeyre F, Boudou A (1990) Mercury contamination levels and distribution in tissues and organs of delphinids (*Stenella attenuata*) from the Eastern Tropical Pacific, in relation to biological and ecological factors. Mar Environ Res 30: 43–72.
36. Das K, Debacker V, Bouquegneau JM (2000) Metallothioneins in marine mammals. Cell Mol Biol 46.
37. Holsbeek L, Siebert U, Joiris CR (1998) Heavy metals in dolphins stranded on the French Atlantic coast. Sci Total Environ 217: 241–249.
38. Caurant F, Navarro M, Amiard JC (1996) Mercury in pilot whales: possible limits to the detoxification process. Sci Total Environ 186: 95–104.
39. Cáceres-Saez I, Dellabianca NA, Goodall RNP, Cappozzo HL, Guevara SR (2013) Mercury and Selenium in Subantarctic Commerson's Dolphins (*Cephalorhynchus c. commersonii*). Biol Trace Elem Res 151: 195–208.

40. Peterson SA, Ralston NV, Peck DV, Sickle JV, Robertson JD, et al. (2009) How might selenium moderate the toxic effects of mercury in stream fish of the western US? Environ Sci Technol 43: 3919–3925.

41. Sørmo EG, Ciesielski TM, Øverjordet IB, Lierhagen S, Eggen GS, et al. (2011) Selenium Moderates Mercury Toxicity in Free-Ranging Freshwater Fish. Environ Sci Technol 45: 6561–6566.

42. Palmisano F, Cardellicchio N, Zambonin P (1995) Speciation of mercury in dolphin liver: a two-stage mechanism for the demethylation accumulation process and role of selenium. Mar Environ Res 40: 109–121.

43. Yang J, Kunito T, Tanabe S, Miyazaki N (2007) Mercury and its relation with selenium in the liver of Dall's porpoises (*Phocoenoides dalli*) off the Sanriku coast of Japan. Environ Pollut 148: 669–673.

44. Seixas TG, Kehrig HdA, Fillmann G, Di Beneditto APM, Souza CM, et al. (2007) Ecological and biological determinants of trace elements accumulation in liver and kidney of *Pontoporia blainvillei*. Sci Total Environ 385: 208–220.

8

Dose Schedule Optimization and the Pharmacokinetic Driver of Neutropenia

Mayankbhai Patel, Santhosh Palani, Arijit Chakravarty, Johnny Yang, Wen Chyi Shyu, Jerome T. Mettetal*

Drug Metabolism and Pharmacokinetics, Takeda Pharmaceuticals International Co., Cambridge, Massachusetts, United States of America

Abstract

Toxicity often limits the utility of oncology drugs, and optimization of dose schedule represents one option for mitigation of this toxicity. Here we explore the schedule-dependency of neutropenia, a common dose-limiting toxicity. To this end, we analyze previously published mathematical models of neutropenia to identify a pharmacokinetic (PK) predictor of the neutrophil nadir, and confirm this PK predictor in an *in vivo* experimental system. Specifically, we find total AUC and C_{max} are poor predictors of the neutrophil nadir, while a PK measure based on the moving average of the drug concentration correlates highly with neutropenia. Further, we confirm this PK parameter for its ability to predict neutropenia *in vivo* following treatment with different doses and schedules. This work represents an attempt at mechanistically deriving a fundamental understanding of the underlying pharmacokinetic drivers of neutropenia, and provides insights that can be leveraged in a translational setting during schedule selection.

Editor: Junxuan Lu, Texas Tech Univ School of Pharmacy, United States of America

Funding: All authors were employees of Takeda Pharmaceuticals International Co. at the time of these studies and therefore had a role in study design, data collection and analysis, decision to publish, and preparation of the manuscript.

Competing Interests: All authors are employees of Takeda Pharmaceuticals International Co.

* Email: mettetal@alum.mit.edu

Introduction

Balancing antitumor efficacy with toxicity remains a fundamental challenge in the development of antineoplastic agents, both for traditional chemotherapeutics and for the newer generation of targeted therapies. Therefore, a better understanding of the relationship between schedule and toxicity assumes a critical role in development of novel agents; as such an understanding would permit the rational selection of dosing schedules during the early clinical development of oncology drugs that could decrease the likelihood of adverse events while maintaining drug exposure and efficacy.

A common side-effect for many oncology drugs, (including both chemotherapeutic as well as targeted therapies), is hematological toxicity or myelosuppression [1–5]. In many cases, this hematological toxicity is clearly mechanism-related, as bone marrow stem cells represent a rapidly dividing population of cells that is vulnerable to antineoplastic agents that interfere with cell division and survival. Of the hematological toxicities, neutropenia is one of the most common reasons for chemotherapy delay and dose reduction [6,7]. A significant drop in absolute neutrophil counts (ANC) has been demonstrated to be linked to the incidence of serious adverse events (such as sepsis, febrile neutropenia and other life-threatening infections). While neutropenia is serious, it is also easily monitored and anticipated. There is often a strong schedule-dependent component to neutropenia, for example with taxanes in breast cancer, where weekly administration of drug resulted in a reduced toxicity profile relative to once-every-three weeks administration [8–12]. The active design of dosing

schedules to limit the incidence of neutropenia, therefore, holds the potential of significant impact in the development of novel antineoplastic agents.

Much research has been focused on understanding the underlying PK driver of neutropenia in the clinic. A variety of model forms have been used to describe the relationship between neutropenia and overall drug exposure, such as linear [13–15], log-linear [16], nonlinear [17–19], and logistic regression [20–24] models. However, capturing the underlying relationship between pharmacokinetics (PK) and toxicity can often be challenging, as patient data is often analyzed from a single dose schedule and exposure metrics derived from these studies, such as AUC (Area Under the Curve) or C_{max} (maximum concentration of drug during the treatment period), are typically highly correlated with one another on any fixed schedule. This complexity often makes it complicated to extract a single simple PK parameter directly from empirical models of induction of neutropenia that have been described in the clinic [9,11,12,25].

Here we take an alternative approach to mitigate the issue of correlations between PK parameters on experimentally tested schedules by utilizing prior knowledge built into semi-mechanistic models. These models have been successfully applied to predict not only the probability of occurrence, but also the time-course of neutropenia. These models work by combining a model of drug PK and compound specific myelosuppression potential with a model of the underlying biology of the blood-cell life cycle [26–34]. The semi-mechanistic models represent an advance over exposure metrics, as they provide a more complete description of

ANC kinetics, and permit the comparison of different schedules for their potential to induce neutropenia. Interestingly, it is has been shown that models for chemotherapy-induced neutropenia can be based primarily on systemic (patient-specific) parameters for the bone marrow hematopoietic cascade, with a limited number of drug-specific parameters [26].

In this work we seek to identify an underlying PK parameter that predicts the degree of neutropenia by analyzing the dynamic and severity of neutropenia derived from the semi-mechanistic models of neutropenia in response to a variety of dosing schedules [26,35–39]. First, we sought to determine whether there were any schedules that were less likely to induce neutropenia. Next, we analyzed the schedules to determine which PK parameter was most closely linked to the severity of neutropenia nadir. Finally, we tested the identified PK parameter on a set of *in vivo* neutrophil counts to demonstrate the validity and utility of the approach, independent of the model. The approach presented here is a natural extension of the foundational work done on semi-mechanistic models of neutropenia, and represents a mechanistic insight into the behavior of these models with practical implications for clinical study design and interpretation.

Results

Effect of Dosing Schedules on Docetaxel Induced ANC-nadir

Clinical observations have shown that even for constant total dose per cycle, different dose schedules (e.g. frequency of dosing or infusion time) can lead to very distinct neutrophil dynamics and incidence of neutropenia [22,27,34,36,39–42]. Therefore, we used the Friberg model of neutropenia to study in detail how drug plasma time course correlated with incidence or severity by employing previously published semi-mechanistic population PK-PD models (Figure 1a) built from clinical ANC profiles following treatment with docetaxel [26,34].

First, a range of different schedules were generated over an interval of eighty-four days keeping the total dose of docetaxel fixed (to match total exposure). The schedules tested were of the form of days-on/days-off, where an interval of continuous dosing (days-on) is followed by a holiday (days-off) before repeating the cycle on a fixed period. For example Q3W (once every three weeks) dosing can be expressed as one day of dosing within a 21 day period. Figure 1b illustrates several examples of the PK and ANC dynamics that result from various dosing schedules for a fixed total dose (equivalent to 100 mg/m^2 given every three weeks).

ANC profiles were then simulated for a virtual population of 1000 patients for these schedules. Two different total dose levels, representing a high and low clinical dose range, were tested (Table 1). The results are shown in Figure 2a and 2c as a heat map of median ANC nadir (minimal absolute neutrophil count) for the simulated patient population under docetaxel treatment on a variety of schedules. Points along the diagonal in the plot (y = x) represent schedules with constant (QD) dosing. As can be seen in Figures 2a and 2c, the points in the upper left corner (e.g. a larger and less frequent dose) have a more severe ANC nadir compared to frequent dosing, and this trend is conserved both for low (Figure 2a) and high (Figure 2c) total dose.

The probability of an individual patient developing grade-4 neutropenia (defined as neutrophil count below $0.5 \times 10^9/\text{L}$) is shown in Figure 2b and 2d with similar trends as neutropenia nadir. Median ANC nadir is a good predictor of incidence of grade-4 neutropenia within the virtual population with an $R^2 = 0.91$ ($p < 0.0001$). Since both the ANC nadir and the probability of developing grade-4 neutropenia show similar schedule-dependent trends, we next asked what correlation existed between the two measures across schedules.

PK driver of neutropenia

Based on the prediction that frequent low doses of docetaxel would induce less neutropenia than infrequent large doses, we hypothesized the existence of a PK parameter for each schedule that would correlate directly with the simulated ANC nadir. To this end, we first examined two common PK parameters, C_{max} and total cycle AUC, for correlation with the median ANC nadir. The schedule-dependent C_{max} correlates poorly with the median ANC nadir ($R^2 = 0.10$, $p < 0.05$; Figure 3a). The total cycle AUC was also tested to see if it could explain the schedule-to-schedule differences in ANC nadir. The very low correlation between total cycle AUC and the median ANC nadir ($R^2 = <0.01$, $p > 0.75$) suggests that AUC alone is not fully accounting for the neutropenia effect. It is not surprising that AUC is not correlated, since total cycle AUC should be constant for linear PK and a fixed total dose.

Since total cycle AUC and C_{max} are not strongly associated with neutropenia at a fixed totally cycle dose, we sought another PK parameter that would be a better predictor of neutropenia. We examined the model under simplified linear conditions and found that the circulating neutrophil counts over time could be approximated analytically by a weighted moving average of the drug concentration over time (see Methods S1). We therefore tested a PK parameter ($c_{avg,ndays}$) based on the moving average concentration, which only considers concentrations over a set window of time (n_{days}). At each point in time, the moving average concentration is simply the average concentration over a set preceding interval of time, and is related to AUC over n_{days}. The moving average is therefore capturing drug exposure occurring in the recent past (set by n_{days}) but not exposures in the very distant past.

To assess the ability of this parameter to predict the neutropenia nadir, however, we must determine the duration over which the moving average is calculated, n_{days}. To accomplish this, we assessed the correlation between median neutropenia nadir (maximal neutropenia) and $\max(c_{avg,ndays})$ over all schedules. The time-interval over which the moving average was calculated, n_{days}, was varied from 1 day to 28 days. The correlation is plotted in Figure 3b, showing that the parameter correlates best with a moving average window set to 16 days. In Figure 3c the median ANC nadir is compared with $\max(c_{avg,16days})$ for all tested schedules, and is found to be a good predictor of the incidence of grade 4 neutropenia ($R^2 = 0.86$, $p < 0.01$). As a further test, we also examined the ability of $\max(c_{avg,16days})$ to predict the degree of neutropenia within the high and low total dose levels separately, and this again shows a strong correlation ($R^2 = 0.77$ ($p < 0.01$) and $R^2 = 0.85$ ($p < 0.01$) for high and low total dose respectively). This strong correlation suggests that the moving average is a good predictor of the neutropenia nadir.

This result suggests that the neutrophil system has a 'memory' of roughly two weeks in duration (10–20 days), meaning that this is roughly the amount of time needed for the stem cell compartment to have recovered sufficiently in response to a single bolus drug exposure. This parameter provides a quick and easy principle for direct ranking of different dosing schedules based on the expected neutropenia effect. For example, schedules which have the greatest maximal exposure over a two week period will be expected to produce the most severe neutropenia nadir.

A)

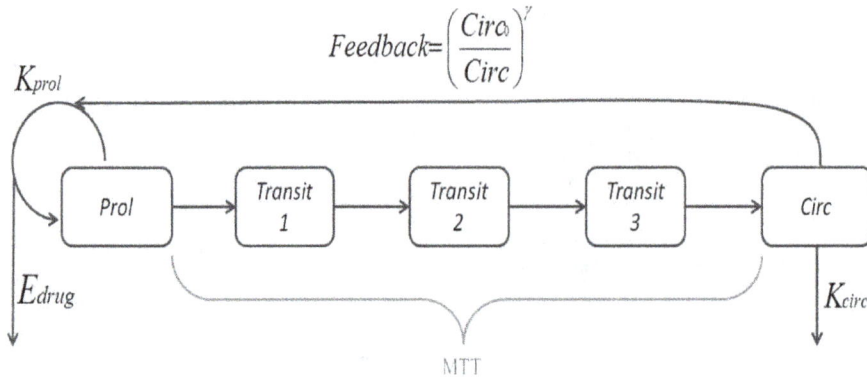

B)

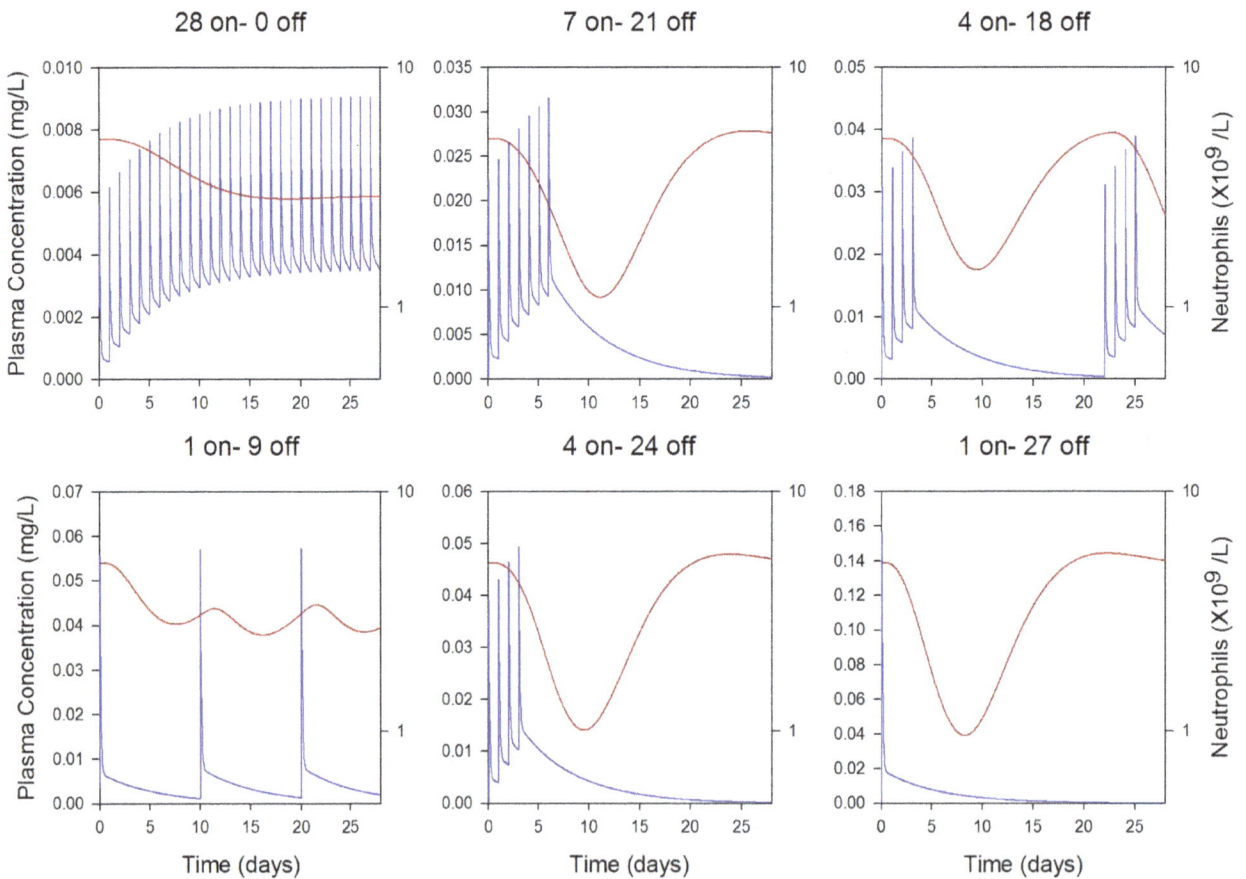

Figure 1. Model structure and simulated ANC time-course. (A) The structure of semi-mechanistic pharmacokinetic-pharmacodynamic Friberg model (from ref [26]) used to describe cytotoxic effect of drugs on proliferating neutrophils. Drug PK was linked to the semi-mechanistic PD model for neutrophil kinetics and unique PK-ANC profile for given drug at various schedules was generated. (B) Docetaxel PK-ANC simulation was carried out at an equivalent total dose to 100 mg/m² every 21 days. The plots show the plasma PK profile (blue lines) and ANC upon treatment (red lines) for schedules of 28 on-0 off, 7 on-21 off, 4 on-18 off, 1 on-9 off, 4 on–24 off and 1 on-27off.

Generalization of findings to other drugs

Having identified a PK parameter, $\max(c_{avg,16days})$, that highly correlates with the severity of neutropenia induced by docetaxel, we then sought to demonstrate that this parameter was an intrinsic property of the neutrophil system and not specific to docetaxel. The analysis was therefore extended to include both etoposide and topotecan (Figures S1, S2, and S3). To test if the moving average concentration, $\max(c_{avg,16days})$, is a property of the neutrophil

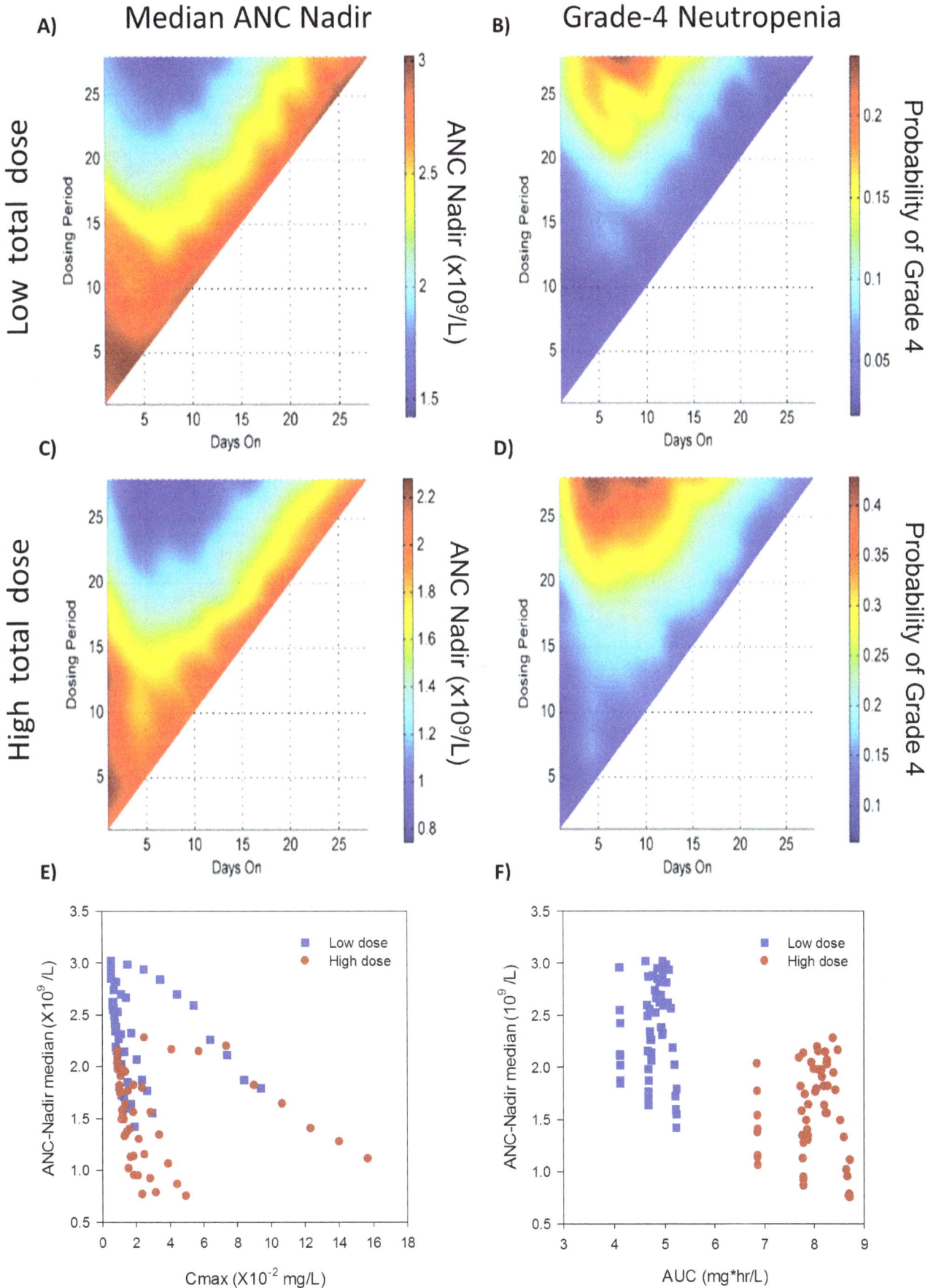

Figure 2. Effect of schedule on docetaxel induced neutropenia. Summary of population simulation of PK-ANC model for 1000 virtual individuals at two total dose levels of docetaxel shows constant dosing induces a less severe nadir than punctuated dosing. Population median ANC nadir for low (A) total dose and high (C) total dose as well as probability of grade 4 neutropenia (nadir $<0.5\times109/L$) are shown for low (B) and high (D) dosing total dose levels. Each plotted captures schedules with the "days-on/days-off" format with number of consecutive days on in given treatment period shown on the X-axis and treatment period (sum of days on and days off) on the Y axis. Population estimation of median ANC nadir and probability of grade-4 neutropenia compared with common PK parameters across variety of schedules for low (blue) and high (red) total dose. (E) C_{max} plotted against median ANC nadir for each of the schedules tested and shows weak correlation of -0.32 ($R^2=0.10$, $p<0.01$). (F) Total cycle AUC over all schedules shows overall correlation of -0.64 ($R^2=0.41$, $p<0.01$) with median ANC nadir, but the correlation is mainly driven by the differences in total dose as it loses ability to predict neutropenia at a fixed total dose level ($R^2<0.01$ and $p>0.75$ at low and high total dose).

system alone, we tested if this parameter was a good predictor independent of the drug inducing the neutropenia. For topotecan, which has a linear drug-effect model [26,34], the moving average of concentration is strongly predictive for ANC nadir ($R^2=0.79$, $p<0.01$; Figure 4a and Figure S1). On the other hand, compared to clinically relevant plasma exposures, etoposide was found to have a highly nonlinear relationship between drug concentration and effect on the stem cell compartment [26,34]. To account for the nonlinearity, we therefore used the moving average of concentration below IC_{50} of the drug (see methods) and the moving average of this parameter again is strongly predictive ($R^2=0.84$, $p<0.01$; Figure 4b and Figure S2).

In vivo ANC analysis

We next sought to determine if the PK parameter determined from the model was appropriate for analyzing *in vivo* data. To this end, we measured ANC levels in rats after administration of TAK-960, an investigational inhibitor of Polo-Like Kinase (PLK), a target known to induce neutropenia [43]. A variety of schedules and dose levels were tested to study the correlation between ANC nadir and PK in this system, each giving a different C_{max} and AUC which were calculated from a rat PK model (Figure S4). The time-course of circulating neutrophils was then assessed and normalized to control (Figure 5a). From this, the PK-ANC correlation was tested for AUC (Figure 5b) and C_{max} (Figure 5c), and shows a weak correlation for both ($R^2=0.18$ ($p=0.40$) and $R^2=0.09$ ($p=0.55$)), respectively. Since rat neutrophil development has a different timescale than in human [36] we again adjusted the n-days over which we tested the maximal moving average correlation with neutrophil nadir. For n-day values between 3 and 6, the correlation is strong ($R^2=0.70$) and statistically significant ($p<0.05$) (Figure 5d-5e). The ~3- fold difference between the nadir-predictive moving average between human (16 days) and rat (3–6 days) can be explained by the differences in the mean transit time in the human and rat neutropenia models [26,36].

Discussion

Identifying the PK parameter related to a pharmacological effect is important for schedule optimization, as well as for assessing dose-response relationships in the clinic. Often, when looking at clinical data, one has only one or two schedules to compare, which can make it difficult to decouple the effect of PK parameters which are often highly correlated between tested schedules. In this work we have attempted to bridge this gap by using a hybrid approach based on systems pharmacology and dose-response analysis. First we identified a potential PK driver by probing and mathematically analyzing the dynamic models built from clinical time-course of pharmacodynamic endpoints, and then validated the PK parameter retrospectively from experimental *in vivo* data. The result is a PK parameter that can be prospectively applied to analyze and select between alternative dosing schedules.

We found that the relationship between neutropenia nadir and schedule was not well explained by either total cycle AUC or C_{max}. For AUC, this parameter is often more closely related to the total cycle dose and number of dosing cycles, than it is to the schedule of administration. For example, a patient undergoing treatment for two cycles would have twice the total cycle AUC of a patient undergoing a single cycle of treatment, but would not necessarily be expected to endure twice the nadir depth as a patient exposed to a single cycle. Similarly, C_{max} can often correlate more closely with the size of the dose more than with the schedule of administration. With regard to neutropenia, a second dose given before the stem cell compartment has fully recovered will be expected to induce a more severe nadir than a second dose given after stem cell compartment has fully recovered to pretreatment levels.

On the other hand neutrophil counts will eventually return to baseline sometime after drug has been cleared from the system, so at any point in time the system response is likely determined by drug exposures experienced in the recent past (e.g. a few days ago) but not in the distant past (e.g. over a year ago). Neutropenia can therefore be thought of as a transient response, which 'remembers' events up to some point in the past but 'forgets' events that occurred prior to that. In this context, it is not surprising, then that C_{max} and AUC did not faithfully capture the severity of neutropenia induced by various schedules. C_{max}, for example, is a parameter with an infinitely short 'memory' and only represents the maximal instantaneous concentration (see Equation 2). On the other hand total AUC has an infinitely long 'memory', treating drug exposure from the recent past equally as strongly as drug exposures that occurred in the very distant past (see Equation 3).

Instead, based on an analytical analysis of the Friberg model of the transient neutrophil response to drug, we introduced a PK

Table 1. Equivalent total dose used in generation of simulated dosing schedules.

Dose Strength	Docetaxel	Topotecan	Etoposide
Low Dose	60 mg/m2 every 3 week	1.5 mg/m2 given as 30 min infusion on day 1,3 and 5 repeated 3 week	50 mg/m2 given as 30 min infusion for 5 days every 3 week
High Dose	100 mg/m2 every three week	4 mg/m2 given as 30 min infusion on day 1,3 and 5 repeated 3 week	100 mg/m2 given as 30 min infusion for 5 days every 3 week

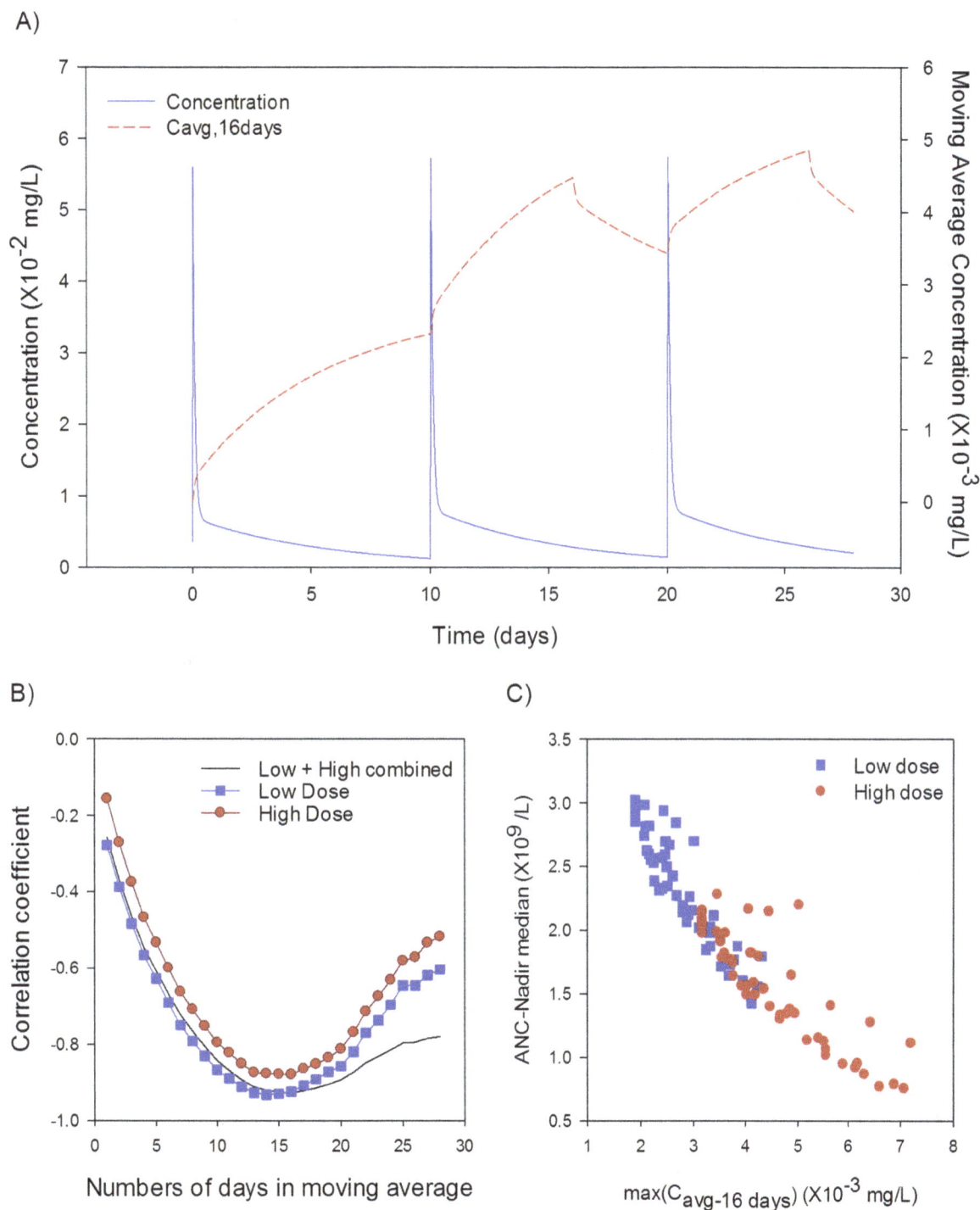

Figure 3. Moving average of PK describes neutropenia. The maximum of the moving average concentration over the dosing interval was examined for its ability to predict the simulated median ANC nadir. (A) Example of the 16-day moving average calculated from concentration profile from 1on-9off dosing schedule. (B) The correlation between maximal moving average concentration and ANC nadir was calculated for sliding windows of 1 day to 28 days for low dose (blue squares), high dose (red circles), and combination (black line). The maximum ability to predict neutropenia for the combined low and high total doses occurs when the moving average is calculated over 16 days. (C) The maximum of the moving average concentration, max($C_{avg,16day}$), accounts for most of the variability in median ANC nadir across total dose and schedule ($R^2 = 0.86$, $p < 0.01$).

parameter based on the moving average concentration which captures the timescales inherent in the development and recovery of neutropenia. This parameter is related to the AUC that the system sees over a specific time period, rather than over the entire

treatment duration, and it provides a quick and easy method for comparing dosing schedules. For example, it suggests that schedules with a lower total exposure given over a two week

A)

Topotecan

B)

Etoposide

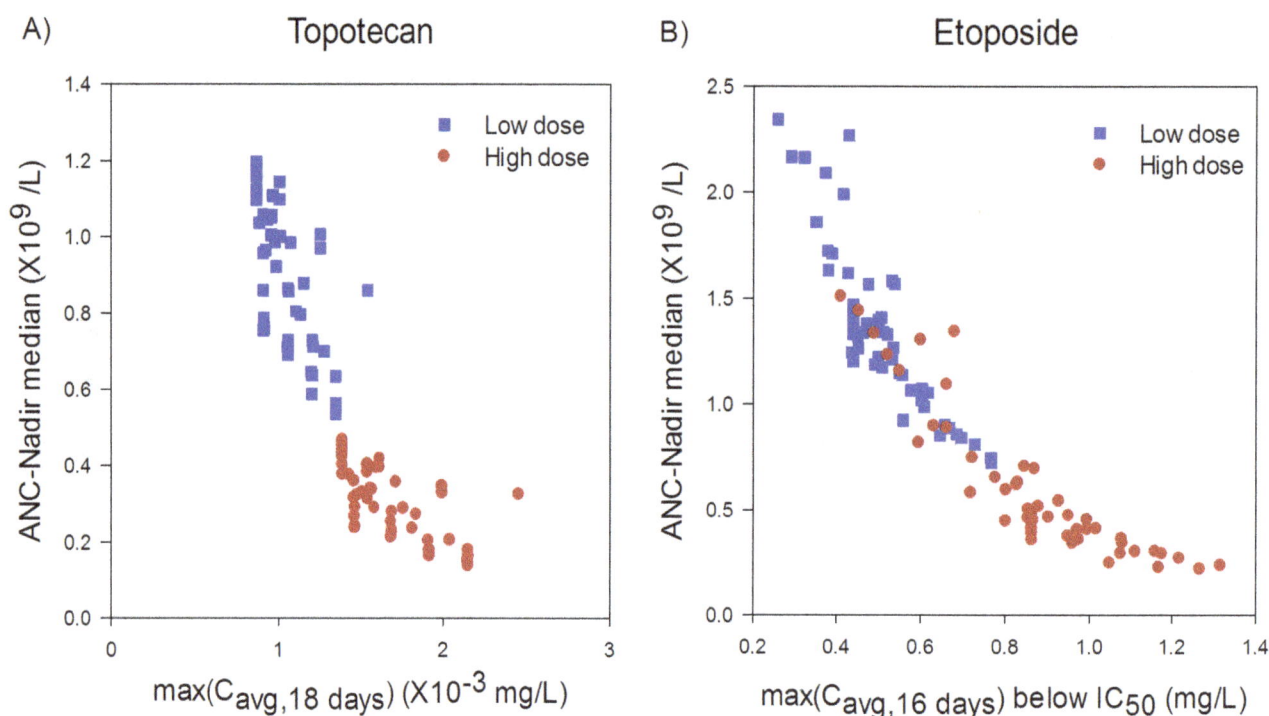

Figure 4. Consistency of moving average of PK in describing severity of neutropenia across drugs. The maximum of the moving average concentration over the dosing interval was examined for its consistency to predict neutropenia across different drugs. Topotecan induced neutropenia was simulated using linear drug effect model while in case of Etoposide, simulation was carried out using nonlinear drug effect (E_{max}) model. (A) The maximum of moving average concentration over 18 days, $\max(C_{avg,18day})$, turns out to be a good predictor of Topotecan induced median ANC nadir($R^2 = 0.79$, $p < 0.01$). While in case of Etoposide the maximum of moving average concentration below threshold over 16 days i.e IC_{50}, $\max(C_{avg,16day} < IC_{50})$, shows maximum ability to predict Etoposide induced median ANC nadir across total dose and schedules($R^2 = 0.84$, $p < 0.01$).

interval tend to produce less severe neutropenia nadirs and therefore lower probability of neutropenia incidence.

This model-derived insight differs from the conventional wisdom on the dosing schedule development for agents that induce neutropenia, where the goal is typically to space doses apart widely to provide enough time for the bone marrow to recover. Our work demonstrates that in many cases lower dose levels with more frequent administration of drug induced less neutropenia than larger infrequent doses, which is consistent with the published literature on taxanes [8–12,25]. This finding has both a clinical and biological relevance for the future development of agents that induce neutropenia. Findings such as this also point to the value of a simplified PK parameter (such as the moving average) in decision-making, as it provides a simple way to assess clinical exposure-response data for homeostatic processes like production of circulating neutrophils.

When evaluating any model, it is especially important to keep in mind the assumptions that went into constructing it. One assumption that went into this analysis, is that inter-patient variability is constant across schedules being tested. For example, interpretation of results from clinical trials with different formulations [44] can be complicated by differences in magnitude and inter-individual variability of the bioavailability between the two formulations [45]. Similarly, it is worth noting the shape of the antiproliferative concentration-effect relationship for a compound. Based on previous model fitting exercises which assessed the best model fit for neutropenia, docetaxel and etoposide were both simulated using an E_{max} model for concentration effect rather than the simple linear concentration-effect relationship that was found

to fit best for topotecan. At the low, clinically relevant, concentrations, docetaxel effectively had a nearly linear relationship since concentrations spent little time above IC_{90}. To demonstrate how to correct for highly nonlinear compounds, we used the example of etoposide which had a low IC_{50} relative to plasma concentration, resulting in a different rank order of schedules for the compound (Figure S5). Here instead, we examined average concentration below IC_{50}, and found the moving average was still able to accurately capture the variability between schedules.

Clinical utility is a combination of safety and efficacy, and the goal of this study was to identify the predominant schedule effects driving neutropenia, a common safety endpoint. In many cases, total cycle exposure is likely to be an important determinant of efficacy. For example, dose fractionation of taxanes in the clinic have led to sustained efficacy (8, 10), and preclinical work often shows linear or saturating efficacy with increased concentration (46). In these scenarios, directly comparing schedules with equivalent total exposure as done in this study is appropriate, as schedules that maintain total exposure would not be expected to reduce efficacy even when resulting in a lower C_{max}. Even for compounds when total cycle exposure is not the key determinant, the results we present with respect to identification of PK driver of neutropenia can still be used in conjunction with a similar PK determinant of efficacy to identify an optimal schedule. These results provide guidance for prioritization of schedules from a physiological perspective, and would therefore need to be verified directly in the clinic. Any decisions of clinical utility of an

A)

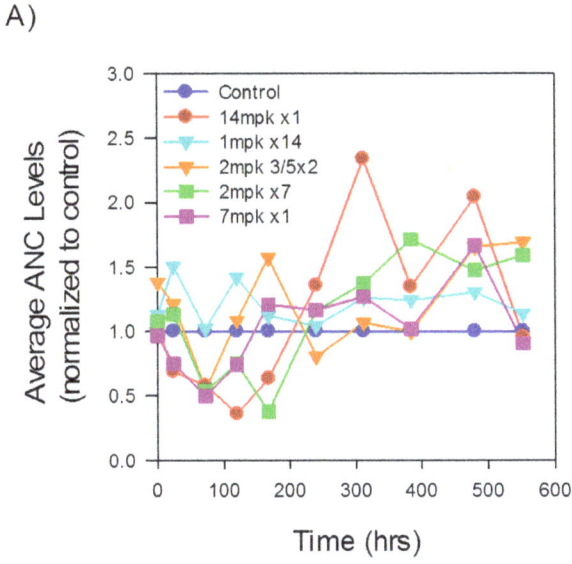

B)

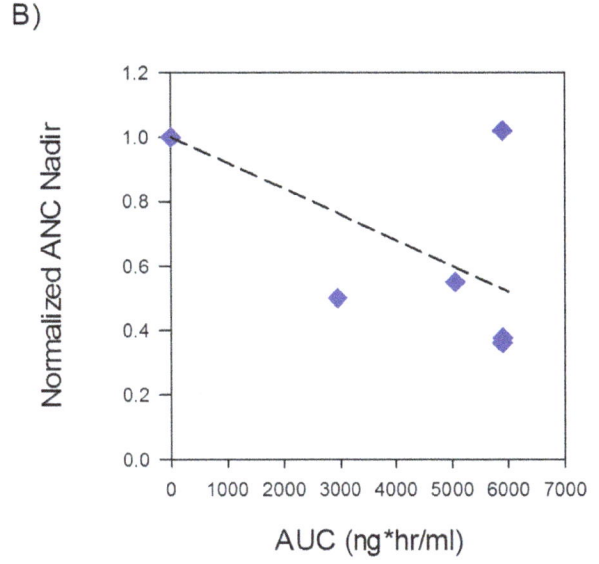

C)

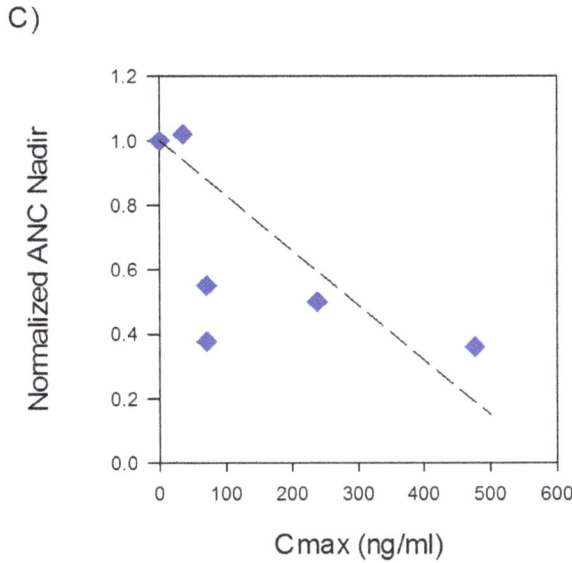

D)

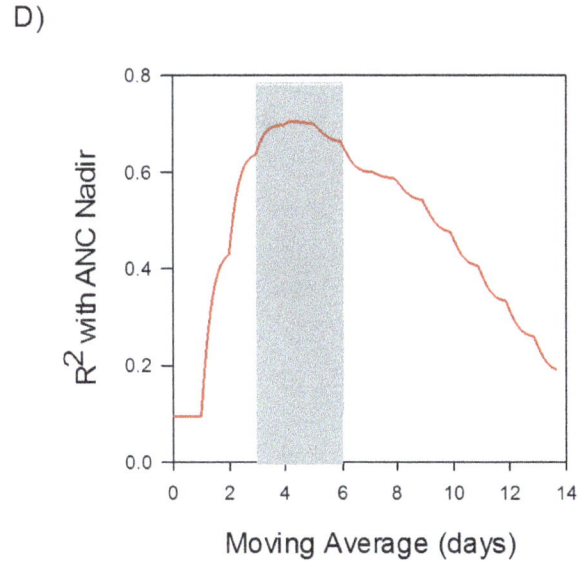

E)

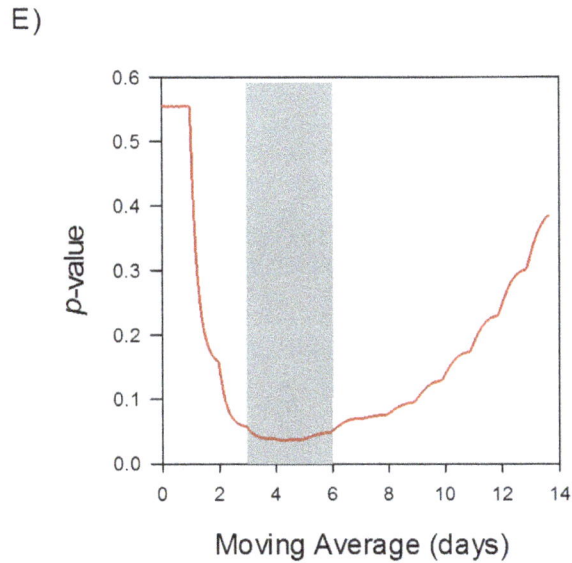

F)

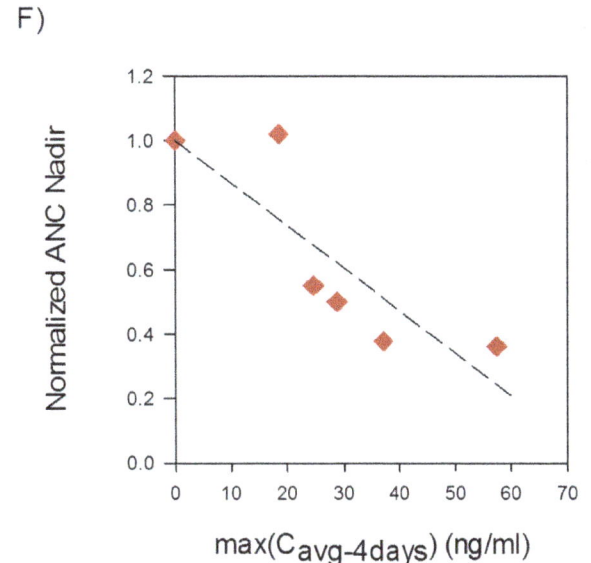

Figure 5. Moving average PK describes rat neutrophil counts. Rat neutrophil counts were measured response to the investigational PLK inhibitor TAK-960 and the relationship between plasma PK and neutrophil nadir was assessed. A) Absolute Neutrophil Count (ANC) normalized to control group plotted over the course of 21 days on a variety of dosing regimens. B) Normalized ANC nadir plotted versus total cycle AUC for each schedule tested. C) Normalized ANC nadir plotted versus the C_{max} for each schedule tested. D) R^2 plotted for $C_{avg,ndays}$ for n-days from 1 to 14 days. E) The corresponding p-values of the $C_{avg,ndays}$ correlation showing correlation. F) Normalized ANC nadir is highly correlated with $max(C_{avg,4days})$ with $R^2 = 0.70$ ($p < 0.05$), a better correlation than either C_{max} or AUC.

optimized schedule would need to then be considered from a cost-benefit analysis before implementation.

The moving average concentration has the inherent ability to capture a wide variety of timescales and can elicit properties of either C_{max} or AUC depending on the timescale over which the average is calculated. For example when the moving average window is very short compared to the PK of the compound (e.g. n_{days} on the order of hours) the $max(c_{avg,ndays})$ closely reflects C_{max} respond acutely to instantaneous concentration of drug. On the other hand, for a longer moving average window (e.g. n_{days} on the order of weeks or months), $max(c_{avg,ndays})$ more closely correlates with a total cycle AUC, and would therefore reflect the entire history of drug exposure.

It is likely that the concept of moving average concentration could be applicable to other types of toxicity beyond neutropenia. As with neutropenia, the moving average timescale could be taken to represent the inherent time over which any toxic endpoint is induced and transiently recovers. The moving average is a feature of the memory of such a system, and would therefore apply to cases where homeostatic mechanisms bring the system back to baseline sometime after pharmacological intervention is removed. Once the timescale (n_{days}) for a particular toxicity is understood, it can become much easier to develop optimal dosing schedules to avoid inducing toxic events. We thus expect that the moving average concentration concept introduced here may have broad applicability as a PK parameter in analysis of many types of pharmacological activities, regardless of the timescale over which they develop and dissipate.

Methods

Ethical Statement

This study was performed in strict accordance with the recommendations in the Guide for the Care and Use of Laboratory Animals to ensure good science and animal care and welfare through compliance with internal policies as well as external regulatory agencies. The protocol was reviewed and approved for compliance with these regulations prior to study initiation by Millennium's Institutional Animal Care and Use Committee IACUC Committee (Protocol Number: 08-009, Study # DSD-01321). All animal were sacrificed at end of experiment using surgery using pentobarbital (iv) with accepted American Veterinary Medical Association (AVMA) guidelines, and every effort was made to minimize suffering.

Neutropenia Model

The semi-mechanistic PK-PD model described by Friberg et al. [26], has been used in the current study and is shown in Figure 1a. The population PK-PD simulation was carried out using parameters in references [26,34] with inter-individual variability incorporated on Circ0, MTT and drug effect parameters Slope or EC_{50}. Here non-linear drug effect (E_{max}) model was used to simulated ANC profiles upon docetaxel and etoposide administration, while topotecan induced myelosuppression was simulated using linear drug effect model (Table 2). Plasma concentration time profiles for all three drugs were simulated using published

clinical PK models [27,30,46]. Using the PK-PD model, overall effect of drug fractionation on neutrophil counts was simulated for various schedules by keeping the total dose constant. All simulations were done for 84 days (corresponding to 28 days/cycle ×3 dosing cycles). The pharmacokinetics (PK) of topotecan, etoposide and docetaxel were simulated using typical population PK model parameters (Table S1). PK profiles were simulated for a wide range of schedules maintaining clinical recommended total doses (high dose and low dose, Table 1). Docetaxel was dosed as an IV bolus while topotecan and etoposide were dosed as short 30 minute infusions. Population PK-PD simulation was carried out using NONMEM Ver 7.1 for populations of 1000 virtual patients. Population simulations were analyzed with MATLAB (Mathworks, Natick, MA) and ANC nadir (median), ANC Nadir (90th percentile), probability of grade-3 neutropenia (ANC less than 1×10^9 neutrophils/liter) and probability of grade-4 neutropenia (ANC less than 0.5×10^9 neutrophils/liter) were estimated. Probability of grade-4 neutropenia for more than seven continuous days was also calculated for each schedule from population simulations (Figure S6). The AUC of plasma concentration time profile for all drugs was calculated by noncompartmental analysis using the linear trapezoidal rule. The Pearson correlation coefficient was calculated in excel to measure correlation between two arrays of interest. Linear regression analysis was performed using graphpad PRISM (GraphPad Software, Inc., CA).

Rat PK and ANC measurements

Single dose of TAK-960 was administered via oral gavage to male Sprague Dawley rats (n = 3), 8–10 weeks of age, at 7 mg/kg and 14 mg/kg to estimate the PK profile. Blood samples were collected at 0, 0.5, 1, 2, 4, 8 and 24 hours. All blood samples were centrifuged to obtain plasma and freeze at $\leq -70°C$ till analysis. A one-compartmental extravascular PK model adequately described the concentration-time profile of TAK-960 in rats (Figure S4). The PK model fitting and PK simulations were performed using Phoenix (Pharsight).

A repeat-dose hematological toxicity study of TAK-960 administered via oral gavage was performed on male Sprague Dawley rats. Six study groups with six rats per group were given the following PO schedules: vehicle (0.5% methylcellulose 1500 cps), 1 mg/kg QD days 1–14, 2 mg/kg QD days 1–7, 2 mg/kg 3on/4off 2 cycles, 7 mg/kg single dose and 14 mg/kg single dose. C_{max} and AUC estimates from the PK model for each schedule are provided in the Table S2. Blood samples were collected periodically to estimate the absolute neutrophil count.

Comparison of PK Parameters: Maximal Moving Average, Total Cycle AUC, and Cmax:

The moving average concentration is defined over a time interval, n_{days}, using the formula in Eq. 1 and was calculated from simulated concentration profiles. Pretreatment concentrations (t < 0) are assumed to be zero.

Table 2. Pharmacodynamic model parameters used in the simulation of ANC kinetics.

DRUG	Circ0 ($\times 10^9$/L)	MTT (hours)	Drug Effect (E_{drug})	γ	Reference
Docetaxel	5.05	88.7	Emax Model	0.161	Friberg et al. 2006
			$I_{max} = 83.9$		
			$IC_{50} = 7.17$ uM		
Topotecan	5.02	137	Linear Model	0.101	Kloft et al. 2006
			Slope $= 60.8$ uM^{-1}		
Etoposide	5.45	135	Emax Model	0.174	Friberg et al. 2006
			$I_{max} = 1.57$		
			$IC_{50} = 5.2$ uM		

$$c_{avg,n_{days}}(t) = \frac{1}{n_{days}} \int_{t-n_{days}}^{t} c(t)dt \qquad \text{(Eq.1)}$$

The parameter $\max(c_{avg,ndays})$ can be thought of as blending properties of both C_{max} and AUC. For example, in the limit where n_{days} is very small compared to the half-life of the molecule, $\max(c_{avg,ndays})$ is roughly equivalent to c_{max} on any given schedule(Eq. 2).

$$\max\left(c_{avg,n_{days}}(t)\right) \cong \frac{1}{n_{days}} \max\left(c(t) \int_{t-n_{days}}^{t} dt\right) = \qquad \text{(Eq.2)}$$

$$\max(c(t)) = c_{max}$$

On the other hand, when n_{days} is very large compared to the duration of treatment, the parameter $\max(c_{avg,ndays})$ will be more related to the total cycle AUC for each schedule (Eq. 3).

$$\max\left(c_{avg,n_{days}}(t)\right) = \frac{1}{n_{days}} \max\left(\int_{0}^{t} c(t)dt\right) \cong \frac{AUC}{n_{days}} \qquad \text{(Eq.3)}$$

For Etoposide, the C_{max} was in some cases much larger than IC_{50}. To account for this higher degree of nonlinearity we used the moving average of the concentration below IC_{50} defined by:

$$c_{avg,IC50,n_{days}}(t) = \frac{1}{n_{days}} \int_{t-n_{days}}^{t} \min(c(t),IC_{50})dt \qquad \text{(Eq.4)}$$

Supporting Information

Figure S1 Effect of schedule on topotecan induced neutropenia. Population estimation of median ANC nadir and

probability of grade 4 neutropenia (nadir $<0.5 \times 10^9$/L) from PK-PD simulation for topotecan shows similar patterns across schedules. The top row (A-B) represents median ANC nadir and probability of grade 4 neutropenia for all different schedules at low total dose while the bottom row (C-D) represents same for high total dose. Frequent dosing (schedules where 'days-on' is close to or equal the dosing period, such as 7on/0off) is associated with less probability of grade 4 neutropenia.

Figure S2 Effect of schedule on etoposide induced neutropenia. Population simulation of etoposide induced neutropenia was carried our using non-linear drug effect (Emax) model. The top row (A-B) represents median ANC nadir and probability of grade 4 neutropenia for all different schedules at low total dose while the bottom row (C-D) represents same for high total dose. Here intermittent dosing is associated with low probability of grade 4 neutropenia and higher ANC nadir.

Figure S3 C_{max} and AUC are weak predictor of severity of neutropenia. Common PK parameters were tested for its correlation with median ANC nadir and probability of grade-4 neutropenia across variety of schedules and dose for topotecan and etoposide. (A-C) C_{max} plotted against median ANC nadir for each of the schedules tested and shows weak correlation of -0.29 ($R^2 = 0.08$, $p = 0.002$) and -0.31 ($R^2 = 0.09$, $p = 0.001$) for topotecan and etoposide respectively. (B-D) Total cycle AUC over all schedules shows overall good correlation (CC $= -0.82$ ($R^2 = 0.67$) and -0.72 ($R^2 = 0.50$, $p < 0.01$) for topotecan and etoposide respectively) with median ANC nadir, but the correlation is mainly driven by the differences in total dose as it loses ability to predict neutropenia at a fixed total dose level ($R^2 < 0.05$ at low and high total dose for both drugs).

Figure S4 Rat plasma PK model fits and model parameters. One compartment pharmacokinetic model adequately describes TAK-960 plasma disposition/elimination after IV administration. Model fits and model parameters are shown in figure S4.

Figure S5 Moving average concentration predicts neutropenia across drugs. Maximal moving average concentration of n days, $\max(c_{avg,n\text{-}days})$, was found to predict degree of neutropenia precisely except highly nonlinear drug effect model of etoposide. In case of etoposide maximum moving concentration below threshold i.e. IC_{50} for 16 days, $max(C_{avg,16days} < IC_{50})$ turn out to be a good predictor of median ANC nadir and probability of grade-4 neutropenia. The median ANC nadir (top row) and probability of grade-4 neutropenia (bottom row) was plotted against moving average concentration, $max(c_{avg,n\text{-}days})$.

Figure S6 Schedule-dependence of grade-4 neutropenia for greater than seven days. Probability of an individual presenting with grade-4 neutropenia continuously for seven days or more derived from PK-PD simulation for all three drugs is shown. The upper row (A-C) represents probability of grade-4 neutropenia continuously for seven days over all schedules tested at low total dose and lower row (D-F) represents same for high total dose of each drug. This parameter tends to favor dosing schedules with some dose holiday (e.g. 7on/7off). However, as with probability of a grade-4 event, schedules such as 1on/27off are suboptimal under this analysis.

References

1. Amadori S, Stasi R, Martelli AM, Venditti A, Meloni G, et al. (2012) Temsirolimus, an mTOR inhibitor, in combination with lower-dose clofarabine as salvage therapy for older patients with acute myeloid leukaemia: results of a phase II GIMEMA study (AML-1107). Br J Haematol 156: 205–212.
2. DuBois SG, Shusterman S, Reid JM, Ingle AM, Ahern CH, et al. (2012) Tolerability and pharmacokinetic profile of a sunitinib powder formulation in pediatric patients with refractory solid tumors: a Children's Oncology Group study. Cancer Chemother Pharmacol 69: 1021–1027.
3. Witzig TE, Reeder CB, LaPlant BR, Gupta M, Johnston PB, et al. (2011) A phase II trial of the oral mTOR inhibitor everolimus in relapsed aggressive lymphoma. Leukemia 25: 341–347.
4. Oosterhuis B, ten Berge RJ, Sauerwein HP, Endert E, Schellekens PT, et al. (1984) Pharmacokinetic-pharmacodynamic modeling of prednisolone-induced lymphocytopenia in man. J Pharmacol Exp Ther 229: 539–546.
5. Fetterly GJ, Tamburlin JM, Straubinger RM (2001) Paclitaxel pharmacodynamics: application of a mechanism-based neutropenia model. Biopharm Drug Dispos 22: 251–261.
6. Silber JH, Fridman M, DiPaola RS, Erder MH, Pauly MV, et al. (1998) First-cycle blood counts and subsequent neutropenia, dose reduction, or delay in early-stage breast cancer therapy. J Clin Oncol 16: 2392–2400.
7. Link BK, Budd GT, Scott S, Dickman E, Paul D, et al. (2001) Delivering adjuvant chemotherapy to women with early-stage breast carcinoma: current patterns of care. Cancer 92: 1354–1367.
8. Tabernero J, Climent MA, Lluch A, Albanell J, Vermorken JB, et al. (2004) A multicentre, randomised phase II study of weekly or 3-weekly docetaxel in patients with metastatic breast cancer. Ann Oncol 15: 1358–1365.
9. Qi M, Li JF, Xie YT, Lu AP, Lin BY, et al. (2010) Weekly paclitaxel improved pathologic response of primary chemotherapy compared with standard 3 weeks schedule in primary breast cancer. Breast Cancer Res Treat 123: 197–202.
10. Huang TC, Campbell TC (2012) Comparison of weekly versus every 3 weeks paclitaxel in the treatment of advanced solid tumors: a meta-analysis. Cancer Treat Rev 38: 613–617.
11. Bria E, Cuppone F, Ciccarese M, Nistico C, Facciolo F, et al. (2006) Weekly docetaxel as second line chemotherapy for advanced non-small-cell lung cancer: meta-analysis of randomized trials. Cancer Treat Rev 32: 583–587.
12. Socinski MA (1999) Single-agent paclitaxel in the treatment of advanced non-small cell lung cancer. Oncologist 4: 408–416.
13. Egorin MJ, Van Echo DA, Tipping SJ, Olman EA, Whitacre MY, et al. (1984) Pharmacokinetics and dosage reduction of cis-diammine(1,1-cyclobutanedicarboxylato)platinum in patients with impaired renal function. Cancer Res 44: 5432–5438.
14. Duffull SB, Robinson BA (1997) Clinical pharmacokinetics and dose optimisation of carboplatin. Clin Pharmacokinet 33: 161–183.
15. Arakawa A, Nishikawa H, Suzumori K, Kato N (2001) Pharmacokinetic and pharmacodynamic analysis of combined chemotherapy with carboplatin and paclitaxel for patients with ovarian cancer. Int J Clin Oncol 6: 248–252.
16. Jakobsen P, Bastholt L, Dalmark M, Pfeiffer P, Petersen D, et al. (1991) A randomized study of epirubicin at four different dose levels in advanced breast cancer. Feasibility of myelotoxicity prediction through single blood-sample measurement. Cancer Chemother Pharmacol 28: 465–469.
17. Ando M, Minami H, Ando Y, Sakai S, Shimono Y, et al. (1999) Pharmacological analysis of etoposide in elderly patients with lung cancer. Clin Cancer Res 5: 1690–1695.
18. Jodrell DI, Egorin MJ, Canetta RM, Langenberg P, Goldbloom EP, et al. (1992) Relationships between carboplatin exposure and tumor response and toxicity in patients with ovarian cancer. J Clin Oncol 10: 520–528.
19. Testart-Paillet D, Girard P, You B, Freyer G, Pobel C, et al. (2007) Contribution of modelling chemotherapy-induced hematological toxicity for clinical practice. Crit Rev Oncol Hematol 63: 1–11.
20. van Groeningen CJ, Pinedo HM, Heddes J, Kok RM, de Jong AP, et al. (1988) Pharmacokinetics of 5-fluorouracil assessed with a sensitive mass spectrometric method in patients on a dose escalation schedule. Cancer Res 48: 6956–6961.
21. Gianni L, Kearns CM, Giani A, Capri G, Vigano L, et al. (1995) Nonlinear pharmacokinetics and metabolism of paclitaxel and its pharmacokinetic/pharmacodynamic relationships in humans. J Clin Oncol 13: 180–190.
22. Henningsson A, Sparreboom A, Sandstrom M, Freijs A, Larsson R, et al. (2003) Population pharmacokinetic modelling of unbound and total plasma concentrations of paclitaxel in cancer patients. Eur J Cancer 39: 1105–1114.
23. Huizing MT, Keung AC, Rosing H, van der Kuij V, ten Bokkel Huinink WW, et al. (1993) Pharmacokinetics of paclitaxel and metabolites in a randomized comparative study in platinum-pretreated ovarian cancer patients. J Clin Oncol 11: 2127–2135.
24. Karlsson MO, Molnar V, Bergh J, Freijs A, Larsson R (1998) A general model for time-dissociated pharmacokinetic-pharmacodynamic relationship exemplified by paclitaxel myelosuppression. Clin Pharmacol Ther 63: 11–25.
25. Walker LG, Eremin JM, Aloysius MM, Vassanasiri W, Walker MB, et al. (2011) Effects on quality of life, anti-cancer responses, breast conserving surgery and survival with neoadjuvant docetaxel: a randomised study of sequential weekly versus three-weekly docetaxel following neoadjuvant doxorubicin and cyclophosphamide in women with primary breast cancer. BMC Cancer 11: 179.
26. Friberg LE, Henningsson A, Maas H, Nguyen L, Karlsson MO (2002) Model of chemotherapy-induced myelosuppression with parameter consistency across drugs. J Clin Oncol 20: 4713–4721.
27. Sandstrom M, Lindman H, Nygren P, Lidbrink E, Bergh J, et al. (2005) Model describing the relationship between pharmacokinetics and hematologic toxicity of the epirubicin-docetaxel regimen in breast cancer patients. J Clin Oncol 23: 413–421.
28. Troconiz IF, Garrido MJ, Segura C, Cendros JM, Principe P, et al. (2006) Phase I dose-finding study and a pharmacokinetic/pharmacodynamic analysis of the neutropenic response of intravenous diflomotecan in patients with advanced malignant tumours. Cancer Chemother Pharmacol 57: 727–735.
29. Latz JE, Karlsson MO, Rusthoven JJ, Ghosh A, Johnson RD (2006) A semimechanistic-physiologic population pharmacokinetic/pharmacodynamic model for neutropenia following pemetrexed therapy. Cancer Chemother Pharmacol 57: 412–426.
30. Leger F, Loos WJ, Bugat R, Mathijssen RH, Goffinet M, et al. (2004) Mechanism-based models for topotecan-induced neutropenia. Clin Pharmacol Ther 76: 567–578.
31. Zandvliet AS, Siegel-Lakhai WS, Beijnen JH, Copalu W, Etienne-Grimaldi MC, et al. (2008) PK/PD model of indisulam and capecitabine: interaction causes excessive myelosuppression. Clin Pharmacol Ther 83: 829–839.
32. van Kesteren C, Zandvliet AS, Karlsson MO, Mathot RA, Punt CJ, et al. (2005) Semi-physiological model describing the hematological toxicity of the anti-cancer agent indisulam. Invest New Drugs 23: 225–234.
33. Brain EG, Rezai K, Lokiec F, Gutierrez M, Urien S (2008) Population pharmacokinetics and exploratory pharmacodynamics of ifosfamide according to continuous or short infusion schedules: an n = 1 randomized study. Br J Clin Pharmacol 65: 607–610.
34. Kloft C, Wallin J, Henningsson A, Chatelut E, Karlsson MO (2006) Population pharmacokinetic-pharmacodynamic model for neutropenia with patient subgroup identification: comparison across anticancer drugs. Clin Cancer Res 12: 5481–5490.

Table S1 Pharmacokinetic model parameters used in simulation of concentration time profiles.

Table S2 PK parameters, AUC and C_{max} on each of the schedules tested.

Acknowledgments

We would like to thank Shu-Wen Teng, Vivek Kadambi, and Karthik Venkatakrishnan for helpful discussion and critique of the manuscript.

Author Contributions

Conceived and designed the experiments: JM. Performed the experiments: MP SP JY. Analyzed the data: MP SP JY. Contributed reagents/materials/analysis tools: MP. Wrote the paper: MP SP AC WCS JM.

35. Friberg LE, Freijs A, Sandstrom M, Karlsson MO (2000) Semiphysiological model for the time course of leukocytes after varying schedules of 5-fluorouracil in rats. J Pharmacol Exp Ther 295: 734–740.

36. Friberg LE, Sandstrom M, Karlsson MO (2010) Scaling the time-course of myelosuppression from rats to patients with a semi-physiological model. Invest New Drugs 28: 744–753.

37. Hansson EK, Friberg LE (2012) The shape of the myelosuppression time profile is related to the probability of developing neutropenic fever in patients with docetaxel-induced grade IV neutropenia. Cancer Chemother Pharmacol 69: 881–890.

38. Hansson EK, Wallin JE, Lindman H, Sandstrom M, Karlsson MO, et al. (2010) Limited inter-occasion variability in relation to inter-individual variability in chemotherapy-induced myelosuppression. Cancer Chemother Pharmacol 65: 839–848.

39. Latz JE, Rusthoven JJ, Karlsson MO, Ghosh A, Johnson RD (2006) Clinical application of a semimechanistic-physiologic population PK/PD model for neutropenia following pemetrexed therapy. Cancer Chemother Pharmacol 57: 427–435.

40. Sandstrom M, Lindman H, Nygren P, Johansson M, Bergh J, et al. (2006) Population analysis of the pharmacokinetics and the haematological toxicity of the fluorouracil-epirubicin-cyclophosphamide regimen in breast cancer patients. Cancer Chemother Pharmacol 58: 143–156.

41. Sandstrom M, Simonsen LE, Freijs A, Karlsson MO (1999) The pharmacokinetics of epirubicin and docetaxel in combination in rats. Cancer Chemother Pharmacol 44: 469–474.

42. Wallin JE, Friberg LE, Karlsson MO (2010) Model-based neutrophil-guided dose adaptation in chemotherapy: evaluation of predicted outcome with different types and amounts of information. Basic Clin Pharmacol Toxicol 106: 234–242.

43. Hikichi Y, Honda K, Hikami K, Miyashita H, Kaieda I, et al. (2012) TAK-960, a novel, orally available, selective inhibitor of polo-like kinase 1, shows broad-spectrum preclinical antitumor activity in multiple dosing regimens. Mol Cancer Ther 11: 700–709.

44. Miller AA, Herndon JE, Hollis DR, Ellerton J, Langleben A, et al. (1995) Schedule dependency of 21-day oral versus 3-day intravenous etoposide in combination with intravenous cisplatin in extensive-stage small-cell lung cancer: a randomized phase III study of the Cancer and Leukemia Group B. J Clin Oncol 13: 1871–1879.

45. Hande KR, Krozely MG, Greco FA, Hainsworth JD, Johnson DH (1993) Bioavailability of low-dose oral etoposide. J Clin Oncol 11: 374–377.

46. Toffoli G, Corona G, Basso B, Boiocchi M (2004) Pharmacokinetic optimisation of treatment with oral etoposide. Clin Pharmacokinet 43: 441–466.

9

In Vitro, In Silico and *In Vivo* Studies of Ursolic Acid as an Anti-Filarial Agent

Komal Kalani[1,5]**, Vikas Kushwaha**[2]**, Pooja Sharma**[3]**, Richa Verma**[2]**, Mukesh Srivastava**[4]**, Feroz Khan**[3,5]**, P. K. Murthy**[2]*****, **Santosh Kumar Srivastava**[1,5]*****

1 Medicinal Chemistry Department, CSIR-Central Institute of Medicinal and Aromatic Plants, Lucknow, 226015 (U.P.) India, **2** Division of Parasitology, CSIR-Central Drug Research Institute, Lucknow, 226001, UP, India, **3** Metabolic & Structural Biology Department, CSIR-Central Institute of Medicinal and Aromatic Plants, Lucknow, 226015 (U.P.) India, **4** Clinical and Experimental Medicine, Biometry section, CSIR-Central Drug Research Institute, Lucknow, 226001, UP, India, **5** Academy of Scientific and Innovative Research (AcSIR), Anusandhan Bhawan, New Delhi, 110 001, India

Abstract

As part of our drug discovery program for anti-filarial agents from Indian medicinal plants, leaves of *Eucalyptus tereticornis* were chemically investigated, which resulted in the isolation and characterization of an anti-filarial agent, ursolic acid (UA) as a major constituent. Antifilarial activity of UA against the human lymphatic filarial parasite *Brugia malayi* using *in vitro* and *in vivo* assays, and *in silico* docking search on glutathione-s-transferase (GST) parasitic enzyme were carried out. The UA was lethal to microfilariae (mf; LC_{100}: 50; IC_{50}: 8.84 µM) and female adult worms (LC_{100}: 100; IC50: 35.36 µM) as observed by motility assay; it exerted 86% inhibition in MTT reduction potential of the adult parasites. The selectivity index (SI) of UA for the parasites was found safe. This was supported by the molecular docking studies, which showed adequate docking (LibDock) scores for UA (−8.6) with respect to the standard antifilarial drugs, ivermectin (IVM −8.4) and diethylcarbamazine (DEC-C −4.6) on glutathione-s-transferase enzyme. Further, *in silico* pharmacokinetic and drug-likeness studies showed that UA possesses drug-like properties. Furthermore, UA was evaluated *in vivo* in *B. malayi-M. coucha* model (natural infection), which showed 54% macrofilaricidal activity, 56% female worm sterility and almost unchanged microfilaraemia maintained throughout observation period with no adverse effect on the host. Thus, in conclusion *in vitro, in silico* and *in vivo* results indicate that UA is a promising, inexpensive, widely available natural lead, which can be designed and developed into a macrofilaricidal drug. To the best of our knowledge this is the first ever report on the anti-filarial potential of UA from *E. tereticornis*, which is in full agreement with the Thomson Reuter's 'Metadrug' tool screening predictions.

Editor: Gnanasekar Munirathinam, University of Illinois, United States of America

Funding: The funding sources are CSIR-network project BSC-0121 and CSIR-SPLENDID and the funders had no role in study design, data collection and analysis, decision to publish, or preparation of the manuscript.

Competing Interests: The authors have declared that no competing interests exist.

* Email: skscimap@gmail.com (SKS); drpkmurthy@gmail.com (PKM)

Introduction

Among the six neglected tropical diseases, lymphatic filariasis (LF) is one of the major health problems in 73 tropical and subtropical countries in Africa, Asia, South and Central America and the Pacific Islands. According to the World Health Organization (WHO) global report, over 120 million people are currently infected with LF [1,2] of which about 40 million people are suffering with chronic disease manifestations: Elephantiasis and hydrocele [3], which cause permanent, long-term disability and economic loss to the nations [3,4]. The LF is caused by the nematode parasites *Brugia malayi*, *B. timori* and *Wuchereria bancrofti* and according to a recent report about 1 billion people (18% of the world's population) are at risk of infection (www.globalnetwork.org). Although, the World Health Organization launched a global filariasis elimination programme [5,6] using diethylcarbamazine (DEC) or ivermectin (IVM), but due to serious technical difficulties the programme is facing problem in the eradication of this endemic disease [4,7–8]. Since, DEC and IVM both are microfilaricides with poor or no activity on adult parasites

[9], the peripheral blood microfilaremia reappears in patients after a certain period of withdrawal of the drug. This depressing perspective demands, an urgent need for new molecular structures associated with macrofilaricidal activity/or sterilizing the adult worms is therefore needed [8–10] as adult parasites not only produce millions of microfilariae (mf) that are picked up by the mosquito vector and transmitted, but are also responsible for the debilitating pathological lesions. Therefore, macrofilaricidal agents are the need of hour, which not only adversely affect the target but should have also very low or no side effect [11].

As a part of our drug discovery program, we recently reported a pentacyclic triterpenoid, glycyrrhetinic acid [9] as a novel class of anti-filarial agent. This prompted us to investigate anti-filarial activity in other pentacyclic triterpenoids, widely available in Indian medicinal plants. For this purpose, in the present study leaves of *Eucalyptus tereticornis* were chemically and biologically investigated in details, which afforded an anti-filarial agent, Ursolic acid (UA, a pentacyclic triterpenoid) as a major constituent. The *in-vitro* activity of UA against the mf and adult worms, *in-silico* docking studies on glutathione-s-transferase (GST)

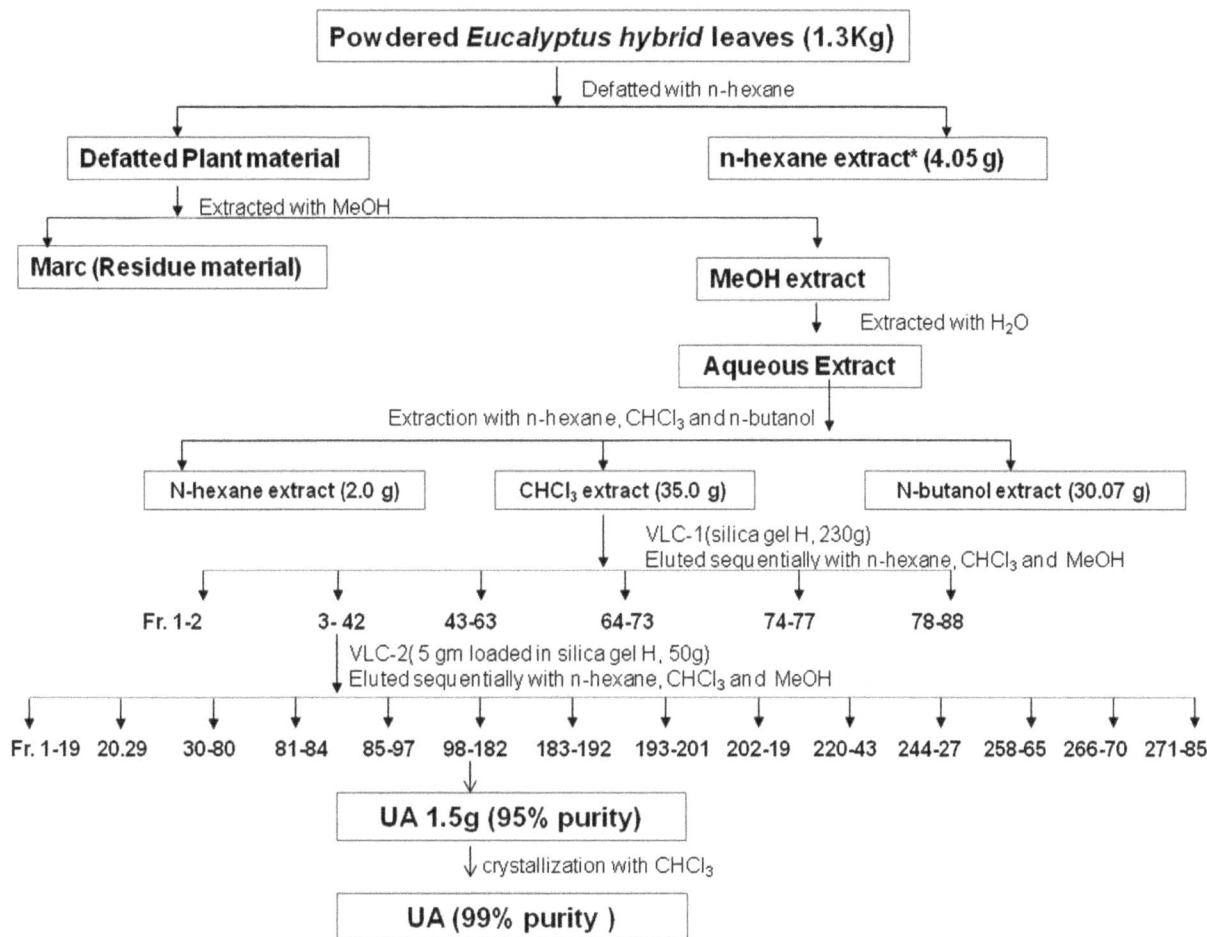

Figure 1. The schematic extraction and fractionation of UA from the leaves of *E. tereticornis.* §Washed with water and the solvent was dried over anhydrous Na$_2$SO$_4$. *Solvent was completely removed under vacuum at 35°C on a Buchi Rota vapour.

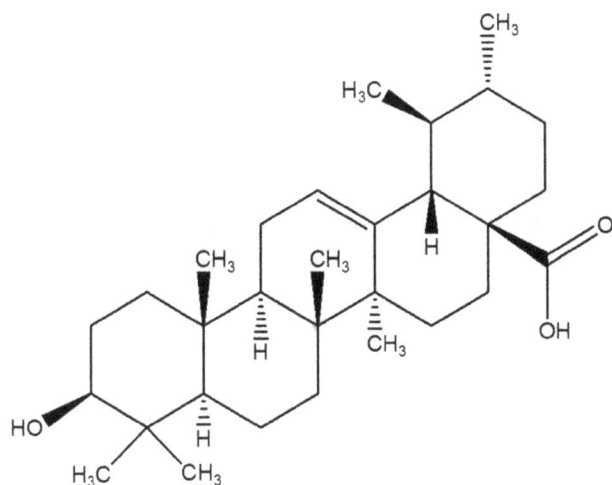

Figure 2. 2D structure of Ursolic Acid (UA).

parasitic enzyme and *in vivo* activity against *B. malayi* in *Meriones unguiculatus* model have been discussed here in detail.

Materials and Methods

General experimental procedure

The ^{1}H and ^{13}C NMR spectra were recorded on a Bruker 300 MHz spectrometer in deuterated pyridine. ESI-MS was carried out on a LCMS-2010 V (Shimadzu, Kyoto, Japan) simultaneously in positive (detector voltage 1.6 KV) ionization under scan mode. The scan speed of the mass analyzer was 2000 m/z per sec within the range of 400–1000 m/z. A positive full scan mode for screening and library assisted identification was used whereas time schedule selected-ion mode (SIM) in +ve ionization mode of the characteristic abundant adduct ions. Purity of UA was assessed by HPLC and was ≥95% [12]. Chemical shifts are in ppm with reference (internal) to tetramethylsilane (TMS) and J values are in hertz. With the Dept pulse sequence, different types of carbons (C, CH, CH$_2$ & CH$_3$) in UA were determined. The vacuum liquid chromatographic separations (VLC) were carried out on TLC grade Silica gel H (average particle size 10 μm) purchased from Merck, (Mumbai, India). All the required solvents and reagents were purchased from Spectrochem (Mumbai, India) and Thomas Baker Pvt. Ltd., India. Pre-coated Silica gel (60F) TLC plates 2.5 mm (Merck) were used to determine the

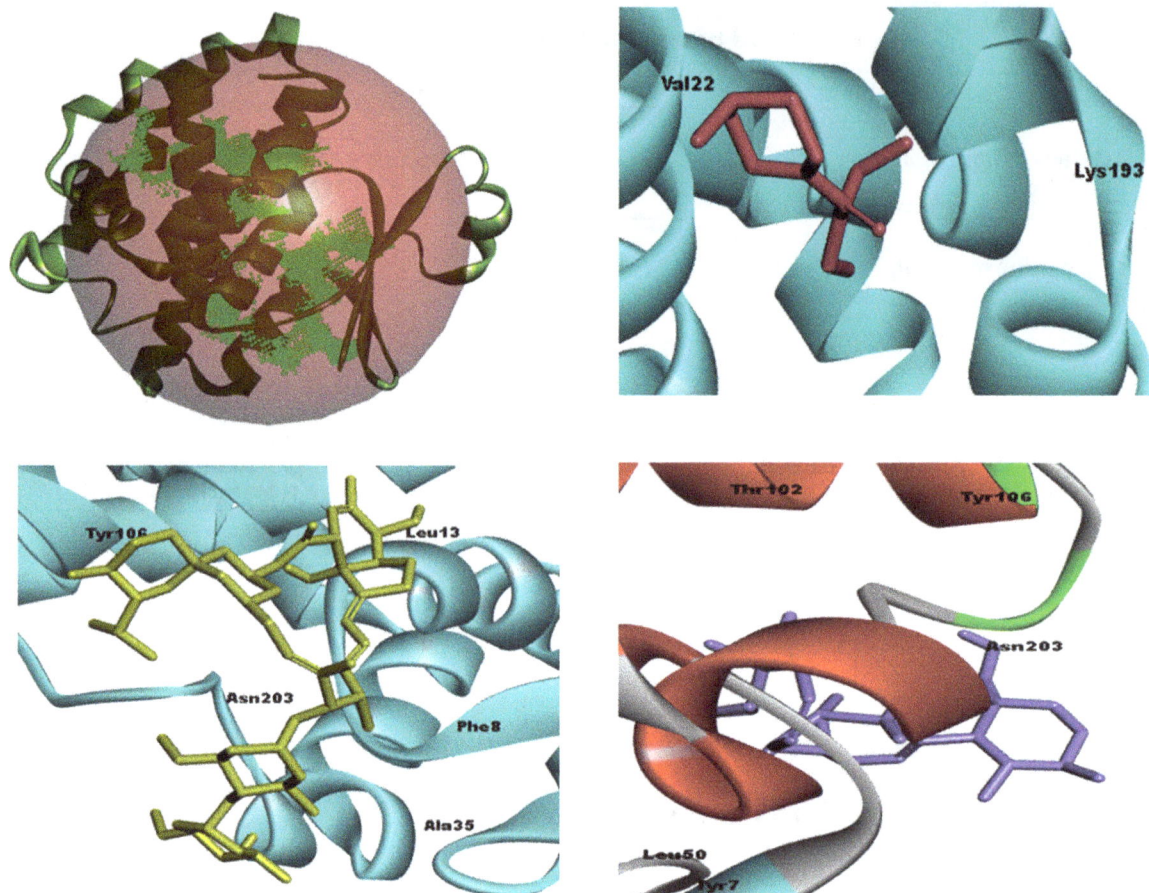

Figure 3. Docking results of studies compounds on *B. malayi* **(Filarial nematode worm) glutathione-S-transferase (***Bm***GST) homology model.** (a) docked standard drug DEC-c (control) on BmGST model active site with docking energy -4.9 kcal mol^{-1}, (b) docked another standard drug Ivermectin (control) with docking energy -8.4 kcal mol^{-1}, (c) docked UA on BmGST model with high docking energy -8.6 kcal mol^{-1}.

profiles of VLC fractions and their purity. The developed TLC plates were first observed at 254 nm in UV and then sprayed with Bacopa reagent [vanillin-ethanol sulphuric acid (1 g: 95 ml: 5 ml)] and spots were visualized after heating the TLC plate at 110°C for 5 minutes.

Plant material

The leaves of *E. tereticornis* were collected from the medicinal farm of Central Institute of Medicinal and Aromatic Plants (CIMAP), Lucknow, Uttar Pradesh, India during the month of January, 2008. A voucher specimen # 12470 was deposited in the Herbarium section of the Botany and Pharmacognosy Department of the institute.

The air dried leaves of *E. tereticornis* (1.3 kg) were powdered and defatted with n-hexane. The defatted leaves were further extracted with MeOH (4×5 L) (Figure 1).The combined MeOH extract was dried under vacuum at 40°C. The MeOH extract so obtained was dissolved in distilled water (2L) and successively fractionated with *n*-hexane, CHCl$_3$ and *n*-BuOH (saturated with H$_2$O) [12,13]. All the fractions were evaluated for anti-filarial activity, of which CHCl$_3$ fraction (35.0 g) was found active hence subjected for chromatographic separation over VLC-1 using silica gel H (260 g). The gradient elution of VLC was carried out with mixture of hexane, CHCl$_3$ and MeOH in increasing order of polarity.

Fractions 3–42 (7.2 g) eluted with hexane- CHCl$_3$ (1:1) to CHCl$_3$ – MeOH (99:1) was a complex mixture. Hence a part of it (5 g) was further chromatographed over VLC-2, using TLC grade silica gel H (50 g). Gradient elution of VLC-2 was carried out with mixture of hexane, CHCl$_3$ and MeOH in increasing order of polarity. Fractions 175–182 (1.5 g) eluted with CHCl$_3$ (100%) afforded a white amorphous compound (95% pure) which on further crystallization with CHCl$_3$ yielded UA (99% pure.). The ^{1}H and ^{13}C NMR and ESI-MS spectra of the homogenous compound (UA) were recorded and the spectroscopic data are presented as below:

ESI-MS m/z 457 [M+H]$^+$, C$_{30}$H$_{48}$O$_3$, ^{1}H NMR (300 MHz, Pyridine): δ 0.77, 0.78, 0.98, 1.09, 1.14 (3H each, all s, 5 x tert. Me) 0.92 & 0.96 (3H each, each d, J = 6.4 and 7.3 Hz, 2 x sec Me), 2.82 (1H, d, J = 9.9 Hz, H-18 β), 3.20 (1H, dd, J = 6.8 & 8.7 Hz, H-3α). ^{13}C NMR (75.5 MHz, Pyridine): C1- 39.5 (t), C2- 28.3 (t), C3- 78.7(d), C4- 39.9 (q), C5- 56.3 (d), C6- 19.1 (t), C 7- 33.9 (t), C8- 40.4 (q), C9- 47.0 (d), C10- 37.7 (q), C11- 23.9 (t), C12- 126.0 (d), C13- 139.6 (q), C14- 42.9 (q), C15- 28.9 (t), C16- 25.2 (t), C17- 48.5 (q), C18- 54.0 (d), C19- 30.5 (d), C20- 39.7 (d), C21- 31.3 (t), C22- 37.6 (t), C23- 29.0 (s), C24-15.8 (s), C25- 16.4 (s), C26- 17.5 (s), C27- 24.1 (s), C28- 179.7 (q), C29- 17.7 (s), C30- 21.4 (s) (Figure 2).

Table 1. *In vitro* activity of chloroform extract of *E. tereticornis*, its main constituent Ursolic Acid (UA) and reference drugs ivermectin and DEC on microfilariae and female adult worms of *B. malayi*.

Anti-filarial agent	Effect on female adult worm			Effect on microfilariae (Mf)		CC_{50}^{c} (µM)	SI	
	$LC100^{a}$ (µM) in motility assay (% inhibition)	IC_{50}^{b} (µM) in motility assay	Mean % inhibition in MTT	$LC100^{a}$ (µM) in motility assay (% inhibition)	IC_{50}^{b} (µM) in motility assay		w.r.t. motility of Adults	w.r.t. motility of Mf
$CHCl_3$ extract	>100	-	8.55	>100	-	-	-	-
UA	100 (100)	35.36	86.12	25 (90)	8.84	300	8.48	33.94
IVM	5	3.05	5.80	2.5	1.57	250	81.96	159.23
DEC-c*	1000 (100)	314.98	62.54	500 (100)	297.30	8926	28.34	30.02

^{a}LC100 = 100% reduction in motility indicates death of parasite;
^{b}IC$_{50}$ = 50% concentration of the agent at which 50% inhibition in motility is achieved;
^{c}CC$_{50}$ = concentration at which 50% of cells are killed; SI = Selectivity Index (CC$_{50}$/IC$_{50}$); w.r.t. = with respect to; *Diethylcarbamazine citrate.

In vitro evaluation of UA/drugs against filarial parasites

Animals: The study was approved by the Institute's Animal Ethics Committee (IAEC) [approval no. 86/09/Para/IAEC; 27/4/09] of CSIR-Central Drug Research Institute, Lucknow, India, under the provisions of CPCSEA (Committee for the Purpose of Control and Supervision on Experiments on Animals), Government of India. All the experiments in animals were conducted in compliance with the IAEC guidelines for use and handling of animals. Throughout the study, jird and *M. coucha* were kept in climate (23±2°C; RH: 60%) and photoperiod (12hr light-dark cycles) controlled animal room. They were fed standard rodent chow supplemented with dried shrimps (*M. coucha*) and had free access to drinking water.

B. malayi infection in animals: The human sub-periodic strain of *B. malayi* was cyclically maintained in *M. coucha* [14] and jirds (*Meriones unguiculatus*) [15] through black-eyed susceptible strain of *Aedes aegypti* mosquitoes. Infective larvae of *B. malayi* isolated from experimentally infected *A. aegypti* mosquitoes which were fed on microfilaraemic *M. coucha* (150–200 mf/10 µl blood), were washed thoroughly with insect saline (0.6%). Each animal was inoculated with 100 (*M. coucha*) or 200 L3 (jirds), through subcutaneous (s.c.) and intraperitonial (i.p.) routes, respectively.

Isolation of parasites: Mf and adult worms (female parasites) isolated freshly from peritoneal cavity (p.c.) of jirds harboring 5–6 month old *B. malayi* infection were washed thoroughly in medium Hanks Balanced Salt Solution (HBSS; pH 7.2) containing mixture of antibiotics (penicillin: 100 U/mL; streptomycin: 100 µg/mL) and used for the present study.

In vitro anti-filarial efficacy evaluation

Primary evaluation. *In vitro* assays: Based on viability of the parasites, two *in vitro* motility and 3-(4, 5-dimethylthiazol-2-yl)-2,5 diphenyltetrazolium bromide (MTT) reduction assays [16] were carried out for UA. IVM and Diethylcarbamazine-citrate (DEC-C) were used as reference drugs. Incubation medium used was HBSS; pH 7.2 containing mixture of antibiotics as above. For incubation of mf and adult worms cell culture plate (Nunc, Denmark) were used.

The UA and IVM were dissolved in DMSO whereas DEC-C was prepared in sterile triple distilled water (STDW). The antifilarial agents were used at 2-fold serial dilutions ranged from 15.63–1000 µM (DEC), 1.56–100 µM (UA) and 0.31–20 µM (IVM). The final conc. of DMSO in the incubation medium was kept below 0.1%. DMSO (<0.1%) was used in place of test agents solution for control.

Motility assay: Efficacy of the UA and reference drugs was assessed *in vitro* on mf and adult worms of *B. malayi* (as target parasites) using motility (Mf and adult parasite) and MTT (adult parasite only) reduction assay [16,17]. Duplicate wells containing 40–50 mf/100 µl/well (of 96 well plates) and 1 female worm/ml/well (of 48-well plate) were used. UA (100 µM) or reference drugs IVM (20 µM), or DEC-C (1000 µM) were added to duplicate wells and incubated. Wells with the test compound and DEC were incubated for 24 hr and those with IVM were incubated for 24 and 48 hr as it has a slow action on the parasites. This is the standard protocol followed in our lab [16,17,18]. All incubations were at 37°C in 5% CO_2 atmosphere. The effect on motility of the parasite stages was examined under microscope and scored. The experiment was repeated twice. In case of mf, only motility assay was used.

Motility assessment: Parasite motility was assessed under a microscope after 24/48 h exposure to test substance and scored as: 0 = dead; 1–4 = loss of motility (1 = 75%; 2 = 50%; 3 = 25% and 4 = no loss of motility). Loss of motility is defined as the inability of

Table 2. Details of Docking energy, active site pocket residues and H-bonds revealed by molecular docking of DEC, IVM and UA on *BmGST* of *B. malayi*.

S. No.	Receptor	Anti-filarial agent	Binding Affinity (kcal/mol)	Interacting Residues	No of H-bonds
1	1SJO	DEC *	-4.9	VAL-22, ILE-26, LYS-189, GLU-190, LYS-193, ARG-195	2.9 = LYS-193
2	1SJO	IVM*	-8.4	PHE-8, LEU-13, ASN-34, ALA-35, LEU-50, TYR-106, ASN-203, ASN-205	2.7 = ASN-203 3.1 = TYR-106
3	1SJO	UA	-8.6	TYR-7, PHE-8, LEU-13, GLN-49, LEU-50, THR-102, TYR-106, ASN-203	3.0 = TYR-106

the worms to regain pretreatment level of motility even after incubating in fresh medium *minus* the test agent at 37°C for 1 h. and was expressed as percentage (%) inhibition of control.

MTT- formazan colorimetric assay for viability of worms: The same female worms used in motility were then gently blotted and transferred to 0.1 ml of 0.5% MTT in 0.01 M phosphate-buffered saline (pH 7.2) and incubated for 1 h at 37°C. The formazan formed was extracted in 1 ml of DMSO for 1 h at 37°C and its absorbance was measured at 510 nm in spectrophotometer (PowerWaveX, USA). The mean absorbance value obtained from 4 treated worms was compared with the controls. The viability of the treated worms was assessed by calculating per cent inhibition in motility and MTT reduction over DMSO control worms [16].

Criteria for assessment of *in vitro* hits: 100% inhibition in motility of female adults or mf and or ≥50% inhibition in MTT reduction ability of female parasites was considered acceptable antifilarial (microfilaricidal/adulticidal) activity and picked up as hits and subjected to further testing *in vivo* [17].

Secondary evaluation. Determination of IC_{50}: For IC_{50} (the concentration at which the parasite motility was inhibited by 50%) determination of the parasites were incubated with two fold serial dilutions from 1.56–100 (UA), 0.31–40 (IVM) and 15.63–1000 µM (DEC-C) using triplicate wells of cell culture plate. Experiments were run in duplicate and incubations were carried out in replicates for 24/48 hr as above. After incubation, inhibition in motility (mf and female worm) and MTT reduction potential of the parasites were assessed as above. The experiment was repeated twice.

Determination of Cytotoxic concentration 50 (CC_{50}): The cytotoxicity assay of the test substances was carried out broadly following the method of Pagé et al. [19] with some modifications [20]. Briefly, VERO Cell line C1008 (African green monkey kidney cells) was plated in 96-well plates (Nunc, Denmark) at 0.1×10^6 cells/ml (100 µl per well) in DMEM supplemented with 10% heat inactivated FBS. A three-fold serial dilution of the test substances (starting from >20 x LC100 conc. of the test agent) in test medium was added. The plates with a final volume of 100 µl/well were incubated in 5% CO_2 atmosphere at 37°C. After 72 h

incubation 10 µl of 0.025% Resazurin in phosphate buffered saline (PBS; pH 7.2) was dispensed as indicator for viability followed by an additional incubation for 4 h and the plate was then read in a fluorescence reader (Synergy HT plate reader, Biotek, USA) at excitation wavelength of 530 nm and an emission wavelength of 590 nm. The assay was run in replicates in each of two independent experiments.

Data of IC_{50} and CC_{50} transferred to a graphic program (Excel) were calculated as described by Page et al. [19] and Mosmann [20] by linear interpolation between the two concentrations above and below 50% inhibition [21].

Selectivity Index (SI) of the UA was computed by the formula as:

$$SI = \frac{CC_{50}}{IC_{50}}$$

Molecular modeling and docking studies against glutathione-S-transferase (*BmGST*) enzyme

Molecular modeling and geometry cleaning of the UA was performed through ChemBioDraw-Ultra-v12.0 (Cambridge Soft, UK). The 3D structure was subjected to minimized the energy by using molecular mechanics-2 (MM2) force field until the root mean square (RMS) gradient value became smaller than 0.100 kcal mol^{-1} Å. Re-optimization was done by MOPAC (Molecular Orbital Package) method until the RMS gradient attained a value smaller than 0.0001 kcal mol^{-1} Å. The 3D chemical structure of known drugs DEC-c (CID:15432) and IVM (CID: 6321424) were retrieved from PubChem compound database (NCBI, USA). The theoretically solved structure of *B. malayi* glutathione-S-transferase (*BmGST*) was selected as the potential target for molecular docking simulation studies. The *BmGST* crystallographic protein 3D structure was retrieved from Protein Data Bank (PDB ID: 1SJO). The Ligsite program was used to identify the potential active site of *BmGST* model for molecular

Table 3. Predicted ADME parameters (DS v3.5, Accelrys, USA).

Anti-filarial agent	Aqueous solubility	Blood brain barrier penetration	CYP2D6 binding	Hepatotoxicity	Intestinal absorption	Plasma protein binding
DEC	4	2(Medium)	False (non-inhibitor)	True (toxic)	0 (Good)	False (Poorly bounded)
IVM	3	4 (Undefined)	False (non-inhibitor)	True (toxic)	3 (very poor)	False (Poorly bounded)
UA	1	0 (very high penetrant)	False (non-inhibitor)	False (non-toxic)	1 (moderate)	True (Highly bounded)

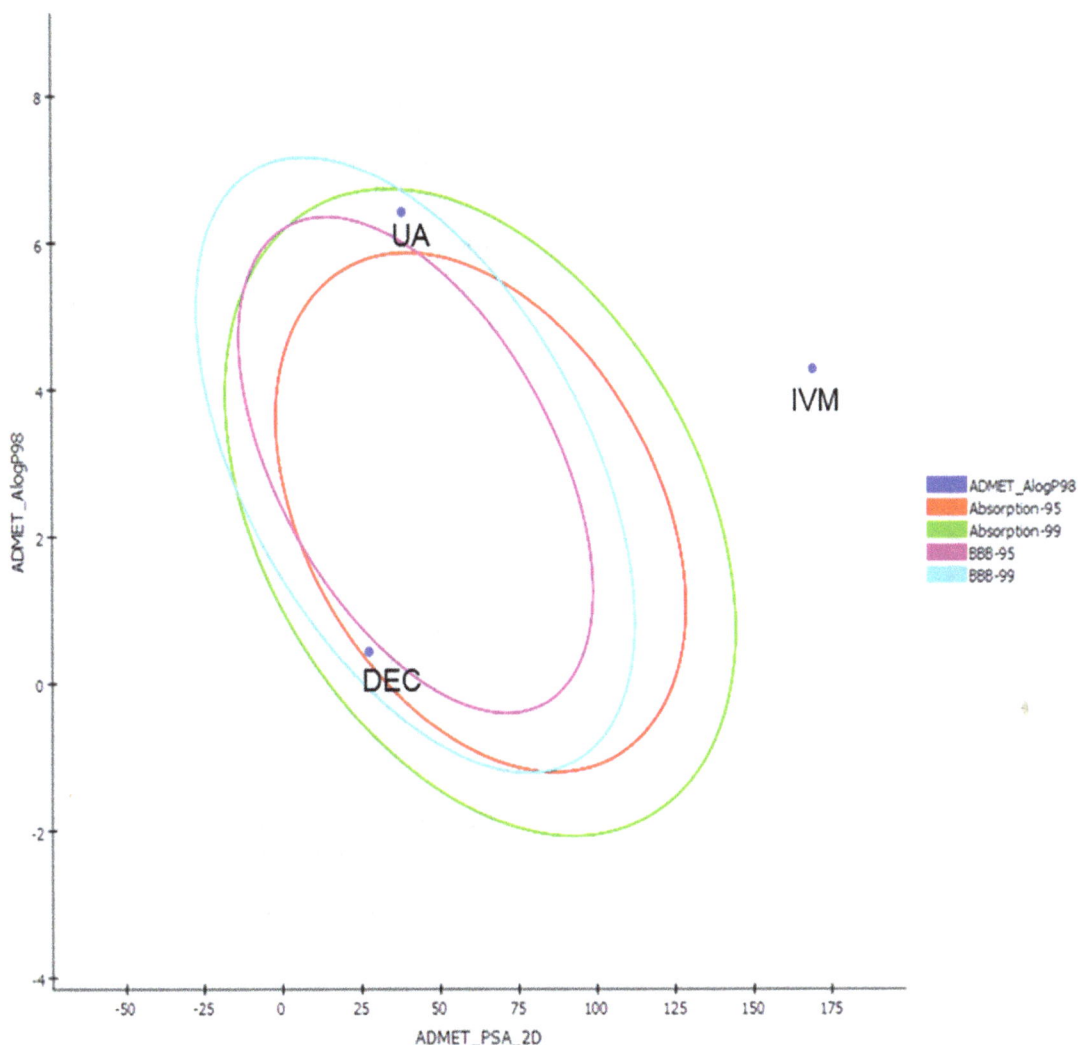

Figure 4. Adsorption model of Ursolic Acid (UA) and the standard antifilarial drugs.

docking studies and was then cross-checked with template active site as shown in Figure 3 [22]. The visualization studies were executed through Discovery Studio v3.5 (Accelrys Inc., USA, 2013).

In vivo efficacy

Administration of UA and the reference drugs: The finely powdered UA was suspended in 0.1% Tween-80 prepared in sterilized tap water. Solution of DEC was made in plain STW. *M. coucha* was administered with UA and DEC-c at 100 and 50 mg/kg body weight respectively through i.p. route for 5 consecutive days. The suspensions/solutions of UA/DEC-c were prepared daily before administration to the animals. Control animals received vehicle only.

B. malayi -*M. coucha* model: Animals harboring 5–7 months old *B. malayi* infection and showing progressive increase in microfilraemia were used in this study. UA and reference drug treated groups and an equal number of infected untreated animals kept as vehicle treated control, consisted of 5 animals each in two experiments were used.

Mf count in 10 μl blood drawn from tail of the animals between 12:00 noon and 1:00 PM [14] was assessed just before initiation of

treatment (day 0), on days 7/8 and 14 post initiation of treatment (p.i.t.) and thereafter at fortnightly intervals till day 84 p.i.t. [17]. The animals were killed on day 91 p.i.t.

Assessment of microfilaricidal efficacy: Microfilaricidal efficacy of UA was evaluated on day 7/8 and 14 p.i.t. and expressed as percent reduction in mf count over pretreatment level [23–25].

Assessment of macrofilaricidal and worm sterilization efficacy: Adult worms were recovered from heart, lungs and testes of treated and control animals [14]. Tissues were teased gently and the parasites recovered were then examined under microscope for status of the motility, cell adherence on their surface, dead or calcified worms [23,24]. Number of worms recovered from the treated and untreated animals was recorded. Macrofilaricidal efficacy of UA and DEC-C was assessed and expressed as percent change in adult worm recovery in treated group over control animals.

All the surviving females were teased individually in a drop of saline to examine condition of intrauterine mf stages of the parasite [23,24]. Number of sterile female worms recovered from the treated animals was compared with that of control animals and percent sterilization of female worms was determined in treated or

Table 4. Compliance of Dec, IVM & UA to the theoretical parameters of oral bioavailability and drug likeness properties.

Anti-filarial agent	Pharmacokinetic properties (ADME) dependent on chemical descriptors								
	ADM	AE	ADME	AD					
				H-bond donor			H-bond acceptor		Lipinski's rule of 5 violation
	Oral bioavailability: TPSA (Å²)	MW	logP	NH_2 group count	-N- group count	OH group count	N atom count	O atom count	
DEC	26.785	199	0.881	0	0	0	3	1	0
IVM	170.095	861	4.076	0	0	3	0	14	2
UA	57.527	456	6.789	0	0	1	0	3	1

Note: A = absorption, D= distribution, M= metabolism, and E= excretion; TPSA = topological polar surface area; MW = molecular weight; Log P= octanol/water partition coefficient.

control groups over total live female worms recovered from the respective groups.

Statistical analysis

Statistical analyses were carried out using Statistica version 7/ GraphPad Prism 3.0 version software. Results were expressed as mean ± S.D. of data from 5–6 animals in two experiments. The data were subjected to One-way ANOVA analysis and the significance of the difference between means were determined by Newman-Keuls Multiple Comparison Test. $P<0.05$ was considered significant and marked as *, $P<0.01$ as highly significant and marked as **, and $P<0.001$ was very highly significant and marked as ***. The trend analysis was done by fitting the simple regression model (Y = A+BX) using the method of least squares. The slopes of the line were compared by Analysis of Variance.

Drug likeness screening studies for ADME/Tox compliance. The ADME/Toxicity parameters compliance was evaluated by screening through Metadrug[TM], a commercial tool of MetaDiscovery (Thomson Reuters, USA) (http://www. genego.com) [26]. MetaDrug is a system pharmacology or system chemical biology and toxicology platform designed for the assessment of would-be therapeutic indications, off-target effects and potential toxic end points of novel small molecule compounds. In the studied work, this database/tool was used to predict and evaluate the human metabolism compliance, toxicity risk assessment and mode of action by using standard experimental data.

Results

The leaves of *E. tereticornis* were extracted and fractionated, according to the scheme given in Figure 1.

Worm motility and MTT reduction assay

Of the three extracts tested *in vitro* using worm motility assay, the $CHCl_3$ extract killed adult female worms (LC_{100}: 400 μM) and mf (LC_{100}: 200 μM) (Table 1). The $CHCl_3$ extract was subjected to repeated chromatographic separations over VLC using TLC grade silica gel H, which finally resulted in the isolation of a major compound. This major compound on further crystallization with $CHCl_3$ afforded 99% pure white crystals. The ^1H, ^{13}C NMR and ESI-MS spectroscopic data of these crystals confirmed that this is a pentacyclic triterpene, ursolic acid (UA) (Figure 1). Finally, UA was tested for its anti-filarial activity against *B. malayi* using *in vitro* assays.

Further, UA was tested against mf and female adult worms of *B. malayi* using motility and or MTT assays and the results are summarized in Table 1. Like chloroform extract UA was also found to be more effective in killing mf (LC_{100}: 50 μM) than adult worms (LC100: 100 μM) and its IC_{50} values were 35.36 and 8.84 μM against the respective parasite stages. UA exerted >86% inhibition in MTT reduction ability of the adult worms. It reduced the viability of female parasite in a gradual dose dependent manner as assessed by MTT reduction assay (**Figure S1**). The CC_{50} (>300 μM) and SI (>10) values of UA demonstrated that it is safe for carrying out *in vivo* screening (Table 1).

The time point studied for the standard drug IVM was 24 hr and 48 hr as IVM has slow action on the parasites. After 48 hr post incubation IVM was effective in inhibiting motility of female adult worm and mf at a minimum conc. of 5.0 μM and 2.5 μM (LC_{100}), respectively. Its IC_{50} against adult worms was 3.05 μM and that of mf was 1.49 μM. However IVM was less effective when parasites were incubated for 24 hr. IVM failed to inhibit MTT reduction ability of female worms even after 48 hr incubation (Table 1). On the other hand DEC-C required much

Table 5. Details of computational toxicity risk parameters of DEC, IVM and UA calculated by OSIRIS.

Compound	Toxicity risk parameters			
	MUT	**TUMO**	**IRRI**	**REP**
DEC	High Risk	No risk	No risk	High Risk
IVM	No risk	No risk	No risk	No risk
UA	No risk	No risk	No risk	No risk

Note: MUT = Mutagenicity, TUMO = Tumorogenicity, IRRI = Irritation, REP = Reproduction.

higher concentration to kill the female worms (LC_{100}: 1000 µM) and mf (LC_{100}: 500 µM); it inhibited MTT reduction skill of the adult parasite to the tune of 62.55%. The IC_{50} of DEC against the respective parasite stages were found to be 353.55 µM and 297.30 µM.

Concentration-dependent' LC_{100} and IC_{50} of UA, ivermectin and DEC for microfilariae and adult parasites of *B. malayi* in motility and MTT assays are shown in Figures S1–S3. After 24 h incubation UA (**Figure S1**) and DEC-C (**Figure S2**) caused concentration dependent decrease in viability of the parasites. However, in case of IVM the viability was time and conc. dependent (**Figure S3**).

In summary, *in vitro* findings revealed that $CHCl_3$ extract of *E. tereticornis* was microfilaricidal and macrofilaricidal, active against human filarial worm *B. malayi* and the active principal was localized to UA.

Molecular docking of UA on *Bm*GST

The current status of filaria have paved the way for investigating new lead compounds, which could be useful for the development of anti-filarial agents as there is a persistent urge for a lead to

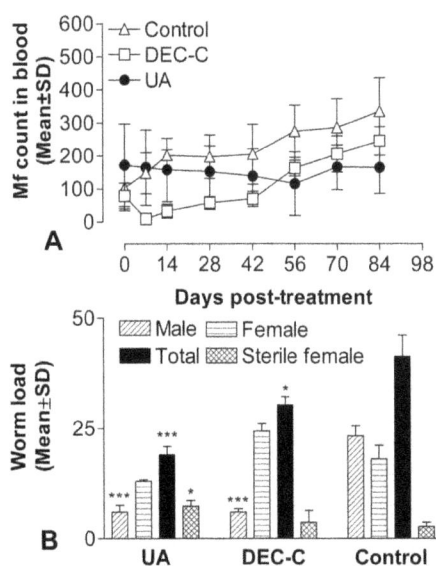

Figure 5. Micro-(A) and macrofilaricidal (B) activity of UA and reference drug diethylcarbamazine-citrate (DEC-C) against *Brugia malayi* in *Mastomys coucha*. Values are mean ± S.D. of 5 animals from two experiments. (A) No alteration in Microfilarial count in treated animals at each time point post initiation of treatment over day 0. Statistics: Student's 't' test. Significance level (B) *P<0.05 (vs sterilized female worm of control animals).

become candidate drug. The enzyme glutathione-s-transferase (GST) is playing a significant role in the long-term existence of filarial worms in mammalian host. The GST enzyme is a well known potential molecular target to inhibit filarial parasite's growth [27,28]. Therefore, the *Bm*GST theoretical protein structure 3D model was retrieved from PDB crystallographic database and later used for molecular docking simulation studies of UA, to explore the possible mechanism of action within the filarial worm (Table 2). The docking results showed high binding affinity (i.e., low docking energy; −8.6 kcal mol^{-1}) similar to that of reference drugs, DEC-c (−4.9 kcal mol^{-1}) and IVM (−8.4 kcal mol^{-1}). Docking results of UA also showed formation of H-bond (length 3.0 Å) with aromatic hydrophobic residue TYR-106, this may be the reason of high binding affinity, stability and activity of UA. The other binding site amino acid residues within a selection radius of 4 Å from the bound UA against *Bm*GST protein structure model were nucleophilic (polar, hydrophobic) e.g., threonine (THR-102), aromatic (hydrophobic) e.g., phenylalanine (PHE-8), tyrosine (TYR-7, TYR-106), polar amide e.g., asparagine (ASN-203), glutamine (GLN-49), hydrophobic e.g., leucine (LEU-13, LEU-50) (Figure 3). These results suggest that UA interacted well with the conserved hydrophobic amino acid residues of *Bm*GST. The molecular docking results showed that UA had significant similarity with respect to interacting amino acid residues and hydrogen bonds to that of the reference drug IVM, while the second reference drug Dec-c showed almost different interacting amino acid residues and hydrogen bond pattern. On the basis of docking binding affinity studies, it may be suggested that UA can be used as a potential lead against lymphatic filarial parasites by targeting GST.

ADME/Tox parameters evaluation

Since, docking results showed that UA may act as a potential anti-filarial lead, therefore *in silico* ADME/Tox parameters screening study was performed through Discovery Studio v3.5 molecular modeling & drug discovery software (Accelrys, USA). The UA, DEC and IVM were evaluated with standard descriptors and all the chemical descriptors and parameters of ADME were calculated (Table 3). The ADME results showed that there was no predictive hepatotoxicity and UA was comparable to standard range.

The ADME 2-D graph was plotted against Alogp98 versus PSA_2D (polar surface area) (Figure 4), which showed that the UA and Dec-c were inside the confidence limit ellipses of 99% for the blood brain barrier penetration and human intestinal absorption models compliance. On the other hand, IVM fallen outside the ellipse (undefined) showing very poor absorption and blood brain barrier penetration. Although, UA showed less water solubility, moderate intestinal absorption, but exhibited high plasma protein binding.

Table 6. Predicted therapeutic activity of UA against various reported diseases.

Property	Model description	Value/(TP)
Allergy	Potential antiallergic activity. Cutoff is 0.5. Values higher than 0.5 indicate potentially active compounds. Training set consists of approved drugs. Model description: Training set N = 258	0.50 (60.67)
Arthritis	Potential activity against arthritis. Cutoff is 0.5. Values higher than 0.5 indicate potentially active compounds. Training set consists of approved drugs.	0.72 (58.72)
Cancer	Potential activity against cancer. Cutoff is 0.5. Values higher than 0.5 indicate potentially active compounds. Training set consists of approved drugs. Model description: Training set N = 886	0.69 (64.84)
Hyperlipidemia	Potential antihyperlipidemic activity. Cutoff is 0.5. Values higher than 0.5 indicate potentially active compounds. Training set consists of approved drugs. Model description: Training set N = 185	0.91 (66.67)
Inflammation	Potential anti-inflammatory activity. Cutoff is 0.5. Values higher than 0.5 indicate potentially active compounds. Training set consists of approved drugs. Model description: Training set N = 598	0.50 (79.31)
Migraine	Potential activity against migraine. Cutoff is 0.5. Values higher than 0.5 indicate potentially active compounds. Training set consists of approved drugs	0.62 (97.37)
Obesity	Potential activity against obesty. Cutoff is 0.5. Values higher than 0.5 indicate potentially active compounds. Training set consists of approved drugs	0.94 (97.37)
Osteoporosis	Potential anti-osteoporosis activity. Cutoff is 0.5. Values higher than 0.5 indicate potentially active compounds. Training set consists of approved drugs	0.80 (97.37)
Skin Diseases	Potential activity against skin diseases. Cutoff is 0.5. Values higher than 0.5 indicate potentially active compounds. Training set consists of approved drugs. Model description: Training set N = 255	0.94 (53.04)

Although, ADME results showed that UA violates Lipinski's rule of five due to high logP value (logP>5), hence may cause problem in absorption through biological membranes or intestinal absorption, but it still falls within the acceptable limit of rule of five, when compared with the reference drugs, DEC and IVM (Table 4).

Toxicity risk assessment

The toxicity risk assessment at high doses and/or long term use was evaluated through the OSIRIS web server for the reference drugs, DEC, IVM and the studied compound UA (Table 5). In this screening four important toxicity risk parameters *viz.*, mutagenicity, tumorogenicity, skin irritation and reproductive/developmental toxicity parameters were evaluated for high doses or long term use toxicity. The toxicity screening results showed that UA and the reference drug IVM showed no features of risk of tumorogenicity, mutagenicity, reproductive toxicity and skin irritation, therefore UA is safe for human use, whereas DEC yielded a high risk of mutagenicity and reproductive toxicity.

In vivo anti-filarial efficacy

Brugia malayi - M. coucha **model.** Microfilaricidal activity: Figure 5A shows anti-filarial efficacy of UA against *B. malayi* in *M. coucha* at 100 mg/kg s.c. for 5 consecutive days. UA produced 4–33% lower microfilaremia (statistically not significant) than 0 day throughout the post treatment observation period (Figure 5A). In other words, the microfilaremia in UA treated animals remained below (4–33%) the pretreatment (0 day) level throughout the observation period, while in the untreated control it was (progressively) higher than the pretreatment level and never equaled the 0 day level. This clearly shows that UA possesses considerable antifilarial efficacy. DEC-C (50 mg/kg, s.c. x 5 days), which is principally a microfilaricide, caused >85% reduction in microfilarial count on day 7 p.i.t. which progressively increased and relapsed on day 49 p.i.t.; the count further increased rapidly and crossed the pretreatment level by day 56 p.i.t. The trend of microfilaremia from day 7 to day 84 p.i.t. in the three groups (control untreated, UA treated and DEC treated) against time

(post treatment) was determined and compared among each other using linear trend analysis. The baseline of each group was subjected to equality and the observations were converted to show percent change at each time point. The baseline adjusted data was fitted to straight line. The analysis showed that while the mf count in the DEC-treated animals after an initial dramatic drop on day 7 p.i.t., increased gradually over time, it remained almost unchanged with time in UA treated group (trend not significant). Thus UA was found to be better than DEC in controlling microfilaremia. The details are given in File S1: '*In vivo* antifilarial efficacy in *Brugia malayi -M. coucha* model: Microfilaricidal activity'.

Macrofilaricidal and embryostatic activity: UA (100 mg/kg, s.c. for 5 days) caused around 54% (P<0.001) adulticidal action over the untreated control. A moderate embryostatic effect of UA (56.15%; P<0.05) was also noticed in female worms (Figure 5B). DEC-C treatment (50 mg/kg, s.c. x 5 days) resulted in 26.47% reduction (P<0.05) in adult worms but did not exert any significant embryostatic effect on female worms when compared to that of untreated control animals (Figure 5B). The general behavior of the treated animals was found normal during entire observation period indicating that UA is safe.

Together, the results of UA showed promising antifilarial activity *in vitro* and *in vivo* with no adverse affect on health and general behavior of the treated animals.

ADME/Tox compliance

The compound UA was evaluated through MetaDrug tool (Thomson Reuters, USA) for compliance to the standard ADME/Tox parameters. Results showed the information of metabolites, QSAR based prediction of ADME/Tox properties, therapeutic activities, information of analogues, pathways, potential targets and signaling pathway map by leveraging an extensive database of chemical structures and pharmacological activities and visualized in the context of pathways, cell processes, toxicity and disease networks that are perturbed by the compound and its metabolites. These results for UA are briefly discussed below:

Prediction of therapeutic activities for UA: Large numbers of therapeutic activities for the compound UA were identified

Table 7. The reported interaction between UA and target.

S. No.	Target	Type	Drug	Interactions	Similarity	Effect	Pubmed/Patent ID
1	COX-2 (PTGS2)	§	Ursolic acid	€	100	Inhibition	12444669
2	OATP-C	¥	Ursolic acid	£	100	Inhibition	12871156
3	DNA ligase I	§	(1S, 2R, 4aS, 6aS, 6bR, 10S, 12aR)-10-Hydroxy-1, 2, 6a, 6b, 9, 9, 12a-heptamethyl-1, 3, 4, 5, 6, 6a, 6b, 7, 8, 8a, 9, 10, 11, 12, 12a, 12b, 13, 14b-octadecahydro-2H-picene-4a-carboxylic acid	€	100	Unspecified	15519169
4	DNA polymerase beta	§	10-Hydroxy-1, 2, 6a, 6b, 9, 9, 12a-heptamethyl-1, 3, 4, 5, 6, 6a, 6b, 7, 8, 8a, 9, 10, 11, 12, 12a, 12b, 13, 14b-octadecahydro-2H-picene-4a-carboxylic acid (1)	€	100	Inhibition	15974441
5	ACAT2	§	(1S, 2R, 4aS, 6aS, 6bR, 8aR, 10S, 12aR, 12bR, 14bS)-10-Hydroxy-1, 2, 6a, 6b, 9, 9, 12a-heptamethyl-1, 3, 4, 5, 6, 6a, 6b, 7, 8, 8a, 9, 10, 11, 12, 12a, 12b, 13, 14b-octadecahydro-2H-picene-4a-carboxylic acid	€	100	Inhibition	16462051
6	SOAT1	§	(1S, 2R, 4aS, 6aS, 6bR, 10S, 12aR)-10-Hydroxy-1, 2, 6a, 6b, 9, 9, 12a-heptamethyl-1, 3, 4, 5, 6, 6a, 6b, 7, 8, 8a, 9, 10, 11, 12, 12a, 12b, 13, 14b-octadecahydro-2H-picene-4a-carboxylic acid	€	100	Inhibition	16462051
7	SOAT2	§	(1S, 2R, 4aS, 6aS, 6bR, 10S, 12aR)-10-Hydroxy-1, 2, 6a, 6b, 9, 9, 12a-heptamethyl-1, 3, 4, 5, 6, 6a, 6b, 7, 8, 8a, 9, 10, 11, 12, 12a, 12b, 13, 14b-octadecahydro-2H-picene-4a-carboxylic acid	€	100	Inhibition	15974441
8	ACAT1	§	(1S, 2R, 4aS, 6aS, 6bR, 8aR, 10S, 12aR, 12bR, 14bS)-10-Hydroxy-1, 2, 6a, 6b, 9, 9, 12a-heptamethyl-1, 3, 4, 5, 6, 6a, 6b, 7, 8, 8a, 9, 10, 11, 12, 12a, 12b, 13, 14b-octadecahydro-2H-picene-4a-carboxylic acid	€	100	Inhibition	11794520

§ = Generic enzymes; € = Unspecified; £ = Inhibition is done with unspecified mechanism; ¥ = Transporter.

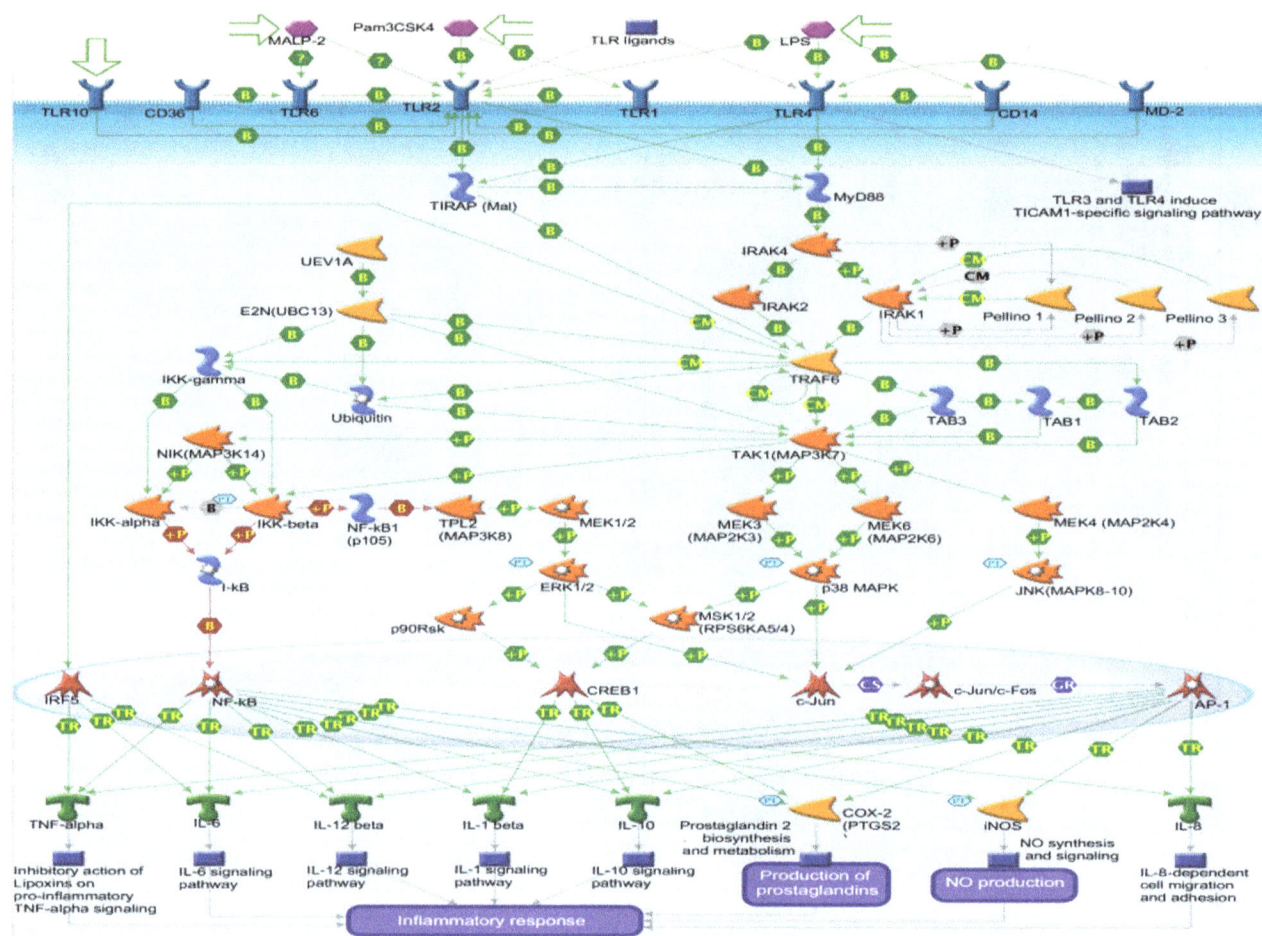

Figure 6. Signaling pathway map screened by Metadrug.

through MetaDrug tool (Thomson Reuters, USA). The evaluated therapeutic activities for UA were; allergy, Alzheimer, angina, arthritis, asthma, bacterial, cancer, depression, diabetes, HIV, heart failure, hyperlipidaemia, obesity, migraine, osteoporosis and many more. The predicted activities for UA were classified as active or non-active based on calculated values. The predicted properties of UA were calculated on the basis of Tanimoto Percentage [TP] values (standard cut-off ≥0.5) (Table 6).

Prediction of analogues, pathways and potential targets for UA: The chemical structures and the name of some known similar compounds or analogues were predicted by MetaDrug tool related to UA on the basis of structural similarity (in the range of 98–100%). MetaDrug tool also detected the potential biological pathways and the targets with experimentally known prior mode of action for UA (Table 7).

Prediction of metabolic signaling pathway map for UA: Immune response through TLR2 and TLR4 signaling pathways identified through MetaDrug tool on the basis of -lopP value i.e., 1.834e-8 (7.736) with six network objects. TLR2 and TLR4 induce MyD88/IRAK/TRAF6-dependent pathway in target cells, leading to activation of transcription factors NF-kB, AP-1, CREB1 and IRF5, which induce production of various proinflammatory mediators including cytokines, chemokines, nitric oxide (NO) and prostaglandins, leading to inflammatory response (Figure 6).

Discussion

There are only a few medicinal plant extracts and the isolated molecules, which have shown good anti-filarial activity. The literature showed that some secondary metabolites such as triterpenoids and coumarins showed significant activity against filarial parasites. Our recent finding on the antifilarial activity of pentacyclic triterpenoid, glycyrrhetinic acid (GA) has given us advantage of exploring anti-filarial activity in UA, having similar pentacyclic triterpenoid chemical structure [9,29]. The UA isolated from the leaves of E. tereticornis was in full agreement with the ^{1}H, ^{13}C NMR and ESI-MS spectroscopic data with the commercially available UA (SIGMA-ALDRICH).

The in vitro anti-filarial activity of UA against mf and the adult worms, prompted us to carry out it's in silico studies to investigate its possible mechanism of action. It is well known that filarial nematode's detoxify GST enzymes, which play a significant role in the survival of the parasites inside the host's body. This enzyme has effective ability to neutralize the reactive oxygen species (ROS) attack on membrane that acts as cytotoxic products and protect the helminths inside the host [30–32]. With this background, the in silico molecular docking binding affinity of UA against the GST enzyme was studied. The docking experiments were performed, which showed high binding affinity of UA with BmGST enzyme.

It was observed that for killing the life stages of parasites in vitro, 10 times less concentration of UA was required than the drug DEC. Similarly, in vivo, UA treatment afforded 4–33% drop in microfilaraemia over 0 day throughout the post treatment observation period. While in the untreated control it was (progressively) higher than the pretreatment level and never equaled the 0 day level. The analysis trend in the DEC-treated animals showed that the mf count after an initial dramatic drop, increased gradually over time, while in UA treated animals microfilaraemia remained almost static. This clearly shows that UA was better than DEC in controlling microfilaraemia. Further UA exhibited 54% adulticidal and 56% embryostatic effect with static microfilaraemia while DEC produced ~26% macrofilaricidal, 15% embryostatic and >85% microfilaricidal effect (on day 7 p.i.t.). These results indicate that UA is clearly superior to DEC with respect to macrofilaricidal and embryostatic effect though not with respect to microfilaricidal effect. It may be mentioned here that macrofilaricidal and embryostatic effect of UA were probably responsible for the low and static microfilaraemia. Thus, UA is better than DEC both *in vitro* and *in vivo* in its antifilarial activity. Further UA being a natural compound, has the possibility of lead optimization by QSAR approach. Thus, in view of potential antifilarial activity, absence of toxicity and favorable pharmacokinetics UA may be considered as a suitable lead for designing and development of a safe and effective antifilarial agent.

Supporting Information

Figure S1 LC$_{100}$ and IC$_{50}$ of Ursolic acid (UA) for microfilariae and adult parasites of *Brugia malayi*. After incubation with UA for 24 h the viability of parasite was assessed

in motility assay using mf (**A**) and adult female worms (**B**) and in MTT reduction assay using adult female worms (**C**).

Figure S2 LC$_{100}$ and IC$_{50}$ of diethylcarbamazine citrate (DEC-C) for microfilariae and adult parasites of *B. malayi*. After incubation with DEC-C for 24 h the viability of parasite was assessed in motility assay using mf (**A**) and adult female worms (**B**) and in MTT reduction assay using adult female worms (**C**).

Figure S3 LC$_{100}$ and IC$_{50}$ of ivermectin for microfilariae and adult parasites of *B. malayi*. After incubation with ivermectin for 24 h (**A–C**) and 48 h (**D–F**) the viability of parasite was assessed in motility assay using mf (**A, D**) and adult female worms (**B, E**) and in MTT reduction assay using adult female worms (**C, F**).

Acknowledgments

The authors thank the Directors, CSIR-CIMAP and CSIR-CDRI, Lucknow, for their keen interest and encouragement during the course of this work.

Author Contributions

Conceived and designed the experiments: SKS PKM FK. Performed the experiments: KK VK RV PS MS. Analyzed the data: SKS PKM FK. Contributed reagents/materials/analysis tools: SKS PKM FK. Wrote the paper: SKS PKM FK.

References

1. WHO, 2012. Global Programme to Eliminate Lymphatic Filariasis. Weekly Epidemiological Record. Available: http://apps.who.int/iris/bitstream/10665/78611/1/WHO_HTM_NTD_PCT_2013.5_eng.pdf. Accessed 16 July 2014.
2. Molyneux DH, Zagaria N (2002) Lymphatic filariasis elimination: Progress in global programme development. Ann Trop Med Parasitol 96: 15–40.
3. WHO, 2006. Global programme to eliminate lymphatic filariasis. Weekly epidemiological record, Geneva. Available: http://www.who.int/lymphatic_filariasis/resources/wer/en/. Accessed 22 January 2013.
4. Ottesen EA (2000) The global programme to eliminate lymphatic filariasis. Trop Med Int Hlth 5: 591–594.
5. WHO, 2005. Global programme to eliminate lymphatic filariasis. Weekly epidemiological record. Available: http://www.who.int/lymphatic_filariasis/resources/wer/en/. Accessed 22 April 2014.
6. Molyneux DH, Bradley M, Hoerauf A, Kyelem D, Taylor MJ (2003) Mass drug treatment for lymphatic filariasis and onchocerciasis. Trends Parasitol 19: 516–22.
7. Dadzie Y, Neira M, Hopkins D (2003) Final report of the conference on the eradicability of Onchocerciasis. Filaria J 2: 2.
8. Burkot TR, Durrheim DN, Melrose WD, Speare R, Ichimori K (2006) The argument for integrating vector control with multiple drug administration campaigns to ensure elimination of lymphatic filariasis. Filaria J 5: 10.
9. Kalani K, Kushwaha V, Verma R, Murthy PK, Srivastava SK (2013) Glycyrrhetinic acid and its analogs: A new class of antifilarial agents. Bioorg Med Chem Lett 23: 2566–2570.
10. Murthy PK, Joseph SK, Murthy PS (2011) Plant products in the treatment and control of filariasis and other helminth infections and assay systems for antifilarial/antihelmintic activity. Planta Med 77: 647–61.
11. Kushwaha V, Saxena K, Verma SK, Lakshmi V, Sharma RK, et al. (2011) Antifilarial activity of gum from Moringa oleifera Lam. on human lymphatic filaria *Brugia Malayi*. Chronicles of Young Scientists 202–06.
12. Maurya A, Srivastava SK (2012) Determination of ursolic acid and ursolic acid lactone in the leaves of *Eucalyptus tereticornis* by HPLC. J Braz Chem Soc 23: 468–472.
13. Kalani K, Yadav DK, Khan F, Srivastava SK, Suri N (2012) Pharmacophore, QSAR, and ADME based semisynthesis and *in vitro* evaluation of ursolic acid analogs for anticancer activity. J Mol Model 18: 3389–413.
14. Murthy PK, Tyagi K, Roy Chowdhury TK, Sen AB (1983) Susceptibility of Mastomys natalensis (GRA strain) to a sub periodic strain of human *Brugia malayi*. Indian J Med Res 77: 623–630.
15. Murthy PK, Murthy PSR, Tyagi K, Chatterjee RK (1997) Fate of infective larvae of *Brugia malayi* in the peritoneal cavity of Mastomys natalensis and Meriones unguiculatus. Folia Parasitol (Praha) 44: 302–304.
16. Murthy PK, Chatterjee RK (1999) Evaluation of two *in vitro* test systems employing *Brugia malayi* parasite for screening of potential antifilarials. Curr Sci 77: 1084–1089.
17. Lakshmi V, Joseph SK, Srivastava S, Verma SK, Sahoo MK, et al. (2010) Antifilarial activity in vitro and in vivo of some flavonoids tested against *Brugia malayi*. Acta Trop 116: 127–133.
18. Sashidhara KV, Rao KB, Kushwaha V, Modukuri RK, Verma R, et al. (2014) Synthesis and antifilarial activity of chalcone-thiazole derivatives against a human lymphatic filarial parasite, *Brugia malayi*. Eur J Med Chem 81: 473–80.
19. Page C, Page M, Noel C (1993) A new fluorimetric assay for cytotoxicity measurements *in vitro*. Int J Oncol 3: 473–476.
20. Mosmann T (1983) Rapid colorimetric assay for cellular growth and survival: application to proliferation and cytotoxicity assays. J Immunol Methods 65: 55–63.
21. Huber W, Koella JC (1993) A comparison of three methods of estimating EC$_{50}$ in studies of drug resistance of malaria parasites. Acta Trop 55: 257–261.
22. Hendlich M, Rippmann F, Barnickel G (1997) LIGSITE: automatic and efficient detection of potential small molecule-binding sites in proteins. J Mol Graph Model 15: 359–63.
23. Chatterjee RK, Fatma N, Murthy PK, Sinha P, Kulshreshtha DK, et al. (1992) Macrofilaricidal activity of the stem bark of Streblus asper and its major active constituents. Drug Develop Res 26: 67–78.
24. Gaur RL, Dixit S, Sahoo MK, Khanna M, Singh S, et al. (2007) Antifilarial activity of novel formulations of albendazole against experimental brugian filariasis. Parasitology 134: 537–544.
25. Lämmler G, Wolf E (1977) Chemo prophylactic activity of filaricidal compounds on Litomosoides carinii infection of Mastomys natalensis. Tropen Med Parasitol 28: 205–225.
26. Bugrim A, Nikolskaya T, Nikolsky Y (2004) Early prediction of drug metabolism and toxicity: systems biology approach and modeling. Drug Discov Today 9: 127–135.
27. Yadav D, Singh SC, Verma RK, Saxena K, Verma R, et al. (2013) Antifilarial diarylheptanoids from Alnus nepalensis leaves growing in high altitude areas of Uttarakhand, India. Phytomedicine 20: 124–132.

28. Azeez S, Babu RO, Aykkal R, Narayanan R (2012) Virtual screening and *in vitro* assay of potential drug like inhibitors from spices against glutathione-S-transferase of filarial nematodes. J Mol Model 18: 151–63.

29. Kalani K, Yadav DK, Singh A, Khan F, Godbole MM, et al. (2014) QSAR guided semi-synthesis and *in-vitro* validation of anticancer activity in ursolic acid derivatives. Curr Top Med Chem 14: 1005–13.

30. Lanham A, Mwanri L (2013) The Curse of Lymphatic Filariasis: Would the Continual Use of Diethylcarbamazine Eliminate this Scourge in Papua New Guinea? American Journal of Infectious Diseases and Microbiology 1: 5–12.

31. Sommer A, Nimtz M, Conradt HS, Brattig N, Boettcher K, et al. (2001) Structural analysis and antibody response to the extracellular glutathione S-transferases from Onchocerca volvulus. Infect Immun 69: 7718–28.

32. Brophy PM, Pritchard DI (1994) Parasitic helminth glutathione S-transferases: an update on their potential as targets for immuno- and chemotherapy. Exp Parasitol 79: 89–96.

10

Identification of Reference Proteins for Western Blot Analyses in Mouse Model Systems of 2,3,7,8-Tetrachlorodibenzo-P-Dioxin (TCDD) Toxicity

Stephenie D. Prokopec[1], John D. Watson[1], Raimo Pohjanvirta[2,3], Paul C. Boutros[1,4,5]*

1 Informatics and Bio-computing Program, Ontario Institute for Cancer Research, Toronto, Ontario, Canada, 2 Laboratory of Toxicology, National Institute for Health and Welfare, Kuopio, Finland, 3 Department of Food Hygiene and Environmental Health, University of Helsinki, Helsinki, Finland, 4 Department of Medical Biophysics, University of Toronto, Toronto, Ontario, Canada, 5 Department of Pharmacology & Toxicology, University of Toronto, Toronto, Ontario, Canada

Abstract

Western blotting is a well-established, inexpensive and accurate way of measuring protein content. Because of technical variation between wells, normalization is required for valid interpretation of results across multiple samples. Typically this involves the use of one or more endogenous controls to adjust the measured levels of experimental molecules. Although some endogenous controls are widely used, validation is required for each experimental system. This is critical when studying transcriptional-modulators, such as toxicants like 2,3,7,8-tetrachlorodibenzo-p-dioxin (TCDD).To address this issue, we examined hepatic tissue from 192 mice representing 47 unique combinations of strain, sex, *Ahr*-genotype, TCDD dose and treatment time. We examined 7 candidate reference proteins in each animal and assessed consistency of protein abundance through: 1) TCDD-induced fold-difference in protein content from basal levels, 2) inter- and intra- animal stability, and 3) the ability of each candidate to reduce instability of the other candidates. Univariate analyses identified HPRT as the most stable protein. Multivariate analysis indicated that stability generally increased with the number of proteins used, but gains from using >3 proteins were small. Lastly, by comparing these new data to our previous studies of mRNA controls on the same animals, we were able to show that the ideal mRNA and protein control-genes are distinct, and use of only 2–3 proteins provides strong stability, unlike in mRNA studies in the same cohort, where larger control-gene batteries were needed.

Editor: Xuejiang Guo, Nanjing Medical University, China

Funding: This study was conducted with the support of the Academy of Finland (grant nos. 123345 and 261232 to RP), the Canadian Institutes of Health Research (grant no. MOP-57903 to ABO and PCB), and the Ontario Institute for Cancer Research to PCB through funding provided by the Government of Ontario. Dr. Boutros was supported by a Terry Fox Research Institute New Investigator Award and a CIHR New Investigator Salary Award. The above funding sources had no involvement in the study design, in the collection, analysis and interpretation of data, in the writing of the document, or in the decision to submit the work for publication.

Competing Interests: The authors have declared that no competing interests exist.

* Email: Paul.Boutros@oicr.on.ca

Introduction

2,3,7,8-tetrachlorodibenzo-*p*-dioxin (TCDD) is a member of a class of environmental contaminants, known as dioxins, and is primarily produced through industrial processes including incineration and manufacture of herbicides and pesticides [1,2] as well as electronics recycling [3]. Exposure to TCDD evokes a wide range of toxicities in laboratory animals, including wasting syndrome and death [4]. In humans, short-term exposure to high levels of TCDD often presents as liver damage and chloracne, while low-dose long-term exposure has been linked to immune deficiency [5], diabetes [6], and various cancer types [2,7].

TCDD is an exogenous ligand for the aryl hydrocarbon receptor (AHR) [8]. Upon cell entry, TCDD binds cytoplasmic AHR, leading to the formation of a ligand-receptor complex which translocates into the nucleus, dimerizes with the AHR nuclear translocator (ARNT) and binds to DNA to regulate transcription of target genes [9]. Previous studies have shown that TCDD exposure results in the dysregulation of hundreds of genes in numerous models [10,11,12,13,14]. While specific changes to the transcriptome resulting from TCDD-mediated regulation have been identified across a wide range of experimental models, downstream effects on the proteome which may prove causative of toxicities, remain unclear. Complete examination of various –omics data will be required to identify the specific molecules responsible for the severe toxic effects induced by TCDD.

Animal models have been, and will continue to be, crucial to understanding the mechanisms described above [15]. In particular, the varying sensitivities to TCDD of different species and strains of rodent greatly contribute to our understanding of TCDD-mediated toxicities. For example, the Long-Evans rat strain (*Turku/AB*; L-E) displays a very low tolerance for TCDD ($LD_{50} = 10$ µg/kg) while the Han/Wistar rat (*Kuopio*; H/W) is resistant to TCDD-induced lethality ($LD_{50} > 9600$ µg/kg) [16]. This difference in sensitivity is caused by a point mutation in the H/W *Ahr*, resulting in expression of multiple isoforms of the AHR [17], leading to differential regulation of a subset of genes in H/W animals [18]. These differentially abundant transcripts, and any ensuing changes to the proteome, may lead to strain-specific TCDD toxicities. Similarly, in mice, both the C57BL/6 and DBA/2 strains exhibit TCDD-mediated toxic effects, however DBA/2 mice are much more resistant (approximately 10 to 20 times) than the C57BL/6 strain [19]. This resistance is caused by a point mutation within the ligand binding domain of the *Ahr* in the DBA/2 mice [20]. TCDD-toxicity also varies between male and female animals within a species. Female rats are more sensitive to TCDD-lethality than male rats, while in mice this relationship is reversed [21].

Analysis of protein content is the general end-point for many biological experiments. While mass spectrophotometry is a highly sensitive and specific technique, both the data generation and analysis steps are highly complex [22]. As such, western blot has become the standard method of use, as it allows for the sensitive and specific detection of target proteins with accurate relative quantitation of protein content in a relatively simple and inexpensive manner [23]. However, as in transcriptomic studies, accurate assessment of protein abundance by western blot requires thorough normalization of the data prior to the interpretation of results. This normalization typically involves the use of total protein or one or more endogenous loading controls in order to account for technical variability and to determine relative target abundance, thereby allowing multiple samples to be compared. While measurement of total protein is a relatively simple approach, it leads to complications downstream [24]. Specifically, coomassie stained gels cannot be transferred to membrane for subsequent analysis and thereby requires the assumption that simultaneously run gels are loaded with identical amounts of protein [25]. The use of endogenous controls bypasses the need for additional steps, thereby reducing the number of gels and amount of sample used. Ideal endogenous control proteins maintain consistent levels of abundance regardless of environmental conditions, and thus often perform functions essential for cell survival [26]. Glyceraldehyde-3-phosphate dehydrogenase (GAPDH) and beta-actin (ACTB) have frequently been used as reference genes for both

mRNA expression measured by qPCR [26,27] and western blot analyses of protein content [28]. However, studies have shown that the stability of these widely used reference genes is not always consistent under different experimental conditions [29,30]. Factors such as tissue-type [30], organism (between and within species) [31], experimental manipulation [32] and even reagents used [33] can affect the abundance of candidate reference molecules. For these reasons, it is essential that endogenous reference proteins be thoroughly evaluated prior to experimental use.

Investigations into TCDD-induced proteomic changes are necessary to further our understanding of dioxin toxicity. Before these studies can proceed, candidate reference proteins must be carefully validated for use in western blot within the model systems used. Several reference genes have been previously validated for use in transcriptomic studies in rat [34] and mouse models [31] of TCDD toxicity. Currently, reference proteins for use in proteomic studies within these animal models have yet to undergo thorough validation. Since the transcriptomic responses differ dramatically across animal models [14,35], it is unclear whether these validated transcriptomic reference genes will translate to proteomic studies in either species. While it is not necessary to use the same controls for assessments of both gene and protein abundance, it is generally accepted that stably expressed genes may result in consistent abundance of protein [36,37]. We therefore chose to examine those genes previously identified as suitable references for transcriptomic studies of TCDD-toxicity [31], in addition to ACTB, to determine their validity for proteomic studies. Seven candidate proteins (*i.e.* ACTB, EEF1A1, GAPDH, HPRT, PGK1, PPIA and SDHA) were tested in hepatic tissue from multiple mouse models of TCDD-toxicity. This allows us to experimentally verify the idea that similar controls can be used at the RNA and protein levels, which would reduce the workload inherent in establishing controls.

Table 1. Experimental Design.

Study	Strain	Sex	Genotype	Treatment (TCDD μg/kg)	Time of tissue harvest (hours)	Number of animals
1	C57BL/6	Male	WT	0, 500	6	4, 5
	C57BL/6	Female	WT	0, 500	6	4, 5
2	C57BL/6	Male	rWT	0, 5, 500	19	4, 4, 4
	DBA/2J	Male	Ala375Val	0, 5, 500	19	4, 4, 4
3	C57BL/6	Male	WT	0, 500	24	4, 5
	C57BL/6	Female	WT	0, 500	24	3, 5
4	C57BL/6	Male	WT	0, 500	72	4, 5
	C57BL/6	Female	WT	0, 500	72	4, 5
5	C57BL/6	Male	WT	0, 500	144	3, 4
	C57BL/6	Female	WT	0, 500	144	3, 5
6	C57BL/6	Male	WT	0, 125, 250, 500, 1000	96	4, 4, 4, 4, 4
7	C57BL/6	Male	DEL	0, 125, 250, 500, 1000	96	5, 4, 3, 3, 4
8	C57BL/6	Male	INS	0, 125, 250, 500, 1000	96	5, 4, 4, 4, 5
9	C57BL/6	Male	rWT	0, 125, 250, 500, 1000	96	5, 3, 1, 4, 3
10	C57BL/6	Female	WT	0, 125, 250, 500, 1000	96	5, 5, 4, 4, 5

Animals analyzed (n = 192) varied in strain, sex, *Ahr*-allele, TCDD-treatment and time-point at which tissue was collected.

Table 2. Summary of analysis methods.

| | Student's t-test | NormFinder | | Normalization Method |
		Training	Validation	
ACTB	6/28	0.092	0.060	996.59
EEF1A1	11/28	0.112	0.050	278.40
GAPDH	5/31	0.072	0.077	316.07
HPRT	**1/31**	0.078	**0.046**	306.46
PGK1	6/29	0.144	0.081	**259.58**
PPIA	8/31	0.140	0.066	366.06
SDHA	10/26	**0.071**	0.056	286.62

Three analysis methods were used to evaluate the abundance consistency of each individual candidate protein; values in bold indicate the top ranked score for each method. 1) The difference between treated and untreated animals for each experimental condition was assessed by Student's t-tests; a p-value <0.05 was deemed significant. 2) The variation of each candidate was assessed using the NormFinder algorithm in two separate cohorts; a lower score indicates greater stability. 3) The comparative normalization method was used to evaluate the ability of each candidate to remove variation from a dataset; the average standard deviation for each pairwise comparison is reported.

Methods

Ethics Statement

All study plans were approved by the Finnish National Animal Experiment Board (Eläinkoelautakunta, ELLA; permit code: ESLH-2008-07223/Ym-23).

Animal Handling

Animal models and handling have been described previously [31]. Briefly, mouse colonies were maintained at the National Public Health Institute (today National Institute for Health and Welfare), Division of Environmental Health, Kuopio, Finland. Male and female C57BL/6 wild-type mice [21], male transgenic mice [38] and male DBA/2J mice [21] were studied. Wild-type animals were 12–15 weeks old and transgenic mice ranged up to 23 weeks. Animals were housed singly to avoid aggressive social behaviour, with environmental conditions maintained at $21 \pm 1°C$ with a relative humidity of $50 \pm 10\%$ on a 12 hour light cycle (12 hours of light followed by 12 hours of dark). Housing consisted of suspended, wire-mesh stainless-steel cages or Makrolon cages with aspen chip bedding (Tapvei Oy, Kaavi, Finland) and animals were provided with Altromin 1314 pellet feed (Altromin Spezialfutter GmbH & Co. KG, Lage, Germany) and water available *ad libitum*. The microbiological status of the animal facilities was regularly monitored in compliance with the recommendations of the Federation of European Laboratory Animal Science (FELASA), but individual mice were not tested in this regard. All experimental animals were drug and test naïve. Initial body weights for each animal are provided in Table S6.

Animals were stratified according to age such that groups contained a similar age-range, followed by randomization into experimental groups. Mice were treated in a group-wise manner, starting with the control in order to minimize the chance of human error. In most cases, the administration for a group was accomplished within an hour. Mice were treated with TCDD or corn oil vehicle alone and assessed following both timecourse and dose-response studies as described previously [31]. A total of 192 mice were used distributed across 47 separate experimental conditions (Table 1, Figure S1). TCDD was dissolved in corn oil and administered by oral gavage (10 mL/kg). Mice treated with corn oil alone acted as controls in each experiment.

Briefly, animals in the timecourse study were treated with a single dose of TCDD (500 μg/kg) or corn oil alone at time zero, followed by euthanasia at different time points (animals with tissue collected at the 19 hour time point received either 0, 5 or 500 μg/kg TCDD). Animals in the dose-response study received a single dose of 0, 125, 250, 500 or 1000 μg/kg TCDD followed by euthanasia 96 hours post-treatment. Although some of these doses were above the LD_{50} level of the exposed animals, the exposure time was in all cases maximally about 50% of the shortest time-to-death for these strains and genetic models as recorded in previous studies [21,33], and no mortality was therefore expected. However, all animals were carefully observed at least twice daily throughout the experimental period and, should signs consistent with severe suffering have been detected, those animals would have been euthanized immediately, as per the approved animal study plans.

Mouse livers were excised and snap-frozen in liquid nitrogen following euthanasia by carbon dioxide exposure. Tissue was shipped on dry ice to the analytical laboratory and stored at −80°C or colder. All animal handling and reporting comply with ARRIVE guidelines [39].

Western analysis

Protein levels for candidate genes were determined by quantitative western blot. Each experiment was assessed on a single western blot to ensure identical analysis conditions between treated and control animals. Total protein was isolated from mouse liver using Tissue Extraction Reagent I (Life Technologies, Burlington, ON) supplemented with cOmplete protease inhibitor cocktail (Roche, Laval, QC). Protein extract, diluted 1/10 and 1/20 with 1XPBS, was quantified by Bradford assay and diluted to a final concentration of 10 μg/μL. A total of 65 μg protein [40,41] was loaded into each well of a Novex 4–12% Bis-Tris midi-gel system to ensure sufficient material would be available for the detection of low abundance targets [42]. Prepared gels were then electrophoresed for 40 minutes at 200V with MES running buffer (Life Technologies). Protein was transferred to PVDF membrane with the iBlot system using program P0 for 7 minutes (Life Technologies). The Colloidal Blue Staining Kit (Life Technologies) was used to observe total protein before and after electrophoresis and Ponceau staining was performed on the transferred membrane to ensure sufficient protein transfer (Figure S4). While there is some variation between samples, protein transfer appears consistent. Primary antibodies were purchased from Santa Cruz (Santa Cruz Biotechnology Inc.,

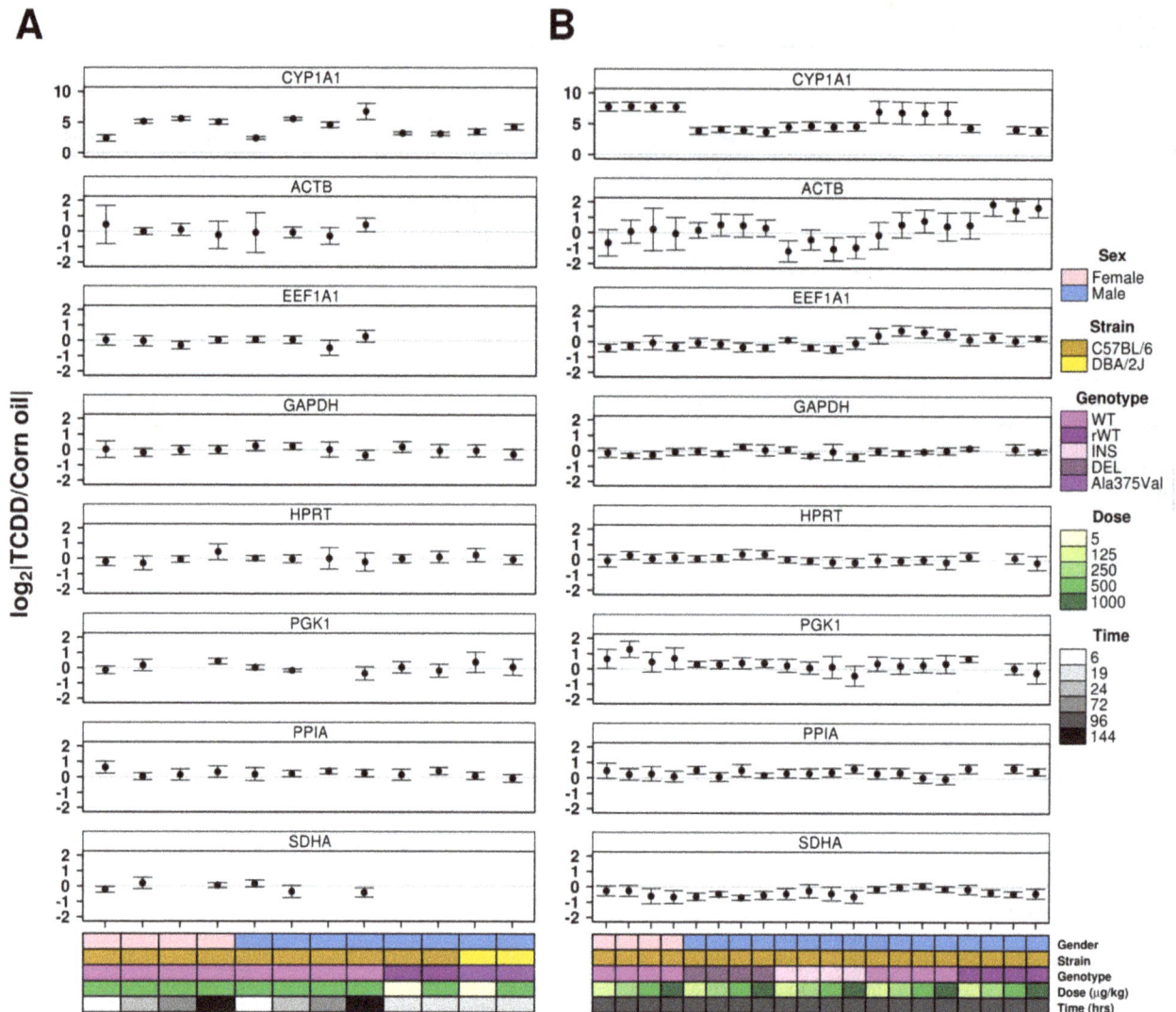

Figure 1. Timecourse and Dose-response by Treatment Group. The fold-differences in protein abundance between treated and control animals were calculated and results compared across all conditions. (**A**) Timecourse and (**B**) dose-response studies were visualized. Points represent the fold change in abundance (in log₂ space) and error bars indicate the standard deviation for each experimentally unique group.

Dallas, TX) or Abcam (Abcam Inc., Toronto, ON) and were diluted at the recommended concentrations in Li-Cor blocking buffer supplemented with 0.1% Tween-20, with overnight incubation at 4°C. Blots were washed three times with PBS supplemented with 0.1% Tween-20 at room temperature for 5 minutes each. The Li-Cor IRDye-labelled secondary antibodies (Mandel Scientific, Guelph, ON) were used at a dilution of 1:10,000 in Li-Cor blocking buffer supplemented as above with 0.01% SDS and incubated at room temperature for 1 hour (ordering information and optimal dilutions for all antibodies are provided in Table S1). After washing as described, blots were scanned and analyzed with the Odyssey quantitative western blot near-infrared system (Li-Cor Biosciences, Lincoln, NE, USA) using default settings. Antibodies were initially tested individually and then grouped based on banding patterns in order to reduce the number of blots required [43]. Average band intensities were normalized by subtraction of background levels. Background normalized values are provided in Table S2 and scanned images in Figure S2. Primary and secondary antibodies were initially

tested individually to identify optimal concentrations for the reduction of nonspecific banding patterns. Antibodies were then grouped where possible such that desired bands did not overlap.

Statistical Analyses and Visualization

Data were loaded in the R statistical environment (v3.0.3) for all analyses. Protein content was aggregated across biological replicates to obtain a mean abundance with standard for each candidate protein. Aggregation into biological replicates resulted in 47 separate experimental conditions. The ratio between treated and control abundances provided the fold-difference (M) in expression. Individual proteins and all possible combinations of multiple proteins were assessed. Visualizations were produced using the lattice (v0.20–29) and latticeExtra (v0.6–26) R packages.

Protein content was assessed across timecourse and dose-response studies. Animals treated with TCDD were compared to control animals of the same experimental group resulting in 26–31 comparisons (some comparisons were not done due to unsatisfactory loading patterns and/or lack of sufficient sample). Differential

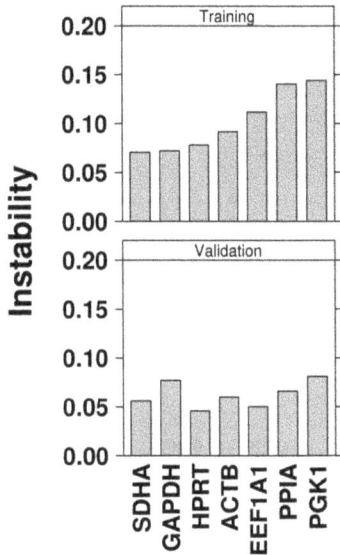

Figure 2. Univariate Analysis of Candidate Stability. Animals were separated into training and validation cohorts based on experiment, ensuring similar treatment conditions and animal numbers appeared in both sets. Within each cohort, animals were categorized as either TCDD-treated or control. Candidate proteins were analyzed using the NormFinder algorithm to determine stability across all treatment groups. A lower value indicates less variance across all experimental conditions.

abundance resulting from exposure to TCDD was evaluated for each candidate using an unpaired, two-tailed Student's t-test with Welch's adjustment for heteroscedasticity. Results were visualized as M $\pm$ standard-deviation for all experimental conditions.

Protein stability was evaluated using the NormFinder algorithm, which estimates the overall variation of a dataset by analysing its variance both within an experimental group and across experimental conditions [44]. Prior to analysis, animals were categorized into one of two groups (TCDD-treated or control) to estimate variance within experimental groups. Experiments were then split into 2 cohorts, labelled training (including experiments 1, 4, 6, 8 and 9) and validation (consisting of experiments 2, 3, 5, 7 and 10), such that each cohort contained similar types and number of animals and each cohort was analysed independently of the other. For each combination of candidates, the geometric mean of the background-normalized protein levels was calculated for each animal. For interpretation, a lower score indicates higher consistency of input across experimental groups signifying a potentially good loading control. Stability scores are available in Table S3. Linear modelling was performed to identify the contribution of each candidate protein [$Y_{OS} = \alpha_{ACTB} + \alpha_{EEF1A1} + \alpha_{GAPDH} + \alpha_{HPRT} + \alpha_{PGK1} + \alpha_{PPIA} + \alpha_{SDHA} + \varepsilon$] where Y_{OS} represents the overall stability of each combination of candidates and each protein is a Boolean variable indicating presence/absence in the combination while epsilon represents any error in the observations not explained by the model.

The comparative normalization method was used to contrast abundance levels between pairs of candidate molecules for each sample (adapted for use with protein abundance data from the comparative ΔC_q method [45]). The ability of each candidate to remove variability from other proteins was assessed and the mean standard deviation across comparisons provided a measure of stability.

mRNA analysis of candidate reference genes was reported previously for these animals and C_q data were downloaded (Supplementary Table 2, [31]); protein abundance and mean C_q data are provided in Table S4 for each animal. The correlation between protein levels and mean C_q values for each gene was assessed using Spearman's correlation using the AS89 method to assess statistical significance. NormFinder-generated stability scores were compared using the Spearman's correlation metric as the ordering of the scores is more meaningful than the magnitude (data available in Table S5).

Results

Quantitation of protein abundance by western blot is an essential technique widely used in the scientific community. In the past, this was typically performed using chemiluminesence. However, the Odyssey Infrared Imaging System is a well-documented alternative that provides many benefits over earlier methods, including an enhanced dynamic range of detection. Additionally, this system has the capacity for multiplexed reactions; specifically, antibodies are conjugated to IR fluorophores that can be detected at different wavelengths. As such, this system is ideal for detecting multiple targets [46].

Univariate Analysis

A good reference gene is one whose abundance is consistent across a wide range of conditions. This is most easily detected through analysis of the fold-difference (M) in expression from basal levels across specific treatment conditions. Candidate abundance was compared across conditions. Moderate correlations were observed between HPRT and PGK1 (Pearson's correlation, $R = 0.6$) as well as EEF1A1 and SDHA ($R = 0.49$), while the remaining candidates were weakly correlated (Figure S3).

To better understand this variation, each experimental group was examined individually (Figure 1). Of the 31 different experiment groups and 192 animals for which protein data were obtained (and for which mRNA data were obtained previously), HPRT was significantly altered by TCDD in only one group and GAPDH (5/31 conditions significantly altered) was also consistent, while the remainder of targets displayed less consistency, with greater than 20% of conditions altered (Table 2). To verify our samples and approach, the prototypical Ahr-regulated gene, CYP1A1, was examined as above and was determined to be significantly altered by TCDD at the protein level across all 31 conditions, as expected (Figure 1).

As this evaluation of differences in TCDD-altered abundance only accounts for variation within a single treatment, individual candidate stability across all experimental conditions was assessed using the NormFinder algorithm [44]. Briefly, NormFinder estimates the overall numerical stability of a molecule based on variability within a single treatment condition, variation within and between multiple conditions and systemic variation between experimental runs. Lower stability scores indicate less variation while higher scores indicate greater instability across experiments. As with our previous analysis of reference genes for transcriptomic analysis [31], experiments were organized into training and validation sets, thereby evaluating protein stability in two independent cohorts (Figure 2, Table 2). Although the cohorts differed in the magnitudes of stability scores, HPRT and SDHA were consistently amongst the most stable of the candidates, while PGK1 and PPIA were consistently the most unstable of the proteins evaluated.

To ensure that our results are not confounded by a shift in abundance caused by technical variation and independent of

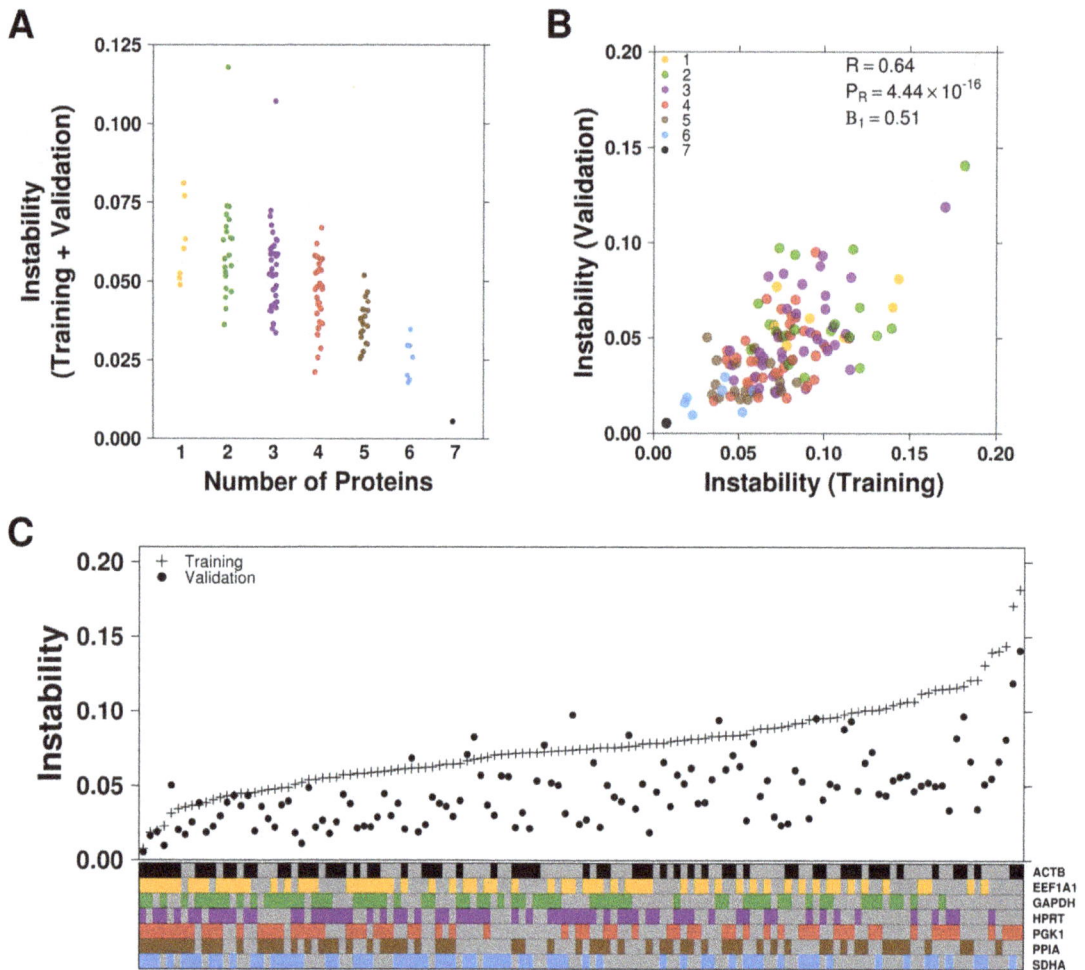

Figure 3. Multivariate Analysis of Candidate Stability. Animals were categorized as either TCDD-treated or control and separated into training and validation cohorts. All possible combinations of candidates were analyzed using the NormFinder algorithm. A lower value indicates less variance across all experimental conditions. (**A**) Combinations of candidates were organized according to the number of proteins included, in order to determine the optimal number of proteins used. (**B**) Stability results for each combination of candidates were compared between the training and validation sets to assess concordance. (**C**) Results for each combination of gene(s) were plotted for both the training (+) and validation (●) cohorts. Combinations are organized according to performance in the training set.

TCDD-treatment, we applied an alternate univariate analysis technique. Under typical experimental settings, it would be the purpose of the reference gene to normalize abundance levels for this shift. To this end, abundances of 6 proteins from each animal were normalized using the 7th, and the variance across technical replicates evaluated. This process was repeated using each protein as the normalization candidate. Using this approach, a lower score indicated greater stability across a dataset resulting from normalization with the given candidate protein (Table 2). By this method, PGK1 and EEF1A1 were determined to be the most stable of candidate proteins while ACTB was responsible for increased variation, likely due to the difference in magnitude of the intensity values between targets (intensity values for ACTB are significantly higher than for other candidates). Surprisingly, while PGK1 was identified as one of the more variable candidates both by analysis of fold-differences and the NormFinder algorithm, it was among the most stable candidates by this normalization method.

Multivariate Analysis

It has previously been shown that the use of multiple reference genes can improve normalization [31,47]. Although this generally applies to more high-throughput technologies capable of analyzing a large number of genes simultaneously, we evaluated the usefulness of utilizing multiple controls for western blot studies. The normalization capabilities of each possible combination of our candidate proteins were tested using the NormFinder algorithm, as described above. In general, including more control genes improved stability; however, specific pairs of candidates, and even some individual candidates, showed greater stability than some larger combinations (Figure 3A). Within each subset of samples, candidate combinations generally performed similarly; however, the training cohort demonstrated slightly more variance among samples (Pearson's correlation $= 0.64$) (Figure 3B). Despite this, the combination of all 7 candidates displayed the greatest stability in both cohorts (Figure 3C).

As a greater instability score appeared to primarily result from the inclusion of select candidates, linear modeling was performed to examine the contribution of each candidate to overall stability.

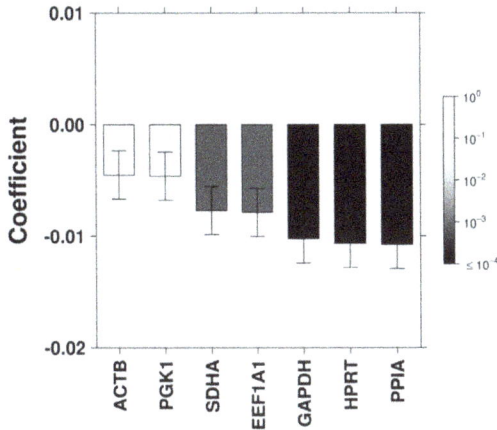

Figure 4. Linear Modelling of Multivariate Results. Linear modelling was performed to identify the contribution of each candidate to stability as determined by NormFinder across the complete dataset bars are coloured according to FDR-corrected p-value; error bars indicate standard error within the model; negative values are representative of decreased variation (increased stability).

ACTB and PGK1 decreased stability while GAPDH, HPRT and PPIA significantly increased stability (Figure 4).

Comparison with mRNA

As a similar analysis on the mRNA abundance of these candidates had been previously conducted in the liver of these animals, we thus compared the mRNA and protein abundances for each candidate. Spearman's correlation was used to determine whether protein abundance was concordant with mRNA levels. In general, there was little to no correlation between these molecules, possibly indicating differential regulation of translational mechanisms or variation in stability of the protein (Table 3, Figure 5A). To verify this, stability scores for each dataset generated by

NormFinder were combined, and the overlapping gene combinations compared (Figure 5B). Interestingly, while the abundance patterns of these candidates varied, combinations of candidates generally demonstrated similar stability (Spearman's correlation $= 0.5$, $p = 3.65 \times 10^{-5}$). Among the candidates (independently or in combination) that overlapped between studies, HPRT was among the most stable individual genes while the partnership of HPRT and GAPDH was consistently the most stable pair of candidates. Beyond this, the order of combination stability varied, sometimes dramatically, between data types. For example, the combination of EEF1A1, GAPDH and PPIA proved highly stable within the mRNA data, but was among the most unstable within the protein dataset. Alternatively, the pair-wise combination of EEF1A1 and PGK1 was among the most stable within the protein data and among the least stable in the mRNA data (Table S5).

Discussion

Thorough validation of reference genes is essential prior to any quantitative experimentation. Whether for evaluation of mRNA or protein abundance, all experimental methods are prone to some variation; the general rule is that each step in a process will introduce some error. This error may not be noticeable throughout the process, and only becomes apparent in downstream analyses, such as molecule quantitation. To ensure accurate interpretation, it is imperative to account for this technical variation. Estimation of target values relative to a reference molecule, whether internal or exogenous spike-in control is a proven method across technologies [48,49]. In the case of an endogenous molecule reference, careful validation must first occur as it has been shown that even classically-used controls can differ in abundance across different sample types or even by sample handling methods. For example, *Gapdh* was found to be less stable over time in FFPE breast tumour samples by qRT-PCR [50] whereas it was deemed a suitable reference gene for use in lung tumour FFPE samples [51]. In a proteomic analysis, multiple species of GAPDH were identified within human platelet samples; of these, the most abundant of species was highly variable across

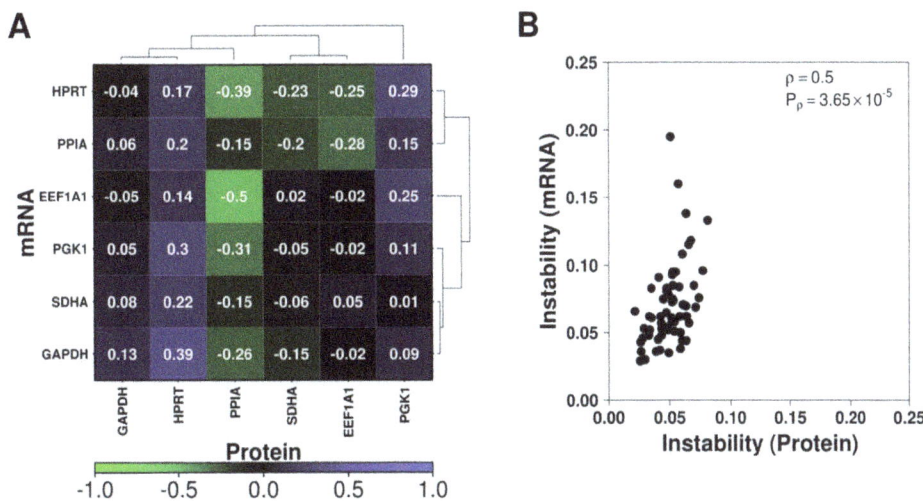

Figure 5. Comparison of candidate mRNA and protein abundances. mRNA and protein abundances as determined by qPCR and quantitative western blot were compared for each candidate. (**A**) Spearman's correlation was used to compare mean C_q values across technical replicates for qPCR and protein intensity for candidate genes and visualized in a heatmap organized using divisive clustering: blue indicates perfect correlation, green indicates inverse correlation and black indicates little or no correlation. Note that an increasing mRNA abundance results in a lower C_q; hence an inverse correlation indicates similarity between molecule abundances. (**B**) Spearman's correlation was used to assess similarity in candidate combination stability calculated by NormFinder for each data type.

Table 3. Comparison between mRNA and protein abundances.

	Spearman's correlation	
	ρ	p-value
EEF1A1	−0.02	0.79
GAPDH	0.13	0.08
HPRT	0.17	0.02
PGK1	0.11	0.14
PPIA	−0.15	0.04
SDHA	−0.06	0.46

Spearman's correlation was used to evaluate concordance between mRNA and protein abundances as determined by qPCR (mean C_q of technical replicates) and western blot (log_2 of the protein intensity). Note that an increasing mRNA abundance results in a lower C_q; hence an inverse correlation indicates similarity between molecule abundance.

both age and sex [52]. This indicates that particular effort must be made when validating loading controls for western blot, as different antibodies may target different species.

Exposure to TCDD has been shown to have a dramatically different effect on transcriptomic regulation across various animal models. This has been shown to result from ligand activation of the AHR by TCDD-binding [8] while the degree of toxicity is directly related to the *Ahr*-genotype within rodents. While studies into the specific transcriptomic changes responsible for overall toxicity are still ongoing, progress has been made in the identification of candidate lists within various animal models, including strains of rats [53,54] and mice [55]. However, as toxicity likely results from subsequent changes in the proteome, further studies are required to verify which of these candidate genes are concomitantly altered at the protein level. While validation of reference genes for RNA quantitation in various mouse models has been completed [31], there is no reason to expect similar results to be obtained at the level of the proteome.

Here, we have evaluated the protein abundance of 7 reference genes for use in toxico-proteomic analyses of TCDD-induced toxicity within a wide range of mouse models. In particular, we have assessed the effect of TCDD exposure on protein abundance within mouse models of various strains, *Ahr*-genotype and sex across both a timecourse and dose-response approach. Protein abundance was assessed by quantitative western blot analysis and each candidate's suitability as a reference control was evaluated using 3 analysis methods: 1) the fold-difference in protein content from basal levels, 2) the NormFinder algorithm [44], which is an assessment of target stability and 3) the ability of each candidate to reduce instability of the others [45].

As TCDD is known to have a significant impact on transcriptional regulation, and has been shown to affect the proteome [56], the protein abundance of our candidates was first assessed using biologically similar animals that were treated with either TCDD (at various doses) or corn oil alone. HPRT was identified as the protein least affected by TCDD while EEF1A1 and SDHA showed significant variability across multiple experimental conditions (Figure 1, Table 2). The suitability of this method is proven through the evaluation of CYP1A1; a protein involved in the detoxification of xenobiotics known to be significantly induced by TCDD. As well, since data for both treated and control animals were generated on a single western blot (experiencing identical experimental settings), this metric was arguably the most appropriate for our goals. Next, as the purpose of a reference gene is to efficiently remove technical variation from the quantified results, we sought to characterize the residual

variability among the remaining proteins after normalization with each candidate. An assumption of this method is that all candidate proteins demonstrate consistent expression over experimental conditions and that increased variation indicates decreased stability of the candidate in question [47]. Here we identified EEF1A1 and PGK1 as the most consistently expressed candidate genes while PPIA was again determined to be the least stable candidate (Table 2). The high instability of ACTB should be interpreted with caution as it does not follow the above assumption. One limitation of this approach is its disregard for technical considerations; since each western blot contained a separate experiment, and were performed one at a time, some technical variation would be inherent across the entire study. Finally, unlike the above comparative method, the NormFinder algorithm considers variation both within and between experiments in its assessment of candidate stability [44]. While the specific order of stability varied, NormFinder analysis identified HPRT, ACTB and SDHA as the most stable candidates in all cohorts examined (training, validation and overall). Similarly, PGK1 and PPIA were always deemed the most unstable candidates. The consistency in stability scores for each candidate protein verifies that NormFinder is a robust and reproducible method for identifying good reference proteins.

A major finding of our previous study of reference gene stability in qPCR studies was that greater stability was obtained through increasing the number of reference genes used. This finding was consistent with other reference gene validation studies [47,57]. In order to determine whether this finding was consistent with proteomic analysis, NormFinder analysis was applied as above. In general, the trend of increasing stability was consistent with the inclusion of an increasing number of candidates (Figure 3). However, due to the low-throughput nature of any western blot analysis, increasing the number of reference proteins is largely impractical. Therefore, careful selection of 2 or 3 candidates with good stability would prove ideal. In some cases, even a single reference gene could provide a more stable normalization factor than a larger, less consistently expressed group of candidates. To this effect, linear modelling of the multivariate analysis indicated that 2 of the 3 most stable candidates identified in the univariate analysis (HPRT and SDHA) each contributed significantly to increased stability when included in combinations of any number of candidates (Figure 4) while PGK1 contributed less.

The availability of both mRNA and protein abundances collected from the same 192 animals presented an interesting opportunity, as an in-depth comparison of these molecules for these candidate genes across such a wide range of conditions has yet to be performed. We sought to determine whether targets selected as optimal reference genes at the level of mRNA would be suitable for normalization of protein abundance data. A comparison of abundance levels suggested little or no correlation between molecules (Table 3). The largest correlation coefficient, though showing an inverse relationship in abundance, was observed for HPRT. While analysis of the fold-changes identified HPRT as most stable univariate candidate at the protein level, it was much less stable at the level of mRNA abundance. However, it consistently ranked among the most stable genes across all analysis methods in each study. Alternatively, the least stable gene identified in the RNA study, *Sdha*, ranked among the most stable in the current protein analysis and did not show correlation between molecules. As such, the optimal reference gene for studies of mRNA abundance may not be optimal for studies of protein abundance and should be validated prior to use. Conversely, multivariate analysis by NormFinder generated stability scores that were moderately correlated between data types and, in general, these scores improved with the addition of an increased number of genes. Even so, the practicality of using a larger number of genes is limited by the technology used and must be taken into consideration. As such, while using a larger number of genes is encouraged for studies easily multiplexed (such as qPCR), careful selection of fewer genes is required for low-throughput methods such as western blot.

For any type of quantitative analysis, data must be thoroughly normalized in order to account for the technical variation inherent in any experiment and to ensure reliable and reproducible results. The use of multiple controls is ideal for generation of a normalization factor; however, a carefully selected group of fewer candidates can prove sufficient when larger numbers are impractical. Here we have identified and suggested specific combinations of loading controls, such as HPRT alone or combined with ACTB or GAPDH, for use in western blot analysis of various mouse models of TCDD toxicity.

Supporting Information

Figure S1　Experimental Design. Mice were treated with either 0, 5, 125, 250, 500 or 1000 μg/kg TCDD dissolved in corn oil vehicle and euthanized at 6, 19, 24, 72, 96 or 144 hours post-exposure. Timecourse experiments followed male (blue) and female (pink) wild-type C57BL/6 mice treated with 500 μg/kg TCDD. Male DBA/2J and ratonized-WT mice were collected at 19 hours post-exposure following treatment with either 5 or 500 μg/kg TCDD. Dose-response experiments followed male (blue) wild-type or ratonized mice and female (pink) wild-type mice treated with a single dose of TCDD and euthanized 96 hours following exposure.

Figure S2　Western blots. Western blots were scanned and analyzed with the Odyssey quantitative western blot near-infrared

system using default settings. Each blot was scanned twice as two groups of antibodies were used. Wells with unusual loading patterns (noted by the *) were not used in the downstream analysis.

Figure S3　Correlation of Candidate Proteins. The fold-difference in abundance between treated and control groups were calculated for each experimental condition and Pearson's correlations applied. Correlation results were visualized using a heatmap and organized by divisive clustering. Blue indicates perfect correlation; green represents inverse correlations while black indicates little or no correlation. Pearson's correlations are shown in white for each pair-wise comparison.

Figure S4　Ponceau Stain. Total protein abundance was assessed in a representative gel using Colloidal Blue Stain pre-(A) and post-transfer (B). Total protein was quantified and background-normalized intensity values were visualized for both gels (C). Transferred protein was also visualized on the membrane (D) using Ponceau stain. Lanes labelled in black indicate untreated samples, while blue labels are TCDD-treated (500 μg/kg) samples. The first four lanes show increasing amounts of loaded protein.

Table S1　Antibody Information.

Table S2　Protein Abundances.

Table S3　NormFinder Stability Scores.

Table S4　Comparison of mRNA and Protein Abundances.

Table S5　Comparison of mRNA and Protein Stability Scores.

Table S6　Animal Information.

Acknowledgments

The authors thank Arja Moilanen, Virpi Tiihonen, Janne Korkalainen and Susanna Lukkarinen for performing all animal experiments and sample preparation, as well as Herman Cheung for invaluable technical assistance.

Author Contributions

Conceived and designed the experiments: RP PCB. Performed the experiments: SDP. Analyzed the data: SDP. Contributed reagents/materials/analysis tools: SDP. Wrote the paper: SDP. Sample preparation: SDP JW.

References

1. Schecter A, Birnbaum L, Ryan JJ, Constable JD (2006) Dioxins: an overview. Environ Res 101: 419–428.
2. Marinkovic N, Pasalic D, Ferencak G, Grskovic B, Stavljenic Rukavina A (2010) Dioxins and human toxicity. Arh Hig Rada Toksikol 61: 445–453.
3. Shen C, Chen Y, Huang S, Wang Z, Yu C, et al. (2009) Dioxin-like compounds in agricultural soils near e-waste recycling sites from Taizhou area, China: chemical and bioanalytical characterization. Environ Int 35: 50–55.
4. Seefeld MD, Corbett SW, Keesey RE, Peterson RE (1984) Characterization of the wasting syndrome in rats treated with 2,3,7,8-tetrachlorodibenzo-p-dioxin. Toxicol Appl Pharmacol 73: 311–322.

5. Weisglas-Kuperus N, Patandin S, Berbers GA, Sas TC, Mulder PG, et al. (2000) Immunologic effects of background exposure to polychlorinated biphenyls and dioxins in Dutch preschool children. Environ Health Perspect 108: 1203–1207.
6. Longnecker MP, Michalek JE (2000) Serum dioxin level in relation to diabetes mellitus among Air Force veterans with background levels of exposure. Epidemiology 11: 44–48.
7. Bertazzi PA, Zocchetti C, Guercilena S, Consonni D, Tironi A, et al. (1997) Dioxin exposure and cancer risk: a 15-year mortality study after the "Seveso accident". Epidemiology 8: 646–652.
8. Okey AB, Riddick DS, Harper PA (1994) The Ah receptor: mediator of the toxicity of 2,3,7,8-tetrachlorodibenzo-p-dioxin (TCDD) and related compounds. Toxicol Lett 70: 1–22.

9. Okey AB (2007) An aryl hydrocarbon receptor odyssey to the shores of toxicology: the Deichmann Lecture, International Congress of Toxicology-XI. Toxicol Sci 98: 5–38.

10. Boutros PC, Yao CQ, Watson JD, Wu AH, Moffat ID, et al. (2011) Hepatic transcriptomic responses to TCDD in dioxin-sensitive and dioxin-resistant rats during the onset of toxicity. Toxicol Appl Pharmacol 251: 119–129.

11. Puga A, Sartor MA, Huang MY, Kerzee JK, Wei YD, et al. (2004) Gene expression profiles of mouse aorta and cultured vascular smooth muscle cells differ widely, yet show common responses to dioxin exposure. Cardiovasc Toxicol 4: 385–404.

12. Hanlon PR, Zheng W, Ko AY, Jefcoate CR (2005) Identification of novel TCDD-regulated genes by microarray analysis. Toxicol Appl Pharmacol 202: 215–228.

13. Kim S, Dere E, Burgoon LD, Chang CC, Zacharewski TR (2009) Comparative analysis of AhR-mediated TCDD-elicited gene expression in human liver adult stem cells. Toxicol Sci 112: 229–244.

14. Boverhof DR, Burgoon LD, Tashiro C, Sharratt B, Chittim B, et al. (2006) Comparative toxicogenomic analysis of the hepatotoxic effects of TCDD in Sprague Dawley rats and C57BL/6 mice. Toxicol Sci 94: 398–416.

15. Pohjanvirta R, Korkalainen M, Moffat ID, Boutros PC, Okey AB (2011) Role of the AHR and its Structure in TCDD Toxicity. In: Pohjanvirta R, editor. The AH Receptor in Biology and Toxicology. Hoboken, NJ, USA: John Wiley & Sons, Inc.

16. Pohjanvirta R, Unkila M, Tuomisto J (1993) Comparative acute lethality of 2,3,7,8-tetrachlorodibenzo-p-dioxin (TCDD), 1,2,3,7,8-pentachlorodibenzo-p-dioxin and 1,2,3,4,7,8-hexachlorodibenzo-p-dioxin in the most TCDD-suscep-tible and the most TCDD-resistant rat strain. Pharmacol Toxicol 73: 52–56.

17. Pohjanvirta R, Wong JM, Li W, Harper PA, Tuomisto J, et al. (1998) Point mutation in intron sequence causes altered carboxyl-terminal structure in the aryl hydrocarbon receptor of the most 2,3,7,8-tetrachlorodibenzo-p-dioxin-resistant rat strain. Mol Pharmacol 54: 86–93.

18. Franc MA, Moffat ID, Boutros PC, Tuomisto JT, Tuomisto J, et al. (2008) Patterns of dioxin-altered mRNA expression in livers of dioxin-sensitive versus dioxin-resistant rats. Arch Toxicol 82: 809–830.

19. Chapman DE, Schiller CM (1985) Dose-related effects of 2,3,7,8-tetrachloro-dibenzo-p-dioxin (TCDD) in C57BL/6J and DBA/2J mice. Toxicol Appl Pharmacol 78: 147–157.

20. Poland A, Palen D, Glover E (1994) Analysis of the four alleles of the murine aryl hydrocarbon receptor. Mol Pharmacol 46: 915–921.

21. Pohjanvirta R, Miettinen H, Sankari S, Hegde N, Linden J (2012) Unexpected gender difference in sensitivity to the acute toxicity of dioxin in mice. Toxicol Appl Pharmacol 262: 167–176.

22. Kislinger T, Gramolini AO, MacLennan DH, Emili A (2005) Multidimensional protein identification technology (MudPIT): technical overview of a profiling method optimized for the comprehensive proteomic investigation of normal and diseased heart tissue. J Am Soc Mass Spectrom 16: 1207–1220.

23. Gerk PM (2011) Quantitative immunofluorescent blotting of the multidrug resistance-associated protein 2 (MRP2). J Pharmacol Toxicol Methods 63: 279–282.

24. Zeng L, Guo J, Xu HB, Huang R, Shao W, et al. (2013) Direct Blue 71 staining as a destaining-free alternative loading control method for Western blotting. Electrophoresis 34: 2234–2239.

25. Eaton SL, Roche SL, Llavero Hurtado M, Oldknow KJ, Farquharson C, et al. (2013) Total protein analysis as a reliable loading control for quantitative fluorescent Western blotting. PLoS One 8: e72457.

26. Li X, Bai H, Wang X, Li L, Cao Y, et al. (2011) Identification and validation of rice reference proteins for western blotting. J Exp Bot 62: 4763–4772.

27. Suzuki T, Higgins PJ, Crawford DR (2000) Control selection for RNA quantitation. Biotechniques 29: 332–337.

28. Weldon S, Ambroz K, Schutz-Geschwender A, Olive DM (2008) Near-infrared fluorescence detection permits accurate imaging of loading controls for Western blot analysis. Anal Biochem 375: 156–158.

29. Deindl E, Boengler K, van Royen N, Schaper W (2002) Differential expression of GAPDH and beta3-actin in growing collateral arteries. Mol Cell Biochem 236: 139–146.

30. Ferguson RE, Carroll HP, Harris A, Maher ER, Selby PJ, et al. (2005) Housekeeping proteins: a preliminary study illustrating some limitations as useful references in protein expression studies. Proteomics 5: 566–571.

31. Prokopec SD, Buchner NB, Fox NS, Chong LC, Mak DY, et al. (2013) Validating reference genes within a mouse model system of 2,3,7,8-tetrachlo-rodibenzo-p-dioxin (TCDD) toxicity. Chem Biol Interact 205: 63–71.

32. Greer S, Honeywell R, Geletu M, Arulanandam R, Raptis L (2010) Housekeeping genes; expression levels may change with density of cultured cells. J Immunol Methods 355: 76–79.

33. Linden J, Ranta J, Pohjanvirta R (2012) Bayesian modeling of reproducibility and robustness of RNA reverse transcription and quantitative real-time polymerase chain reaction. Anal Biochem 428: 81–91.

34. Pohjanvirta R, Niittynen M, Linden J, Boutros PC, Moffat ID, et al. (2006) Evaluation of various housekeeping genes for their applicability for normaliza-tion of mRNA expression in dioxin-treated rats. Chem Biol Interact 160: 134–149.

35. Boutros PC, Yan R, Moffat ID, Pohjanvirta R, Okey AB (2008) Transcriptomic responses to 2,3,7,8-tetrachlorodibenzo-p-dioxin (TCDD) in liver: comparison of rat and mouse. BMC Genomics 9: 419.

36. Kislinger T, Cox B, Kannan A, Chung C, Hu P, et al. (2006) Global survey of organ and organelle protein expression in mouse: combined proteomic and transcriptomic profiling. Cell 125: 173–186.

37. Gygi SP, Rochon Y, Franza BR, Aebersold R (1999) Correlation between protein and mRNA abundance in yeast. Mol Cell Biol 19: 1720–1730.

38. Pohjanvirta R (2009) Transgenic mouse lines expressing rat AH receptor variants – a new animal model for research on AH receptor function and dioxin toxicity mechanisms. Toxicol Appl Pharmacol 236: 166–182.

39. Kilkenny C, Browne WJ, Cuthill IC, Emerson M, Altman DG (2010) Improving bioscience research reporting: the ARRIVE guidelines for reporting animal research. PLoS Biol 8: e1000412.

40. Zhu M, Yu P, Jiang B, Gu Y (2012) Investigation of the influence of Arg555Trp and Thr538Pro TGFBI mutations on C-terminal cleavage and cell endoplasmic reticulum stress. Mol Vis 18: 1156–1164.

41. Hoene V, Fischer M, Ivanova A, Wallach T, Berthold F, et al. (2009) GATA factors in human neuroblastoma: distinctive expression patterns in clinical subtypes. Br J Cancer 101: 1481–1489.

42. Hinson JA, Michael SL, Ault SG, Pumford NR (2000) Western blot analysis for nitrotyrosine protein adducts in livers of saline-treated and acetaminophen-treated mice. Toxicol Sci 53: 467–473.

43. Anderson LV, Davison K (1999) Multiplex Western blotting system for the analysis of muscular dystrophy proteins. Am J Pathol 154: 1017–1022.

44. Andersen CL, Jensen JL, Orntoft TF (2004) Normalization of real-time quantitative reverse transcription-PCR data: a model-based variance estimation approach to identify genes suited for normalization, applied to bladder and colon cancer data sets. Cancer Res 64: 5245–5250.

45. Silver N, Best S, Jiang J, Thein SL (2006) Selection of housekeeping genes for gene expression studies in human reticulocytes using real-time PCR. BMC Mol Biol 7: 33.

46. Schutz-Geschwender A, Zhang Y, Holt T, McDermitt D, Olive DM (2004) Quantitative, Two-Color Western Blot Detection With Infrared Fluorescence. LI-COR Biosciences.

47. Vandesompele J, De Preter K, Pattyn F, Poppe B, Van Roy N, et al. (2002) Accurate normalization of real-time quantitative RT-PCR data by geometric averaging of multiple internal control genes. Genome Biol 3: RESEARCH0034.

48. Karge WH 3rd, Schaefer EJ, Ordovas JM (1998) Quantification of mRNA by polymerase chain reaction (PCR) using an internal standard and a nonradio-active detection method. Methods Mol Biol 110: 43–61.

49. Geiss GK, Bumgarner RE, Birditt B, Dahl T, Dowidar N, et al. (2008) Direct multiplexed measurement of gene expression with color-coded probe pairs. Nat Biotechnol 26: 317–325.

50. Tramm T, Sorensen BS, Overgaard J, Alsner J (2013) Optimal reference genes for normalization of qRT-PCR data from archival formalin-fixed, paraffin-embedded breast tumors controlling for tumor cell content and decay of mRNA. Diagn Mol Pathol 22: 181–187.

51. Walter RF, Mairinger FD, Wohlschlaeger J, Worm K, Ting S, et al. (2013) FFPE tissue as a feasible source for gene expression analysis – A comparison of three reference genes and one tumor marker. Pathol Res Pract.

52. Baumgartner R, Umlauf E, Veitinger M, Guterres S, Rappold E, et al. (2013) Identification and validation of platelet low biological variation proteins, superior to GAPDH, actin and tubulin, as tools in clinical proteomics. Journal of Proteomics 94: 540–551.

53. Yao CQ, Prokopec SD, Watson JD, Pang R, P'ng C, et al. (2012) Inter-strain heterogeneity in rat hepatic transcriptomic responses to 2,3,7,8-tetrachlorodi-benzo-p-dioxin (TCDD). Toxicol Appl Pharmacol 260: 135–145.

54. Watson JD, Prokopec SD, Smith AB, Okey AB, Pohjanvirta R, et al. (2013) TCDD dysregulation of 13 AHR-target genes in rat liver. Toxicol Appl Pharmacol.

55. Boverhof DR, Burgoon LD, Tashiro C, Chittim B, Harkema JR, et al. (2005) Temporal and dose-dependent hepatic gene expression patterns in mice provide new insights into TCDD-Mediated hepatotoxicity. Toxicol Sci 85: 1048–1063.

56. Pastorelli R, Carpi D, Campagna R, Airoldi L, Pohjanvirta R, et al. (2006) Differential expression profiling of the hepatic proteome in a rat model of dioxin resistance: correlation with genomic and transcriptomic analyses. Mol Cell Proteomics 5: 882–894.

57. Teste MA, Duquenne M, Francois JM, Parrou JL (2009) Validation of reference genes for quantitative expression analysis by real-time RT-PCR in Saccharo-myces cerevisiae. BMC Mol Biol 10: 99.

11

Clinically Approved Iron Chelators Influence Zebrafish Mortality, Hatching Morphology and Cardiac Function

Jasmine L. Hamilton[1], Azadeh Hatef[2], Muhammad Imran ul-haq[1], Neelima Nair[2], Suraj Unniappan[2]*, Jayachandran N. Kizhakkedathu[1,3]*

1 The Centre for Blood Research, Department of Pathology and Laboratory Medicine, Life Sciences Institute, The University of British Columbia, Vancouver, British Columbia, Canada, 2 Veterinary Biomedical Sciences, Laboratory of Integrative Neuroendocrinology, Western College of Veterinary Medicine, University of Saskatchewan, Saskatoon, Saskatchewan, Canada, 3 Department of Chemistry, The University of British Columbia, Vancouver, British Columbia, Canada

Abstract

Iron chelation therapy using iron (III) specific chelators such as desferrioxamine (DFO, Desferal), deferasirox (Exjade or ICL-670), and deferiprone (Ferriprox or L1) are the current standard of care for the treatment of iron overload. Although each chelator is capable of promoting some degree of iron excretion, these chelators are also associated with a wide range of well documented toxicities. However, there is currently very limited data available on their effects in developing embryos. In this study, we took advantage of the rapid development and transparency of the zebrafish embryo, *Danio rerio* to assess and compare the toxicity of iron chelators. All three iron chelators described above were delivered to zebrafish embryos by direct soaking and their effects on mortality, hatching and developmental morphology were monitored for 96 hpf. To determine whether toxicity was specific to embryos, we examined the effects of chelator exposure via intra peritoneal injection on the cardiac function and gene expression in adult zebrafish. Chelators varied significantly in their effects on embryo mortality, hatching and morphology. While none of the embryos or adults exposed to DFO were negatively affected, ICL -treated embryos and adults differed significantly from controls, and L1 exerted toxic effects in embryos alone. ICL-670 significantly increased the mortality of embryos treated with doses of 0.25 mM or higher and also affected embryo morphology, causing curvature of larvae treated with concentrations above 0.5 mM. ICL-670 exposure (10 µL of 0.1 mM injection) also significantly increased the heart rate and cardiac output of adult zebrafish. While L1 exposure did not cause toxicity in adults, it did cause morphological defects in embryos at 0.5 mM. This study provides first evidence on iron chelator toxicity in early development and will help to guide our approach on better understanding the mechanism of iron chelator toxicity.

Editor: Dimas T. Covas, University of Sao Paulo - USP, Brazil

Funding: This research was funded by grants from Canadian Institutes of Health Research (MOP-130408 & MOP-97833) to JNK. The research using zebrafish was partly supported by a Discovery grant and Discovery Accelerator award from the Natural Sciences and Engineering Research Council (NSERC) of Canada, and an Establishment Grant from the Saskatchewan Health Research Foundation (SHRF) to SU. The funders had no role in study design, data collection and analysis, decision to publish, or preparation of the manuscript.

Competing Interests: The authors have declared that no competing interests exist on the work presented in the manuscript in the form of grants, patents or copyrights or any other form.

* Email: jay@pathology.ubc.ca (JNK); suraj.unniappan@usask.ca (SU)

Introduction

Iron chelators are used to treat transfusion associated iron overload in patients with β-thalassemia (TM), sickle-cell anemia (SCD) and myelodysplastic syndromes (MDS) [1–2], and for the treatment of metal poisoning in children [3]. Due to ineffective erythropoiesis, patients with TM and to a lesser extent, SCD, must be treated with red blood cell (RBC) transfusions to ameliorate anemia. RBC transfusions also reduce the risk of stroke in patients with SCD and are used as supportive care for treating anemia in MDS [2,4]. However, due to the high iron content in RBCs and the inability of man to actively excrete iron, transfusion therapy inevitably leads to the development of iron overload. The long term adverse consequences of iron overload are numerous; ranging from growth retardation in children to iron induced cardiac dysfunction, the life-limiting complication of severe iron

overload [5]. Thus, the degree of iron loading is correlated to life expectancy.

Iron chelation therapy (ICT) is used to manage iron overload [6]. Iron chelators bind iron to form non-toxic complexes that are then excreted from the body, enabling safer body iron levels [6–7]. There are 3 chelators currently approved for treating transfusion associated iron overload (**Figure 1**). Desferrioxamine (DFO), the oldest iron chelator, has been used in clinical practice since the 1960s and has drastically improved survival in TM patients who comply with therapy [8]. Deferiprone (L1), the second iron chelator to be licensed and the first orally active chelator to become available is indicated for use when chelation with DFO alone does not work well enough [9]. Unlike DFO, which has a very low cellular permeability, L1 is reported to have an ability to enter cardiac cells and has proven to be efficacious in enhancing iron excretion when used in combination with DFO [10].

Desferasirox (ICL-670) is the second orally active iron chelator to become available and the most recent to be approved for use [11–12]. Like L1, studies suggest that ICL-670 can also penetrate cells to access intracellular iron pools and has positively contributed to patient adherence to therapy [12]. Further details regarding the properties of DFO, L1 and ICL-670 are given in **Table 1**.

Iron chelators can reduce complications such as cardiomyopathy, the major cause of death from iron overload. Further, iron chelation therapy can slow the progression of liver fibrosis and reduce glucose intolerance in transfusion dependent patients [5–6]. However, a wide range of chelator-induced toxicities have also been reported. The use of DFO at high doses may cause neurological disturbances, growth retardation, peripheral neuropathies, vision changes, endocrine dysfuction and bone deformities [13–14]. Severe toxicities associated with L1 include agranulocytosis and neutropenia [14–16]. Gastrointestinal disturbances, arthropathy and increased liver-enzyme levels were also reported [15]. ICL-670 can cause severe renal impairment, and failure, increase in serum creatinine level as well as gastrointestinal hemorrhage in some patients [17–18].

While toxicities of iron chelators are well documented, there is currently very limited data regarding the toxicity of DFO, ICL-670 and L1 in developing embryos. A few studies have been conducted in mice and show that DFO caused developmental toxicity only in the presence of maternal toxicity and that L1 can cause toxicity in rat embryos [19–21]. Thus, in this study we took advantage of the optical transparency and ex-utero development of zebrafish embryos to directly assess the functional, morphological and behavioral effects of clinically approved iron chelators on embryos in the absence of interference from maternal factors.

Zebrafish (*Danio rerio*) are increasingly used as a cost-effective *in vivo* model and have been shown to be useful in evaluating chemical toxicity [22–24]. The toxicity data obtained in zebrafish correlates well with developmental toxicity data from rat *in vivo* studies and previous studies have demonstrated that the prediction success rate for some drugs can be as high as 100% in zebrafish [25–26]. Further advantages of zebrafish include the rapid rate of organogenesis and the large number of embryos obtained per spawn, which allows throughput screening [27].

In this study, we exposed developing zebrafish embryos to various concentrations of DFO, L1 and ICL-670 and assessed their effects on mortality, hatching and morphology in embryos. To determine whether the effects were specific to embryos and to probe possible underlying mechanisms of the observed toxicities, we investigated the effects of chelator exposure on the cardiac function and gene expression in adults. Since the toxicity of iron chelators can result from sequestration of iron required for biological processes, we investigated the change in expression of hepcidin, ferroportin (FPN) and DMT-1, three genes directly involved in iron transport and recycling [28–31]. This study improves our understanding of the differences in potential effects of clinically approved iron chelators at the earlier stages of embryonic development. Results will guide our approach in

further understanding the effect of iron chelation in vertebrates during development, and will provide clues on the possible organ systems perturbed by iron depletion in developing embryos.

Materials and Methods

Chemicals

Desferrioxamine (>99%), deferiprone (1, 2-dimethyl, 3-hydroxy, pyrid-4-one) and 100% cell culture grade DMSO were obtained from Sigma-Aldrich Canada Ltd. (Oakville, ON). Desferasirox (4-[3, 5-bis (2-hydroxyphenyl)-1,2,4-triazol-1-yl]benzoic acid) was synthesized in house according to established protocols [32]. The analysis and characterization of the final product are shown in supplementary materials (Figures S1 and S2 in File S1). Aquacalm was obtained from Syndel Laboratories Ltd. (British Columbia, Canada).

Zebrafish Husbandry

All experiments complied with the Canadian Council of Animal Care guidelines and the animal care protocol (2012-0082), which was approved by the University of Saskatchewan Animal Research Ethics Board. Zebrafish were obtained from (Aquatic Imports, Calgary) and were maintained in a recirculating, light and temperature controlled facility on a standard 14:10 h light:dark cycle in standard system fish water. Embryos were maintained at 28°C throughout all experiments. Embryos were washed and healthy, non-coagulated embryos were selected for exposure to chelators.

Chelator Exposure to Zebrafish Embryos

Embryos were grown in 6-well plates (Corning, Life sciences) containing 4 mL of chelator solution in DMSO and serial dilutions were done using fish water. DMSO was used as control. Chelator solutions were replenished every day and seven concentrations of chelator (0.015, 0.03, 0.06, 0.125, 0.25, 0.5 and 1 mM) were used. The maximum DMSO concentration for DFO and ICL-670 was 0.45%. The maximum concentration tested for L1 was 0.5 mM, with a DMSO concentration range of 0.02–1% as shown in supplementary materials (Figure S5 in File S1). All embryos were derived from the same spawn of eggs to allow statistical comparison. After fertilization, embryos were collected and transferred to 6-well plates; 15 embryos per well and 3 wells per concentration (n = 45) for a treatment period of 96 h post fertilization (hpf). This study was repeated twice after an initial optimization study and the final concentration of DMSO present in each solution was noted and is given in supplementary materials (Figure S3–S5 in File S1).

Mortality, Hatching and Morphology Readings

Mortality, hatching and morphology were assessed and recorded every 24 h using a CCD digital camera (OLYMPUS DP70, Japan) mounted on a microscope (Olympus, BX51, Japan) every 24 h from 6 hpf to 96 hpf. Morphology, mortality and

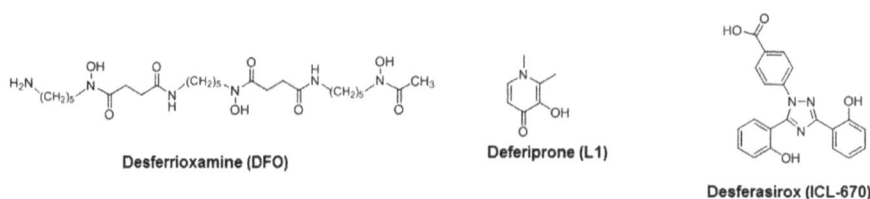

Figure 1. The chemical structures of clinically approved iron chelators.

Table 1. Summary of the properties of iron chelators in clinical use.

Property of Chelator	Desferrioxamine (DFO)	Deferiprone (L1)	Desferasirox (ICL-670)
Date of approval for clinical use[1,8,14]	1970s	1999 in Europe and Asia, 2012 in the USA	2005
Usual dose[1]	20–50 mg/kg/day	75–100 mg/kg/day	20–40 mg/kg/day
Molecular weight	560	139	373
Fe binding log stability constant[6,7,32]	30.6	35	38
Chelator: Iron[39]	1:1 (Hexadentate)	3:1 (Bidentate)	2:1 (Tridentate)
Potential toxicities[11,13,16]	Reaction at the infusion site, neurotoxicity, bone abnormalities	Neutropenia, agranulocytosis, arthralgia, elevation of liver enzyme	Gastrointestinal, rash, renal and liver

hatching rate were determined. Other parameters such as defects in swim behavior were also monitored. Percentage of hatch (% hatch success) was defined as: (the number of larvae/initial number of embryos)×100.

Chelator Exposure and Ultrasound Analysis in Adult Zebrafish

Adult fish were anesthetized with 28 mg/L aquacalm solution. Stock solutions were prepared in DMSO and serial dilutions were prepared before each experiment using saline (0.15 M NaCl). The final concentration of DMSO present in each solution was noted and is given in supplementary materials (Figure S3 in File S1). Male and female zebrafish were used and emphasis was placed on identifying the gender of each fish and balancing the number of males and females in each group. The fish used in our experiments were approximately 1 year old. Six adult zebrafish were injected intraperitoneally (*i.p.*) with 10 µL of 100 µM of each chelator and subjected to ultrasound monitoring using a VEVO 660 high frequency ultrasound machine (VisualSonics, Markham, ON), 30 minutes post injection. Each zebrafish was removed from fish water and placed in 28 mg/L aquacalm until they succumbed to the anesthetic. Once sufficiently anesthetized, they were positioned ventral side up and secured in a 3% agarose gel with minutien pins (Fine Science Tools, Vancouver, BC). The probe (A RMV 708B), attached to the machine is kept at startup mode so that the probe is already moving. The probe is then lowered above the horizontally placed zebrafish and adjusted as the view is needed. The ultrasound monitoring was carried out using the VisualSonics software (Markham, ON). Three short axis views; A1 (towards the gills), A2 (slightly away from the gills) and A3 (towards the tail), were taken. One long axis view of the ventricle was also taken by placing the fish in a vertical position. All these readings were measured both at the systole and diastole using the VisualSonics Software. Calculations were conducted as follow: Stroke Volume (SV) = EDV (end diastolic volume) − ESV (end systolic volume). Heart Rate = heart rate/10 sec×6 and cardiac output = stroke volume×heart rate.

Quantitative PCR

Six adult zebrafish from each group were injected *i.p.* with 10 µL of 100 µM of chelators and sacrificed 24 h after injection. Liver, heart and gut were harvested for RNA extraction. Total RNA was extracted using the TRIzol RNA isolation reagent (Invitrogen, Canada).

The purity of extracted RNA was assessed by optical density absorption ratio (OD 260 nm/OD 280 nm) using the nanodrop (ND 100, NanoDrop Technologies Inc. Wilmington, DE, USA).

One microgram of RNA was used for iScript cDNA synthesis as directed by the manufacturer (BioRad, Canada). cDNAs were diluted 1:3 before qRT-PCR using a CFX connect (BioRad Laboratories Inc. Canada) with iQSYBR Green supermix (BioRad, Canada). The cDNAs were amplified using the forward and reverse primers shown in Table 2 (Sigma-Aldrich Canada Ltd). For each sample, qRT-PCR was run in duplicate to ensure consistency. The thermal profile for all reactions was 3 min at 95°C and 40 cycles of 10 s at 95°C, and 30 s at 60°C. The specificity of the amplified product in the quantitative PCR assay was determined by analyzing the melting curve to discriminate target amplicon from primer dimer and other nonspecific products. A single melt curve was observed for each primer set in all quantitative PCR reactions. Fluorescence monitoring occurred at the end of each cycle. Relative expression levels were determined by normalizing to the β-actin housekeeping gene. Results were determined using method of Livak and Schmittgen [33]. The genes investigated were hepcidin, ferroportin (FPN) and the divalent metal transporter (DMT-1) [28–31,34]. Primers and accession numbers can be found in **Table 2**.

Statistical Analysis

Statistical analysis was performed using SPSS 19.0 software. Data were expressed as means ± SEM. Comparisons between groups were made using one-way analysis of variance (ANOVA) followed by Turkey post hoc analysis for multiple comparisons. Homogeneity of variance was tested for all data using Levene's test. Data for non-homogeneous were log transformed to meet assumptions of normality and homoscedasticity. P values less than 0.05 were considered statistically significant.

Results

Effects of Clinically Used Iron Chelators on Mortality, Hatching Success and Morphology of Zebrafish Embryos

Iron chelators (DFO, L1, ICL-670) differed significantly in their effects in developing zebrafish embryos. The mortality of zebrafish embryos exposed to different iron chelators at different time points are shown in **Figure 2**. The mortality of DFO-treated embryos did not differ significantly (p = 0.961) from the control regardless of exposure duration and drug concentration (**Figure 2**). In contrast, the mortality of ICL-670 varied significantly from controls (p << 0.05) in a dose and time-dependent manner (**Figure 2**); while the mortality of embryos exposed to L1 caused a slight but insignificant increase in mortality at 0.5 mM. The percentage mortality was highest in ICL-670 treated embryos; with more than 80% mortality occurring above 0.25 mM of ICL-670. The onset

Table 2. The forward and reverse primers used for real-time qPCR.

Gene	Primer	Accession No. Gen Bank	Amplicon size, bp
Hamp 1	F: 5'-CCGAGCAGAAGACAAGTAGAT-3' R: 5'-GCAGCCAGAAACACGTTAGA-3'	NM_205583.1	104
DMT-1	F: 5'-ACCGCAGCAATAAGAAGGAG-3' R: 5'-TTGGTTTTCCCGTAGAAGGC-3'	NM_001040370.1	136
Ferroportin	F: 5'-ATTTACTTTGCCCGAGCCTT-3' R: 5'-CAGCGAGGTTTCTTTGATGC-3'	NM_131629.1	104
β-Actin	F: 5'-TTCAAACGAACGACCAACCT-3' R: 5'-TTCCGCATCCTGAGTCAATG-3'	NM_131031.1	93

of mortality in embryos exposed to ICL-670 varied from 24 hpf for 1 mM treated embryos to 72 hpf and 96 hpf in embryos treated with 0.5 mM and 0.25 mM, respectively. L1-treated embryos did not differ significantly from control although there was a slight increase in mortality at 0.5 mM after 96 hpf exposure. Control experiments with different concentrations DMSO used for dissolving the different iron chelators suggest that there is no interference from DMSO in this study (Figure S3 in File S1). The morphology of zebrafish embryos after 48 hpf in presence of different concentrations of chelators in given in Figure S6 and Figure S7 (in File S1).

DFO, L1 and ICL-670 also differed significantly in their effect on zebrafish embryo morphology upon hatching. Similar to the mortality, DFO-treated embryos did not show any differences in hatching when compared to control, up to concentrations of

1 mM (**Figure 3**). While all the embryos treated with L1 hatched into larvae successfully, the hatching rate was reduced in ICL-670 treated embryos due to increased mortality; embryos treated with 1 mM of ICL-670 did not survive to hatch.

We next looked at the morphological deformities of the hatched larvae at different concentrations after exposure to iron chelators (**Figure 3B**). The percentage of deformities was highest for ICL-670. The deformities increased with increasing exposure time (**Figure 3C**). Representative optical images of zebrafish embryos after exposure to iron chelators and control are shown in **Figure 4**. Bent bodies (BB) of larvae were the most commonly observed defects for ICL-670 and L1. However, DFO at the doses tested, did not cause any deformities compared to controls. ICL-670 samples showed deformities at much lower concentrations than L1. Signs of rapid breathing and change in the swimming

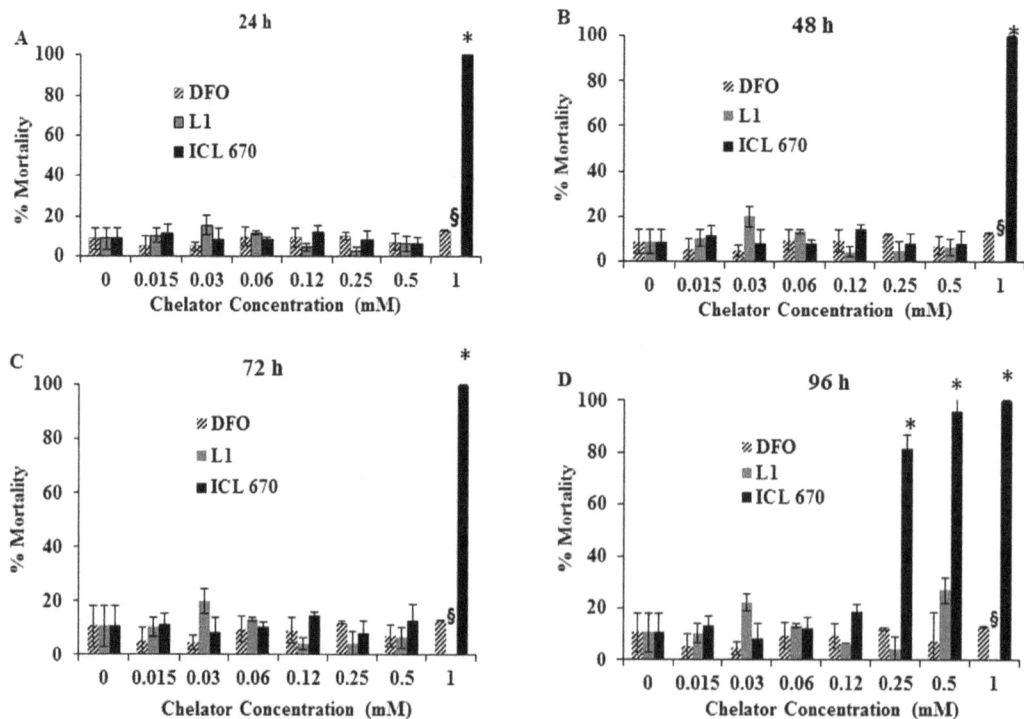

Figure 2. Mortality of zebrafish embryos exposed to iron chelators. The mortality of DFO and L1-treated embryos did not vary significantly from control after 96 hpf of exposure (A–D). The mortality of ICL-670-treated embryos increased in a dose and time-dependent manner and was significantly higher than control embryos; death occurred within 24 hpf of exposure to 1 mM ICL-670 (A) and 96 hpf for 0.25 and 0.5 mM treated embryos (D). § denotes missing bar for L1 at 1 mM; the DMSO content would have exceeded 1.5% thus, this concentration was omitted. The concentration of chelator for which mortality was significantly different from control is denoted by *.

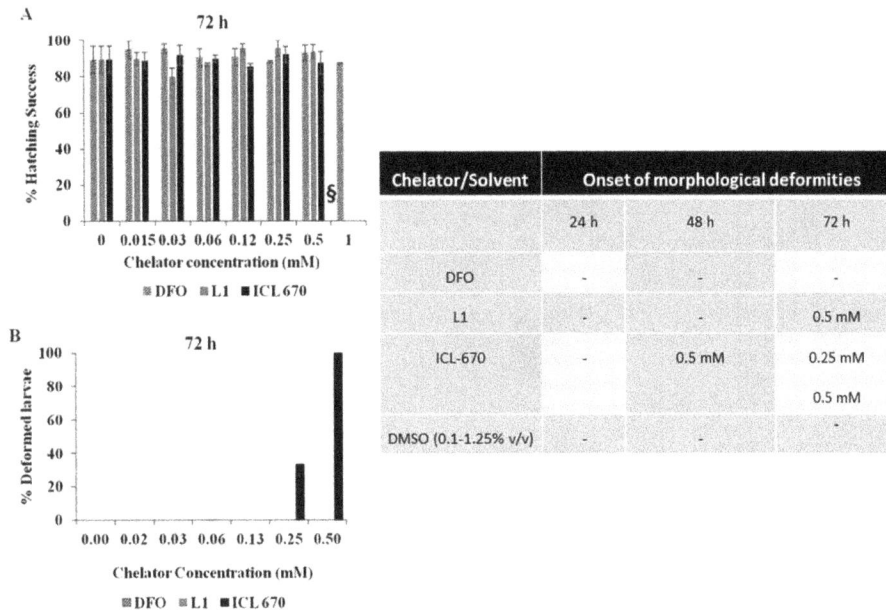

Figure 3. Hatching rate and morphological alterations of zebrafish embryos. DFO and L1-treated embryos hatched successfully, while ICL-670-treated embryos hatched less successfully than control due to high mortality (A). Bars missing at 1 mM are due to the death of embryos prior to hatching. § denoted the concentration of L1 that was excluded due to high DMSO content. There were no significant defects observed in DFO treated embryos. However, the percentage of embryos demonstrating behavioral and morphological defects increased in a time and concentration dependent manner in L1 and ICL-670-treated embryos (B). The time of onset of morphological and behavioral alterations is outlined in the figure as a separate panel. Swimming behavior was affected and bent bodies (**Figure 5**) were observed at concentrations above 0.25 mM for ICL 670-treated embryos and at 0.5 mM for L1 treated embryos.

behavior were also observed. The ICL-670-treated larvae exhibited lethargy and often moved only when a small stimulus was provided. Edema was also observed in ICL-670 treated larvae. Similar but less abundant morphological defects occurred in embryos exposed to L1 at 0.5 mM (**Figures 4A and B**). Drug dose and duration of exposure were the two most important factors influencing the toxicity.

Acute Exposure to Iron Chelators on Cardiac Output and Heart Rate in Adult Zebrafish

To enhance our understanding of iron chelator-induced toxicities in zebrafish, we investigated the effects of DFO, ICL-670 and L1 on the cardiac function of adult zebrafish. Adult fish were injected with 10 µL of 100 µM of chelators and subjected to ultrasound 30 minutes after treatment. We chose a lower concentration of the chelators that was not lethal and would allow us to determine more subtle changes. The heart rate, cardiac output, stroke volume, end systolic volume and end diastolic volume were measured and are shown in **Figure 5**. We used DMSO as a vehicle control and saline treated zebrafish to confirm that the vehicle solvent did not have an adverse effect on the zebrafish and that observed effects from chelator treated fish were real. DMSO and saline treated zebrafish controls did not show any difference in heart function with aquacalm treatment. Therefore, we believe there was no unwanted effect from the anesthetic.

ICL-670 but not L1 nor DFO caused a significant increase in the heart rate and cardiac output of zebrafish (**Figure 5A and B**). The average heart rate increased from 102 to 138 beats per minute and cardiac output increased from 12 µL/min in controls compared to 30 µL/min in ICL-670, ($p < 0.05$; $P_{heart\ rate} = 0.001$; $P_{cardiac\ output} = 0.01$). Interestingly, there was a significant difference in heart rate between L1 treated and ICL-670 treated fish.

The heart rate of DFO treated fish did not differ significantly from control. Chelators did not significantly affect the end-diastolic volume, end-systolic volume and stroke volume in adult zebrafish (**Figure 5C–E**) ($P_{end\ diastolic\ volume} = 0.3421$; $P_{end\ systolic\ volume} = 0.25$; $P_{stroke\ volume} = 0.1137$).

Acute Exposure to Iron Chelators on the Expression of Hepcidin, Ferroportin and DMT-1 Genes in Adult Zebrafish

Hepcidin, FPN and DMT-1 are genes involved in iron regulation in zebrafish and changes in iron status have been shown to influence their expression levels [28–31]. Thus, we investigated the effect of different chelators on mRNA levels in adult fish in the gut, liver and heart tissue. Hepcidin is a multifunctional peptide and the chief iron regulatory hormone in vertebrates [29–30]. One of its functions is to bind to FPN, which is located on the basolateral surface of the enterocyte, and prevent iron absorption. Upon binding to FPN, hepcidin causes it to be broken down when the body's iron supplies are adequate. DMT-1 functions as an iron transporter in vertebrates. It can also transport other divalent metals [28]. Adult fish were injected i.p. with 10 µL of 100 µM chelators and the gene expression at 24 h post-treatment was measured.

None of the iron chelators tested significantly altered the levels of hepcidin in the liver or heart. DFO and L1 caused a down-regulation of hepcidin expression in the gut. While ICL-670 also down-regulated hepcidin in the gut, its effect was less than that of DFO and L1 (**Figure 6**). Chelators did not significantly alter FPN expression in the gut. L1 and ICL-670 down-regulated, while DFO up-regulated FPN expression in the liver. All chelators caused a slight up-regulation of FPN in the heart with ICL-670 showing a significant difference from control. DFO, L1 and ICL-

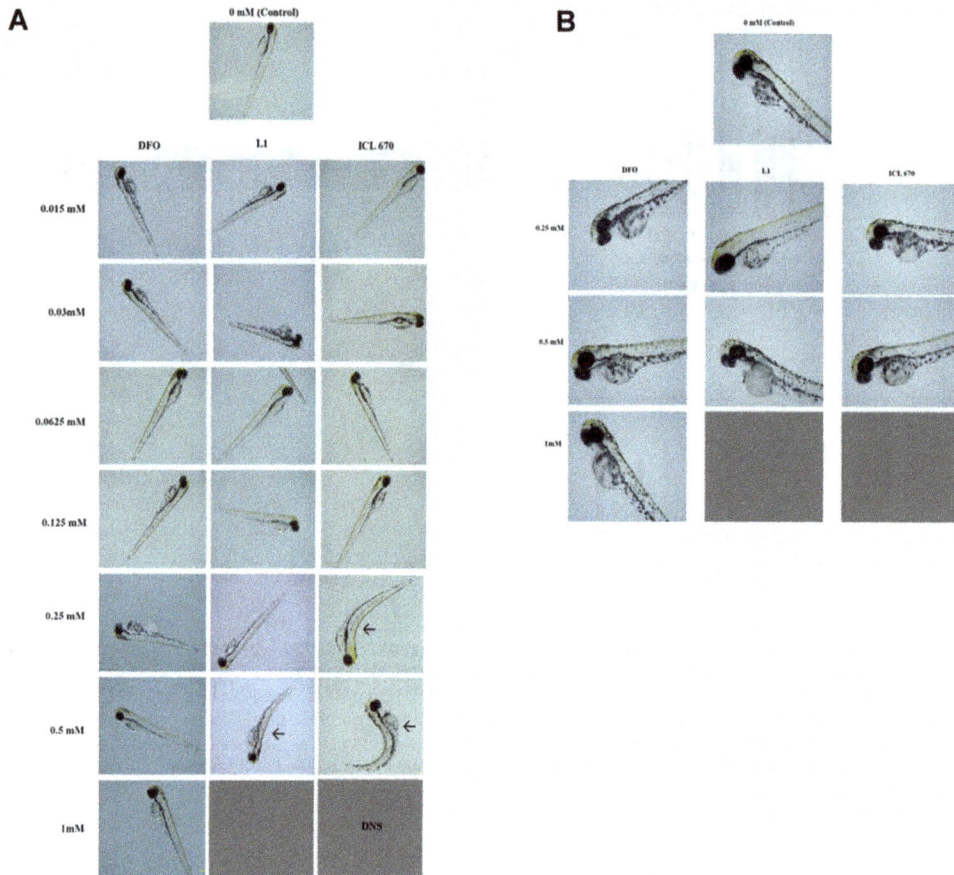

Figure 4. Zebrafish larvae morphology after 72 hpf of exposure to iron chelators. A: Representative optical images of zebrafish morphology after 72 hpf exposure to DFO, L1 and ICL 670. Zebrafish kept in DMSO was used as control. Embryos treated with 1 mM ICL-670 did not survive to hatch (DNS); while those treated with 0.25 mM and 0.5 mM hatched abnormally and had bent bodies (shown with arrows). Images were captured at 2X magnification. **B:** Representative optical images of zebrafish morphology after 72 hpf exposure to DFO, L1 and ICL 670. Higher magnification (4X) shows edema in L1 and ICL-670 treated embryos. No abnormalities were observed in DFO treated embryos up to concentrations of 1 mM. Images were captured at 4X magnification.

670 caused a down regulation of DMT-1 in the gut with L1 causing the strongest change. However, none of the iron chelators significantly altered DMT-1 expression in the liver and heart.

Discussion

Iron chelators are used to reduce iron levels in patients that are susceptible to iron overload. Although a wide range of toxicities have been reported to occur, information on the effect of iron chelators in embryo development is lacking. Thus we investigated the effects of iron chelator exposure on mortality, hatching and morphology of zebrafish embryos. We also investigated possible mechanisms of toxicity by measuring the changes in cardiac function and the expression of hepcidin, FPN and DMT-1, genes anticipated to be sensitive to iron status.

Different chelators (DFO, L1, ICL-670) exerted distinct effects in zebrafish embryos and differed in the extent of toxicity exerted (**Figures 2 to 5**). While DFO treated embryos did not differ from control in any of the parameters measured; ICL-670 treated embryos exerted a range of toxicity which increased with increasing dose and longer duration of exposure. Exposure to L1 was associated with small changes to morphology.

The chemical properties of pharmacological agents and the characteristics of the zebrafish chorion may have separate, additive or synergistic effects on the chelator-induced toxicities. The size, polarity and specificity of each chelator for cations may vary and may influence the ability of chelators to permeate the zebrafish embryo, thus influencing the observed toxicities. The notable differences in size of chelators (DFO-560 Da, L1-139 Da and ICL-670-373 Da) and polarity may also be important factors influencing the intensity of chelator exposure in embryos [35–37]. Moreover, the hydrophilic nature of DFO may prevent it from readily entering cells to elicit this pattern of toxicity. A direct correlation has been reported for the rate of cellular uptake of a drug and its potential toxicity [37]. Direct injection might overcome this barrier compared to the soaked solutions as reported in a recent study on the evaluation of cardiotoxic drugs in zebrafish embryos [25], however the generality of this approach is not well-documented, and continuous exposure (up to 96 hpf in our case) may not be generated in the case of single direct injection. Further experimentation is needed to probe this.

Another important aspect of toxicity in relation to iron chelation therapy may be the removal or displacement of iron or essential other metals. In the absence of iron overload, iron chelators can interfere with zinc, copper and other micronutrient binding although the binding constants for these chelators to other metal ions are relatively small compared to Fe (III) (the log cumulative stability constant of DFO-Fe (III) is 30.6 versus 11.1 for DFO-

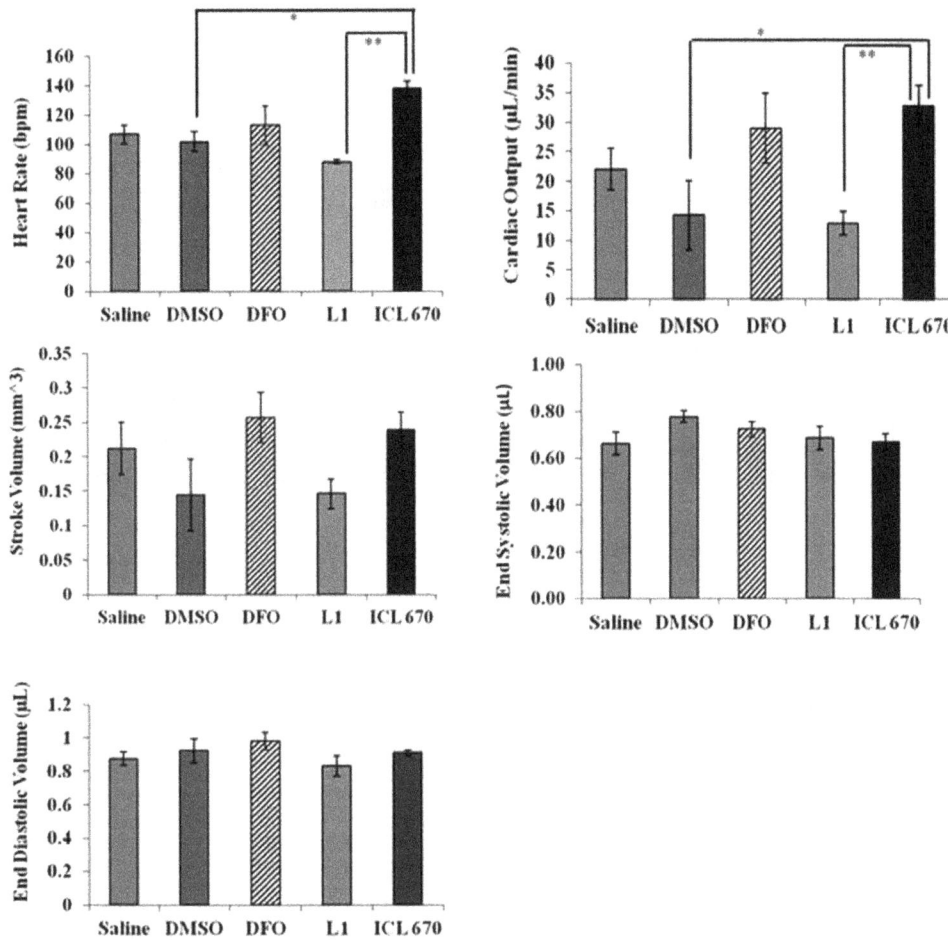

Figure 5. Iron chelator exposure significantly influences heart rate and cardiac output in adult zebrafish. Six adult zebrafish were injected with 10 µL of 100 µM of each chelator and subjected to analysis by ultrasound 30 min after injection. The heart rate of fish treated with ICL-670 differed significantly from controls. There was also a significant difference in heart rate between L1 and ICL-670 treated fish. Similarly, the cardiac output of fish exposed to ICL-670 differed significantly from control and L1-treated fish. However, DFO and L1 treated fish did not vary significantly from controls in any of the measurements obtained. DFO, L1 and ICL-670 did not significantly affect the end-diastolic volume, end-systolic volume or the stroke volume compared to the saline or 0.1% DMSO controls.

Zn^{2+}) [38]. Additionally, reducing essential iron in the cell can result in reduced cell proliferation by inhibiting intracellular ribonucleotide reductase [39]. Although the precise daily iron requirements of teleost fish are unknown, the daily loss of iron is comparable to that in humans [40]. It has also been shown that developing fish embryos receive sufficient iron from maternal stores in the yolk and that iron acquisition by fish embryos is generally limited, while studies show that mature teleost fish can become iron limited [41]. Roeder and Roeder showed that retarded growth results when swordtail and platyfish were fed iron poor foods, with growth rates returning to normal when the diet was supplemented with iron salts [42]. Thus, although the effects of chelators were less pronounced in adults the significant change in heart function observed upon treatment with ICL-670 (**Figure 5**) may have resulted due to the depletion of essential cardiac iron or perturbation of metal balance (other essential metal ions) in heart tissue. Furthermore, the higher lipophilicity of ICL-670 has been shown to cause accumulation in some tissues and related organ damage in humans [43].

The seemingly mild effects of chelators on mRNA expression (**Figure 6**) are likely due to the short duration of exposure. Hepcidin is a multifunctional peptide with a key role in iron

metabolism. FPN exports iron to the blood stream during absorption while DMT-1 functions as a carrier for most divalent metals across the apical surface of the cell. DFO produced a slight but insignificant increase in FPN expression after 24 h of exposure while gene expression in L1 and ICL-670 treated fish did not differ from control. Because DFO is known to be efficient at hepatocellular iron removal this finding is not surprising [1]. This may mean that DFO caused a reduction in the zebrafish liver iron causing an iron poor state.

DFO and L1 also induced the greatest change in hepcidin expression in the gut; causing a significant down-regulation of the gene compared to control, while ICL-670 did not appear to significantly affect hepcidin expression. When iron levels fall in the body, hepcidin levels are also decreased and more FPN is available to bring iron into the body and to release it from storage. Down regulation of hepcidin implies that cells are iron poor and causes enhanced iron absorption through increased FPN expression. This would be expected if these iron chelators chelate significant amounts of iron. Thus, it is likely that increasing the dose of chelator would result in a corresponding down regulation in hepcidin with the effect being increased iron absorption. Interestingly, ICL-670 did not have the same effect.

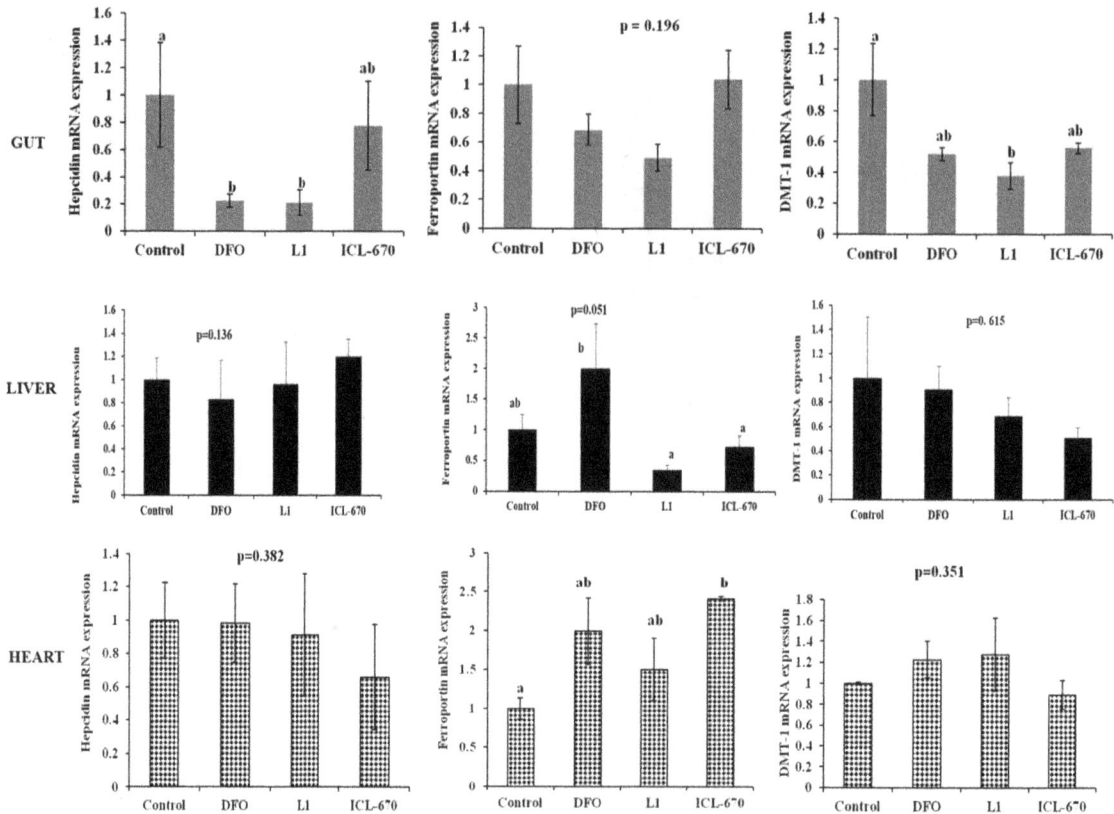

Figure 6. Gene expression of hepcidin, ferroportin (FPN) and divalent metal transporter (DMT-1) in the gut, liver and heart tissues of adult zebrafish after 24 h exposure to 100 µM (10 µL injection) of iron chelators. Hepcidin expression in the liver and heart tissue of adult zebrafish did not differ significantly from control. However, DFO and L1 significantly down-regulated hepcidin expression in the gut. There was no change in FPN expression in the gut upon chelator exposure. However, L1 and ICL-670 down-regulated, while DFO upregulated FPN in the liver and all chelators upregulated FPN in the heart. Treatment with DFO, L1 and ICL-670 resulted in a down-regulation of gut DMT-1. Gene expression values were normalized to β-actin and are presented as means ± SEM. Treatments that do not share a common letter are significantly different from each other, n = 6 for all treatments.

DMT-1 functions as an iron transporter in vertebrates. It can also transport other divalent metals. For example, rat DMT-1 has been shown to transport a range of divalent metal cations, including Fe, Pb, Zn, Cu and Cd [44]. DMT-1 has a critical function in iron metabolism as it allows the entrance of iron through the duodenal enterocyte, and enables the utilization of iron by cells via the transferring receptor mediated iron uptake. DMT-1 is also required for transporting iron out of the endosome and into the cytosol where it is incorporated into proteins or stored in ferritin [27].

The response of zebrafish to chemicals such as small molecules, drugs and environmental toxicants can be similar to that of mammals, however, it is important to conduct further studies that are aimed at determining how the effect of different iron chelator concentrations in zebrafish are related to those of mammalian models. This is especially relevant as the exposure to drugs in fish embryos is static, and internal concentrations are established by partition equilibrium. While in mammals, drugs are administered by single or repeat doses, and the exposure is not static. Thus, it is important to appropriately translate all findings obtained in experimental models. Koren and Ito [45] provide an excellent review regarding this.

Not surprisingly, juvenile zebrafish were more susceptible to toxic effects than adults. This may have resulted from the longer duration of chelator exposure (96 hpf) in the embryos compared to the single dose given to adult zebrafish. The short duration of

exposure in adults may also account for the mild alterations in gene expression observed in adults in the organs tested. This study provides information on the feasibility, potential doses of interest and time effects for testing chelator toxicity in zebrafish. Further studies of gene expression which take advantage of increased exposure time in adults (chronic exposure) would help to improve our understanding.

Conclusions

This study demonstrates that clinically approved iron chelators vary in their ability to induce toxicity in zebrafish embryos and adults, and that the time and dose of exposure are major factors influencing toxicity. DFO exposure did not induce any toxicity; there was no change in mortality, morphology, or hatching rate. L1 did not significantly affect mortality but caused morphological alterations at higher concentrations. While ICL-670 caused significant morphological deformities and hatching problems in zebrafish embryos above certain concentrations such that these iron chelators are influencing the development into larvae. Unlike other chelators, ICL-670 caused significant change in the heart rate and cardiac output in adult zebrafish when injected at a concentration of 100 µM (10 µL). Changes in expression of hepcidin, FPN and DMT-1 genes were observed in adults, however, the effect are not pronounced as in embryos.

It is most likely that a combination of factors including the differential permeability of the components of the embryo; the size, lipophilicity and chemical structure of DFO, L1 and ICL-670 influenced their ability to induce toxic effects in zebrafish. Studies focused on characterizing the permeability barriers in the zebrafish chorion will further elucidate the factors that influence the observed chelator toxicity. Additionally, future studies which investigate the method of chelator exposure, as well as the absorption, metabolism and excretion profile of each chelator in zebrafish are recommended. Such studies can elucidate scaling factors which may allow more suitable and accurate comparisons and correlation to rodents, and other relevant experimental models.

Acknowledgments

Authors acknowledge the funding from Canadian Institutes of Health Research (CIHR) for funding. JLH acknowledges the Canadian Blood Services for Graduate Fellowship Award and the Center for Blood Research for Collaborative Scholarship. JNK acknowledges Career Investigator Scholar award from Michael Smith Foundation for Health Research (MSFHR). SU is a CIHR New Investigator. The research using zebrafish was partly supported by a Discovery grant and Discovery Accelerator award from the Natural Sciences and Engineering Research Council (NSERC) of Canada, and an Establishment Grant from the Saskatchewan Health Research Foundation (SHRF) to SU. AH is a recipient of postdoctoral fellowships from the CIHR and SHRF. The authors acknowledge Jith Thomas, PhD candidate of the University of Saskatchewan for assistance with obtaining zebrafish embryos and Benjamin Lai of the University of British Columbia for providing administrative support.

Author Contributions

Conceived and designed the experiments: JLH SU JNK. Performed the experiments: JLH AH MI NN. Analyzed the data: JLH AH MI NN SU JNK. Contributed to the writing of the manuscript: JLH SU JNK.

References

1. Hershko C, Link G, Konijn AM, Cabantchik ZI (2005) Objectives and mechanisms of iron chelation therapy. Ann N Y Acad Sci 1054: 124–135.
2. Gattermann N, Finelli C, Della Porta M, Fenaux P, Ganser A, et al. (2010) Deferasirox in iron-overloaded patients with transfusion-dependent myelodysplastic syndromes: Results from the large1-year EPIC study. Leuk Res 34: 1143–1150.
3. Robotham JL, Lietman PS (1980) Acute Iron Poisoning. Am J Dis Child 134: 875–879.
4. Adams RJ, Brambilla D, The optimizing primary stroke prevention in sickle cell anemia (STOP 2) Trial investigators (2005) Discontinuing prophylactic transfusions used to prevent stroke in sickle cell disease. N Engl J Med 353: 2769–2778.
5. Olivieri NF, Nathan DG, MacMillan JH, Wayne AS, Liu PP, et al. (1994) Survival in medically treated patients with homozygous β-thalassemia. N Engl J Med 331: 574–578.
6. Olivieri NF, Brittenham GM (1997) Iron-chelating therapy and the treatment of thalassemia. Blood 89: 739–761.
7. Crisponi G, Remelli M (2008) Iron chelating agents for the treatment of iron overload. Coord Chem Rev 252: 1225–1240.
8. Modell CB, Beck J (1974) Long-term desferrioxamine therapy in thalassemia. Ann N Y Acad Sci 232: 201–210.
9. Kontoghiorghes GJ, Aldouri MA, Hoffbrand AV, Barr J, Wonke B, et al. (1987) Effective chelation of iron in beta thalassaemia with the oral chelator 1, 2-dimethyl-3-hydroxypyrid-4-one. Br Med J (Clin Res Ed) 295: 1509–1512.
10. Link G, Konijn AM, Breuer W, Cabantchik ZI, Hershko C (2001) Exploring the "iron shuttle" hypothesis in chelation therapy: Effects of combined desferrioxamine and deferiprone treatment in hypertransfused rats with labeled iron stores and iron-loaded rat heart cells in culture. J Lab Clin Med 38: 130–138.
11. Capellini MD (2005) Iron chelation therapy with the new oral agent ICL670 (Exjade) Best Pract Res Clin Haematol 18: 289–298.
12. Galanello R, Campus S, Origa R (2012) Desferasirox: pharmacokinetics and clinical experience. Expert Opin Drug Metab Toxicol 8: 123–134.
13. Levine JE, Cohen A, MacQueen M, Martin M, Giardina PJ (1997) Sensorimotor neurotoxicity associated with high-dose deferoxamine treatment. J Pediatr Hematol Oncol 19: 139–41.
14. Kontoghiorghes GJ, Pattichi K, Hadjigavriel M, Kolnagou A (2000) Transfusional iron overload and chelation therapy with deferoxamine and deferiprone (L1). Transfus Sci 23: 211–223.
15. Hoffbrand AV, Cohen A, Hershko C (2003) Role of deferiprone in chelation therapy for transfusional iron overload. Blood 102: 17–24.
16. Cohen AR, Galanello R, Piga A, De Sanctis V, Tricta F (2003) Safety and effectiveness of long-term therapy with the oral iron chelator deferiprone. Blood 102: 1583–1587.
17. Wei HY, Yang CP, Cheng CH, Lo FS (2011) Fanconi syndrome in a patient with B-thalassemia major after using desferasirox for 27 months. Transfusion 51: 949–954.
18. Sánchez-González PD, López-Hernandez FJ, Morales AI, Macías-Nu~nez JF, López-Novoa JM (2011) Effects of deferasirox on renal function and renal epithelial cell death. Toxicol Lett 203: 154–161.
19. Bosque MA, Domingo JL, Corbella J (1995) Assessment of the developmental toxicity of deferoxamine in mice. Arch Toxicol 69: 467–471.
20. Berdoukas V, Bentley P, Frost H, Schnebli HP (1993) Toxicity of oral iron chelator L1. The Lancet 341: 1088.

21. Domingo JL (1998) Developmental toxicity of metal chelating agents. Reprod Toxicol 12: 499–510.
22. Peterson RT, Macrae CA (2012) Systematic approaches to toxicology in the zebrafish. Annu Rev Pharmacol Toxicol 52: 433–453.
23. Hill AJ, Teraoka H, Heidman W, Peterson RE (2005) Zebrafish as a model vertebrate for investigating chemical toxicity. Toxicol Sci 86: 6–19.
24. Zon LI, Peterson RT (2005) In vivo drug discovery in the zebrafish. Nat Rev Drug Discov 4: 35–44.
25. Zhu JJ, Xu YQ, He JH, Yu HP, Huan CJ, et al. (2014) Human cardiotoxic drugs delivered by soaking and microinjection induce cardiovascular toxicity in zebrafish. J Appl Toxicol 34: 139–148.
26. Tan JL, Zon LI (2011) Chemical screening in zebrafish for novel biological and therapeutic discovery. Methods in Cell Biology 105: Chapter 21, 493–516.
27. Haldi M, Harden M, D'Amico L, DeLise A, Seng WL (2012) Developmental toxicity in zebrafish. In Zebrafish: Methods for assessing drug safety and toxicology. (McGrath, P. Ed.) John Wiley & Sons, 15–25.
28. Donovan A, Brownlie A, Dorschner MO, Zhou Y, Pratt SJ, et al. (2002) The zebrafish mutant gene chardonnay (cdy) encodes divalent metal transporter 1 (DMT1). Blood 100: 4655–4659.
29. Nemeth E, Tuttle MS, Powelson J, Vaughn MB, Donovan A, et al. (2004) Hepcidin regulates cellular iron efflux by binding to ferroportin and inducing its internalization. Science 306: 2090–2093.
30. Shike H, Shimizu C, Lauth X, Burns JC (2004) Organization and expression analysis of the zebrafish hepcidin gene, an antimicrobial peptide gene conserved among vertebrates. Dev Comp Immunol 28: 747–754.
31. Fraenkel PG, Traver D, Donovan A, Zahrieh D, Zon LI (2005) Ferroportin1 is required for normal iron cycling in zebrafish. J Clin Invest 115: 1532–1541.
32. Steinhauser S, Heinz U, Bartholomä M, Weyhermüller T, Nick H, et al. (2004) Complex formation of ICL670 and related ligands with Fe III and Fe II. Eur J Inorgan Chem 4177–4192.
33. Livak KJ, Schmittgen TD (2001) Analysis of relative gene expression data using real-time quantitative PCR and the 2[-Delta Delta C (T)] method. Methods 25: 402–408.
34. Craig PM, Galus M, Wood CM, McClelland GB (2009) Dietary iron alters waterborne copper-induced gene expression in soft water acclimated zebrafish (Danio rerio). Am J Physiol Regul Integr Comp Physiol 296: R362–R373.
35. Walter A, Gutknecht J (1986) Permeability of Small Nonelectrolytes through Lipid Bilayer Membranes. J Membr Biol 90: 207–217.
36. Kansy M, Senner F, Gubernator K (1998) Physicochemical High Throughput Screening: Parallel Artificial Membrane Permeation Assay in the Description of Passive Absorption Processes. J Med Chem 41: 1007–1010.
37. Camenisch G, Alsenz J, van de Waterbeemd H, Folkers G (1998) Estimation of permeability by passive diffusion through Caco-2 cell monolayers using the drugs' lipophilicity and molecular weight. Eur J Pharm Sci 6: 313–319.
38. Zhou T, Ma Y, Kong X, Hider RC (2012) Design of Iron Chelators with Therapeutic Applications. Dalton Trans 41: 6371–6389.
39. Cooper CE, Lynagh GR, Hoyes KP, Hider RC, Cammack R, et al. (1996) The Relationship of Intracellular Iron Chelation to the Inhibition and Regeneration of Human Ribonucleotide Reductase. J Biol Chem 271: 20291–20299.
40. Bury N, Grosell M (2003) Iron acquisition by teleost fish. Comp Biochem Physiol Phamacol 135: 97–105.
41. Andersen O (1997) Accumulation of waterborne iron and expression of ferritin and transferring in early developmental stages of brown trout (Salmo trutta). Fish Physiol Biochem 16: 223–231.

42. Roeder M, Roeder RH (1966) Effect of iron on the growth rate of fishes. J Nutr 90: 86–90.

43. Kontoghiorghes GJ, Kolnagou A, Peng C-T, Shah SV, Aessopos A (2012) Safety issues of iron chelation therapy in patients with normal range iron stores including thalassemia, neurodegenerative, renal and infectious diseases. Expert Opin Drug Saf 9: 201–206.

44. Gunshin H, Mackenzie B, Berger UV, Gunshin Y, Romero MF, et al. (1997) Cloning and characterization of a mammalian proton-coupled metal-ion transporter. Nature, 388: 482–488.

45. Koren G, Pastuszak A, Ito S (1998) Drugs in pregnancy. N Engl J Med 338: 1128–1137.

12

Phytoavailability of Cadmium (Cd) to Pak Choi (*Brassica chinensis* L.) Grown in Chinese Soils: A Model to Evaluate the Impact of Soil Cd Pollution on Potential Dietary Toxicity

Muhammad Tariq Rafiq[1,2]⦾, Rukhsanda Aziz[1]⦾, Xiaoe Yang[1], Wendan Xiao[1], Peter J. Stoffella[3], Aamir Saghir[4], Muhammad Azam[5], Tingqiang Li[1]*

1 Ministry of Education Key Laboratory of Environmental Remediation and Ecological Health, College of Environmental and Resource Sciences, Zhejiang University, Hangzhou, China, 2 Department of Environmental Science, International Islamic University, Islamabad, Pakistan, 3 Indian River Research and Education Center, Institute of Food and Agricultural Sciences, University of Florida, Fort Pierce, Florida, United States of America, 4 Institute of Statistics, Zhejiang University, Hangzhou, China, 5 College of Agriculture and Biotechnology, Zhejiang University, Hangzhou, China

Abstract

Food chain contamination by soil cadmium (Cd) through vegetable consumption poses a threat to human health. Therefore, an understanding is needed on the relationship between the phytoavailability of Cd in soils and its uptake in edible tissues of vegetables. The purpose of this study was to establish soil Cd thresholds of representative Chinese soils based on dietary toxicity to humans and develop a model to evaluate the phytoavailability of Cd to Pak choi (*Brassica chinensis* L.) based on soil properties. Mehlich-3 extractable Cd thresholds were more suitable for Stagnic Anthrosols, Calcareous, Ustic Cambosols, Typic Haplustalfs, Udic Ferrisols and Periudic Argosols with values of 0.30, 0.25, 0.18, 0.16, 0.15 and 0.03 mg kg^{-1}, respectively, while total Cd is adequate threshold for Mollisols with a value of 0.86 mg kg^{-1}. A stepwise regression model indicated that Cd phytoavailability to Pak choi was significantly influenced by soil pH, organic matter, total Zinc and Cd concentrations in soil. Therefore, since Cd accumulation in Pak choi varied with soil characteristics, they should be considered while assessing the environmental quality of soils to ensure the hygienically safe food production.

Editor: Wenju Liang, Chinese Academy of Sciences, China

Funding: This study was supported by the Ministry of Environmental Protection of China (grant no. 2011467057), the ministry of Science and Technology of China (grant no. 2012AA100605), and by the Fundamental Research Funds for the Central Universities of China. The funders had no role in study design, data collection and analysis, decision to publish, or preparation of the manuscript.

Competing Interests: The authors have declared that no competing interests exist.

* Email: litq@zju.edu.cn

⦾ These authors contributed equally to this work.

Introduction

Cadmium (Cd) is an important environmental pollutant toxic to animals and human beings. It is one of the most mobile elements, among all the toxic heavy metals [1]. Cadmium is not required for plants growth or reproduction, however its bioaccumulation and subsequent accrual in the food chain surpasses all other trace elements due to its high mobility in soil [2]. It is the most toxic element in the environment and even at low concentrations is very toxic to living cells and considered as carcinogenic [3]. In humans, Cd exposure can result in multiple adverse effects, such as testicular damage, renal and hepatic dysfunction, etc. [3]. Moreover, Cd is implicated in the development of cancer, phytotoxic at higher levels of concentrations [4] and classified as a type I carcinogen by the International Agency for Cancer Research [5]. Significant quantities of Cd can be transferred from contaminated soil to plants [6]. Therefore, crops produced from Cd contaminated soils may be unsuitable or even detrimental for animal and human consumption [7].

Vegetables are an important component of human diet since they contain proteins, carbohydrates as well as minerals and vitamins [8]. The proportion of vegetables consumed in the total diet has been increased with the improvement of living standards. However, vegetables are also one of the most important pathways through which heavy metals enter the food chain and affect human health. Leafy vegetables can accumulate higher concentrations of Cd than other crops [9,10]. Leafy vegetables are known to accumulate higher concentrations of Cd in the edible parts even when grown in soils containing low concentrations of Cd [11]. Pak choi (*Brassica chinensis* L.), also known as Chinese cabbage, is a popular leafy vegetable, grown and consumed worldwide. Therefore, it is imperative to control Cd concentrations in Pak choi, especially in its edible parts to ensure food safety. To limit the transfer of soil Cd into the edible parts of Pak choi, an understanding of its accumulation characteristics is required. Currently, there is an elevated concern over Cd accumulation in food and its potential risks to human health [12]. Cadmium accumulation and distribution varies among vegetable cultivars and tissues [13]. However, the accumulation and distribution of Cd in vegetables grown in a diversity of soil types were rarely studied [14].

About one fifth of agricultural land is contaminated by Cd, lead (Pb) and arsenic (As) in China [15]. Moreover, it was reported that about 20% of farm lands in China are contaminated with heavy metals and Cd contamination accounts for more than 1.3×10^5 ha of the total affected area [16,17]. Cadmium uptake by rice (*Oryza sativa* L.) and vegetables from soil is the initial source of exposure for human beings [18,19]. Therefore, there are environmental concerns of soils, food safety and human health for the present and future agricultural and environmental sustainability of world vegetable supplies. As, only a small fraction of total trace metals in soil is available for plant absorption, it is widely accepted that the total metal content in soils is neither a viable indicator of phytoavailability nor an adequate tool to assess the potential risk of dietary toxicity [12]. Tracy and Sheila [20] reported that extractable Cd content in soil may be an improved indicator of bioavailability and toxicity than the total contents and toxicity and availability of metals differed among soils types. Metal uptake and translocation studies were conducted for different crops under varying soil conditions, to further understanding uptake and the transport mechanisms [21,22].

To ensure the food safety and environmental quality of soils, guidelines for permissible concentrations of Cd in agricultural soils need to be established. Due to limited number of studies, the soil environmental quality guidelines for heavy metals in farmland soils developed and applied in the world are still based on total metal contents of soil. Minimal attention has been focused on metal accumulation differences among the edible parts of crops, and the relationship between total concentration and phytoavailability of heavy metals in different soil types [4]. Developing the linkage between the bioavailability of Cd in soil and its transfer into the edible plant parts is a key to improving existing soil environmental quality standards. Information is vital on the degree of translocation of heavy metals from soils to plants, which are used as food crops, and absorption of metals in food plants to concentration that does not cause phytotoxicity symptoms [23]. This study was conducted in seven Chinese soil types to establish direct relationship of Cd level in such contaminated soils and Cd uptake in Pak choi. The main objectives were to establish soil Cd thresholds for representative Chinese soils based on human dietary toxicity and to determine the relationships between several soil properties and Cd accumulation in Pak choi. This information will be useful in establishing soil protection guidelines to produce hygienically safe vegetables.

Materials and Methods

Ethics Statement

The soils used in this study were agricultural soils. No specific permissions were required for the described locations. We confirm that the field studies did not involve endangered or protected species.

Soil Collection and Analysis

Seven Chinese soils were selected for this study. Udic Ferrisols, Mollisols, Periudic Argosols, Typic Haplustalfs, Ustic Cambosols, Calcaric Regosols and Stagnic Anthrosols were collected from Chinese cities of Guilin (104°40′–119°45′E, 24°18′– 25°41′N), Harbin (125°42′– 130°10′E, 44°04′–46°40′N), Huzhou (119°14′–120°29′E, 30°22′–31°11′N), Zhanjiang (110°08′–110°77′E, 20°33′–21°62′N), Qufu (116°51′–117°13′E, 35°29′–35°49′N), Ya'an (102°37′–103°12′E, 29°23′–30°37′N) and Jiaxing

(120°7′–121°02′E, 30°5′–30°77′N), respectively. Soils samples were taken at a depth of up to 20 cm from the upper horizon. Each sample was air-dried, ground, and screened through two mm sieve before laboratory analysis. Soil pH, cation exchange capacity, organic matter contents, and particle size density were measured by using previously described methods [24–27]. Physicochemical properties of these soils are reported (Table 1).

Cadmium Spiking and Aging

Soil samples of Mollisols, Periudic Argosols, Stagnic Anthrosols and Ustic Cambosols were spiked with Cd as $Cd(NO_3)_2$ in an aqueous solution at loading rates of 1.0, 2.0, 4.0, 6.0 and 8.0 mg Cd kg^{-1} soil along with an untreated control (Ck), the background values of Cd concentration was below 0.50 mg kg^{-1} in these soil. However, the Udic Ferrisols, Typic Haplustalfs and Calcaric Regosols soil samples, with the background values of Cd concentration above 0.50 mg kg^{-1}, were spiked with Cd to establish the contamination levels of 2.0, 4.0, 6.0 and 8.0 mg Cd kg^{-1} soil along with the untreated control (Ck). Soil moisture was maintained up to 70% of its water-holding capacity by using distilled water. All the spiked soils were aged for one year subsequent to greenhouse experimentation. After one year aging period, the concentrations of total Cd, and Mehlich-3 extractable Cd were determined in each of the spiked soils.

Containerized Experiment

A containerized experiment was performed in greenhouse by growing Pak choi (*Brassica chinensis* L.) during March – April, 2012 at Zhejiang University, Hangzhou, China. Seed of Pak choi was obtained from the Zhejiang Seed Co. Hangzhou, China. Seeds were washed with distilled water and air-dried prior to sowing. Seeds were germinated in dark at 25°C and transplanted into quartz sand bed to establish seedlings. Four healthy, uniform and 21-day-old seedlings were transplanted into plastic containers with a diameter of 18 cm and height of 17 cm. Each container had 3 kg of soil. Fertilizers were applied at the rates of 0.4 g of N as CO $(NH_2)_2$ and 0.2 g P as KH_2PO_4 per kg of soil. The experiment was carried out in a completely randomized design (CRD). Treatments were established in triplicate, and the containers were randomly arranged in a greenhouse bench under controlled conditions of 16 h of light at 30°C and 8 h of dark at 22°C. Plants were monitored daily and watered as necessary.

Plant Sample Collection

Pak choi was harvested after 30 days from transplanting. The plants of Pak choi were removed from each container and separated into root and shoots (including stems and leaves). Roots and shoots of Pak choi were first washed with tap water and then with ultrapure distilled water, to remove all visible soil particles. Clean plant samples were first blotted dry, and then dried at 70°C for 72 h in an oven. Dry shoot weight of samples was recorded. Dry plant samples were ground to pass through a 60 mm sieve using an agate mill prior to Cd concentration analysis.

Total Cd of Soil and Plant

For determination of total Cd concentration in soil, 0.20 g of soil samples was digested with HNO_3–HF–$HClO_4$ (5:1:1) [4]. For plant samples, 0.20 g of shoots for each treatment was digested with HNO_3–H_2O_2 (5:1). After cooling the digest was transferred to a volumetric flask, diluted with distilled water to 50 mL [28]. The concentrations of Cd in the filtrate were determined using inductively coupled plasma–mass spectrometry (ICP-MS, Agilent, 7500a, CA, USA). The ICP-MS was operated at the following

Table 1. Basic Chemical and Physical Characteristics of Seven Chinese soils.

Soil Types	Mollisols	Ustic Cambosols	Stagnic Anthrosols	Periudic Argosols	Typic Haplustalfs	Udic Ferrisols	Calcaric Regosols
pH	7.23±0.08	7.80±0.02	6.49±0.03	4.85±0.06	5.16±0.05	4.43±0.07	8.02±0.04
OM (g kg⁻¹)	32.2±0.32	7.54±0.20	21.4±0.34	11.6±0.17	6.37±0.56	19.1±0.15	21.8±0.14
CEC (cmol kg⁻¹)	34.0±2.51	15.8±1.62	20.2±1.41	12.6±1.52	8.33±2.14	17.3±1.96	25.5±1.46
Total Cd (mg kg⁻¹)	0.51±0.02	0.59±0.06	0.79±0.04	0.47±0.02	0.92±0.01	1.06±0.09	0.96±0.06
Total Zn (mg kg⁻¹)	31.18±1.47	26.93±0.43	41.36±1.71	15.17±0.88	25.3±1.44	24.6±0.23	28.59±1.38
Sand (%)	20.6±1.54	21.6±1.29	11.4±0.26	24.8±0.65	37.4±0.96	32.75±1.65	31.6±0.57
Silt (%)	60.2±2.21	65.4±2.62	73.0±2.41	58.2±1.04	40.8±1.66	39.8±1.26	44.0±1.26
Clay (%)	19.2±1.24	13.0±1.05	15.6±1.17	17.0±0.34	21.8±0.82	49.6±1.19	24.4±1.32

conditions: the radio frequency power at the torch 1.2 kW, the plasma gas flow 15 L min⁻¹, the auxiliary gas flow 0.89 L min⁻¹, and the carrier gas flow 0.95 L min⁻¹ [28]. The same procedure without samples was used as control and three replications were conducted for each sample.

Mehlich-3 Extractable Cd in Soils

Mehlich-3 extractable Cd in soils was determined following the extraction method described by Mehlich [29]. Briefly, 5 g (0.2 mm sieved) of dry soil was shaken with 50 mL of Mehlich-3 solution (0.2 mol L⁻¹ CH_3COOH, 0.25 mol L⁻¹ NH_4NO_3, 0.015 mol L⁻¹ NH_4F, 0.013 mol L⁻¹ HNO_3, 0.001 mol L⁻¹ EDTA) for 5 min (200 rpm) at 25°C. The suspension was centrifuged at 5000 rpm for 10 min and filtered through 0.45 μm filter paper. The same procedure without samples was used as control and three replications were conducted for each soil sample. The Cd concentration in the filtrate was analyzed by inductively coupled plasma–mass spectrometry (ICP-MS, Agilent 7500a, CA, USA).

Quality Control for Cd Analysis

Quality assurance and quality control (QA/QC) for Cd in soil and Pak choi were conducted by determining Cd contents in the certified reference materials (soil GSBZ 50013-88 and plant GBW-07402) respectively, approved by General Administration of Quality Supervision, Inspection and Quarantine of the People's Republic of China (AQSIQ) and National Center for Reference Materials. The analytical results showed a recovery rate of 97.3% and 102.1% respectively.

Derivation of Soil Cd Thresholds for Potential Dietary Toxicity in Pak choi

For ensuring the environmental and food safety for human beings, an effort has been made to develop guidelines for acceptable concentrations of potentially harmful Cd in seven agricultural soils types of China. In this context, the amounts of Cd in Pak choi above than threshold level of food safety are adversely affecting humans are critical. Since, Cd bioavailability differed among soil types, the focus was on the development of soil Cd thresholds for representative Chinese soils based on food safety, Provisional Tolerable Weekly Intake (PTWI) of Cd recommended by FAO/WHO Joint Expert Committee on Food Additives, is 7 μg kg⁻¹ of body weight [30]. Estimated daily intake of metal (EDIM) was determined by the following equation.

$$\text{EDIM} = \frac{C_{cadmium} \times C_{factor} \times D_{daily\ intake}}{B_{average\ weight}}$$

Where, Cc_{admium}, C_{factor}, $D_{food\ intake}$ and $B_{average\ weight}$ represent average Cd concentration in Pak choi (mg kg⁻¹), conversion factor, daily consumption of Pak choi (g) and average body weight (kg) of the adult consumers, respectively. Average daily consumption of Pak choi for adults was considered to be 0.345 kg person⁻¹ d⁻¹ [31] and a conversion factor 0.085 was used to convert fresh Pak choi weight to dry weight [32]. Average body weight of adult was considered to be 60 kg as motioned in previous reports [30]. According to the above equation of EDIM, the provisional tolerable daily tolerable intake of Cd for Pak choi was 2.04 mg kg⁻¹ on a dry weight basis. Soil Cd threshold levels for potential dietary toxicity from Pak choi were calculated according to the tolerable daily dietary intake level of Cd (2.04 mg kg⁻¹) and the regression equations.

Statistical Analysis

Stepwise multiple regression analysis, single linear regression and one-way analysis of variance (ANOVA) were performed using the statistical software package SPSS (version 18.0). All values reported in this work are means of three independent replications. Treatment means were separated by least significant difference (LSD) test, at 5% level.

Results

Characteristics of Soils

Soils evaluated were representative of most of Chinese soil types, pH range of soils were strongly acidic to mild alkaline. Chemical and physical characteristics varied among the seven soils. Highest total Cd and Zn concentrations (background value) were observed in Udic Ferrisols and Stagnic Anthrosols respectively. Mollisols contained the highest amount of organic matter and exhibited an elevated cation exchange capacity as well (Table 1).

Mehlich-3 Extractable Cd in Soils after Aging of 1 Year

Mehlich-3 extractable Cd content increased significantly with increasing Cd spiking levels in all the seven soils. Mehlich-3 extractable Cd ranged from 0.16–3.95 mg kg^{-1} in these soils under different Cd levels (Table 2). The Cd contents varied significantly among these soils, decreasing in order: Periudic Argosols> Typic Haplustalfs> Udic Ferrisols> Stagnic Anthrosols> Mollisols> Ustic Cambosols> Calcaric Regosols. Mehlich-3 extractable Cd concentration was greater at higher rates of Cd spiking in each soil. These results indicated that minimum and maximum extractability of Cd was found in Calcaric Regosols and Periudic Argosols, respectively under the highest (8 mg kg^{-1}) level of Cd spiked. Mehlich-3 extractable concentrations were dependent on total Cd in each soil, however the extractability was significantly higher in low pH soils as compared to the medium and high pH soils (Table 2).

Biomass Yield of Pak choi

Generally, Pak choi had tolerance to Cd toxicity in Mollisols, Stagnic Anthrosols and Calcaric Regosols soils, indicating low phytoavailability of Cd in these soils. Shoot biomass of Pak choi under different Cd treatments of these soils did not decrease significantly as compared with their respective controls. However, the shoot biomass of Pak choi grown in Ustic Cambosols, Udic Ferrisols, Periudic Argosols and Typic Haplustalfs decreased significantly as compared with the control indicating higher phytoavailability of Cd in these soils (Table 3). The stimulating effect of Cd on shoot biomass of Pak choi occurred at 1 mg kg^{-1} and 2 mg kg^{-1} in Ustic Cambosols and Mollisols respectively, whereas in Stagnic Anthrosols, it occurred at 4 mg kg^{-1}. The dry weight of Pak choi shoots at 8 mg kg^{-1} Cd generally decreased in order of: Calcaric Regosols> Mollisols, Stagnic Anthrosols> Ustic Cambosols> Udic Ferrisols> Periudic Argosols> Typic Haplustalfs (Table 3).

Accumulation and Distribution of Cadmium in Pak choi

Cadmium concentration in the shoots and roots of Pak choi varied significantly among soils at different Cd levels and soil types. Roots exhibited the higher Cd contents as compared with Pak choi shoots. The content of Cd enhanced with increasing Cd loading rate in the soils. Cd concentration was high in the roots (2.42 to 169. 95 mg kg^{-1} DW), while low in the shoot (0.48 to 89.21 mg kg^{-1} DW) (Table 4). Cd uptake in Pak choi tissues was affected by soil type, primarily due to the variation in Cd

Table 2. Mehlich-3 Extractable Cd Contents (mg kg^{-1}) in Seven Chinese Soils at the onset of Containerized Experiment after Aging of 1 year.

Cd conc. (mg kg^{-1})	Mollisols	Ustic Cambosols	Stagnic Anthrosols	Periudic Argosols	Typic Haplustalfs	Udic Ferrisols	Calcaric Regosols
Ck	0.19±0.05c	0.17±0.07c	0.22±0.08d	0.16±0.06e	0.31±0.12d	0.42±0.09d	0.29±0.07c
1	0.21±0.04c	0.19±0.06c	0.30±0.04d	0.41±0.13e	-	-	-
2	0.62±0.04bc	0.48±0.10c	0.56±0.27d	0.99±0.29d	0.69±0.17d	0.65±0.11d	0.35±0.06c
4	1.19±0.08b	1.05±0.90bc	1.17±0.24c	1.79±0.54c	1.52±0.26c	1.46±0.60c	0.71±0.10bc
6	2.21±0.91a	2.13±0.90b	2.01±0.47b	2.98±0.46b	2.44±0.64b	2.39±0.90b	1.38±0.29ab
8	2.89±1.04a	3.28±0.84a	3.29±0.73a	3.95±0.41a	3.58±0.53a	3.47 ±0.70a	2.01±0.94a

Mean values followed by different letters within the same column are significantly different at $P < 0.05$.

Table 3. Dry Biomass (g plant⁻¹) of Pak choi Shoots Grown on Seven Chinese Soils with Different Loading Rates of Cd.

Cd conc. (mg kg⁻¹)	Mollisols	Ustic Cambosols	Stagnic Anthrosols	Periudic Argosols	Typic Haplustalfs	Udic Ferrisols	Calcaric Regosols
Ck	1.95±0.18a	1.54±0.13a	1.13±0.31a	0.84±0.29a	0.73±0.20a	0.95±0.11a	2.07±0.46a
1	1.91±0.37a	1.66±0.59a	1.10±0.30a	0.63±0.35ab	-	-	-
2	2.22±0.58a	1.02±0.49a	1.14±0.53a	0.59±0.47ab	0.54±0.41ab	0.79±0.23ab	1.98±0.11a
4	1.89±0.49a	1.47±0.08a	1.25±0.28a	0.51±0.03ab	0.43±0.38ab	0.58±0.06abc	1.95±0.06a
6	1.86±0.48a	1.35±0.13ab	1.09±0.09a	0.36±0.02ab	0.38±0.11ab	0.50±0.24bc	1.90±0.15a
8	1.54±0.28a	0.95±0.15b	1.11±0.51a	0.17±0.06b	0.10±0.01b	0.39±0.29c	1.75±0.17a

Mean values followed by different letters within the same column are significantly different at $P < 0.05$.

bioavailability. The lowest and highest Cd concentrations in the Pak choi tissues were at the highest (8 mg kg⁻¹) level of Cd in Calcaric Regosols and Periudic Argosols, respectively. Cadmium concentrations in Pak choi followed an order of: Periudic Argosols> Typic Haplustalfs> Udic Ferrisols> Ustic Cambosols> Mollisols> Stagnic Anthrosols> Calcaric Regosols at 8 mg kg⁻¹ soil Cd level (Table 4).

Relationship between Mehlich-3 Extractable Cd in Soils and Pak choi Cd Content

Cadmium concentrations in shoots of Pak choi were significantly correlated to total Cd and Mehlich-3 extractable Cd contents in soils ($R^2 = 0.95$ to 0.99, and 0.97 to 0.99 respectively). Cadmium concentrations in Pak choi shoots were best related to total Cd content in Mollisols ($R^2 = 0.99$). Whereas, the Cd concentrations of Pak choi shoots were best correlated to Mehlich-3 extractable Cd in Ustic Cambosols, Stagnic Anthrosols Periudic Argosols, Udic Ferrisols, Typic Haplustalfs and Calcaric Regosols with $R^2 = 0.97$, 0.99, 0.99,0.98,0.99 and 0.98, respectively (Table 5).

Soil Cd Thresholds for Potential Dietary Toxicity in Pak choi

Total soil Cd thresholds for potential dietary toxicity from the consumption of Pak choi conformed to an order of: Calcaric Regosols> Stagnic Anthrosols> Ustic Cambosols> Mollisols> Udic Ferrisols> Typic Haplustalfs> Periudic Argosols, and were 1.25, 1.16, 1.02, 0.86, 0.72, 0.70 and 0.12 mg kg⁻¹, respectively. Mehlich-3 extractable Cd thresholds were 0.30, 0.25, 0.23, 0.18, 0.16, 0.15 and 0.03 mg kg⁻¹ and decreased in the following order of: Stagnic Anthrosols> Calcareous> Mollisols> Ustic Cambosols> Typic Haplustalfs> Udic Ferrisols>Periudic Argosols, respectively (Table 6).

Discussion

Biomass Yield of Pak choi

Dry weight of Pak choi did not decrease significantly under different Cd levels (Ck to 8.0 mg kg⁻¹) in Mollisols, Stagnic Anthrosols and Calcaric Regosols and even increased at 1, 2 and 4.0 mg kg⁻¹of treatment levels. Similar stimulatory responses of biomass to Cd exposure have also been reported in several plant species [33,34]. The stimulatory effect of Cd on plant biomass may be explained by various mechanisms, for examples, metal ions can serve as enzyme activators in cytokinins metabolism, which stimulates the growth of plants, [35] and a low dose of metal exposure may cause changes in cytokinins and plant hormones that regulate growth and development of plants [36]. Kaminek [36] reported that cytokinins may delay senescence by maintaining chlorophyll production and photosynthetic activity in plant leaves.

Cd exposure may cause changes to various physiological and biochemical processes in plant tissues, such as, reduction in dry biomass may be due to the negative effects of Cd on the roots, and plants could not take up nutrients to continue their normal activities. It has been well reported that Cd can reduce plant growth and development by interfering in various metabolic processes, such as, inhibition of the proton pump, reduction in root elongation, and damage to photosynthetic activity [37,38]. The excess amount of Cd in soil may be responsible for causing disturbances in mineral nutrition and carbohydrate metabolism [39].

Shoot biomass of Pak choi grown in Ustic Cambosols, Udic Ferrisols, Periudic Argosols and Typic Haplustalfs decreased significantly as compared with the control. The inhibitory effect of

Table 4. Cd Concentration (mg kg^{-1} DW) in Pak choi Grown under Different Cd Levels in Seven Chinese Soils.

Cd (mg kg^{-1})	Mollisols		Ustic Cambosols		Stagnic Anthrosols		Periudic Argosols		Typic Haplustalfs		Udic Ferrisols		Calcaric Regosols	
	Root	Shoot	Root	Shoot	Root	Shoot	Root	Shoot	Root	Shoot	Root	Shoot	Root	Shoot
Ck	3.41±0.64e	1.00±0.28e	2.42±0.45f	0.48±0.22e	2.73±0.28e	0.85±0.12e	7.26±1.10f	1.84±0.56f	12.35±1.68e	4.37±1.02e	11.81±0.78e	6.77±0.92e	3.11±0.66e	1.92±0.58b
1	5.09±0.91e	2.53±0.76e	6.69±0.65e	2.06±0.98e	4.12±0.75e	1.92±0.94e	21.3±2.01e	11.00±1.57e	-	-	-	-	-	-
2	8.92±1.09d	4.31±0.54d	9.30±1.29d	4.77±0.22d	8.34±1.11d	3.94±0.83d	39.33±3.86d	28.51±2.61d	25.41±1.79d	12.09±1.34d	19.41±1.27d	10.06±1.10d	4.24±0.99d	2.70±0.99b
4	14.21±0.90c	8.34±1.11c	14.00±1.43c	9.01±1.06c	13.21±1.55c	7.06±1.06c	68.43±3.71c	39.12±3.06c	39.11±2.28c	32.51±2.51c	33.55±1.71c	20.89±1.46c	10.37±1.21c	3.46±1.10b
6	21.24±1.20b	11.75±1.17b	24.36±1.11b	17.23±1.50b	20.21±1.80b	11.63±1.54b	117.76±6.53b	68.21±4.08b	68.00±3.96b	41.11±3.01b	55.53±2.67b	31.45±2.48b	14.41±1.03b	6.57±0.93a
8	38.96±1.39a	18.11±1.12a	43.21±2.21a	22.22±1.51a	28.56±1.42a	17.63±1.37a	169.95±8.11a	89.21±5.70a	118.21±6.24a	69.21±4.11a	85.32±4.28a	53.73±2.88a	18.73±1.54a	8.13±0.87a

Mean values followed by different letters within the same column are significantly different at $P < 0.05$.

Cd on shoot growth is consistent with earlier reports of three Chinese cabbage cultivars exposed to different soil Cd levels of 1, 2.5 and 5 mg kg^{-1}. A significant decrease in the shoot biomass was observed at 2.5 and 5 mg kg^{-1} levels of Cd as compared to their respective controls [40]. Shentu et al. [4] found a 46% reduction in root dry weight of radish at 6.31 mg kg^{-1} Cd exposure in red yellow soil, which is in accordance with our results as we also noticed a shoot dry weight reduction of 58.9%, 79.7%, and 86.3% in Udic Ferrisols, Periudic Argosols and Typic Haplustalfs respectively at 8 mg kg^{-1} level of soil Cd as compared to their respective controls.

Accumulation and Distribution of Cadmium in Pak choi

Variations of Cd accumulation in Pak choi grown in different soils with different pH may be due to the difference in bioavailability of Cd in each soil. Liang et al. [13] stated that Cd content of spinach plants was highly dependent upon the soil pH being highest at pH 5.3. Lai and Chen [41] reported that Cd concentration in Pak choi shoots was up to 85 mg kg^{-1} DW with an application of soil Cd up to 20 mg kg^{-1}. Moreover, it was observed that accumulation of the Cd in rice shoot ranged from 67.9 to 241.7 µg/pot in different rice genotypes at 5 mg kg^{-1} soil Cd level [42].

Relationship between Mehlich-3 Extractable Cd in Soils and Pak choi Cd Content

Mehlich-3 extraction technique appeared efficient to assess Cd phytoavailability to Pak choi, grown in seven textured soils, as evidenced by high correlation coefficients ($R^2 > 0.97$). This is in agreement with our previous studies, [43,28] which reflected a high linear correlation ($R^2 > 0.98$) between Mehlich-3 Cr and Cr contents in Pak choi and rice grown under six different textured soils. These results are similar to those reported in which extractable soil metal was an improved indicator for Cd phytoavailability in several vegetable crops [4]. Mehlich-3 extraction method is applicable to a large range of soil types, from acidic to alkaline, and makes it ideal for application at a wide scale [44]. Generally, the extraction techniques are assumed to have a relationship between the extractable fraction of metals and the phytoavailability of the metals to plants, and these metals such as exchangeable, soluble, and loosely adsorbed metals are labile and thus readily available to plants [12,45]. The efficiency of Mehlich-3 extraction method was compared with the EPA 3050 B method (a strong acid digestion method) to assess the predictive capabilities through a lettuce (green specie) bioassay. Mehlich-3 extraction was positively correlated with the more costly EPA test, and could be developed as a less expensive and easily conduct able technique [46].

Soil Cd Thresholds for Potential Dietary Toxicity in Pak choi

Cadmium concentrations in the shoots of Pak choi were significantly correlated to total Cd and Mehlich-3 extractable Cd contents in soils, with R^2 values of 0.95 to 0.99, and 0.97 to 0.99, respectively. From this investigation, Cd contents in Pak choi shoots were correlated to total Cd content in Mollisols (R^2 values of 0.99). Cadmium concentrations of Pak choi shoots were highly correlated to Mehlich-3 extractable Cd in Ustic Cambosols, Stagnic Anthrosols, Periudic Argosols, Udic Ferrisols, Typic Haplustalfs and Calcaric Regosols with R^2 values of 0.97, 0.99, 0.99, 0.98, 0.99 and 0.98, respectively. Total Cd threshold levels for potential dietary toxicity conformed to an order of: Calcaric Regosols> Stagnic Anthrosols> Mollisols> Ustic Cambosols>

Table 5. Regression Correlation between Cd Contents in the Edible Shoots of Pak choi and Different Forms of Cd in Various Soils.

Soil type	Form of Soil Cd	Regression equation	R^2
Mollisols	Total Cd	y = 2.1706x +0.1669	0.99
	Mehlich-3 extractable Cd	y = 5.7207x +0.7037	0.98
Ustic Cambosols	Total Cd	y = 2.9358x −0.9586	0.96
	Mehlich-3 extractable Cd	y = 7.0409x +0.7648	0.97
Stagnic Anthrosols	Total Cd	y = 2.2344x −0.5651	0.98
	Mehlich-3 extractable Cd	y = 5.3848x +0.4458	0.99
Periudic Argosols	Total Cd	y = 11.061x +0.6961	0.98
	Mehlich-3 extractable Cd	y = 22.326x +1.3968	0.99
Typic Haplustalfs	Total Cd	y = 8.7318x −4.0825	0.97
	Mehlich-3 extractable Cd	y = 19.123x −0.8046	0.98
Udic Ferrisols	Total Cd	y = 6.6697x −2.7793	0.97
	Mehlich-3 extractable Cd	y = 14.873x −0.3773	0.99
Calcaric Regosols	Total Cd	y = 0.8936x +0.924	0.95
	Mehlich-3 extractable Cd	y = 3.5937x +1.1512	0.98

Typic Haplustalfs> Udic Ferrisols> Periudic Argosols and were 1.25, 1.16, 1.02, 0.86, 0.72, 0.70 and 0.12 mg kg^{-1}, respectively. Mehlich-3 extractable Cd thresholds decreased in the following order of: Stagnic Anthrosols> Calcareous> Mollisols> Ustic Cambosols> Udic Ferrisols>Typic Haplustalfs> Periudic Argosols and were 0.30, 0.25, 0.23, 0.18, 0.16, 0.15 and 0.03 mg kg^{-1}, respectively (Table 6).

Cadmium concentrations in Pak choi shoots, were highly correlated to total Cd content in Mollisols with the threshold levels of 0.86 mg kg^{-1} with a $R^2 = 0.99$. However, the Cd concentrations of Pak choi shoots were best related to Mehlich-3 extractable Cd in Stagnic Anthrosols, Calcaric Regosols, Mollisols, Ustic Cambosols, Typic Haplustalfs and Periudic Argosols with thresholds values of 0.30, 0.25, 0.23, 0.18, 0.16, 0.15 and 0.03 mg kg^{-1}, (R^2 values of 0.97, 0.99, 0.99, 0.98, 0.98 and 0.98), respectively. Based on the wide range of applicability and the simplicity of extraction method, it is proposed that Mehlich-3 extractable Cd is more suitable to be used as soil Cd thresholds for potential dietary toxicity in Pak choi. Our previous study evaluated the phytoavailability of Cd to rice, and demonstrated the suitability of Mehlich-3 extraction method in different textured soils [47]. Similar to our results, Murakami et al. [48] reported that Mehlich-3 extractable Cd was an improved indicator than total soil Cd and HCl-

extractable Cd to predict the grain Cd content of japonica rice varieties. Our results are also in agreement with Shentu et al. [4] who also concluded that extractable Cd was a better soil test index for Cd phytoavailability of several vegetables and could be used as soil Cd thresholds for food safety. Among the predicted thresholds (total soil Cd) the lowest value (0.12 mg kg^{-1}) was observed for the Periudic Argosols, an acidic soil. Bioavailability and uptake of Cd are very high in this soil. The leafy vegetables like Pak choi can accumulate large quantities of Cd as compared to other crops [9,10]. Therefore the predicted threshold is even lower than background value of Cd in soil; it means that there is a risk for dietary toxicity from Pak choi grown on it, even with the background value of total Cd in soil. This kind of information has been reported in our previous study. The threshold of total soil Cd for rice was 0.21 mg kg^{-1} which was also lower than background value of total Cd in soil [47].

Cd levels (Ck, 1, 2, 4, 6, 8 mg kg^{-1}) used in this investigation represented uncontaminated, lightly contaminated, and moderately Cd polluted soils. Therefore, these levels of Cd contamination are realistic, comparable to those applied in other soil safety risk assessment studies, and thus, the results are applicable in field conditions as well.

Table 6. Soil Cd Threshold Levels for Potential Dietary Toxicity in Edible Part of Pak choi Calculated from the Permissible Limit of Cd (2.04 mg kg^{-1} DW) in Leafy Vegetables and Regression Equations.

Soil Type	Total Cd (mg kg^{-1})	Mehlich-3 extractable Cd (mg kg^{-1})
Mollisols	0.86	0.23
Ustic Cambosols	1.02	0.18
Stagnic Anthrosols	1.16	0.30
Periudic Argosols	0.12	0.03
Udic Ferrisols	0.72	0.16
Typic Haplustalfs	0.70	0.15
Calcaric Regosols	1.25	0.25

Table 7. Stepwise Regression Model for Predicting Cd Concentration (Y) in Edible Part of Pak choi based on Soil Properties.

Stepwise regression model	R^2	F value	T value and R^2 of partial regression coefficient		
				T value	R^2
Y = −39.256−15.516 pH−0.944 Zn_T−0.379 OM +26.752 Cd_T	0.977	138.808*	pH	−18.682**	0.964
			Zn_T	−3.788**	0.524
			OM	−3.652*	0.376
			Cd_T	2.67*	0.354

[a]Cd_T and Zn_T refer to the total Cadmium and Zinc concentrations.
[b]Superscripts * and ** indicate significant levels of probability at 0.05 and 0.01, respectively.

Stepwise Regression Model for Predicting Cd Phytoavailability to Pak choi

Many physicochemical properties of soils can influence the heavy metal accumulation in vegetables. For example, the amount of heavy metal uptake from soils was influenced by soil pH, organic matter (OM) content, cation exchange capacity (CEC) and soil texture [49]. The combinations of basic soil properties may explain Cd uptake by plants [50]. By considering this aspect, soil pH, OM, CEC, total soil Cd, total Zn and clay contents were integrated to simulate the combined effects of soil environment on Cd phytoavailability to Pak choi. Stepwise linear regression was conducted and four independent variables pH, total Zn, OM and total Cd significantly influenced the accumulation of Cd in Pak choi plants (Table 7). Both the multiple correlation and partial regression coefficients reached the statistically significant levels at least the 0.05. For multiple linear regression analyses, R^2 values could be used to explain variation of the dependents [12]. It was found that R^2 value was above 0.97, which means that more than 97% of variation in Cd concentration in Pak choi shoots could be attributed to soil pH, total Zinc, OM and total Cd contents in soils (Table 7).

The influence of each factor on Cd concentration of Pak choi (Y) shoots could be further explained by the values of each coefficient [12]. Stepwise regression model revealed that Cd concentration in the Pak choi was enhanced by lower soil pH (negative coefficients showed negative effect and vice versa), total Zinc, OM contents and higher total soil Cd. Lower soil pH, zinc, OM and higher soil total Cd are among the factors which enhance the bioavailability Cd contents in soils. Therefore, these three variables had the contradictory effect on Cd phytoavailability to Pak choi. Wang et al. [12] reported that soil characteristics (e.g. pH, CEC and OM) affected the phytoavailability of different heavy metals in soils, and such influences could be considered in the assessment of phytoavailability of heavy metals. There are four parameters involved in this model and then interactions between them were obvious (e.g. Cd concentration in the extractable fraction was correlated with lower soil pH, soil zinc and OM content). Furthermore, the coefficients obtained in the present model can regulate these cross effects and result in an improved model fitting. For example, there was a negative correlation between the soil pH, Zinc and OM, these factors had an inverse effect on Cd phytoavailability and soil Cd was the leading factor influencing Cd phytoavailability to Pak choi (coefficient of soil Cd was greater than those of pH, Zinc and OM). Our results about soil Cd and pH are in accordance with our recent study which developed an empirical model to correlate the Cd phytoavailability to rice with several soil properties. Soil pH and bioavailable soil Cd were major influencing factors which (pH negatively and soil Cd positively) correlate with the Cd phytoavailability, however

total Zn and OM were not included in our previously developed model [47]. Eriksson and Soderstrom [51] reported that the Cd concentration of wheat grain grown on non-calcareous soils of Sweden was positively correlated to soil total Cd and negatively to extractable Zn. A study was conducted on Cd contaminated soils in Taiwan, whereas regression equation was developed to predict Cd concentrations in rice roots by available fractions of Cd and Zn in soil [52]. The negative coefficient of Zn indicated that soil Zn suppressed the uptake of Cd by rice roots in all varieties as Zn has an antagonistic effect on Cd uptake by root [53]. Oliver et al. [54] also observed a significant decrease of Cd up to 50% in wheat grain when 2.5–5.0 kg Zn ha^{-1} was applied to Cd contaminated Australian soils.

Organic matter content was negatively correlated with the accumulation of Cd in Pak choi shoots (Table 7). Organic matter plays an important role in determining the bioavailability and mobility of heavy metals in soils. Organic matter is involved in supplying organic chemicals to the soil solution, which may act as chelates and increase metal bioavailability to plants [55]. However, OM could reduce the bioavailability of heavy metals in soils by adsorption or forming stable complexes with humic substances [56]. Halim et al. [57] reported that addition of humic acid demonstrated a decrease in extractable heavy metal fraction in metal contaminated soils. This could partially explain the negative correlation of organic matter contents and Cd uptake observed in our present study.

Conclusions

The present study concludes that Cd concentration in Pak choi tissues was dependent on soil type. To establish the soil Cd thresholds of potential dietary toxicity from Pak choi, both Cd bioavailability in garden soils and Pak choi tissues should be taken into consideration. The selection of proper soil types for vegetable production can help us to avoid the toxicity of Cd in our daily diet. Stepwise regression model demonstrated that soil pH, organic matter, total Cd and Zinc contents may be the major factors having influence on the phytoavailability of Cd in different textured soils.

Acknowledgments

M.T. Rafiq acknowledges International Islamic University Islamabad Pakistan for providing a PhD scholarship under HEC-IIUI faculty development program.

Author Contributions

Conceived and designed the experiments: MTR XY TL. Performed the experiments: MTR RA WX. Analyzed the data: RA AS MA. Contributed reagents/materials/analysis tools: XY. Wrote the paper: MTR RA PJS.

References

1. Liu JG, Qian M, Cai GL, Yang JC, Zhu QS (2007) Uptake and translocation of Cd in different rice cultivars and the relation with Cd accumulation in rice grain. J Hazard Mater 143: 443–447.

2. Mahler RJ, Bingham FT, Page AL (1978) Cadmium-enriched sewage sludge application to acid and calcareous soils: Effect on yield and cadmium uptake by lettuce and Swiss chard. J Environ Qual 7: 274–281.

3. Stohs SJ, Bagchi D, Hassoun E, Bagchi M (2000) Oxidative mechanisms in the toxicity of chromium and cadmium ions. J Environ Pathol Toxicol Oncol 19: 201–213.

4. Shentu J, He Z, Yang XE, Li TQ (2008) Accumulation properties of cadmium in a selected vegetable –rotation system of south eastern China. J Agric Food Chem 56: 6382–6388.

5. IARC (1993) (International agency for research on cancer), Monographs on the evaluation of the carcinogenic risks to humans beryllium, cadmium, mercury and exposures in the glass manufacturing industry. IARC, Scientific Publications. Lyon, France. 119–238.

6. Li ST, Liu RL, Wang M, Wang XB, Shan H, et al. (2006) Phytoavailability of cadmium to cherry-red radish in soil applied composted chicken or pig manure. Geoderma 136: 260–271.

7. Lebeau T, Bagot D, Jezequel K, Fabr B (2002) Cadmium biosorption by free and immobilized microorganisms cultivated in a liquid soil extract medium: Effects of Cd, pH, and techniques of culture. Sci Total Environ 291: 73–83.

8. Abdola M, Chmtelnicka J (1990) New aspects on the distribution and metabolism of essential trace elements after dietary exposure to toxic metals. Biol Trace Element Res 23: 25–53.

9. Yang JX, Guo HT, Ma YB, Wang LQ, Wei DP, et al. (2010) Genotypic variations in the accumulation of exhibited by different vegetables. J Environ Sci 22: 1246–1252.

10. Yang Y, Zhang FS, Li HF, Jiang RF (2009) Accumulation of cadmium in the edible parts of six vegetable species grown in Cd-contaminated soils. J Environ Manag 90: 1117–1122.

11. Chen HS, Huang QY, Liu LN, Cai P, Liang W, et al. (2010) Poultry manure compost alleviates the phytotoxicity of soil cadmium: Influence on growth of Pak choi (Brassica chinensis L.). Pedosphere 20: 63–70.

12. Wang XP, Shan XQ, Zhang SZ, Wen B (2004) A model for evaluation of the phytoavailability of trace elements to vegetables under field conditions. Chemosphere 55: 811–822.

13. Liang Z, Ding Q, Wei D, Li J, Chen S, et al. (2013) Major controlling factors and predictable equations for Cd transfer factor involved in soil-spinach system. Ecotox Environ Saf 93: 180–185.

14. Ge Y, Murray P, Hendershot WH (2000) Trace metal speciation and bioavailability in urban soils. Environ. Pollut. 107, 137–144.

15. Gu JG, Zhou QX, Wang X (2003) Reused path of heavy metal pollution in soils and its research advance. J Basic Sci Eng 11: 143–151 (in Chinese).

16. Gu JG, Zhou QX (2002) Cleaning up through phytoremediation: A review of Cd contaminated soils. Ecol Sci 21: 352–356. (in Chinese with English abstract)

17. Du TP (2005) Food safety and strategy in China. Productivity Res: 6, 139–141. (in Chinese with English abstract)

18. Franz E, Römkens P, Van Raamsdonk L, Van Der Fels-Klerx I (2008) A chain modeling approach to estimate the impact of soil cadmium pollution on human dietary exposure. J Food Protect: 71, 2504–13.

19. Kobayashi E, Suwazono Y, Dochi M, Honda R, Nishijo M, et al. (2008) Estimation of benchmark doses as threshold levels of urinary cadmium, based on excretion of β_2-microglobulin in cadmium polluted and non-polluted regions in Japan. Toxicol Lett 179: 108–12.

20. Tracy S, Sheila M (2006) Cadmium and zinc accumulation in soybean: A threat to food safety. Sci Total Environ 371: 63–73.

21. Ide G, Becker B (1995) Relationship between the arsenic concentration in soil and in the cropped vegetables. International Conference on Heavy Metal in the Environment, Hamburg, vol. 2, CEP Consultants Ltd, Norwich, UK 302–304

22. Szteke B, Jedrzejczak R (1995) The variability of heavy metal contents in plant and soil samples from fields of one farm. International Conference on Heavy Metal in the Environment, Hamburg, vol. 2, CEP Consultants Ltd., Norwich, UK 228–231.

23. Salvatore M, Carratù G, Carafa A (2009) Assessment of heavy metals transfer from a moderately polluted soil into the edible parts of vegetables. J Food Agric Environ 7: 683–688.

24. Chaturvedi R, Sankar K, (2006) Laboratory manual for the physicochemical analysis of soil, water and plant. Wildlife Institute of India, Dehradun, India.

25. Hendershot WH, Duquette M (1986) A simple barium chloride method for determining cation exchange capacity and exchangeable cations. Soil Sci Soc Am J 50: 605–608.

26. Rashid A, Ryan J, Estefan G (2001) Soil and plant analysis laboratory manual. International center for agricultural research in the dry areas (ICARDA), Aleppo, Syria.

27. Day PR (1965) Particle fractionation and particle-size analysis. In: Klute, A. (eds.), Methods of soil analysis. ASA and SSSA, Madison, WI, pp. 545–567.

28. Xiao W, Yang XE, He Z, Rafiq MT, Hou D, et al. (2013) Model for evaluation of the phytoavailability of chromium (Cr) to rice (Oryza sativa L.) in representative Chinese soils. J Agric Food Chem 61: 2925–2932.

29. Mehlich A (1984) Mehlich-3 soil test extractant a modification of Mehlich-2 extractant. Commun Soil Sci Plan 15: 1409–1416.

30. FAO/WHO (2003) Report of the sixty first meeting of Joint FAO/WHO expert committee on food additives. Rome.

31. Wang XL, Sato T, Xing BS, Tao S (2005) Health risks of heavy metals to the general public in Tianjin, China via consumption of vegetables and fish. Sci Total Environ 350: 28–37.

32. Rattan R, Datta S, Chhonkar P, Suribabu K, Singh A (2005) A Long-term impact of irrigation with sewage effluents on heavy metal content in soils, crops and groundwater: A case study. Agric Ecosyst Environ 109: 310–322.

33. Peter MC (2002) Ecological risk assessment (ERA) and hormesis. Sci Total Environ 288: 131–140.

34. Liu X, Peng K, Wang A, Lian CL, Shen ZG (2010) Cadmium accumulation and distribution in populations of Phytolacca Americana L. and the role of transpiration. Chemosphere 78: 1136–1141.

35. Peter N, Karoly B, Laszlo G (2003) Characterization of the stimulating effect of low-dose stressors in maize and bean seedlings. J Plant Physiol 160: 1175–1183.

36. Kaminek M (1992) Progress in cytokinin research. TIBTECH 10: 159–162.

37. Ali B, Tao QJ, Zhou YF, Gill RA, Ali S, et al. (2013) 5-aminolevolinic acid mitigates the cadmium-induced changes in Brassica napus as revealed by the biochemical and ultra-structural evaluation of roots. Ecotox Environ Safe 92: 271–280.

38. Ali B, Wang B, Ali S, Ghani MA, Hayat MT, et al. (2013) 5-Aminolevulinic acid ameliorates the growth, photosynthetic gas exchange capacity and ultrastructural changes under cadmium stress in Brassica napus L. J Plant Growth Regul 32: 604–614.

39. Moya JL, Ros R, Picazo I (1993) Influence of cadmium and nickel on growth, net photosynthesis and carbohydrate distribution in rice plants. Photosyn Res 36: 75–80.

40. Weitao L, Zhou Q, Ana J Suna Y, Liu R (2010) Variations in cadmium accumulation among Chinese cabbage cultivars and screening for Cd-safe cultivars. J Hazard Mater 173: 737–743.

41. Lai HY, Chen BC (2013) The dynamic growth exhibition and accumulation of cadmium of Pak choi (Brassica campestris L. ssp. chinensis) grown in contaminated soils. Int J Environ Res Public Health 10: 5284–5298.

42. Cui YJ, Zhu YG, Smith SA, Smith SE (2004) Cadmium uptake by different rice genotypes that produce white or dark grains. J Environ Sci 16: 962–967.

43. Xiao W, Yang XE, Zhang Y, Rafiq MT, He Z, et al. (2013) Accumulation of chromium in Pak choi (Brassica chinensis L.) grown on representative Chinese soils. J Environ Qual 42: 758–765.

44. De Villiers S, Thiart C, Basson NC (2010) Identification of sources of environmental lead in South Africa from surface soil geochemical maps. Environ Geochem Health 32: 451–459.

45. Kabata-Pendias A, Pendias H (2001) Trace Elements in Soils and Plants. Boca Raton, FloridaCRC Press.

46. Laura W, Wander M, Phillips E (2011) Testing and educating on urban soil lead: A case of Chicago community gardens. J Agric Food Sys Comm Develop, ISSN: 2152–0801 online.

47. Rafiq MT, Aziz R, Yang XE, Wendan X, Rafiq MK, et al. (2014) Cadmium phytoavailability to rice (Oryza sativa L.) grown in representative Chinese soils. A model to improve soil environmental quality guidelines for food safety. Ecotox Environ Safe 103:101–107.

48. Murakami M, Nakagawa F, Ae N, Ito M, Arao T (2009) Phytoextraction by rice capable of accumulating Cd at high levels: Reduction of Cd content of rice grain. Environ Sci Technol 43: 5878–5883.

49. Jung MC, Thornton I (1996) Heavy metal contamination of soils and plants in the vicinity of a lead-zinc mine, Korea. Appl Geochem 11: 53–59.

50. McBride M (2002) Cadmium uptake by crops estimated from soil total Cd and pH. Soil Sci 15: 84–92.

51. Eriksson JE, Sderstrom M (1996) Cadmium in soil and winter wheat grain in southern Sweden. Factors influencing Cd levels in soils and grain. Acta Agric Scand Sect B 46: 240–248.

52. Romkens PFAM, Guo HY, Chu CL, Liu TS, Chiang CF, et al. (2009) Prediction of cadmium uptake by brown rice and derivation of soil-plant transfer models to improve soil protection guidelines. Environ Pollut 157: 2435–2444.

53. Giordano PM, Mays DA, Behel AD (1979) Soil temperature effects on the uptake of cadmium and zinc by vegetables grown on sludge amended soil. J Environ Qual 8: 232–236.

54. Oliver DP, Hannam R, Tiller KG, Wilhelm NS, Merry RH, et al. (1994) The effects of zinc fertilization on cadmium concentration in wheat grain. J Environ Qual 23: 705–711.

55. McCauley A, Jones C, Jacobsen J (2009) Soil pH and Organic Matter. Nutrient management modules 8, #4449-8. Montana State University Extension Service, Bozeman, Montana, pp. 1–12.

56. Liu LN, Chen HS, Cai P, Liang W, Huang QY (2009) Immobilization and phytotoxicity of Cd in contaminated soil amended with chicken manure compost. J Hazard Mater 163: 563–567.

57. Halim M, Conte P, Piccolo A (2003) Potential availability of heavy metals to phytoextraction from contaminated soils induced by exogenous humic substances. Chemosphere 52: 265–275.

13

Risk of Deaths, AIDS-Defining and Non-AIDS Defining Events among Ghanaians on Long-Term Combination Antiretroviral Therapy

Fred Stephen Sarfo[1,2]*, Maame Anima Sarfo[1], Betty Norman[1], Richard Phillips[1,2], George Bedu-Addo[1,2], David Chadwick[3]

1 Komfo Anokye Teaching Hospital, Kumasi, Ghana, **2** Kwame Nkrumah University of Science and Technology, Kumasi, Ghana, **3** The James Cook University Hospital, Middlesbrough, United Kingdom

Abstract

Combination antiretroviral therapy (cART) has been widely available in Ghana since 2004. The aim of this cohort study was to assess the incidences of death, AIDS-defining events and non-AIDS defining events and associated risk factors amongst patients initiating cART in a large treatment centre. Clinical and laboratory data were extracted from clinic and hospital case notes for patients initiating cART between 2004 and 2010 and clinical events graded according to recognised definitions for AIDS, non-AIDS events (NADE) and death, with additional events not included in such definitions such as malaria also included. The cumulative incidence of events was calculated using Kaplan Meier analysis, and association of risk factors with events by Cox proportional hazards regression. Data were closed for analysis on 31st December, 2011 after a median follow-up of 30 months (range, 0–90 months). Amongst 4,039 patients starting cART at a median CD4 count of 133 cells/mm^3, there were 324 (8%) confirmed deaths, with an event rate of 28.83 (95% CI 25.78–32.15) deaths per 1000-person follow-up years; the commonest established causes were pulmonary TB and gastroenteritis. There were 681 AIDS-defining events (60.60 [56.14–65.33] per 1000 person years) with pulmonary TB and chronic diarrhoea being the most frequent causes. Forty-one NADEs were recorded (3.64 [2.61–4.95] per 1000 person years), of which hepatic and cardiovascular events were most common. Other common events recorded outside these definitions included malaria (746 events) and respiratory tract infections (666 events). Overall 24% of patients were lost-to-follow-up. Alongside expected risk factors, stavudine use was associated with AIDS [adjusted HR of 1.08 (0.90–1.30)] and death (adjusted HR of 1.60 [1.21–2.11]). Whilst frequency of AIDS and deaths in this cohort were similar to those described in other sub-Saharan African cohorts, rates of NADEs were lower and far exceeded by events such as malaria and respiratory tract infections.

Editor: Sarah L. Pett, Faculty of Medicine, Australia

Funding: Funding for setting up the database was provided by the HIV Research Trust, UK. The funder had no role in study design, data collection and analysis, decision to publish, or preparation of the manuscript.

Competing Interests: The authors have declared that no competing interests exist.

* Email: stephensarfo78@gmail.com

Introduction

Combination anti-retroviral therapy (cART) for the long-term management of HIV infection is administered to achieve long-term suppression of virological replication and to maintain CD4 cell counts at a level that reduces the risk of morbidity and mortality. It is encouraging that the effectiveness of cART in developing countries in sub-Saharan Africa has been reported to be similar, and often superior in clinical and immunologic outcomes when compared with those from the developed countries [1–8]. Evidence of the sustainability of these initially favourable immunological and clinical responses is beginning to emerge.

Deaths in the era of cART have largely been due to AIDS-defining clinical events in many such reports from developing countries. But the dynamics of mortality is believed to be changing

in industrialised countries with non-AIDS defining clinical events assuming greater importance as causes of death as patients live longer on potent cART [9–11]. Non-AIDS defining events are classified as cardiovascular, renal, hepatic-related or non-AIDS-defining malignancies that are likely to have an impact on morbidity and mortality [12]. One report from Botswana indicated that the age-standardised incidence rates of non-AIDS defining events were comparable to those in the United States [13]. However, the spectra of disease entities included in this definition is debated [14,15] and does not capture infectious diseases such as malaria which is a common cause of morbidity among patients in sub-Saharan Africa.

Ghana like many other countries in sub-Saharan Africa started cART roll-out in 2004. We have recently published a comparative analysis of the effectiveness and tolerability of nevirapine and efavirenz based cART among a large cohort of Ghanaian HIV-infected patients [16]. The aim of this study is to present a comprehensive analysis of the incidence, causes and risk factors associated with AIDS, non-AIDS clinical events, immunological failure, immune reconstitution inflammatory syndrome, treatment-limiting toxicity, and mortality over the long-term in this Ghanaian cohort.

Methods

Ethical permission for this study was given by the Committee on Human Research Publications and Ethics of the Kwame Nkrumah University of Science and Technology and the Komfo Anokye Teaching Hospital, Kumasi, Ghana (ref: CHRPE/AP/073/13). Our institutional review board waived the need for a written informed consent since this was a retrospective, observational study and anonymised data were collected from patients' records. The study was conducted at the HIV clinic at the Komfo Anokye Teaching Hospital in Kumasi, Ghana, which provides HIV care to a large rural and urban population across central and northern Ghana. Antiretroviral therapy has been administered to patients meeting eligibility criteria since 2004 as has been previously described [16]. Data were extracted from the notes of patients starting ART between January 2004 and December 2010 and was closed for analysis by an intention-to-treat basis on 31st December 2011. For this analysis, AIDS-defining events, non-AIDS defining clinical events, immune reconstitution inflammatory syndrome, loss-to-follow up, death and adherence to therapy were defined as follows. An AIDS-defining clinical event was defined as the occurrence of any opportunistic infections or malignancy according the World Health Organisation (WHO) [17] criteria while the patient was on cART.

The diagnosis of a non-AIDS clinical event was adjudicated by consensus between FSS, BN and RP (BN and RP are Consultants in HIV Medicine at the Komfo Anokye Teaching Hospital). The conditions classified under NADEs included cerebrovascular accident (stroke), cerebral/sub-arachnoid hemorrhage, myocardial infarction, coronary artery disease, congestive cardiac failure, end-stage renal disease, renal failure, cirrhosis of the liver, esophageal varices, hepatic failure, hepatic coma, hepatic encephalopathy, intestinal adenocarcinoma/lymphoma, penile carcinoma, small cell lung carcinoma, malignant melanoma, hepatocellular carcinoma, squamous cell carcinoma, and squamous cell carcinoma of the anus as previously described [14,15]. Severity of specific NADEs in particular liver injury and renal failure were assessed using established Division of AIDS (DAIDS) tables for Grading Severity of Adult Adverse Experiences (NADEs).

Other medical diagnoses that did not fulfil the criteria for AIDS-defining events or serious NADEs were recorded and presented as "medical co-morbidities on cART". These included conditions such as malaria, urinary tract infections, new onset diabetes mellitus or hypertension.

In the present study immune reconstitution inflammatory syndrome (IRIS) was defined as the paradoxical worsening of a previously treated opportunistic infection [18] for which the clinician was able to demonstrate radiological evidence of exacerbation in the cases of tuberculosis or cerebral toxoplasmosis, and fundoscopic evidence of vitreous inflammation in the case of CMV retinitis. Cases of herpes zoster IRIS were defined clinically. Due to the inherent difficulty of differentiating an opportunistic infection with normal presentation and a disorder with presentation that is compatible with unmasking IRIS in our setting, the unmasking type of IRIS was not documented in charts in this cohort. Immunological failure was defined using WHO criteria as

either the return of CD4 counts to pre-therapy baseline, or below and/or more than 50% fall from on-therapy CD4 peak-level (and/or more than 50% fall in CD4), or persistent low CD4 of less than 100 cells/μl after one year of therapy without other concomitant infection to explain the low CD4. Loss to follow up was defined as missing a clinic appointment by at least 3 months of the last scheduled visit to clinic. Death was defined as the demise of a patient from causes related to HIV/AIDS or from toxicity from antiretrovirals or other non-AIDS related causes if known. Confirmation of death was by death certification by medical doctors for patients who died on the wards or by patients' family for those who died outside the hospital. Patient adherence, assessed by pill count, was classified as excellent at each clinic visit if adherence level of ≥95% was achieved. Poor adherence was defined as any documented evidence of <95% of adherence during follow up.

Statistical analysis

Parametric and non-parametric methods were used to compare baseline characteristics of continuous data between patients started on either efavirenz, nevirapine or a protease inhibitor-based ART. A 1-way analysis of variance (ANOVA) or Kruskal-Wallis test was used to compare means or medians respectively. Comparisons of dichotomous data were performed using χ^2 or Fisher's exact test. Crude incidence rates of events were calculated in person-years of follow-up with 95% confidence intervals calculated using Normal approximation to the Poisson distribution. Risk factors associated with death and AIDS-defining events were assessed using multivariable Cox proportional hazards regression with factors attaining a significance level of <0.10 in univariate analyses included in the final model. For these survival analyses, the month in which patients started cART was set as month zero and one day of follow-up was added to patients who did not attend any follow-up visits after initiating therapy. Time to events of interest, namely AIDS-defining events, loss-to-follow up or mortality, was calculated by subtracting the date of the event from the date on which the patient was started on cART. Patients were censored at December 31, 2011 if there were no event of interest. Explanatory variables included in survival analyses were selected on the basis of their well-recognised impact on clinical outcomes such as AIDS-defining events, loss-to-follow up and deaths. The cumulative incidence of loss to follow up and deaths were calculated using the Kaplan Meier methodology. For all analysis, a 2-sided p-value <0.05 was set as the level of statistical significance. All data analyses were conducted using SPSS version 19.

Results

Baseline demographics and laboratory characteristics of study participants

Four thousand and thirty-nine (4,039) patients out of 10,500 (38.5%) patients registered between January 2004 and December 2010 initiated first line therapy. There was a female preponderance in a ratio of 2.1: 1.0 with a median age of patients of 38 years (range of 14–78). As shown in Table 1, 2,376 (58.8%) patients were started on efavirenz based cART compared with 1,623 (40.2%) on nevirapine based cART while 40 (1.0%) were initiated on protease inhibitor based cART because they had HIV-2 mono-infection or HIV-1/2 dual infection: 23 on ritonavir-boosted lopinavir and 17 on nelfinavir. 52.1% were started on an NRTI backbone of stavudine (d4T) and lamivudine (3TC) while 47.7%

Table 1. Baseline demographic, clinical and laboratory characteristics of patients initiating cART.

Characteristic	Efavirenz n = 2,376	Nevirapine n = 1,623	Protease inhibitors n = 40	Total n = 4,039	p-value
Male: female	1,028: 1,348	248: 1,375	11: 29	1,287: 2,752	<0.0001
Median (range) age	40 (14–77)	35 (15–75)	36 (25–65)	38 (14–77)	<0.0001
WHO clinical stage n (%)					0.09
1	165 (6.9)	106 (6.5)	2 (5.0)	273 (6.8)	
2	258 (10.9)	225 (13.9)	6 (15.0)	489 (12.1)	
3	1274 (53.6)	867 (53.4)	25 (62.5)	2166 (53.6)	
4	407 (17.1)	238 (14.7)	10 (10.0)	649 (16.1)	
No data	272 (11.4)	187 (11.5)	3 (7.5)	462 (11.4)	
Mean BMI ± SEM	20.1±0.09	20.5±0.10	21.0±0.62	20.3±0.07	0.0025
BMI categories					
<18.5 kg/m^2	868 (36.5)	543 (33.5)	11 (27.5)	1422 (35.2)	0.0047
18.5–24.5 kg/m^2	1145 (48.2)	804 (49.5)	20 (50.0)	1969 (48.8)	
>24.5 kg/m^2	291 (12.3)	246 (15.2)	6 (15.0)	543 (13.4)	
No data	72 (3.0)	30 (1.8)	3 (7.5)	105 (2.6)	
CD4 count Median (range)	127.5 (1–1085)	140.0 (0–676)	186.0 (1–1134)	134 (0–1134)	0.0006
CD4 categories					
<200 cells/ml	1684 (70.9)	1080 (66.5)	21 (52.5)	2785 (69.0)	<0.0001
200–350 cells/ml	611 (25.7)	495 (30.5)	12 (30.0)	1118 (27.7)	
>350 cells/ml	53 (2.2)	41 (2.5)	7 (17.5)	101 (2.5)	
No data	28 (1.2)	7 (0.5)	0 (0.0)	35 (0.9)	
Median (range) Hemoglobin (g/dl)	10.2 (2.6–19.4)	10.2 (3.2–19.8)	10.9 (6.8–16.3)	10.2 (2.6–19.8)	0.07
Mean ± SEM ALT (U/L)	40.5±0.87	32.0±0.75	39.3±6.64	37.1±0.60	<0.0001
Mean ± SEM AST (U/L)	53.6±0.93	45.2±0.95	51.0±11.6	50.2±0.68	<0.0001
eGFR (ml/min/1.73m^2) Median (IQR), n	64.0 (47.0–83.0) n = 1791	71.0 (54.0–89.0) n = 1240	66.5 (54.5–89.5) n = 32	66.0 (50.0–86.0) n = 3063	<0.0001
eGFR categories					
>60ml/min	1028 (57.4)	849 (68.5)	21 (65.6)	1898 (62.0)	<0.0001
30–59 ml/min	638 (35.6)	345 (27.8)	11 (34.4)	994 (32.5)	
15–29 ml/min	92 (5.1)	35 (2.8)	0 (0.0)	127 (4.1)	
<15ml/min	33 (1.8)	11 (0.9)	0 (0.0)	44 (1.4)	
HBV co-infection Positive/Negative (%)	143/761 15.8%	87/527 14.2%	3/13 18.8%	233/1301 15.2%	>0.05
NRTI backbone					
AZT +3TC	1083 (45.6)	819 (50.5)	23 (57.5)	1925 (47.7)	<0.0001
D4T +3TC	1286 (54.1)	804 (49.5)	13 (32.5)	2103 (52.1)	
Others	7 (0.3)		4 (10.0)	11 (0.2)	

BMI-Body Mass Index; ALT-Alanine transaminitis; AST- Aspartate transaminitis; eGFR- estimated glomerular filtration rate calculated using Cockroft Gault formula; AZT-zidovudine; 3TC- Lamivudine; d4T- stavudine.

were initiated on zidovudine (AZT) plus 3TC with 0.2% commencing other NRTIs.

The characteristics of patients enrolled in the clinic for care, proportion initiating cART, their WHO clinical stages, median CD4 counts and vital status for each calendar year from 2004 to 2010 are shown in Table 2. Overall, the median (IQR) follow-up time on cART for the cohort was 30 (12–54) months. There were 11,236.8 person years of follow up on cART with 2,748 patients (68%) still alive, 967 (24%) lost to follow up and 324 (8%) deaths at the time of closing data for the present analysis.

Immunological responses/events on cART

Changes in CD4 counts with cART. The median (IQR) CD4 count at baseline of 133 (50–218) increased to 314 (204–429) within 6 months of initiation of cART, p<0.0001. This initial increment was sustained at 12 months with a median (IQR) CD4 at 12 months of 355 (244–487), with further increases during follow up to month 90.

Immune reconstitution inflammatory disorders. There were 45 documented cases of IRIS with an overall incidence rate of 4.00 (2.92–5.36) events/1000 person years under follow up. Tuberculosis-associated IRIS was the commonest and manifested clinically as new pulmonary infiltrations (n = 16), lymphadenitis

Table 2. Enrolment, characteristics, follow-up and vital status of patients initiating cART according to calendar year of enrolment.

Year Characteristic	2004	2005	2006	2007	2008	2009	2010	TOTAL	p-value
No. enrolled for ART	1,700	2,020	1,819	1,782	1,738	636	705	10,400	
No. starting ART	769	695	819	658	590	272	236	4039	
% starting ART	45.2	34.4	45.0	36.9	33.9	42.8	33.5	38.8	
WHO Clinical stage, n (%)§									<0.0001
1	52 (7%)	33 (5%)	43 (5%)	47 (7%)	53 (9%)	28 (10%)	16 (7%)	273 (7%)	
2	109 (14%)	80 (12%)	113 (14%)	70 (11%)	63 (11%)	25 (9%)	29 (12%)	489 (12%)	
3	460 (60%)	402 (58%)	420 (51%)	355 (54%)	280 (47%)	134 (49%)	115 (49%)	2166 (54%)	
4	126 (16%)	121 (17%)	145 (18%)	98 (15%)	80 (14%)	38 (14%)	41 (17%)	649 (16%)	
No data	22 (3%)	59 (8%)	98 (12%)	88 (13%)	114 (19%)	47 (16%)	35 (15%)	452 (11%)	
Median (IQR) CD4 count	136 (51–213)	136 (65–211)	133 (51–212)	124 (33–220)	131 (48–228)	128 (41–251)	149 (57–231)	134 (51–218)	0.23
Vital status									<0.0001
Alive*	503 (65%)	426 (61%)	541 (66%)	467 (71%)	438 (74%)	186 (68%)	187 (79%)	2748 (68%)	
Dead	35 (5%)	40 (6%)	50 (6%)	104 (16%)	63 (11%)	14 (5%)	18 (8%)	324 (8%)	
Lost	231 (30%)	229 (33%)	228 (28%)	87 (13%)	89 (15%)	72 (27%)	31 (13%)	967 (24%)	
Person follow up years	3565.1	2531.8	2158.7	1393.8	936.4	455.2	195.8	11236.8	

* And accessing the clinic, § % of patients initiating cART.

Table 3. Frequencies and rates of Non-AIDS defining events (NADEs) and other medical disorders not meeting AIDS-defining or NADEs criteria.

NADEs events	Number of events	Proportion of patients in entire cohort with event (%), n = 4,039	Rate/1000 person years follow up (95% CI)
Hepatic disorders			
Chronic liver disease	13	0.3	1.16 (0.62–1.98)
Hepatitis B virus infection flares*	7	0.2	0.62 (0.25–1.28)
Cardiovascular events			
Stroke	8	0.2	0.71 (0.31–1.40)
Congestive cardiac failure	2	0.1	0.18 (0.02–0.64)
Renal disorders			
Stage 4 or 5 renal impairment	6	0.2	0.53 (0.19–1.16)
Non-AIDS malignancies			
Hepatocellular carcinoma	4	0.1	0.36 (0.10–0.91)
Oesophageal carcinoma	1	0.0	0.09 (0.00–0.05)
Total	41	1.0	3.64 (2.61–4.95)
Medical disorders not meeting NADEs Non-AIDS defining infectious disorders			
Malaria	746	18.5	66.39 (61.71–71.32)
Upper and lower respiratory infections	666	16.5	59.27 (54.85–63.95)
Dermatological infections	364	9.0	32.39 (29.15–35.90)
Gastroenteritis	314	7.7	27.94 (24.94–31.21)
Urinary tract infections	151	3.7	13.43 (11.38–15.76)
Ear nose and throat infections	102	2.5	9.08 (7.40–11.02)
Sepsis	29	0.7	2.58 (1.73–3.71)
Bacterial meningitis	5	0.1	0.45 (0.17–1.01)
Miscellaneous disorders			
Dyspeptic disorders	73	1.8	6.50 (5.09–8.17)
Post-herpetic neuralgia	52	1.3	4.63 (3.46–6.07)
Seizure disorders	24	0.6	2.14 (1.37–3.18)
Paraparesis (unknown cause)	10	0.3	0.88 (0.43–1.64)
Hemiparesis (unknown cause)	9	0.2	0.80 (0.37–1.52)
Monoparesis (unknown cause)	6	0.1	0.53 (0.19–1.16)
Proximal myopathy	3	0.1	0.27 (0.06–0.78)
New onset vascular risk factors			
Hypertension	94	2.3	8.36 (6.76–10.24)
Diabetes mellitus	9	0.2	0.80 (0.37–1.52)

* HBV flare was defined as an elevation of ALT >5X upper limit of normal in a patient with HBSAg sero-positivity.

(n = 2) and pleural effusions (n = 2) over a median of 2 months (range: 2 to 12 months). Others included herpes zoster (n = 13), cerebral toxoplasmosis (n = 9), CMV retinitis (n = 2) and crypto-coccal meningitis (n = 1). The median age of patients experiencing IRIS was 38 years, 33 (73%) were females and the median CD4 count at initiation of cART was 73 (range, 2 to 314) cells/mm^3. At the close of data for analysis, 27 (60%) patients who developed IRIS were alive, 6 (13%) patients died and 12 (27%) were lost-to-follow up.

Incidence and risk factors for immunological failure. Although robust CD4 recovery was noted among most patients on cART, there were 407 immunological failures with a crude event rate of 3.62 (3.28–3.99) per 100 person years. The median (range) time to occurrence of immunological failure on first line cART was 24 (12–78) months. Factors significantly

associated with the risk of immunological failure on multivariable Cox proportional hazards analysis were male sex with an adjusted HR of 1.85 (95% CI of 1.47–2.33), initiating cART below 40 years of age with an adjusted HR of 1.25 (1.01–1.55) and baseline CD4 strata below 200 cells/mm^3 with an adjusted HR of 3.62 (95% CI of 2.59–5.07).

Clinical events on cART

Non-AIDS defining clinical events. There were 41 NADEs with the commonest recorded events being hepatic disorders (n = 20), cardiovascular events (n = 10) and new onset severe renal impairment with eGFR below 30ml/min (n = 6); hepatocellular carcinoma (n = 4) and oesophageal carcinoma (n = 1) were the only non-AIDS defining malignancies. The hepatic disorders noted include liver cirrhosis, hepatitis B transaminitis flares and

Table 4. Frequencies and rates of AIDS-defining conditions.

Condition	Frequency of events n (%) n = 681	Proportion of patients in entire cohort with event (%), n = 4,039	Rate/1000 person years follow up (95% CI)
Pulmonary tuberculosis	179 (26.3)	4.4	15.93 (13.68–18.44)
Chronic diarrhoea	155 (22.8)	3.8	13.79 (11.71–16.14)
Esophageal candidiasis	75 (11.0)	1.9	6.67 (5.25–8.36)
Recurrent pneumonia	58 (8.5)	1.4	5.16 (3.92–6.67)
Oral candidiasis	45 (6.6)	1.1	4.00 (2.92–5.36)
Cerebral toxoplasmosis	38 (5.6)	0.9	3.38 (2.39–4.64)
Extrapulmonary tuberculosis	33 (4.8)	0.8	2.94 (2.02–4.12)
Kaposi sarcoma	31 (4.6)	0.8	2.76 (1.87–3.92)
CMV retinitis	17 (2.5)	0.4	1.51 (0.88–2.42)
HIV encephalopathy	16 (2.5)	0.4	1.42 (0.81–2.31)
Cryptococcal meningitis	12 (1.8)	0.3	1.07 (0.55–1.87)
Intracranial space occupying lesion*	9 (1.3)	0.2	0.80 (0.37–1.52)
Non-Hodgkin's disease	5 (0.7)	0.1	0.44 (0.14–1.04)
HIV wasting syndrome	3 (0.4)	0.1	0.27 (0.05–0.78)
Pneumocystis jirovercii pneumonia	2 (0.3)	0.0	0.18 (0.02–0.64)
CNS lymphoma	1 (0.1)	0.0	0.09 (0.00–0.50)
Herpes esophagitis	1 (0.1)	0.0	0.09 (0.00–0.50)
Invasive cervical carcinoma	1 (0.1)	0.0	0.09 (0.00–0.50)
Total	**681**		**60.60 (56.14–65.33)**

AIDS defining events were defined using WHO clinical criteria. * Causes of Intracranial space occupying lesion on CT scan were not documented but were presumed to be AIDS-defining events.

hepatocellular carcinoma which were all observed in patients with HBsAg sero-positivity. The overall crude NADE incidence rate (95% CI) was 3.64 (2.61–4.95) per 1000 person years as shown in Table 3.

By far, the commonest medical morbidity (not fulfilling AIDS nor NADEs criteria) was from infectious causes of which 2,377 events were documented (Table 3), with malaria being the commonest event. This is followed briefly by upper/lower respiratory tract infections (n = 666). Of the non-infectious medical comorbidities recorded, 94 patients developed hypertension and 9 Type 2 diabetes mellitus while on cART.

Causes and factors associated with AIDS-defining events on cART. Six hundred (600) patients (14.9%) experienced a total of 681 AIDS-defining events during follow up on cART with a crude (95% CI) event rate of 60.60 (56.14–65.33) per 1000 person years of follow up (Table 4). The median (range) time to development of first AIDS-defining event was 6 (2–90) months. Nine patients were documented to have had computed tomographic evidence of an intracranial space occupying lesions, but clinicians did not document the etiology of these mass lesions. For the purposes of the present study, they were judged to be AIDS-defining events. Factors significantly associated with the risk of developing an AIDS-defining event on cART on adjusted analyses were low body mass index below 16 kg/m^2, WHO clinical stages 3 or 4 at baseline and CD4 strata below 200 cells/mm^3 at initiation of therapy (Table 5).

Of the 600 patients who developed AIDS-defining events on cART, 317 (52.8%) were alive as at time of closure of data but 153 (25.5%) were subsequently lost-to-follow up and 130 (21.7%) died of AIDS. The median (range) duration between the first AIDS-defining diagnosis and death was 0.25 months (0 to 72 months) and that for loss-to-follow up was 4 months (0 to 76 months). Patients who developed an AIDS-defining event and were alive at the time of closure of data for analysis survived for a median of 34 months (range of 0 to 88 months).

The incidence, causes and risk factors associated with mortality

There were 324 (8.0%) deaths over the 11,263.8 person follow-up years giving a crude (95% CI) event rate of 28.83 (25.78–32.15) deaths per 1000-person follow up years. The median (range) time to death was 2 months (0–66) by Mann Whitney's U-test. 202 (62.3%) deaths occurred within the first 90-days of initiation of therapy, 88 (27.2%) from month 4 to month 12, 16 (4.9%) within the second year, 9 (2.8%) within the third year, 3 (0.9%) within the fourth year and 6 (1.9%) within the fifth year of follow up. The Kaplan Meier estimated cumulative incidence of mortality at 6, 12, 36, and 72 months were 6.8%, 7.9%, 9.0% and 9.8% respectively and of attrition (including 324 deaths and 958 loss-to-follow ups) from the programme were 17.3%, 20.7%, 27.8%, 34.5% and 36.5% respectively.

As shown in Table 6, significant factors associated with mortality in Cox proportional hazards model were male gender with an adjusted HR (95% CI) of 1.69 (1.29–2.21), advanced HIV disease – Stages 3 or 4 – with an adjusted HR (95% CI) of 2.20 (1.42–3.41), low CD4 strata below 200 cells/mm^3 with an adjusted HR (95% CI) of 2.39 (1.64–3.49), baseline BMI below 16 kg/m^2 with an adjusted HR (95% CI) of 2.60 (1.92–3.53) and starting on an NRTI backbone of d4T plus 3TC with an adjusted HR of 1.60 (1.21–2.11).

Table 5. Univariate and multivariate analysis of factors associated with risk of developing AIDS on cART.

Variable	Person follow-up time (yrs)	Number of events	Crude event rate (/1000 py), 95% CI	Unadjusted HR (95% CI)	p-value	Adjusted HR (95% CI)	p-value
Sex					0.53		–
Male	3467	193	55.67 (48.09–64.10)	1.06 (0.89–1.25)		–	
Female	7770	406	52.25 (47.29–57.59)	1.00		–	
Age					0.90		–
≥40 years	5161	268	51.93 (45.90–58.53)	1.00 (0.94–1.07)		–	
<40 years	6082	331	54.42 (48.72–60.61)	1.00		–	
WHO stage					<0.0001		0.0031
3 or 4	7803	477	61.13 (55.77–66.87)	1.73 (1.37–2.18)		1.45 (1.13–1.86)	
1 or 2	2370	84	35.44 (28.27–43.88)	1.00		1.00	
Baseline CD4 strata					<0.0001		<0.0001
<200	7706	481	62.42 (56.96–68.25)	2.00 (1.64–2.45)		1.87 (1.49–2.35)	
>200	3462	117	33.80 (27.95–40.50)	1.00		1.00	
Baseline BMI					<0.0001		0.0005
<16 kg/m^2	901	99	109.9 (89.3–133.8)	1.91 (1.54–2.38)		1.53 (1.20–1.94)	
≥16 kg/m^2	9189	483	52.56 (47.98–57.47)	1.00		1.00	
Baseline Hb					0.06		0.94
<8g/dl	1176	87	73.98 (59.25–91.25)	0.92 (0.83–1.01)		1.01 (0.78–1.31)	
≥8g/dl	8590	494	57.51 (52.55–62.81)	1.00		1.00	
NRTI backbone					0.04		0.09
D4T plus 3TC	5276	322	61.03 (54.55–68.07)	1.18 (1.01–1.39)		1.08 (0.90–1.30)	
AZT plus 3TC	5940	274	46.13 (40.83–51.93)	1.00		1.00	
NNRTI					0.29		–
Efavirenz	6120	330	53.92 (48.26–60.06)	0.92 (0.78–1.08)		–	
Nevirapine	5013	261	52.06 (45.94–58.78)	1.00		1.00	
Adherence					0.06		0.51
Poor	3835	237	61.80 (54.18–70.18)	1.17 (0.99–1.38)		1.06 (0.89–1.27)	
Excellent	6345	363	57.21 (51.48–63.41)	1.00		1.00	

Table 6. Univariate and multivariate analysis of factors associated with death on cART.

Variable	Patient follow-up time (years)	Number of events	Crude event rate (/1000 person years)	Unadjusted HR (95% CI)	p-value	Adjusted hazard ratio (95% CI)	p-value
Sex							
Male	3467	188	54.23 (46.75–62.56)	1.71 (1.37–2.14)	<0.0001	1.69 (1.29–2.21)	0.0001
Female	7770	136	17.50 (14.69–20.70)	1.00		1.00	
Age							
≥40 years	5161	143	27.71 (23.35–32.64)	0.94 (0.75–1.17)	0.55	–	–
<40 years	6082	180	29.60 (25.43–34.25)	1.00			
WHO stage							
3 or 4	7803	277	35.50 (31.44–39.94)	3.52 (2.34–5.30)	<0.0001	2.20 (1.42–3.41)	0.0004
1 or 2	2370	25	10.55 (6.82–15.57)	1.00		1.00	
Baseline CD4 strata							
<200	7706	276	35.81 (31.72–40.30)	3.13 (2.29–4.29)	<0.0001	2.39 (1.64–3.49)	<0.0001
>200	3462	45	13.00 (9.48–17.39)	1.00		1.00	
Baseline BMI							
<16 kg/m^2	901	88	97.67 (78.33–120.33)	3.79 (2.95–4.85)	<0.0001	2.60 (1.92–3.53)	<0.0001
≥16 kg/m^2	9189	214	23.29 (20.27–26.63)	1.00		1.00	
Baseline Hb							
<8g/dl	1176	76	64.63 (50.92–80.89)	2.43 (1.88–3.16)	<0.0001	1.28 (0.95–1.75)	0.11
≥8g/dl	8590	227	26.43 (23.10–30.10)	1.00		1.00	
NRTI backbone							
D4T plus 3TC	5276	216	40.94 (35.66–46.78)	2.04 (1.62–2.58)	<0.0001	1.60 (1.21–2.11)	0.001
AZT plus 3TC	5940	106	17.85 (14.61–21.58)	1.00		1.00	
NNRTI							
Efavirenz	6120	212	34.64 (30.13–39.63)	1.43 (1.14–1.81)	0.0024	1.15 (0.87–1.51)	0.32
Nevirapine	5013	108	21.54 (17.67–26.01)	1.00		1.00	
Adherence							
Poor	3835	147	38.33 (32.39–45.05)	1.52 (1.22–1.89)	0.0002	1.21 (0.95–1.56)	0.12
Excellent	6345	177	27.90 (23.94–32.32)	1.00		1.00	

Table 7. Causes of death among 188 patients who died in hospital while on first line cART.

Cause of death	Frequency
Pulmonary tuberculosis	37
Gastroenteritis with hypovolemic shock	30
Severe anemia	19
Pneumonia	18
Sepsis	16
Cerebral toxoplasmosis	12
HIV Encephalopathy	7
TB Immune reconstitution inflammatory syndrome	7
Disseminated Kaposi sarcoma	6
Enteric fever	4
End stage kidney failure	4
Lactic acidosis	4
Bacterial meningitis	4
Chronic liver disease	2
Cryptococcal meningitis	2
Steven's Johnsons syndrome due to nevirapine	2
Miscellaneous*	14
TOTAL	188

* Miscellaneous comprises of 1 case each of acute abdomen, amoebic liver abscess, CNS lymphoma, gluteal abscess, hepatocellular carcinoma, HBV flare, high grade non-Hodgkin's lymphoma, hyperglycemic hyperosmolar syndrome, strangulated umbilical hernia, otitis media, *Pneumocystis jirovercii* pneumonia, systemic candidiasis, tuberculous colitis, fulminant vasculitis with gangrene of toes and fingers.

Table 8. Frequencies of specific toxicities and treatment switches among Ghanaian cohort on long-term cART.

Toxicity	Frequency of toxicity among patients who developed any toxicity on ART n (%), n = 1,603	Proportion of patients who developed toxicity n (%)§ n = 4,039	Frequency of treatment switches due to specific toxicity# n (%)	Proportion of patients with treatment switch due to toxicity, (%) n = 4,039
Anemia	675 (42.1)	527 (13.0)	62 (11.8)	1.5
Skin rash	295 (18.4)	281 (7.0)	44 (15.7)	1.1
Neuropsychiatric toxicity	235 (14.7)	218 (5.4)	39 (17.9)	1.1
Peripheral neuropathy	181 (11.3)	181 (4.5)	83 (45.9)	2.1
Severe hepatotoxicity	143 (8.9)	143 (3.5)	8 (5.6)	0.2
Lipoatrophy	40 (2.5)	40 (1.0)	34 (85.0)	0.8
Ptylism	14 (0.9)	14 (0.3)	0 (0.0)	0.0
Gastrointestinal disorders	12 (0.7)	12 (0.3)	0 (0.0)	0.0
Lactic acidosis	4 (0.2)	4 (0.1)	0 (0.0)	0.0
Myalgia	3 (0.2)	3 (0.1)	0 (0.0)	0.0
Hyperpigmentation	3 (0.2)	3 (0.1)	0 (0.0)	0.0
Pancreatitis	1 (0.1)	1 (0.0)	1 (100.0)	0.0
Column total	1,603	1,427 (35.3)	271	6.8

This refers to the number of patients switching treatment due to specific toxicity specified on the row. % was determined by dividing the number of patients switching treatment due to a specific toxicity by the total number of patients with that particular toxicity in question.
§ n(%) n refers to the number of patients who experienced specific toxicity and the % refers to number of patients with toxicity divided by the total number of patients starting ART which was 4,039. An individual patient may experience more than one toxicity during follow up and may experience a specific toxicity more than one episode during follow up.

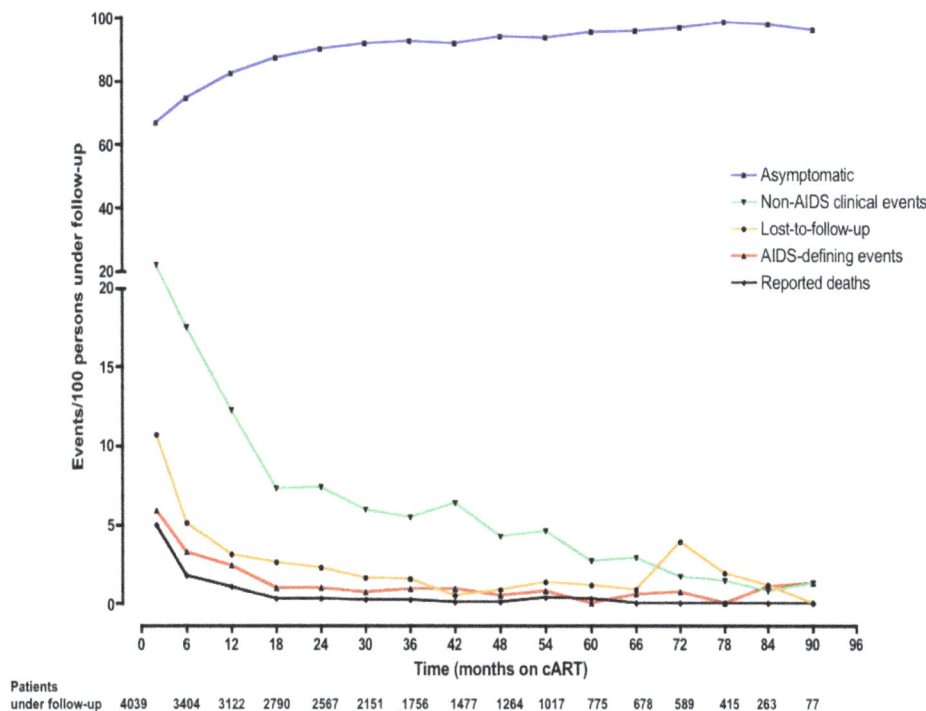

Figure 1. Six monthly incidence rates of Non-AIDS and AIDS events, deaths, loss to follow up and asymptomatic events among Ghanaian HIV-infected patients on long-term cART. Non-AIDS events comprised all medical conditions which are non-AIDS defining by WHO criteria.

In a series of 188 hospital-confirmed deaths, the causes of death are as shown in Table 7. The leading causes of death in this subset of patients were pulmonary tuberculosis, severe diarrhoea with hypovolaemic shock, severe anaemia, pneumonia and sepsis.

Treatment-limiting toxicities. Overall 35.3% (n = 4,039) of patients experienced toxicity during follow up. There were 1,603 documented episodes of cART-related toxicities among patients who started first line cART with an event rate of 14.3 events/100 person-years (95% CI, 13.6 to 15.0/100 person-years). As shown in Table 8, severe anemia, skin rash and neuropsychiatric toxicity were the commonest reported adverse events. 271 patients representing 6.8% of the entire cohort switched therapy due to toxicity.

Rates of major clinical events on cART. Figure 1 depicts the overall decline in the rates of AIDS-defining events, non-AIDS clinical events, mortality and loss to follow up over time on cART. The highest incidence rates of these events were observed within the first two months of initiating cART with rates of 22.1 non-AIDS clinical events per 100 patients, 10.7 lost-to-follow up per 100 patients, 5.9 AIDS defining events per 100 patients and 5.0 deaths per 100 patients under follow-up. One hundred and thirty-five (135) patients (3.3%) starting NNRTI-based first line cART were subsequently switched to a PI-based second line therapy on account of treatment failure at closure of data for analysis.

Discussion

This study is among the largest cohort studies documenting morbidity and mortality in an ART programme in sub-Saharan Africa. The data presented in this paper show that there is a sustained and robust immunological recovery on cART among this cohort of HIV-infected patients. This immune restoration accompanied improvements in morbidity as evidenced the steady decline in the incidence of deaths, losses to follow-up, AIDS-defining and non-AIDS defining clinical events. Attrition from the programme, due mainly to deaths and loss-to-follow up as well as AIDS-defining events, occurred predominantly within the first year of treatment and were predicted by clinical and laboratory indicators of advanced HIV disease at initiation of cART.

Several studies from both developed [19–23] and developing countries [1,24–29] have reported short-, medium- and recently long-term CD4 responses on cART. The findings from this study show that within a programme setting in sub-Saharan Africa, immunological responses to cART are sustainable over the long-term on a limited repertoire of first-line therapy. As expected, the median (IQR) CD4 counts at initiation of therapy of 133 (50–218) cells/mm^3 were low and comparable with those from several cohorts from developing countries [24–34] and serve as an indicator of the advanced stages of immunosuppression at which cART is initiated in these settings [35]. This notwithstanding, cART was associated with a near doubling in median CD4 counts within 6 months of therapy followed by more gradual and sustained increases throughout the period of observation for patients remaining under care. The vigorous restitution of CD4 cell counts within the first six months of therapy was accompanied by the occurrence of IRIS in some patients, of which tuberculosis was the commonest reported cause followed by herpes zoster and cerebral toxoplasmosis. Admittedly, compared with other cohorts where the reported frequency of IRIS has varied between 10% to 25% of all patients initiating cART [18,36–40], the overall frequency of 1.1% of IRIS reported among this cohort is low, and probably reflects the difficulties in the diagnosis of this clinical syndrome within settings of limited diagnostic support. Events were considered as IRIS when clinicians felt they had sufficient clinical and laboratory evidence to support the diagnosis.

For patients who stayed on cART for more than a year, 407 (10.1%) developed immunological failure according to WHO guidelines but only 135 (3.3%) patients in the cohort were switched to second line therapy. The spectra of clinical events classified as IRIS overlaps closely with those diagnosed as AIDS-defining events which occurred at a frequency of 17%. AIDS-defining events on cART occurred at a median time of 6 months, were predicted by low CD4 cell counts, prior AIDS and low BMI at initiation of therapy and were associated with an increased risk of subsequent attrition from the programme. These show that the occurrence of AIDS-defining events in the proximal phases of cART is an indicator of early treatment failure and is representative of progression of HIV disease which cART may be incapable of halting, even when appropriate treatment for opportunistic infections is concurrently commenced. The implication is that cART should be started much earlier, requiring patients to be diagnosed earlier, as has been suggested by others [35,41].

The crude incidence rates of Non-AIDS-defining events of 3.64/1000 person-years is lower compared to that of cohorts from Botswana [13] and the United States [13] of 10.0 py, and 12.4 py, respectively, that of a multicentre Latin American cohort [42] of 8.4/1000 person-years and that of the Eurosida cohort [11] of 17.7 (95% CI of 16.6 to 18.7/1000 py, n = 12,844). The median follow up for the cohorts from Botswana [13], the USA [13], and Latin America [42] were 36 months, 18 months and 30 months respectively which is comparable with the 30 months of follow up of this cohort. However, the retrospective nature of the present study and the relatively short median follow-up in this cohort could have accounted for the lower incidence rates of NADEs. Of the 41 NADEs in this cohort, hepatic disorders (n = 20) were the commonest NADE followed by cardiovascular events (n = 10), end-stage renal disease (n = 6) and non-AIDS malignancies of which hepatocellular carcinoma (n = 4) and one case of oesophageal carcinoma were reported. Overall, 24 of the 41 documented NADEs were associated with HBSAg seropositivity making HBV co-infection an important determinant of NADEs in this cohort. The order of events were different from those in the cohort from Botswana where out of 18 NADEs, 9 were cardiovascular, 4 were renal, five were malignancies and none were of hepatic in etiology [13]. As a composite outcome measure, non-AIDS events are a heterogeneous collection of several end-points with multifactorial aetiologies and risk factors, and also dependent on the presence of chronic hepatitis B co-infection and chronic vascular inflammation due to persistence of HIV viral replication [43–52]. The multidimensional composition of risk factors for NADEs together with the relatively limited observation of events and some missing data restricted analysis of risk factors for these events in this cohort.

Malaria was the leading cause of non-AIDS-defining infectious morbidity on cART and was often treated with artemisinin-based antimalarial therapy. The fact that within this HIV cohort, tuberculosis and malaria were the leading causes of AIDS and non-AIDS infectious morbidity respectively underscores their importance among the most important public health challenges Sub-Saharan Africa is attempting to overcome. Unlike in developed countries where AIDS-related mortality on cART is being superseded by Non-AIDS-related mortality [52], causes of death in this cohort were predominantly driven by AIDS-related events of which tuberculosis was the leading cause followed by gastroenteritis with hypovolemic shock, severe anaemia and pneumonia, as in other cohorts from developing countries. Of the NADEs, end-stage kidney disease and liver-related disease were among the common causes of mortality. It is also noteworthy that 6 deaths were attributed directly to cART-related toxicity: two cases of Stevens Johnson's syndrome from nevirapine and four cases of clinically suspected lactic acidosis from stavudine. cART toxicity is a cardinal factor influencing the durability and therefore the effectiveness of cART and 35.3% of patients experienced one form of toxicity or the other with 6.8% discontinuing therapy on account of toxicity. Use of a stavudine was independently associated with increased risk of death, hence the withdrawal of this antiretroviral from the Ghanaian ART programme is justified. Given the high prevalence of renal impairment among this cohort (38.8%) [53], replacement of stavudine by tenofovir should however be approached with caution due to the well-known association between tenofovir and risk for renal tubular toxicity. It is encouraging that the DART study has provided some reassuring data on the safety of tenofovir among Africans [54]. Furthermore given the high prevalence of hepatitis B co-infection in this cohort, the benefits of tenofovir in slowing the progression of liver disease may outweigh possible renal toxicity.

The analyses presented in this study have limitations worth noting. As over 60% of patients presenting to the clinic did not start cART, and many with advanced HIV/AIDS were lost to follow-up, it is likely there were many deaths in this group. Hence the population studied was skewed towards those patients who survived long enough to start cART, who may have had different causes of death to those not starting cART. The trajectories of CD4 over time reflect those of patients who remained on cART and thus are influenced by survivor bias. Furthermore the sources of ascertainment of causes of deaths in a significant proportion of patients were by verbal autopsy by relatives whose accuracy may be limited. In spite of these the specific causes of death could be verified by medical certification in 188 (58%) out of 324 events. Similarly, the classification of AIDS-defining events, IRIS and NADEs were influenced by availability of data and arrived at by consensus between the authors and local experts.

In summary, cART is effective over the long-term for a substantial proportion of this Ghanaian cohort of HIV-infected patients. Within the constraints of limited resources as it pertains to the ART programme in Ghana, cART was associated with a sustained and durable immunological recovery in most patients, an improvement in morbidity from HIV-infection and trend towards reduction in mortality over the long-term among patients remaining on therapy and in care.

Author Contributions

Conceived and designed the experiments: FSS DC. Performed the experiments: FSS DC. Analyzed the data: FSS MAS. Contributed reagents/materials/analysis tools: FSS BN GBA RP. Wrote the paper: FSS DC.

References

1. Laurent C, Ngom Gueye NF, Ndour CT, Gueye PM, Diouf M, et al. for the ANRS 1215/1290 Study Group (2005) Long-term benefits of highly active antiretroviral therapy in Senegalese HIV-1 infected adults. J Acquir Immune Defic Syndr. 38: 14–17.

2. Desclaux A, Ciss M, Taverne B, Sow PS, Egrot M, et al. (2003) Access to antiretroviral drugs and AIDS management in Senegal. AIDS. 17 (Suppl): S95–S101.

3. Akileswaran C, Lurie MN, Flanigan TP, Mayer KH (2005) Lessons learned from use of highly active antiretroviral therapy in Africa. Clin Infect Dis. 4: 376–385.

4. Braistein P, Brinkhof MW, Dabis F, Schechter M, Boulle A, et al. (2006) Antiretroviral Therapy in Lower Income Countries (ART-LINC) Collaboration; Antiretroviral Therapy Cohort Collaboration (ART-CC) groups. Mortality of

HIV-1-infected patients in the first year of antiretroviral therapy: comparison between low-income and high-income countries. Lancet. 367: 817–824.

5. Coetzee D, Hilderbrand K, Boulle A, Maartens G, Louis F, et al. (2004) Outcomes after two years of providing antiretroviral treatment in Khayelitsha, South Africa. AIDS. 18: 887–895.

6. Severe P, Leger P, Charles M, Noel F, Bonhomme G, et al. (2005) Antiretroviral therapy in a thousand patients with AIDS in Haiti. N Engl J Med. 353: 2325–2334.

7. Wester CW, Kim S, Bussmann H, Avalos A, Ndwapi N, et al. (2005) Initial response to highly active antiretroviral therapy in HIV-1C-infected adults in a public sector treatment program in Botswana. J Acquir Immune Defic Syndr. 40: 336–343.

8. Hawkins C, Achenbach C, Fryda W, Ngare D, Murphy R (2007) Antiretroviral durability and tolerability in HIV-infected adults living in urban Kenya. J Acquir Immune Defic Syndr. 45(3): 304–310.

9. Deeks SG, Phillips AN (2009) HIV infection, antiretroviral treatment, ageing and non-AIDS related morbidity. BMJ. 338: a3172.

10. Phillips AN, Neaton J, Lundgren JD (2008) The role of HIV in serious diseases other than AIDS. AIDS. 22: 2409–2418.

11. Mocroft A, Reiss P, Gasiorowski J, Ledergerber B, Kowalska J, et al. (2010) Serious fatal and nonfatal Non-AIDS-defining illnesses in Europe. J Acquir Immune Defic Syndr. 55: 262–270.

12. Centers for Disease Control (1992) 1993 revised classification system for HIV infection and expanded surveillance case definition for AIDS among adolescents and adults. MMWR Recomm Rep. 41: 1–19.

13. Wester CW, Koethe JR, Shepherd BE, Stinnette SE, Rebeiro F, et al. (2011) Non-AIDS-defining events among HIV-1-infected adults receiving combination antiretroviral therapy in resource-replete versus resource-limited urban setting. AIDS. 25 (12): 1471–1479.

14. Division of AIDS, NIAID (1994) Division of AIDS Table for Grading Severity of Adult Adverse Experiences. Rockville, MD: National Institute of Allery and Infectious Diseases.

15. Division of AIDS, NIAID (2004) Division of AIDS Table for Grading Severity of Adult Adverse Experiences. Rockville, MD: National Institute of Allery and Infectious Diseases; December.

16. Sarfo FS, Sarfo MA, Kasim A, Phillips R, Booth M, et al. (2014) Long-term effectiveness of first-line non-nucleoside reverse transcriptase inhibitor (NNRTI)-based antiretroviral therapy in Ghana. J Antimicrob Chemother. 69(1): 254–261.

17. WHO (2010) Antiretroviral therapy for HIV infection in adults and adolescents, recommendations for a public health approach 2010 revision. Available: http://www.int/entity/hiv/pub/arv/adult2010/en/index.html. Accessed 2012 July 25.

18. Müller M, Wandel S, Colebunders R, Attia S, Furrer H, IeDEA South and Central Africa, et al. (2010) Immune reconstitution inflammatory syndrome in patients starting antiretroviral therapy for HIV infection: a systematic review and meta-analysis. Lancet Infect Dis. 10: 251–261.

19. Wolbers M, Battegay M, Hirschel B, Furrer H, Cavassini M, et al. (2007) CD4+ T-cell count increase in HIV-1-infected patients with suppressed viral load within 1 year after start of antiretroviral therapy. Antivir Ther. 12: 889–897.

20. Moore RD, Keruly JC (2007) CD4+ cell count 6 years after commencement of highly active antiretroviral therapy in persons with sustained virologic suppression. Clin Infect Dis. 44: 441–446.

21. Mocroft A, Phillips AN, Gatell J, Ledergerber B, Fisher M, et al. (2007) Normalisation of CD4 counts in patients with HIV-1 infection and maximum virological suppression who are taking combination antiretroviral therapy: an observational cohort study. Lancet. 370(9585): 407–413.

22. Smith CJ, Sabin CA, Youle MS, Kinloch-de Loes S, Lampe FC, et al. (2004) Factors influencing increases in CD4 cell counts of HIV-positive persons receiving long-term highly active antiretroviral therapy. J Infect Dis. 190: 1860–1868.

23. Gras L, Kesselring AM, Griffin JT, van Sighem AI, Fraser C, et al. (2007) CD4 cell counts of 800 cells/mm^3 or greater after 7 years of highly active antiretroviral therapy are feasible in most patients starting with 350 cells/mm^3 or greater. J Acquir Immune Defic Syndr. 45: 183–192.

24. Sow PS, Otieno LF, Bissagnene E, Kityo C, Bennink R, et al. (2007) Implementation of an antiretroviral access program for HIV-1-infected individuals in resource-limited settings: clinical results from 4 African countries. J Acquir Immune Defic Syndr. 44: 262–267.

25. Charalambous S, Innes C, Muirhead D, Kumaranayake L, Fielding K, et al. (2007) Evaluation of a workplace HIV treatment programme in South Africa. AIDS. 21: S73–8.

26. Stringer JS, Zulu I, Levy J, Stringer EM, Mwango A, et al. (2006) Rapid scale-up of antiretroviral therapy at primary care sited in Zambia: feasibility and early outcomes. JAMA. 296: 782–93.

27. Lawn SD, Myer L, Bekker LG, Wood R (2006) CD4 cell count recovery among HIV-infected patients with very advanced immunodeficiency commencing antiretroviral treatment in Sub-Saharan Africa. BMC Infect Dis 6: 59.

28. Erhabor O, Ejele OA, Nwauche CA (2006) The effects of highly active antiretroviral therapy (HAART) of Stavudine, Lamivudine and nevirapine on the CD4 lymphocyte count of HIV-infected African: the Nigerian experience. Niger J Clin Pract. 9: 128–133.

29. Ferradini L, Jeannin A, Pinoges L, Izopet J, Odhiambo D, et al. (2006) Scaling up of highly active antiretroviral in a rural district of Malawi: an effectiveness assessment. Lancet. 367: 1335–1342.

30. Kilaru KR, Kumar A, Sippy N, Carter AO, Roach TC (2006) Immunological and virological responses to highly active antiretroviral therapy in a non-clinical trial setting in a developing Caribbean country. HIV Med. 7: 99–104.

31. Tuboi SH, Harrison LH, Sprinz E, Albernaz RK, Schechter M (2005) Predictors of virologic failure in HIV-1-infected patients starting highly active antiretroviral therapy in Porto Alegre, Brazil. J Acquir Immune Defic Syndr. 40: 324–328.

32. Marins JR, Jamal LF, Chen SY, Barros MB, Hudes ES, et al. (2003) Dramatic improvement in survival among adult Brazilian AIDS patients. AIDS. 17: 1675–1682.

33. Dai Y, Qiu ZF, Li TS, Han Y, Zuo LY, et al. (2006) Clinical outcomes and immune reconstitution in 103 advanced AIDS patients undergoing 12-month highly active antiretroviral therapy. Chin Med J (Engl). 119: 1677–1682.

34. Srasuebkul P, Ungsedhapand C, Ruxrungtham K, Boyd MA, Phanuphak P, et al. (2007) Predictive factors for immunological and virological endpoints in Thai patients receiving combination antiretroviral treatment. HIV Med. 8: 46–54.

35. Nash D, Katyal M, Brinkhof MWG, Keiser O, May Margaret, et al. (2008) Long-term immunologic response to antiretroviral therapy in low-income countries: Collaborative analysis of prospective studies: The Antiretroviral Therapy in Lower Income Countries (ART-LINC) Collaboration of the International epidemiological Databases to Evaluate AIDS. AIDS. 22(17): 2291–2302.

36. Novak RM, Richardson JT, Buchacz K, Chmiel JS, Durham MD, et al. (2012) Immune reconstitution inflammatory syndrome (IRIS) in the HIV outpatient study (HOPS): incidence and implications. AIDS. 26(6): 721–730.

37. Ratman I, Chiu C, Kandala NB, Easterbrook PJ (2006) Incidence and risk factors for immune reconstitution inflammatory syndrome in an ethnically diverse HIV type-1-infected cohort. Clin Infect Dis. 42: 418–27.

38. French MA, Price P, Stone SF (2004) Immune restoration disease after antiretroviral therapy. AIDS. 18: 1615–1627.

39. Cooney EL (2002) Clinical indicators of immune restoration following highly active antiretroviral therapy. Clin Infect Dis. 34: 224–233.

40. Shelburne SA, Hamill RJ, Rodriguez-Barradas MC, Greenberg SB, Atmar RL, et al. (2002) Immune reconstitution inflammatory syndrome: emergence of a unique syndrome during highly active antiretroviral therapy. Medicine (Baltimore). 81: 213–227.

41. Lawden C, Chene G, Morlat P, Raffi F, Dupon M, et al. (2007) HIV-infected adults with a CD4 cell count greater than 500 cells/mm^3 on long-term combination antiretroviral therapy reach same mortality rates as the general population. J Acquir Immune Defic Syndr. 44: 262–267.

42. Belloso WH, Orellana LC, Grinsztejn B, Madero JS, La Rosa A, et al. (2010) Analysis of serious non-AIDS events among HIV-infected adults at Latin American sites. HIV MED. 11: 554–564.

43. Calza L, Manfredi R, Verucchi G (2010) Myocardial infarction risk in HIV-infected patients: epidemiology, pathogenesis, and clinical management. AIDS. 24(6): 789–802.

44. Kuller LH, Tracy R, Belloso W, deWit S, Drummond F, et al. (2008) Inflammatory and coagulation biomarkers and mortality in patients with HIV infection. PLoS Med. 5: e203.10.1371/journal.pmed.0050203.

45. Lau B, Sharret AR, Kingsley LA, Post W, Palella FJ, et al. (2006) C-reactive protein is a marker for human immunodeficiency virus disease progression. Arch Intern Med. 166: 64–70.

46. Torriani FJ, Komarow L, Parker RA, Cotter BR, Currier JS, et al. (2008) Endothelial dysfunction in human immunodeficiency virus-infected antiretroviral-naïve sujects before and after starting potent antiretroviral therapy. J Am Coll Cardiol. 52: 569–576.

47. Friis-Moller N, Reiss P, Sabin CA, Weber R, Monteforte A, et al. (2007) DAD Study group. Class of antiretroviral drugs and the risk of myocardial infarction. N Engl J Med. 356: 1723–1735.

48. Obel N, Thomsen HF, Kronborg G, Larsen CS, Hilderbrandt PR, et al. (2007) Ischaemic heart disease in HIV-infected and HIV-uninfected individuals: a population-based cohort study. Clin Infect Dis. 44: 1625–1631.

49. Triant VA, Lee H, Hadigan C, Grinspoon SK (2007) Increased acute myocardial infarction rates and cardiovascular risk factors among patients with human immunodeficiency disease. J Clin Endocrinol Metal. 92: 2506–2512.

50. Currier JS (2002) Cardiovascular risk associated with HIV therapy. J Acquir Immune Defic Syndr.(Suppl 1): 31 S16–23. Discussion S4–5.

51. Crum-Cianflone N, Hullsiek KH, Marconi V, Weintrob A, Ganesan A, et al. (2009) Trends in the incidence of cancers among HIV-infected persons and the impact of antiretroviral therapy: a 20-year cohort study. AIDS.23: 41–50.

52. Neuhaus J, Angus B, Kowalska JD, La Rosa A, Sampson J, et al. for the INSIGHT SMART and ESPRIT study groups (2010) Risk of all-cause mortality associated with non-fatal AIDS and serious non-AIDS events among adults infected with HIV. AIDS. 24: 697–706.

53. Sarfo FS, Keegan R, Appiah L, Shakoor S, Phillips R, et al. (2013) High prevalence of renal dysfunction and association with risk of death amongst HIV-infected Ghanaians. J Infect. 67(1): 43–50.

54. Reid A, Stöhr W, Sarah Walker A, Williams IG, Kityo C, et al. (2008) Severe renal dysfunction and risk factors associated with renal impairment in HIV-infected adults in Africa initiating antiretroviral therapy. Clin Infect Dis. 46: 1271–1281.

14

The Importance of Body Weight for the Dose Response Relationship of Oral Vitamin D Supplementation and Serum 25-Hydroxyvitamin D in Healthy Volunteers

John Paul Ekwaru[1], Jennifer D. Zwicker[2], Michael F. Holick[3], Edward Giovannucci[4], Paul J. Veugelers[1]*

1 School of Public Health, University of Alberta, Edmonton, Alberta, Canada, **2** School of Public Policy, University of Calgary, Calgary, Alberta, Canada, **3** Section of Endocrinology, Nutrition and Diabetes, Department of Medicine, Boston University School of Medicine, Boston, Massachusetts, United States of America, **4** Harvard School of Public Health, Departments of Nutrition and Epidemiology, Boston, Massachusetts, United States of America

Abstract

Unlike vitamin D recommendations by the Institute of Medicine, the Clinical Practice Guidelines by the Endocrine Society acknowledge body weight differentials and recommend obese subjects be given two to three times more vitamin D to satisfy their body's vitamin D requirement. However, the Endocrine Society also acknowledges that there are no good studies that clearly justify this. In this study we examined the combined effect of vitamin D supplementation and body weight on serum 25-hydroxyvitamin (25(OH)D) and serum calcium in healthy volunteers. We analyzed 22,214 recordings of vitamin D supplement use and serum 25(OH)D from 17,614 healthy adult volunteers participating in a preventive health program. This program encourages the use of vitamin D supplementation and monitors its use and serum 25(OH)D and serum calcium levels. Participants reported vitamin D supplementation ranging from 0 to 55,000 IU per day and had serum 25(OH)D levels ranging from 10.1 to 394 nmol/L. The dose response relationship between vitamin D supplementation and serum 25(OH)D followed an exponential curve. On average, serum 25(OH)D increased by 12.0 nmol/L per 1,000 IU in the supplementation interval of 0 to 1,000 IU per day and by 1.1 nmol/L per 1,000 IU in the supplementation interval of 15,000 to 20,000 IU per day. BMI, relative to absolute body weight, was found to be the better determinant of 25(OH)D. Relative to normal weight subjects, obese and overweight participants had serum 25(OH)D that were on average 19.8 nmol/L and 8.0 nmol/L lower, respectively (P<0.001). We did not observe any increase in the risk for hypercalcemia with increasing vitamin D supplementation. We recommend vitamin D supplementation be 2 to 3 times higher for obese subjects and 1.5 times higher for overweight subjects relative to normal weight subjects. This observational study provides body weight specific recommendations to achieve 25(OH)D targets.

Editor: Nick Harvey, University of Southampton, United Kingdom

Funding: This is an analysis of secondary data. The data had been collected for the purpose of lifestyle counseling of participants of a preventive health program. None of the authors are involved in the execution of this program neither do they provide financial support for the data collection. PJV holds a Canada Research Chair in Population Health, an Alberta Research Chair in Nutrition and Disease Prevention, and an Alberta Innovates Health Scholarship. The funding for the Canada Research Chair is provided through the Canadian Institutes for Health Research to the University of Alberta. The Alberta Research Chair is awarded by the School of Public Health at the University of Alberta through a thematic research contract with the Pure North S'Energy Foundation. The Health Scholarship is funded by the Alberta provincial government through Alberta Innovates Health Solutions. The funders had no role in study design, data collection and analysis, decision to publish, or preparation of the manuscript.

Competing Interests: The authors have declared that no competing interests exist.

* Email: paul.veugelers@ualberta.ca

Introduction

Vitamin D has been shown to benefit bone health, to prevent rickets, osteomalacia and symptomatic hypocalcaemia, and to reduce the burden of other specific diseases [1–5]. To reduce burden of disease, various institutions recommend defined amounts of vitamin D intake [6–8]. The established proxy for vitamin D status, however, is serum 25-hydroxyvitamin D (25(OH)D) [9,10]. This proxy has been used for definitions of vitamin D deficiency (for example, serum 25(OH)D levels below 50 nmol/L), vitamin D insufficiency (serum 25(OH)D levels between 50 and 75 nmol/L), and vitamin D toxicity (serum

25(OH)D levels exceeding 500 nmol/L) [7], though these definitions are not established. With recommendations based on vitamin D intake and serum 25(OH)D as the best proxy for nutritional status, a good quantification of the dose response relationship between vitamin D intake and serum 25(OH)D is essential. However, this dose response relationship is currently not well documented, particularly not for a wider range and including high levels of vitamin D supplementation.

The Recommended Dietary Allowance (RDA) is the nutrient intake considered to be sufficient to meet the requirements of 97.5% of healthy individuals. The RDA for vitamin D, 600 IU day for individuals 1 to 70 years of age and 800 IU per day for those above the age of 70 years [8]. Although differences in serum 25(OH)D by body mass index (BMI) and by absolute body weight have been reported [11–19], the RDA does not consider either. The Clinical Practice Guidelines by the Endocrine Society do acknowledge body weight differentials and recommended obese subjects be given two to three times more vitamin D to satisfy their body's vitamin D requirement, however they acknowledge that there are no studies that clearly justify this [7,20].

The objectives of the present study are to characterize the dose response relationship of oral vitamin D supplementation and serum 25(OH)D in a large sample of healthy volunteers, and to quantify the extent this dose response relationship is different for BMI and for absolute body weight. As the effect of vitamin D on serum calcium and the risk for hypercalcemia is the most common argument against high doses of vitamin D supplementation, we further studied the relationship between vitamin D supplementation and calcium homeostasis.

Methods

This study is based on information from healthy volunteers participating in a preventive health program provided by the Pure North S'Energy Foundation (PN), a not-for-profit charitable organization providing free services since October 2007. The program and data collection protocol are described elsewhere [21,22]. In brief, PN offers health promotion counseling with an emphasis on vitamin D supplementation as their volunteers mostly reside in the Canadian province of Alberta which is located between the 49th and 60th parallel north. PN asks participants to complete a lifestyle questionnaire, have their height and weight measured, have a medical history, and have blood drawn for the assessment of serum 25(OH)D. Since January 2009 the medical history recorded the question 'how much vitamin D supplementation are you using?' This includes vitamin D from vitamin D supplementation and from multivitamins. Also calcium supplementation was recorded in the medical history. All 22,214 per protocol study visits, that are typically scheduled once a year, prior to June 2013 were included in the present study. All 25(OH)D measurements were assessed with an automated chemiluminescent immunoassay from DiaSorin (LIAISON) which measures the combination of D2 and D3 and which has coefficients of variation ranging from 6.8% to 8.8%.

Various shapes of the relationship between vitamin D intake and 25(OH)D have been proposed [11,23–26]. These include linear, polynominal, bi-phasic, exponential and 'exponential plus linear' relationships [11,23-26]. We therefore sought to identify the regression model that best characterized the relationship by comparing linear, quadratic, cubic, linear-log, exponential and 'exponential plus linear' regression models on the basis of the Akaike Information Criteria (AIC) [27].

We examined the importance of both BMI and absolute body weight for the dose response relationship of oral vitamin D

Table 1. Summary of 22,214 simultaneous assessments of oral vitamin D supplementation and serum 25(OH)D level.

	N	%	Mean	Std
Vitamin D supplementation (IU per day)	22214		2841.6	4022.5
Serum 25(OH)D level nmol/L	22214		90.5	46.5
Albumin corrected calcium (mmol/L)	10940		2.4	0.1
Age (Years)				
<40	7800	35.1		
40 to 49	4766	21.5		
50 to 59	5291	23.8		
60+	4357	19.6		
Gender				
Female	10944	49.3		
Male	11270	50.7		
Weight Status				
Underweight	279	1.3		
Normal weight	7197	33.4		
Overweight	7962	36.9		
Obesity	6131	28.4		
Absolute weight				
<60 kg	2270	10.6		
60 kg to 80 kg	8734	40.8		
80.1 to 100 kg	7232	33.8		
>100 kg	3158	14.8		
season				
Winter	7320	33.0		
Spring	7039	31.7		
Summer	4294	19.3		
Fall	3561	16.0		

Table 2. The relationship between oral vitamin D supplementation and serum 25(OH)D levels estimated with six different parametric regression models.

Parameter	Linear β (95%CI)	Linear p-value	Quadratic β (95%CI)	Quadratic p-value	Cubic β (95%CI)	Cubic p-value	Linear-log β (95%CI)	Linear-log p-value	Exponential β (95%CI)	Exponential p-value	Exponential plus Linear β (95%CI)	Exponential plus Linear p-value
Intercept (Y0)	104.1(100.9,107.2)	<.001	101.8 (98.7,105.0)	<.001	101.1(97.9,104.2)	<.001	18.3(14.5,22.1)	<.001	100.7(97.5,103.8)	<.001	100.8(97.6,103.9)	<.001
Age	0.3(0.3,0.3)	<.001	0.3(0.2,0.3)	<.001	0.3(0.2,0.3)	<.001	0.2(0.1,0.2)	<.001	0.2(0.2,0.3)	<.001	0.2(0.2,0.3)	<.001
BMI	−1.6(−1.7,−1.5)	<.001	−1.6 (−1.7,−1.5)	<.001	−1.6(−1.7,−1.5)	<.001	−1.5(−1.6,−1.4)	<.001	−1.5(−1.6,−1.4)	<.001	−1.5(−1.6,−1.4)	<.001
Sex (male vs female)	−4.6(−5.7,−3.6)	<.001	−4.4 (−5.4,−3.3)	<.001	−4.2(−5.2,−3.1)	<.001	−2.7(−3.8,−1.7)	<.001	−4.0(−5.1,−3.0)	<.001	−4.1(−5.1,−3.0)	<.001
Season												
Spring	1.4(0.2,2.7)	0.023	0.9 (−0.3,2.1)	0.142	0.9(−0.3,2.1)	0.132	2.1(0.9,3.3)	<.001	1.0(−0.2,2.2)	0.105	1.0(−0.2,2.2)	0.116
Summer	4.1(2.7,5.5)	<.001	4.3 (2.9,5.7)	<.001	4.5(3.1,5.9)	<.001	5.3(3.9,6.8)	<.001	4.6(3.2,6.0)	<.001	4.6(3.2,6.0)	<.001
Fall	2.5(1.0,4.1)	<.001	3.0 (1.5,4.5)	<.001	3.1(1.6,4.6)	<.001	3.3(1.8,4.8)	<.001	3.1(1.6,4.6)	<.001	3.1(1.6,4.6)	<.001
Winter	ref.		ref.		ref.		ref.		ref.		ref.	
Vitamin D daily dose (per 1000 IU)	5.9(5.7,6.0)	<.001	8.5 (8.2,8.7)	<.001	9.6(9.2,10.0)	<.001					−1.1(−2.9,0.8)	0.256
Vitamin D daily dose (per 1000 IU)^2			−0.2 (−0.2,−0.2)	<.001	−0.3(−0.4,−0.3)	<.001						
Vitamin D daily dose (per 1000 IU)^3					0.0(0.0,0.0)	<.001						
log10 Vitamin D (per 1000 IU)							34.2(33.4,34.9)	<.001				
A									100.0(94.0,105.9)	<.001	132.1(71.1,193.2)	<.001
B									0.1(0.1,0.1)	<.001	0.1(0.1,0.1)	<.001
AIC	**217424.1**		**216795.0**		**216736.3**		**217725.2**		**216721.8**		**216722.1**	

β: β-coefficient; 95% CI: 95% confidence Interval; ref: reference category; AIC: Akaike Information Criteria; A and B are parameters in the exponential and 'exponential plus linear' regression models. In the exponential model, $Y = Y0 + A*(1 - e^{-BX})$, Y (intercept), Y0 (intercept), Y0 (intercept) denotes serum 25(OH)D, Y denotes serum 25(OH)D in the absence of vitamin D supplementation, and X denotes vitamin D supplementation. The six parametric regression models are compared on the basis of the AIC. The parametric regression model with the lowest AIC value (the exponential model) is the model that best describes the observations.

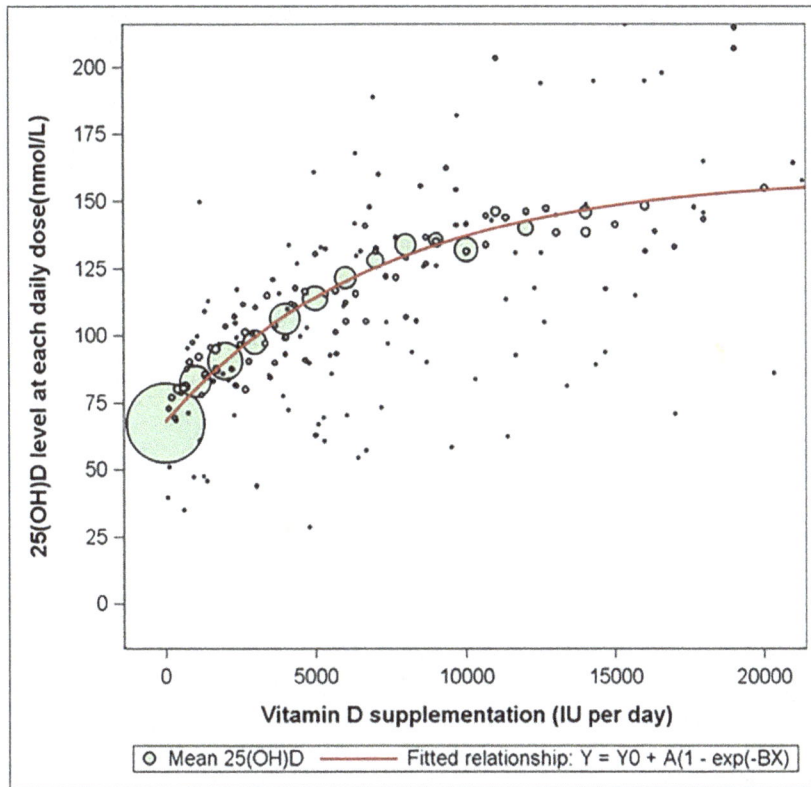

Figure 1. The dose response relationship between oral vitamin D supplementation and serum 25(OH)D levels based on 22,214 observations of healthy volunteers. Footnote: Bubbles represent the mean plasma 25(OH)D level for all reported daily doses. The size of the bubbles is proportional to the number of assessments for each of the reported daily doses. The red line represents the fitted dose response curve.

supplementation and serum 25(OH)D while adjusting for the confounding potential of age, sex and season using multivariable regression models. We compared BMI and absolute body weight both as continuous and categorical variables. When categorized, individuals with a BMI of less or equal than 18.5, more than 18.5 and less or equal than 25, more than 25 and less or equal than 30, and more than 30 were considered underweight, normal weight, overweight and obese, respectively [28]. Weight was categorized as less than 60 kg, 60 kg to 80 kg, more than 80 kg and less or equal to 100 kg, and more than 100 kg.

Assessments of height and weight were missing in 3% of the assessments. These records were excluded in analyses with BMI and absolute body weight as continuous covariates, but were included in analyses with BMI and absolute body weight as categorical covariates by considering missing values as a missing category. Differences in the dose response relationship of oral vitamin D supplementation and serum 25(OH)D by BMI were visualized through plots of model estimated 25(OH)D levels for any given supplementation levels.

As the available data included repeated observations for a subset of 3416 (19.4%) subjects, we included a random intercept in all the exponential regression models. The effects of vitamin D supplementation on calcium levels and probability of hypercalcemia were analyzed using linear regression and logistic regression, respectively.

All analyses were conducted using SAS 9.4 (SAS Institute, Cary NC) and the dose response curves were fitted using PROC NLMIXED, a SAS procedure for fitting nonlinear mixed effect

models. Statistical significance was defined as p-values less than 0.05.

PN anonymized their data prior to forwarding it to the University of Alberta for analyses. The Human Research Ethics Board of the University of Alberta had approved access to and analysis of the PN data for the purpose of the present analyses.

Results

Participants reported vitamin D supplementation ranging from 0 to 55,000 IU per day. Sixty-nine participants (0.3%) reported supplementation above 20,000 IU per day. The participants had serum 25(OH)D levels ranging from 10.1 to 394 nmol/L. Of all participants, 33.4% were normal weight, 1.3% underweight, 36.9% overweight and 28.4% obese (Table 1).

Table 2 depicts characteristics of the linear, quadratic, cubic, linear-log, exponential and 'exponential plus linear' regression models that describe the dose response relationship between oral vitamin D supplementation and serum 25(OH)D. The exponential regression model appeared to describe the dose response relationship best. This conclusion is based on the observation that the AIC for the exponential regression model was lower than for of the other regression models (Table 2).

The dose response relationship between vitamin D supplementation and serum 25(OH)D for supplementation levels of 20,000 IU per day or less is depicted in Figure 1. Bubbles represent the mean serum 25(OH)D level for all reported doses of vitamin D supplementation. The size of the bubbles is proportional to the number of assessments for each of the doses. Though the entire range of supplementation values was included in

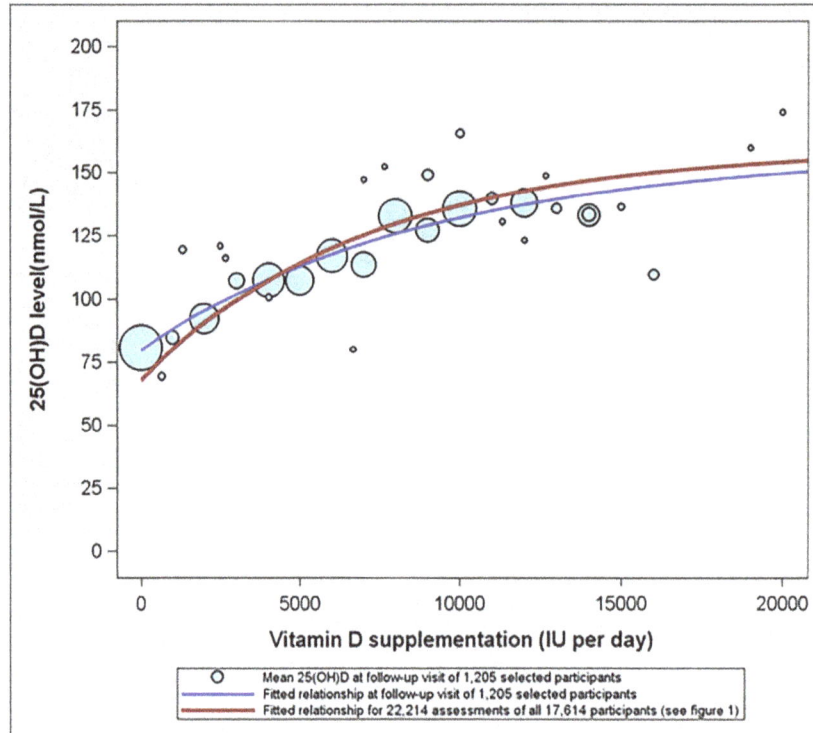

Figure 2. The relationship between oral vitamin D supplementation dose and serum 25(OH)D level at the follow up visits of a subgroup of 1205 healthy volunteers who reportedly did not supplement at their baseline visit. Footnote: Bubbles represent the mean plasma 25(OH)D level for all reported daily doses. The size of the bubbles is proportional to the number of assessments for each of the reported daily doses. The blue line represents the fitted relationship for the subgroup of participants who reportedly did not supplement at their baseline visit. The red line represents the fitted relationship of the entire sample (22,214 observations). Both analytic approaches revealed similar dose response relationships as the red and blue lines are similar.

analyses, the graphs are plotted up to 20,000 IU. The red line represents the fitted exponential dose response curve and confirms the clear impression from the bubbles that the dose response relationship is non-linear and levels off at increasingly higher supplementation levels. The parameter Y0, that represents the average serum 25(OH)D level reached without vitamin D supplementation, was estimated to be 68.0 nmol/L (95% CI: 67.3, 68.7).

For Figure 2 we restricted our analyses to those subjects that had both their baseline visit and a follow up visit between January 2009 and June 2013 and had reported not to supplement with vitamin D at their baseline visit (1205 subjects, 2410 assessments). This analysis mimics a pre-post comparison of an intervention: a comparison of observations prior to introduction to vitamin D supplementation with observations, on average, 0.98 years after the baseline visit. As such, the blue bubbles in figure 2 represent the expected 25(OH)D level of participants who have been taken oral doses of vitamin D for an average of 0.98 year since baseline. The blue line represents the fitted dose response curve for this subset of 1205 subjects. The red line is identical to the red line in Figure 1 representing the fitted dose response curve for the complete sample (22,214 assessments from 17,614 subjects). The red line in Figure 2 (and the observations presented in Figure 1) could be described as a 'snapshot of an ongoing intervention program'. The fact that the red and blue lines in Figure 2 are similar illustrates that a 'pre-post comparison' and a 'snapshot of an ongoing intervention program' reveal similar results.

Both Figure 1 and 2 show that the increase in serum 25(OH)D is leveling off at higher doses of vitamin D supplementation. Serum

25(OH)D levels are estimated to increase on average by 11.98 nmol/L per 1,000 IU in the supplementation interval of 0 to 1,000 IU per day and by 1.13 nmol/L per 1,000 IU in the supplementation of 15,000 to 20,000 IU per day. In addition to supplementation, also age, BMI, absolute body weight, gender and season are associated with serum 25(OH)D levels in a statistically significant manner (Table 3). The differences across BMI categories (Table 3, column 1) are pronounced: obese subjects and overweight subjects had serum 25(OH)D levels that were on average 19.8 nmol/L lower and 8.0 nmol/L lower than those of normal weight subjects, respectively. The differences in serum 25(OH)D levels between underweight and normal weight subjects were not statistically significant. Differences across absolute weight categories were also substantial and statistically significant (Table 3, column 2). In table 3, the AIC values were smaller in models that included BMI relative to models that included absolute body weight regardless of whether they were considered as categorical (213710.6 versus 213990.2; Table 3: columns 1 and 2) or continuous (213602.0 versus 213852.0; Table 3, columns 1 and 2) covariates, suggesting BMI to be a better predictor of 25(OH)D relative to absolute weight. When considering BMI and absolute weight simultaneously (Table 3: columns 3 and 6), BMI appeared to be the better proximate determinant of 25(OH)D. This conclusion is based on the observation that the estimated coefficients for BMI changed only slightly when absolute weight is included in the model (column 3 versus column 1 and column 6 versus column 4), while the coefficients for absolute weight changed substantially when BMI is included (Table 3, column 3 versus 2 and column 6 versus 5).

Table 3. Importance of body mass index and absolute body weight for the relationship between oral vitamin D supplementation and serum 25(OH)D.

| | Categorical BMI and absolute weight | | | | | | Continuous BMI and absolute weight | | | | | |
| | Column 1 BMI | | Column 2 Weight | | Column 3 combined | | Column 4 BMI | | Column 5 Weight | | Column 6 Combined | |
	β (95%CI)	p-value	β (95%CI)	p-value	β (95%CI)	p-value	β (95%CI)	p-value	β (95%CI)	p-value	β (95%CI)	p-value
BMI (continuous)							−1.5(−1.6, −1.4)	<.001			−1.9(−2.2, −1.7)	<.001
Absolute weight (continuous)									−0.4(−0.5, −0.4)	<.001	0.1(0.1,0.2)	<.001
BMI category												
Underweight	1.1(−3.4,5.7)	0.623			0.7(−3.9,5.2)	0.774						
Normal weight	Ref.				Ref.							
Overweight	−8.0(−9.3, −6.7)	<.001			−7.4(−8.9, −6.0)	<.001						
Obesity	−19.8(−21.1, −18.4)	<.001			−18.8(−20.9, −16.8)	<.001						
Absolute weight category												
<60 kg			8.9(7.1,10.7)	<.001	3.8(1.9,5.7)	<.001						
60 kg to 80 kg			Ref.		Ref.							
80.1 to 100 kg			−6.7(−7.9, −5.4)	<.001	1.0(−0.6,2.5)	0.223						
>100 kg			−14.8(−16.4, −3.1)	<.001	−0.7(−3.0,1.6)	0.561						
AIC	213710.6		213990.2				213602.0		213852.0			

Footnote: β: β-coefficient; 95% CI: 95% confidence Interval; ref: reference category; AIC: Akaike Information Criteria; All the estimates are adjusted for age, gender, season and vitamin D supplementation; AIC values are based on models fitted with observations for which both BMI and absolute body weight were not missing.

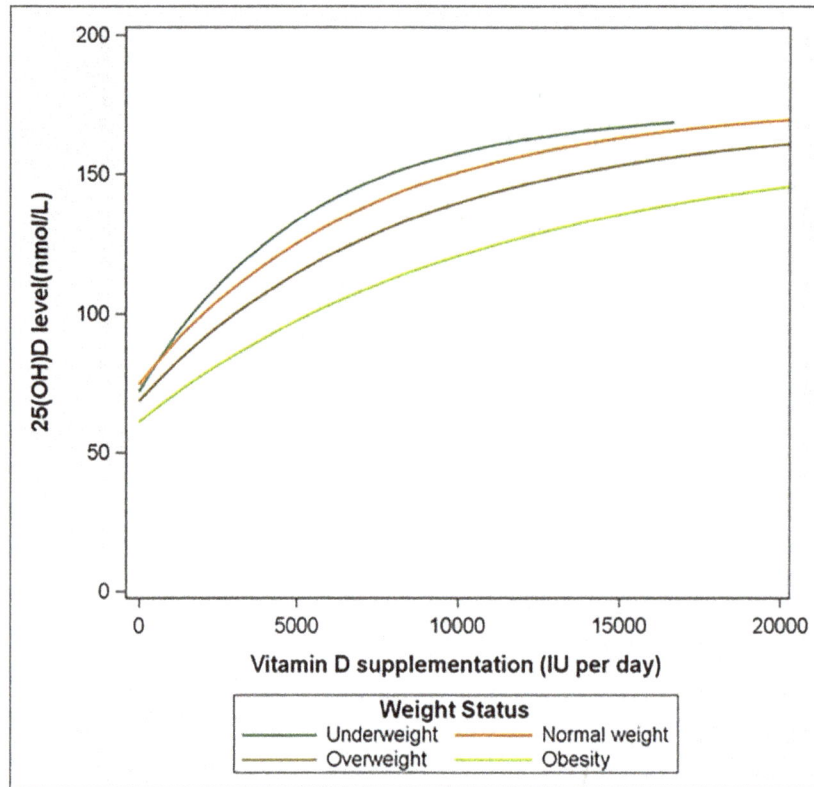

Figure 3. The dose response relationship between oral vitamin D supplementation and plasma 25(OH)D levels by body mass index category. Footnote: the lines are estimated using an exponential plus linear regression model that adjusted for age, gender, and season.

The BMI differences in the dose response relationship are further visualized in Figure 3. Relative to normal weight subjects, obese subjects had lower 25(OH)D values and curved differently. Serum 25(OH)D was estimated to increase at an average rate of 13.1 nmol/L per 1000 IU, 11.5 nmol/L per 1000 IU and 8.6 nmol/L per 1000 IU among normal weight, overweight and obese participant, respectively in the supplementation interval of 0 to 1000 IU per day. The average rates of increase then reduce to 1.3 nmol/L per 1000 IU, 1.5 nmol/L per 1000 IU and 1.9 nmol/L per 1000 IU, respectively in the supplementation interval of 15,000 IU to 20,000 IU per day.

Table 4 provides estimates for the relationship of supplementation and serum 25(OH)D by BMI category. Supplementation with 600 IU per day would achieve average serum 25(OH)D levels of 83, 76 and 66 nmol/L for normal weight, overweight and obese participants, respectively (Table 4). Average serum 25(OH)D levels of 100 nmol/L in normal weight, overweight and obese subgroups, are estimated to require supplementation with 2,080 IU, 3,065 IU and 5,473 IU per day, respectively (Table 4). Relative to normal weight participants, this represents a 1.47 and 2.6 times higher dose for overweight and obese subjects, respectively.

For the 10,940 visits that included assessments for serum calcium, the mean albumin corrected calcium level was 2.35 mmol/L (standard deviation = 0.11) and ranged from 1.79 to 3.23. Figure 4 shows the dose response relationship between vitamin D supplementation and serum calcium levels. In a linear regression model that adjust for age, BMI, gender, season, and calcium supplementation, serum calcium levels did not increase significantly by increasing daily vitamin D supplementation:

0.001 mmol/L per 1000 IU increase in daily vitamin D supplementation, p-value = 0.165 (Table 5).

Of the 10,940 visits that included assessments of serum calcium, 189 (1.7%) had albumin corrected calcium levels exceeding 2.6 mmol/L (hypercalcemia). In a logistic regression model that adjusted for age, BMI, gender, season, and calcium supplementation, there was no statistically significant effect of vitamin D supplementation on the probability of having hypercalcemia (Table 5: Odds ratio = 0.97 per 1000 IU increase in daily vitamin D supplementation, p-value = 0.286). Also, the probability of having hypercalcemia was not statistical significantly different for overweight and obese subjects relative to normal weight subjects. In contrast, female gender and older age appeared important risk factors for hypercalcemia (Table 5).

Discussion

We observed substantial differences in serum 25(OH)D across categories of BMI and absolute body weight, which concurs with observations by others [11–19] and deviates from reports that concluded an absence of body weight differentials [29,30]). The present study suggests that, on statistical grounds, BMI is the better measure relative to absolute body weight to determine which vitamin D doses are needed for which body weight groups to achieve specific serum 25(OH)D targets. The present study also adds to the existing knowledge by revealing that the magnitude of the differences in serum 25(OH)D between normal weight and obese subjects varies by supplementation dose. Furthermore, this study provides detailed recommendations for supplementation to achieve 25(OH)D targets specific for normal weight, overweight

Table 4. Estimated average serum 25(OH)D levels for various vitamin D supplementation doses and the estimated average vitamin D supplementation doses for various serum 25(OH)D levels for normal weight, overweight and obese individuals.

	Underweight		Normal weight		Overweight		Obesity	
	Est.	95% CI	Est.	95% CI	Est.	95% CI	Est.	95% CI
Vitamin D supplementation dose in IU per day	**Serum 25(OH)D level in nmol/L**							
600	83	(78,88)	83	(82,84)	76	(75,77)	66	(65,67)
1000	89	(85,94)	88	(87,89)	80	(79,81)	70	(69,71)
2000	104	(98,109)	99	(98,100)	90	(89,91)	78	(77,79)
4000	125	(117,133)	118	(116,119)	107	(106,109)	91	(90,93)
10000	158	(151,164)	151	(149,152)	140	(138,141)	121	(119,122)
15000	167	(161,173)	163	(160,166)	153	(151,156)	135	(133,138)
Serum 25(OH)D level in nmol/L	**Vitamin D supplementation dose in IU per day**							
75	151	(-,507)	28	(-,115)	534	(450,619)	1663	(1538,1790)
100	1723	(1360,2113)	2080	(1978,2183)	3065	(2928,3204)	5473	(5190,5763)
125	3959	(3142,4923)	4964	(4763,5172)	6733	(6470,7005)	11272	(10701,11874)
150	7871	(6380,9945)	9858	(9389,10360)	13501	(12700,14389)	—	

Footnote: Est: Estimated average; 95% CI: 95% Confidence interval; —: estimate for vitamin D supplementation dose is above 20,000 IU a day.

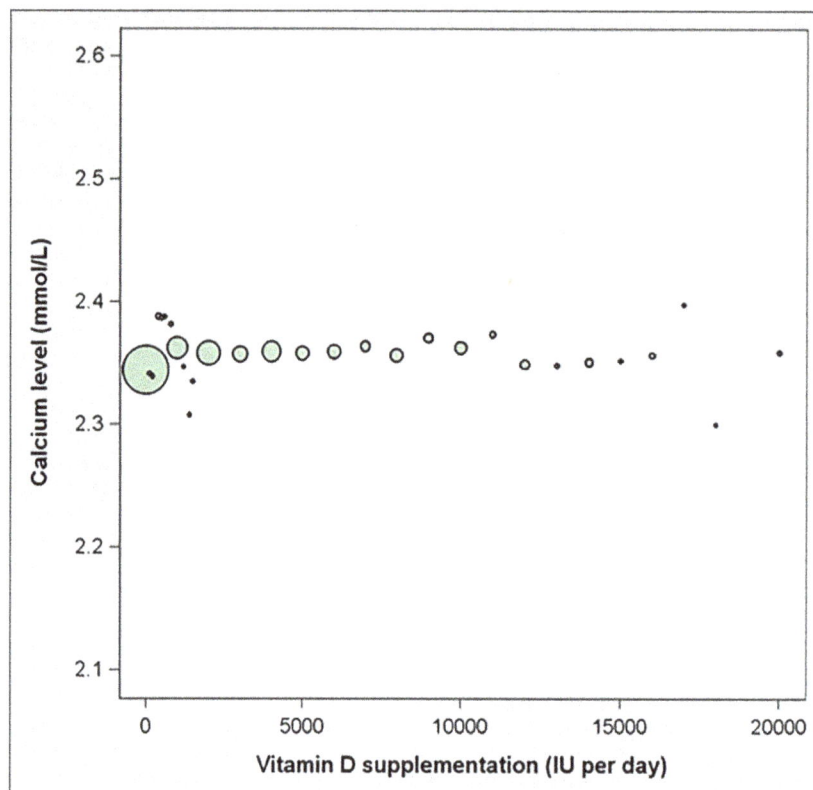

Figure 4. The dose response relationship between vitamin D supplementation and calcium levels. Footnote: Bubbles represent the mean serum calcium level for all reported daily doses. The size of the bubbles is proportional to the number of assessments for each of the reported daily doses. The linear regression line is adjusted for age, gender, BMI, season and calcium supplementation.

and obese individuals (provided in Table 4). These recommendations appeared 2 to 3 times higher for obese participants relative to normal weight subjects, depending on the 25(OH)D target level. This is consistent with the Endocrine Society's recommendation that obese subjects be given two to three times more vitamin D [7,20]. Estimates for overweight individuals appeared approximately 1.5 times higher relative to normal weight subjects. The number of underweight participants was relatively small though do suggest underweight subjects need less vitamin D supplementation relative to normal weight subjects. Others had reported an absence of differences between underweight and normal weight subjects [31]. This study recommends guidelines for vitamin D supplementation be specific for normal weight, overweight and obese individuals, but this study does not recommend specific supplementation levels or specific 25(OH)D target levels.

We observed an exponential dose response relationship whereby serum 25(OH)D levels off with increasing levels of oral vitamin D supplementation. On average, serum 25(OH)D was estimated to increase by approximately 12.0 nmol/L per 1,000 IU in the supplementation interval 0 to 1,000 IU per day and by 1.1 nmol/L per 1,000 IU in the supplementation interval of 15,000 to 20,000 IU per day. Other studies reported that an additional 1,000 IU of vitamin D could increase serum 25(OH)D by approximately 20 to 25 nmol/L [24,32]. The substantial differences may arise from their focus on subjects with low baseline serum 25(OH)D levels, whereas our study had enrolled healthy volunteers. Also Garland et al. [23] and Aloia et al. [11] had reported dose response relationships that leveled off. Garland et al. [23] modeled cross sectional observations of 3,667 US based

community volunteers and Aloia et al. [11] plotted aggregated outcomes of 62 controlled trials. The increase in serum levels per unit increase in supplementation varied across the three studies as a result of, at least in part, differences in study population characteristics. Participants of the present study resided at, on average, a latitude of 53 degrees [21] and had presumably less subcutaneous production of vitamin D by sun exposure. Participants of the present study reportedly without supplemental vitamin D had an average serum level of 68 nmol/L, which approximates the Canadian average of 67.7 nmol/L [33]. Luxwolda et al [34] reported serum 25(OH)D levels ranging from 58 to 171 nmol/L (average 115 nmol/L with 90% having serum 25(OH)D of less than 150 nmol/L) for traditional living populations in East Africa and suggested that this may represent 'natural levels'. The present study shows that on average the upper limit of 171 nmol/L was not reached with oral supplementation of 20,000 IU per day.

The IOM report states that vitamin D toxicity is rare at 10,000 IU per day but more common with regular doses of 50,000 IU per day, suggesting the toxicity range likely starts at 500 nmol/L [8]. In the present study where substantial numbers of participants reported up to 20,000 IU of vitamin D per day, and some even more, the highest serum 25(OH)D value observed was 394 nmol/L. This seems consistent with safety studies that reported an absence of adverse effects from vitamin D doses of up to 50,000 IU per day [35,36]. Our observation that supplementation dose was not associated with hypercalcemia in a statistically significant manner is consistent with an earlier report

Table 5. Determinants of serum calcium and hypercalcemia based on 10,940 assessments from healthy volunteers.

	Serum calcium level		Hypercalcemia	
	β (95%CI)	p-value	OR (95%CI)	p-value
Vitamin D daily dose (per 1000 IU)	0.001(-0.000,0.001)	0.165	0.97(0.91,1.03)	0.286
Calcium supplementation (per 100 mg)	0.003(0.001,0.006)	0.015	1.20(1.03,1.39)	0.023
Age (Years)				
<40	ref.		ref.	
40 to 49	0.003(−0.003,0.009)	0.302	2.09(1.09,4.00)	0.026
50 to 59	0.029(0.023,0.035)	<.001	3.20(1.80,5.67)	<.001
60+	0.044(0.038,0.050)	<.001	5.73(3.32,9.87)	<.001
Gender				
Male	−0.019(−0.024, −0.015)	<.001	0.56(0.39,0.80)	0.001
Female	ref.		ref.	
Weight Status				
Underweight	−0.005(−0.026,0.015)	0.609	1.16(0.28,4.82)	0.837
Normal weight	ref.		ref.	
Overweight	−0.003(−0.009,0.002)	0.239	1.05(0.69,1.59)	0.834
Obesity	0.008(0.002,0.013)	0.009	1.27(0.83,1.93)	0.267
Season				
Spring	−0.024(−0.031, −0.016)	<.001	0.92(0.58,1.47)	0.728
Summer	−0.017(−0.022, −0.011)	<.001	0.57(0.34,0.96)	0.034
Fall	−0.021(−0.027, −0.015)	<.001	0.91(0.59,1.42)	0.682
Winter	ref.		ref.	

Footnote: β: β-coefficient; OR: odds ratio; 95% CI: 95% confidence Interval; ref: reference category; all estimates are adjusted for age, gender, BMI category, season, and supplementation with vitamin D and calcium.

that daily doses of up to 40,000 IU per day are not associated with hypercalcemia [37].

This study represents the first body weight specific characterization of the dose response relationship of a wide range of vitamin D supplementation and serum 25(OH)D levels. The strengths of the study include the large population, the relatively high supplementation dose, and the fact that all serum samples were subjected to the same 25(OH)D assessment methods, with heights and weights measured rather that self-reported. The questions regarding vitamin D supplementation by health professionals may have introduced recall bias and social desirability bias. Information on the duration of using vitamin D supplementation had not been collected. Where participants changed their doses in the months prior to the 25(OH)D assessment, this also may have introduced error. However, we expect the latter error to be small as all participants are aware that the objective of the 25(OH)D assessment is to receive advice on vitamin D supplementation dose, and therefore not likely to changing their supplementation dose in the months prior to the assessment. Although this study included residents of Northern latitude where sun exposure and subcutaneous synthesis of vitamin D are considered limited, and despite our adjustment for season as a proxy of sun exposure, we acknowledge that a precise measure of daily hours of sun exposure may have yielded better estimates. Likewise, where we did adjust for the confounding potential of age, gender, and season, we acknowledge that further adjustment for skin color, physical activity, outdoor activities and dietary intake may have yielded

better estimates. Unlike in blinded trials, confounding by indication, whereby participants whose 25(OH)D levels respond well to vitamin D may lower their dose and participants whose 25(OH)D levels do not respond well may increase their dose, may have biased the estimates of the present study. Lastly, we recommend large randomized controlled trails among healthy subjects be analyzed on BMI differentials in the dose response relationship between vitamin D intake and serum 25(OH)D to confirm the present findings.

In summary, we recommend clinical guidelines for vitamin D supplementation be specific for normal weight, overweight and obese individuals. In this study we provide body weight specific recommendations to reach certain serum 25(OH)D target levels.

Acknowledgments

The authors wish to thank the Pure North S'Energy Foundation for allowing their data to be analyzed for the purpose of this article. They specifically wish to thank the Peter Tran and Ken Fyle for management and validation of the Foundation's data.

Author Contributions

Analyzed the data: JPE. Wrote the manuscript: PJV. Provided feedback and edited the manuscript: JPE JDZ MH EG. Conducted the literature review: JDZ. Conceived and designed the analytic approach: JPE MH EG PJV.

References

1. Cranney A, Horsley T, O'Donnell S, Weiler H, Puil L, et al. (2007) Effectiveness and safety of vitamin D in relation to bone health. Evid Rep Technol Assess (Full Rep) 1–235.

2. Ebeling PR (2014) Vitamin D and bone health: Epidemiologic studies. Bonekey Rep 3: 511.

3. Holick MF (2007) Vitamin D deficiency. N Engl J Med 357: 266–281.

4. Sanabria A, Dominguez LC, Vega V, Osorio C, Duarte D (2011) Cost-effectiveness analysis regarding postoperative administration of vitamin-D and calcium after thyroidectomy to prevent hypocalcaemia. Rev Salud Publica (Bogota) 13: 804–813.

5. Winzenberg T, Jones G (2013) Vitamin D and bone health in childhood and adolescence. Calcif Tissue Int 92: 140–150.

6. Health Canada. Vitamin D and Calcium: Updated Dietary Reference Intakes. Available: http://www.hc-sc.gc.ca/fn-an/nutrition/vitamin/vita-d-eng.php. Accessed 2014 Jan 25.

7. Holick MF, Binkley NC, Bischoff-Ferrari HA, Gordon CM, Hanley DA, et al. (2011) Evaluation, treatment, and prevention of vitamin D deficiency: an Endocrine Society clinical practice guideline. J Clin Endocrinol Metab 96: 1911–1930.

8. Institute of Medicine (2011) Dietary Reference Intakes for Calcium and Vitamin D. The National Academies Press.

9. Heaney RP (2011) Serum 25-hydroxyvitamin D is a reliable indicator of vitamin D status. Am J Clin Nutr 94: 619-20; author reply 620.

10. Holick MF (2010) Vitamin D: Physiology, Molecular Biology, and Clinical Applications. Humana Press.

11. Aloia JF, Patel M, Dimaano R, Li-Ng M, Talwar SA, et al. (2008) Vitamin D intake to attain a desired serum 25-hydroxyvitamin D concentration. Am J Clin Nutr 87: 1952–1958.

12. Blum M, Dallal GE, Dawson-Hughes B (2008) Body size and serum 25 hydroxy vitamin D response to oral supplements in healthy older adults. J Am Coll Nutr 27: 274–279.

13. Chao YS, Brunel L, Faris P, Veugelers PJ (2013) The importance of dose, frequency and duration of vitamin D supplementation for plasma 25-hydroxyvitamin D. Nutrients 5: 4067–4078.

14. Drincic A, Fuller E, Heaney RP, Armas LA (2013) 25-hydroxyvitamin d response to graded vitamin d3 supplementation among obese adults. J Clin Endocrinol Metab 98: 4845–4851.

15. Gallagher JC, Sai A, Templin T, Smith L (2012) Dose response to vitamin D supplementation in postmenopausal women: a randomized trial. Ann Intern Med 156: 425–437.

16. Gallagher JC, Jindal P, Lynette MS (2013) Vitamin D does not Increase Calcium Absorption in Young Women: A Randomized Clinical Trial. J Bone Miner Res.

17. Lee P, Greenfield JR, Seibel MJ, Eisman JA, Center JR (2009) Adequacy of vitamin D replacement in severe deficiency is dependent on body mass index. Am J Med 122: 1056–1060.

18. Tepper S, Shahar DR, Geva D, Ish-Shalom S (2013) Predictors of serum 25(Oh)D increase following bimonthly supplementation with 100,000IU vitamin D in healthy, men aged 25–65 years. J Steroid Biochem Mol Biol.

19. Zittermann A, Ernst JB, Gummert JF, Borgermann J (2013) Vitamin D supplementation, body weight and human serum 25-hydroxyvitamin D response: a systematic review. Eur J Nutr.

20. Holick MF, Binkley NC, Bischoff-Ferrari HA, Gordon CM, Hanley DA, et al. (2012) Guidelines for preventing and treating vitamin D deficiency and insufficiency revisited. J Clin Endocrinol Metab 97: 1153–1158.

21. Chao YS, Brunel L, Faris P, Veugelers PJ (2013) Vitamin D status of Canadians employed in northern latitudes. Occup Med (Lond) 63: 485–493.

22. Heaney RP, French CB, Nguyen S, Ferreira M, Baggerly LL, et al. (2013) A novel approach localizes the association of vitamin D status with insulin resistance to one region of the 25-hydroxyvitamin D continuum. Adv Nutr 4: 303–310.

23. Garland CF, French CB, Baggerly LL, Heaney RP (2011) Vitamin D supplement doses and serum 25-hydroxyvitamin D in the range associated with cancer prevention. Anticancer Res 31: 607–611.

24. Heaney RP, Davies KM, Chen TC, Holick MF, Barger-Lux MJ (2003) Human serum 25-hydroxycholecalciferol response to extended oral dosing with cholecalciferol. Am J Clin Nutr 77: 204–210.

25. Vieth R (2005). The pharmacology of vitamin D, including fortification strategies. In FD, GF, & PJ (Eds.), *Vitamin D* (pp. 995–1015).

26. Vieth R (1999) Vitamin D supplementation, 25-hydroxyvitamin D concentrations, and safety. Am J Clin Nutr 69: 842–856.

27. Akaike H (1973) Information theory as an extension of the maximum likelihood principle. In: Petrov BN, Csaki F. editors. Second International Symposium on Information Theory. Budapest. pp. 267–281.

28. World Health Organization (2006) BMI Classification: The International Classification of adult underweight, overweight and obesity according to BMI.

29. Nelson ML, Blum JM, Hollis BW, Rosen C, Sullivan SS (2009) Supplements of 20 microg/d cholecalciferol optimized serum 25-hydroxyvitamin D concentrations in 80% of premenopausal women in winter. J Nutr 139: 540–546.

30. Shab-Bidar S, Bours SP, Geusens PP, van der Velde RY, Janssen MJ, et al. (2013) Suboptimal effect of different vitamin D3 supplementations and doses adapted to baseline serum 25(OH)D on achieved 25(OH)D levels in patients with a recent fracture: a prospective observational study. Eur J Endocrinol 169: 597–604.

31. Divasta AD, Feldman HA, Brown JN, Giancaterino C, Holick MF, et al. (2011) Bioavailability of vitamin D in malnourished adolescents with anorexia nervosa. J Clin Endocrinol Metab 96: 2575–2580.

32. Vieth R (2006) Critique of the considerations for establishing the tolerable upper intake level for vitamin D: critical need for revision upwards. J Nutr 136: 1117–1122.

33. Langlois K, Greene-Finestone L, Little J, Hidiroglou N, Whiting S (2010) Vitamin D status of Canadians as measured in the 2007 to 2009 Canadian Health Measures Survey. Health Rep 21: 47–55.

34. Luxwolda MF, Kuipers RS, Kema IP, Dijck-Brouwer DA, Muskiet FA (2012) Traditionally living populations in East Africa have a mean serum 25-hydroxyvitamin D concentration of 115 nmol/l. Br J Nutr 108: 1557–1561.

35. Bischoff-Ferrari HA, Shao A, Dawson-Hughes B, Hathcock J, Giovannucci E, et al. (2010) Benefit-risk assessment of vitamin D supplementation. Osteoporos Int 21: 1121–1132.

36. Hathcock JN, Shao A, Vieth R, Heaney R (2007) Risk assessment for vitamin D. Am J Clin Nutr 85: 6–18.

37. Cianferotti L, Marcocci C (2012) Subclinical vitamin D deficiency. Best Pract Res Clin Endocrinol Metab 26: 523–537.

15

Complication Probability Models for Radiation-Induced Heart Valvular Dysfunction: Do Heart-Lung Interactions Play a Role?

Laura Cella[1,2]*, Giuseppe Palma[1], Joseph O. Deasy[3], Jung Hun Oh[3], Raffaele Liuzzi[1,2], Vittoria D'Avino[1], Manuel Conson[1,2], Novella Pugliese[4], Marco Picardi[4], Marco Salvatore[2], Roberto Pacelli[1,2]

1 Institute of Biostructure and Bioimaging, National Council of Research (CNR), Naples, Italy, 2 Department of Advanced Biomedical Sciences, Federico II University School of Medicine, Naples, Italy, 3 Department of Medical Physics, Memorial Sloan Kettering Cancer Center, New York, New York, United States of America, 4 Department of Clinical Medicine and Surgery, Federico II University School of Medicine, Naples, Italy

Abstract

Purpose: The purpose of this study is to compare different normal tissue complication probability (NTCP) models for predicting heart valve dysfunction (RVD) following thoracic irradiation.

Methods: All patients from our institutional Hodgkin lymphoma survivors database with analyzable datasets were included ($n = 90$). All patients were treated with three-dimensional conformal radiotherapy with a median total dose of 32 Gy. The cardiac toxicity profile was available for each patient. Heart and lung dose-volume histograms (DVHs) were extracted and both organs were considered for Lyman-Kutcher-Burman (LKB) and Relative Seriality (RS) NTCP model fitting using maximum likelihood estimation. Bootstrap refitting was used to test the robustness of the model fit. Model performance was estimated using the area under the receiver operating characteristic curve (AUC).

Results: Using only heart-DVHs, parameter estimates were, for the LKB model: $D_{50} = 32.8$ Gy, $n = 0.16$ and $m = 0.67$; and for the RS model: $D_{50} = 32.4$ Gy, $s = 0.99$ and $\gamma = 0.42$. AUC values were 0.67 for LKB and 0.66 for RS, respectively. Similar performance was obtained for models using only lung-DVHs (LKB: $D_{50} = 33.2$ Gy, $n = 0.01$, $m = 0.19$, AUC = 0.68; RS: $D_{50} = 24.4$ Gy, $s = 0.99$, $\gamma = 2.12$, AUC = 0.66). Bootstrap result showed that the parameter fits for lung-LKB were extremely robust. A combined heart-lung LKB model was also tested and showed a minor improvement (AUC = 0.70). However, the best performance was obtained using the previously determined multivariate regression model including maximum heart dose with increasing risk for larger heart and smaller lung volumes (AUC = 0.82).

Conclusions: The risk of radiation induced valvular disease cannot be modeled using NTCP models only based on heart dose-volume distribution. A predictive model with an improved performance can be obtained but requires the inclusion of heart and lung volume terms, indicating that heart-lung interactions are apparently important for this endpoint.

Editor: Roberto Amendola, ENEA, Italy

Funding: This work was partially supported by grants from Ministero dell'Istruzione, dell'Università e della Ricerca (MIUR) in the framework of Fondo per gli Interventi alla Ricerca di Base (FIRB,RBFR10Q0PT_001 and RBNE08YFN3). The funders had no role in study design, data collection and analysis, decision to publish, or preparation of the manuscript.

Competing Interests: The authors have declared that no competing interests exist.

* Email: laura.cella@cnr.it

Introduction

Technological advances in radiation therapy have increased user control over organ-at-risk dose distributions. In a modern radiotherapy setting, radiobiological models potentially play an essential role and normal tissue complication probability (NTCP) modeling may help to identify the optimal plan that minimizes side effects for individual patients.

The toxicity endpoint that have been modeled include radiation-associated cardiac disease [1]. Indeed, late cardiac toxicity is one of the most feared side effects of therapeutic thoracic radiation therapy. Unfortunately, relevant data are limited. Modeling radiation-induced heart disease is hampered both by the relatively low incidence of the complication and the lack of long term results from 3D-based thoracic RT [2–4].

Lyman-Kutcher-Burman (LKB) and Relative Seriality (RS) NTCP heart parameter values have been summarized in the QUANTEC Reports dedicated to radiation-dose volume effects on the heart [1]. Those parameters were estimated for endpoints like pericarditis/pericardial effusion, very delayed cardiac mortality, as well as cardiac perfusion defects. Results were extracted from breast cancer and Hodgkin's lymphoma (HL) patients treated with doses up to 40–50 Gy during the 1970's and the 1980's [5–7]. Importantly, individual dosimetric data were not always available,

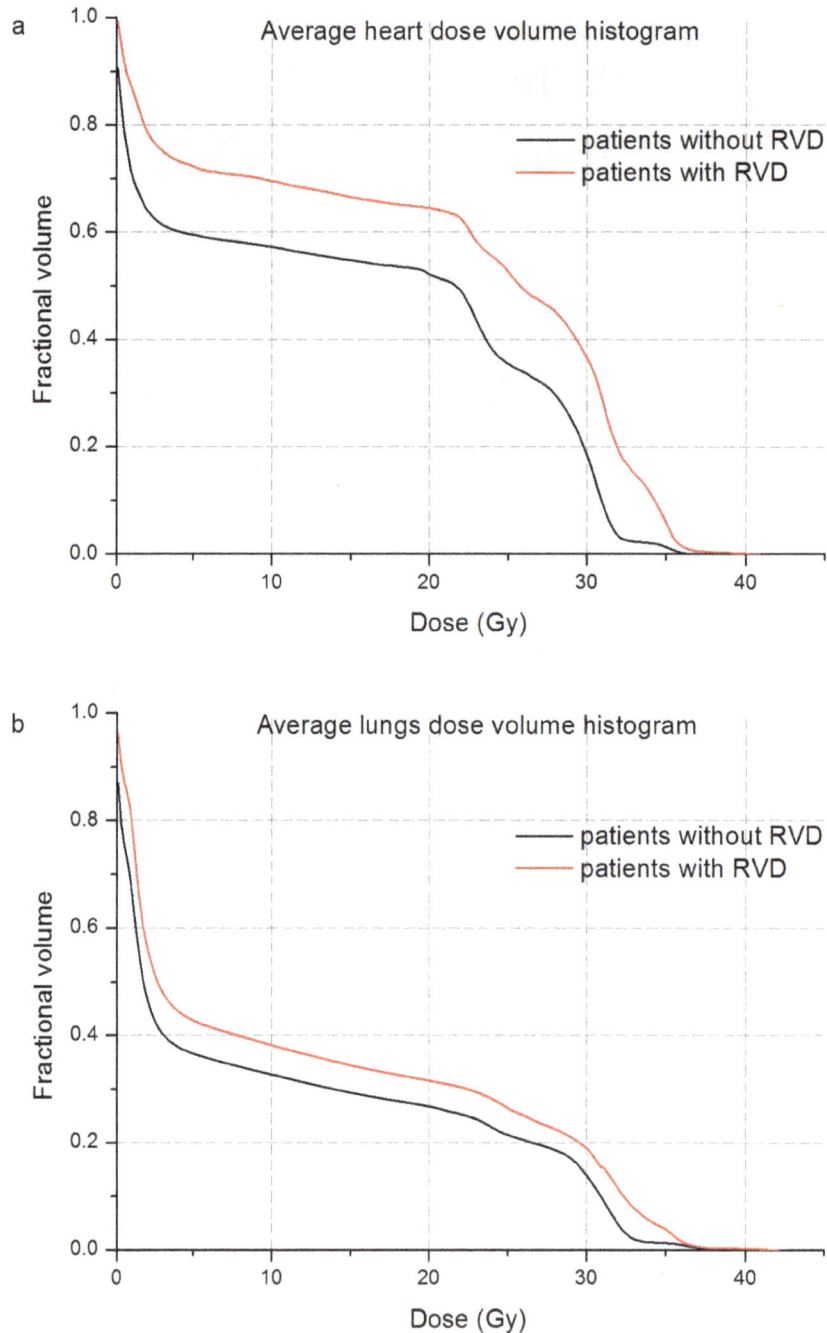

Figure 1. Mean cumulative DVHs for heart (a) and for lung (b). Red line: patients who developed radiation-induced valvular defects; black line: patients who did not develop radiation-induced valvular defects.

and the heart doses were reconstructed as well as possible. Since then, the standard treatment for HL has considerably changed, especially in the last decade [8–10].

An additional, well-recognized effect of chest radiation exposure is the development of valvular abnormalities [11], that represent an important endpoint to analyze due to their role in the progressive development from asymptomatic dysfunction to overt heart failure [12]. Dose-based NTCP models such as the LKB and RS [13,14] models are the most well-known and traditionally accepted methods for predicting toxicity after radiation treatment.

However, to date, no LKB or RS NTCP parameters for this specific radiation-induced heart disease are available.

The mentioned traditional NTCP models use only information about the dose distribution and fractionation. However, it has been reported how RT outcomes may also be affected by multiple factors other than the dose [15]. In a previous study [16], using a different modeling philosophy, we have developed a data-driven multivariate logistic predictive model with a good predictive power for the development of radio-induced valvular defects (RVD) in a population of 56 HL survivors. Besides the heart maximum dose and cardiac volume, that study established the statistical importance of lung volume in the risk prediction of heart toxicity supporting the hypothesis of cardiac damage indirectly caused by additional lung volume irradiation [17–19].

The aim of the present study is to test the predictive power of traditional LKB and the RS NTCP models for the induction of asymptomatic RVDs using a dataset of HL patients, and to compare this to an updated multivariate logistic regression model fit to the current, larger dataset. We proceed by fitting the NTCP model parameters first from heart dose-volume parameters, and separately lung dose-volume parameters, and then with both heart and lung dose-volume parameters. We also update the multivariate logistic NTCP model, using all available parameters, and compare the results.

Methods

Clinical and dosimetric data

The patient dataset reported in this analysis includes all eligible patients from a study of HL survivors [20]. Between 2001 and 2012, 132 total patients entered the clinical study, of whom 90 patients were eligible for the current analysis. Eligibility criteria include availability of complete cardiac toxicity profile before and after RT, lack of any pretreatment cardiac disease, a minimum follow-up of 36 months, and the availability of 3-D treatment dose distributions. The data were analyzed anonymously. Patients and treatment characteristics have been described in detail elsewhere [21,22], although this cohort now includes 90 patients compared to 56 previously reported on. Briefly, all patients received post-chemotherapy supradiaphragmatic involved-field RT at our radiation oncology department, and were retrospectively reviewed for radio-induced valvular defects (RVD). A diagnosis of RVD was based on the presence of regurgitation and/or stenosis (mild, moderate, or severe) in at least one of the aortic, mitral, tricuspid and pulmonary valves. Patients were followed up for a median time of 80 months (range 38–140 months).

All patients were treated with CT-based 3D conformal RT with a median total dose of 32 Gy (range, 21–41 Gy) in 20 daily fractions of 1.5–1.8 Gy. RT was administered with anterior-posterior/posterior-anterior photon fields (energies: 6 to 20 MV). When needed, the segmented field technique was employed to improve dose uniformity [23]. Multigrid superposition dose calculation algorithm that corrects for the presence of heterogeneous tissues was applied. For all patients, the whole heart was retrospectively contoured on the planning CT-images applying the heart atlas proposed by Feng et al. [24]. Total lung tissue was contoured following RTOG 1106 recommendations [25].

For each patient, dose-volume histogram (DVH) extraction from treatment planning data was performed using the CERR open-source available software platform [26]. In this way, individual DICOM RT plans (doses and contoured heart and lungs) were converted into the Matlab/CERR format for further analysis.

All participants gave written informed consent and the patient data were analyzed anonymously, This retrospective study was approved by the local Ethics Committee (Comitato Etico per le Attività Biomediche, Università Federico II di Napoli, n.222-10).

Normal tissue complication probability models

The NTCP models used in this study include the Lyman-Kutcher-Burman (LKB) model [14] and the relative seriality (RS) model [13]. LKB and RS modeling was performed taking into account the irradiation of the heart and at a second step the irradiation of the lungs.

The LKB model

We used the LKB model recast on the concept of generalized equivalent uniform dose ($gEUD$) [27]. This model can be expressed as:

$$NTCP_{LKB} = \int_{-\infty}^{t} \exp\left(\frac{-u^2}{2}\right) du$$

$$t = \frac{gEUD - D_{50}}{mD_{50}}$$

where D_i is the dose and v_i is the relative volume of the i-th bin of the differential DVH. The model contains three parameters (D_{50}, m, n)$_{LKB}$. D_{50} is the uniform dose given to the entire organ volume that results in 50% complication probability, m is a measure of the steepness of the slope of the model curve and n is a parameter describing the volume dependence of the considered tissue. Small values ($<<1$) of n indicate a sensitivity to the highest dose volume, even if small, whereas values closer to 1 indicate that the response is due to an average of effects across the organ.

The RS model

In the relative seriality (RS) model, the probability of a complication after irradiation of a relative volume v_i at a dose D_i is given by:

$$NTCP_{RS} = \left\{ 1 - \prod_i [1 - P(D_i)^s]^{v_i} \right\}^{1/s}$$

$$P(D_i) = 2^{-\exp\left[e\gamma_s\left(1 - \frac{D_i}{D_{50}}\right) \right]}$$

where $P(D_i)$ is the probability of complication due to the irradiation of the relative volume v_i at the dose D_i described by an approximation of Poisson statistics. The model contains three parameters (D_{50}, γ, s)$_{RS}$. D_{50} has the same meaning as for the LKB model, γ is a slope parameter which affects the steepness of the sigmoid shape dose-response curve, and s is a parameter that represents the 'relative seriality' of organ/tissue under consideration (the ratio of serial subunits to all subunits of the organ). Large values (≈ 1) of s indicate a serial structure and small values ($<<1$) indicate a parallel structure.

Correction for fractionation size

The HL patients analyzed in this study were treated with different fraction sizes (1.5 Gy, 1.6 Gy, or 1.8 Gy) other than 2 Gy. In order to compare our results on NTCP parameters estimates with those reported in literature [1] referred to the standard fractionation of 2 Gy, we corrected all heart and lungs DVH bins according to the following equation based on the linear quadratic model [28]:

$$NTD_{2Gy} = D_x \left(\frac{\frac{\alpha}{\beta} + x}{\frac{\alpha}{\beta} + 2} \right)$$

Table 1. Parameters estimates and 95% confidence intervals of LKB and RS NTCP models for heart and lung dose volume histograms fitting.

	D50 (Gy)	m	n	r_s	AUC	LLH
LKB heart	32.8	0.66	0.16	0.27	0.67	−51.6
	(25.9, 44.7)	(0.41, 1)	(0.10, 0.89)		(0.56, 0.78)	
LKB lung	33.2	0.19	0.01	0.28	0.69	−49.7
	(31.3–35.5)	(0.13–0.32)	(0.01–0.03)		(0.58, 0.78)	
	D50 (Gy)	γ	s	r_s	AUC	LLH
RS heart	32.4	0.42	0.99	0.25	0.66	−52.3
	(22.7, 48.5)	(0.24, 0.62)	(0.0–1.0)		(0.55–0.76)	
RS lung	24.4	2.12	0.99	0.26	0.66	−51.1
	(22.3, 26.7)	(0.3–3.8)	(0.67–1.0)		(0.55–0.76)	

Abbreviation- LKB: Lyman-Kutcher-Burman, RS: Relative Seriality, NTCP: Normal Tissue Complication Probability, D_{50}: uniform dose given to the entire organ volume that results in 50% complication probability, r_s: Spearman's correlation coefficient, AUC: the area under the receiver operator characteristic curve, LLH: log-likelihood (LLH).

where NTD_{2Gy} is the normalized total dose to 2 Gy fractions and D_x is the dose for the fractionation scheme x Gy. The α/β ratio was set to 3 Gy for the heart [18] and to 4 Gy for the lungs [29].

Maximum likelihood fitting and confidence intervals

The maximum likelihood (ML) method was employed to find the best fit values for the parameters $(D_{50}, m, n)_{LKB}$ and $(D_{50}, \gamma, s)_{RS}$ of the $NTCP_{LKB}$ and $NTCP_{RS}$, respectively.

The method maximizes the log-likelihood function (LLH):

$$LLH = \sum_{yi=1} \ln NTCP + \sum_{yi=0} \ln(1 - NTCP)$$

for the known binary outcome (heart valvular toxicity), averaged over the patients (y_i) of the available dataset. Fits were made separately considering heart and lung dose-volume histograms.

The LLH function was numerically maximized by the Nelder-Mead Simplex Method (Matlab implementation: FMINSEARCH function) using an in-house developed library for Matlab. Ninety five percent confidence intervals for parameters estimates were obtained using the profile likelihood method [30]. Following this method, each parameter belonging to the set $(D_{50}, m, n)_{LKB}$ (or equivalently to the set $(D_{50}, \gamma, s)_{RS}$) was varied around its ML estimate (optimum LLH) while the other 2 parameters were fixed at their ML estimate. The 95% confidence bounds were determined reducing the maximum LLH by one half of the χ^2 inverse cumulative distribution function associated with a 95% confidence level, so as to obtain the iso-likelihood contours in each Cartesian plane of the parameters space $(D50, m, n)$, or equivalently, of the (D_{50}, γ, s) space.

In correspondence to the parameters values belonging to the iso-likelihood contours, a bundle of NTCP curves was calculated and the 95% confidence region for the model fit was thus estimated [31].

Of note, even if a model fits the available dataset, it may fail to be predictive on a different patient population [32]. The bootstrap method was employed to determine the spread in ML estimation of NTCP parameters. The bootstrap resampling method works by refitting the NTCP model using the ML estimation to many pseudo-datasets, which are created by randomly copying or re-copying individual patient datasets from the input data set (20000 bootstrap resamples were used).

Model evaluation and comparisons

The prediction performance of each NTCP was assessed and the different models were compared. In the comparison, we also included a multivariate logistic NTCP model. In a previous analysis of RVD [16] on a subset (56 patients) of the present HL survivors dataset, we developed a 3-variable logistic regression model consisting of the maximum heart dose (HD$_{max}$), heart volume (HVol), and lungs volume (LVol) given by

$$NTCP_{Logistic} = \frac{1}{1 + e^{-g(x)}}$$

$$g(x) = 0.14 \times HD_{max} + 0.01 \times HVol$$
$$- 0.002 \times LVol - 5.65$$

where HD_{max} was expressed in Gy and $HVol$ and $LVol$ in cc.

For model evaluation, the comparison between mean predicted rates of RVD by each model and the observed rates for patients grouped according to increasing model risk was performed. Patients were binned according to the NTCP model being considered, with a number of patients in each bin as equal as possible.

Model predictive power was assessed by use of Spearman's rank correlation coefficient (r_s). The receiver-operating characteristic (ROC) analysis and the area under the ROC curve (AUC) metrics were employed in order to compare the discriminating ability of each model fit. The discrimination value on the ROC curve, i.e. the cut-off point optimally classifying patients in a binary prediction problem [33], was determined by Youden's J statistic. The ROC curve was created by plotting the fraction of true positives out of the total actual positives (TPR = true positive rate or sensitivity) vs. the fraction of false positives out of the total actual negatives (FPR = false positive rate or 1-specificity), at various probability threshold settings. Youden's index is the difference between the TPR and the FPR. Maximizing this indicates an optimal cut-off point. ROC curve results were compared using a Z test. Statistical analysis was performed with MedCalc version 12.3.

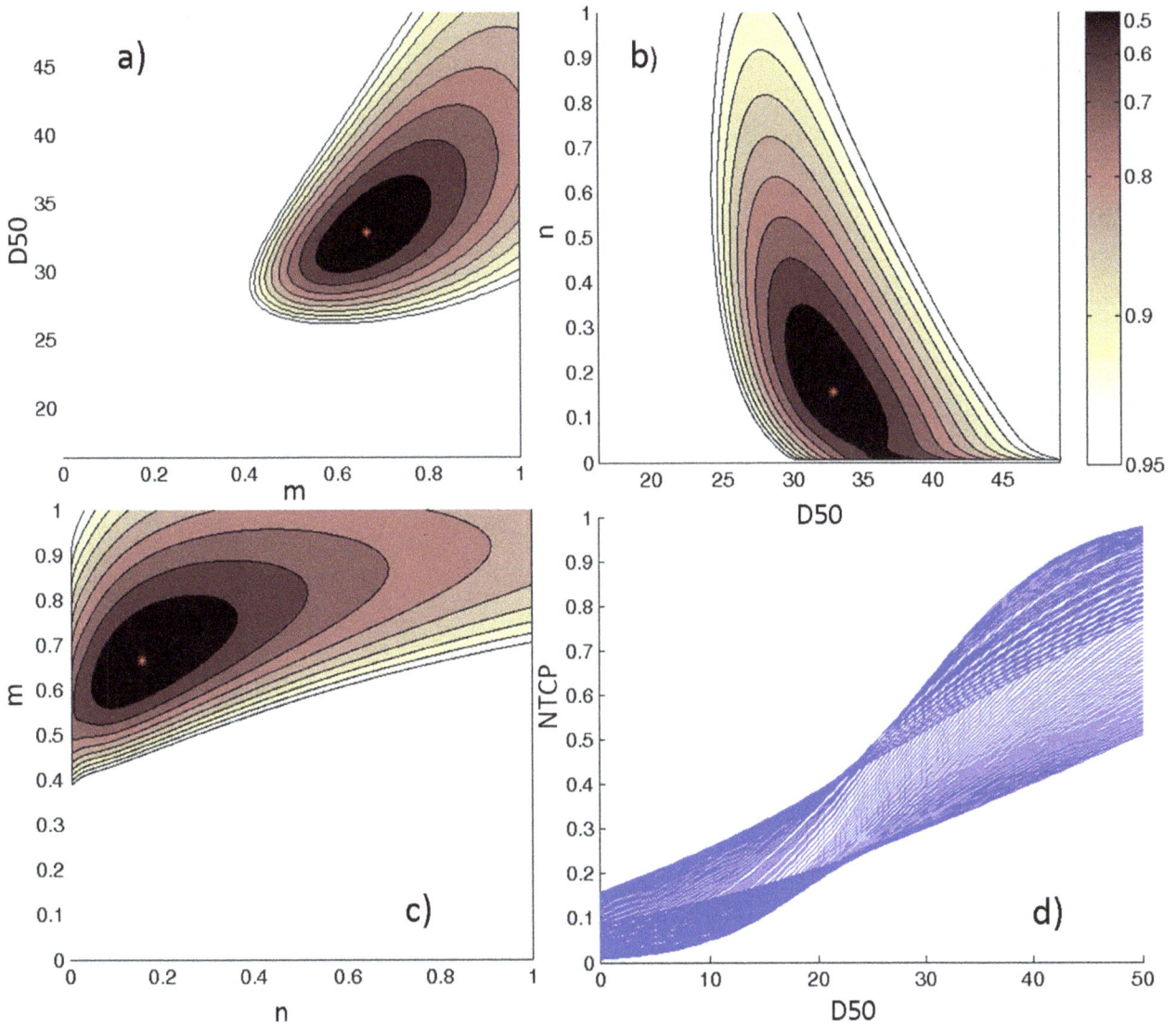

Figure 2. Likelihood estimation values plotted as a function of heart LKB parameters. a) m and D_{50} for a fixed value of $n = 0.16$; b) D_{50} and n for a fixed value of $m = 0.67$; c) n and m for a fixed value of $D_{50} = 32.8$; d) NTCP bundle of curves showing 95% confidence interval region for the model fit. The red point corresponds to the optimum LLH. *Abbreviation*- LKB: Lyman-Kutcher-Burman, D_{50}: uniform dose given to the entire organ volume that results in 50% complication probability, NTCP: Normal Tissue Complication Probability, LLH: Log-likelihood.

Table 2. Summary of mean and standard deviations of LKB and RS NTCP model parameters obtained with maximum likelihood estimation for bootstrap samples.

	D_{50} (Gy)	SD	m	SD	n	SD
LLKB heart	36.1	5.5	0.67	0.11	0.11	0.12
LLKB lung	33.9	1.4	0.22	0.03	0.01	0.02
	D_{50} (Gy)	SD	γ	SD	s	SD
RRS heart	32.7	3.1	0.43	0.07	0.99	0.06
RRS lung	24.3	0.83	2.16	0.56	0.99	0.04

Abbreviation- LKB: Lyman-Kutcher-Burman, RS: Relative Seriality, NTCP: Normal Tissue Complication Probability, D_{50}: uniform dose given to the entire organ volume that results in 50% complication probability, SD: standard deviation.

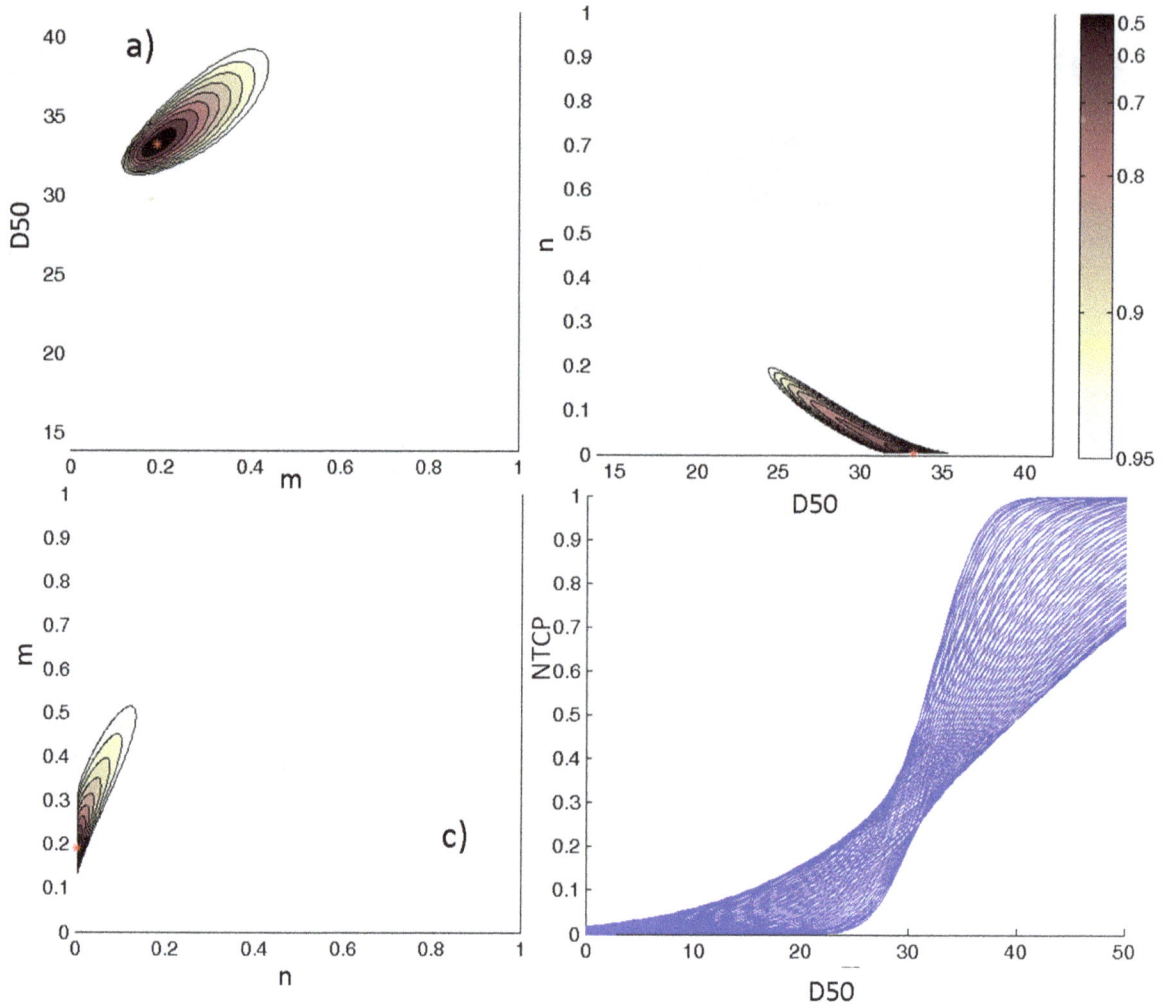

Figure 3. Likelihood estimation values plotted as a function of lung LKB parameters. a) m and D_{50} for a fixed value of $n = 0.01$; b) D_{50} and n for a fixed value of $m = 0.19$; c) n and m for a fixed value of $D_{50} = 33.2$; d) NTCP bundle of curves showing 95% confidence interval for the model fit. The red point corresponds to the optimum LLH. *Abbreviation*- LKB: Lyman-Kutcher-Burman, D_{50}: uniform dose given to the entire organ volume that results in 50% complication probability, NTCP: Normal Tissue Complication Probability, LLH: Log-likelihood.

Results

Twenty-seven out of 90 patients (30%) experienced at least one kind of RVD. The mean cumulative heart DVHs and the mean cumulative lung DVHs for patients who developed complication and complication-free patients are illustrated in figures 1.a and 1.b. Heart and lung clinic- dosimetric variables are reported in Table S1.

LKB and RS model fitting based on heart dose-volume parameters

Maximum likelihood estimation and associated confidence intervals (CIs) for the LKB and RS parameters obtained considering the heart irradiation are provided in Table 1. The LKB and RS models showed similar optimal model fits values: the D_{50} were identical and both volume parameters were consistent with a serial heart architecture ($n = 0.16$ and $s = 0.99$). For the LKB model, the obtained iso-likelihood contours in each Cartesian plane of the parameters space (D_{50}, m, n) are illustrated in figure 2a–c. The corresponding bundle of NTCP$_{LKB}$ curves are plotted in figure 2d. From Table 1, we can observe a large 95%

CI for D_{50} in both LKB and RS models. The volume parameter 95% CI for the LKB model is quite wide while RS model even includes the whole allowed range for the s value, thus suggesting a poor fit of the model to the dataset.

The Spearman's coefficient and the AUC for each model are also reported in Table 1. The discrimination values were 0.36 and 0.33 for NTCP$_{LKB}$ and NTCP$_{RS,}$ respectively.

Table 2 reports the results for bootstrap cohorts showing that the mean values for heart RS parameters are close to the exact fit to the whole patient cohort.

LKB and RS model fits based on lung dose-volume parameters

Maximum likelihood estimations for the LKB and RS parameters obtained using lungs DVHs are provided in Table 1 along with 95% CI. Iso-likelihood contours and NTCP curve bundle for LKB model are illustrated in figure 3a–d.

The LKB and RS models showed similar volume parameters values suggesting a pronounced ($n = 0.01$ or $s = 0.99$) dependence on the high-dose region when the lung is used to model heart toxicity. Of note, there is a difference of about 10 Gy between the

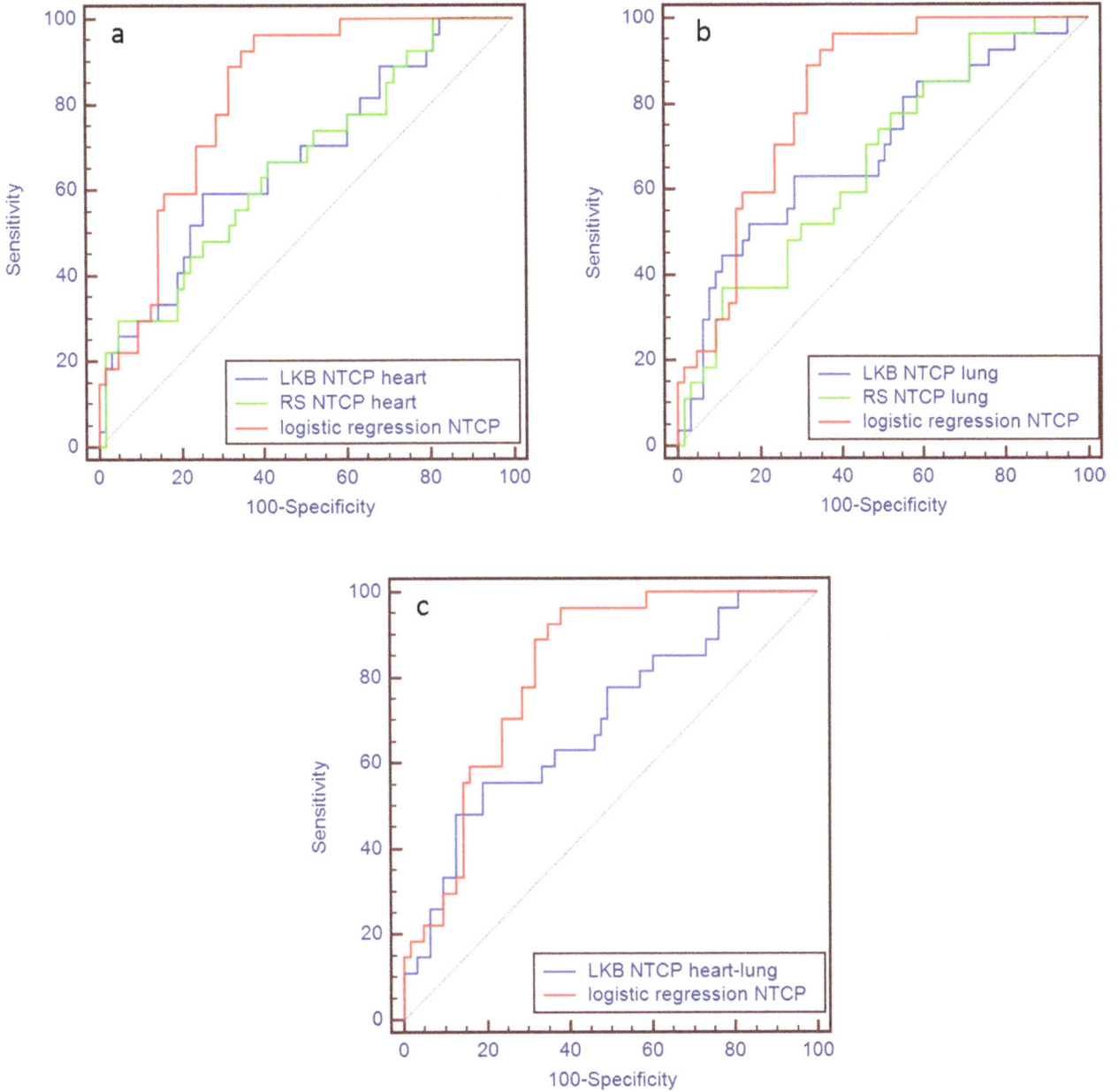

Figure 4. ROC curve comparison. Logistic regression model vs. LKB and RS NTCP model for heart (a) and lungs (b). Logistic regression model vs. combined heart-lung LKB NTCP model (c). *Abbreviation-* ROC: receiver operating characteristic, LKB: Lyman-Kutcher-Burman, RS: Relative Seriality, NTCP: Normal Tissue Complication Probability.

LKB and RS estimates of D_{50}. The 95% CI values obtained for all three parameters of the lung LKB model showed the very good fit result. For the RS model, only two out of three model parameters had narrow CI, being the γ interval of 0.3–3.8.

The r_s coefficient and the AUC values for each model are reported in Table 1. The discrimination values were 0.27 and 0.40 for $NTCP_{LKB}$ and $NTCP_{RS}$, respectively.

Table 2 reports the results for bootstrap cohorts showing the robustness of lung LKB fit procedures.

LKB combined heart-lung fitting

Beyond parameters estimates for NTCP models for heart valve dysfunction, we explored the possible combined contribution of

both heart and lung irradiation to radiation related heart toxicity. In light of the good fitting results obtained for the lung LKB model, we constructed an interaction $gEUD$ variable defined as:

$$gEUD^{int} = \alpha EUD_{heart}$$
$$+ (1-\alpha)EUD_{lung} + \beta EUD_{heart}EUD_{lung}$$
$$\alpha \in [0,1]$$

so as to obtain a LKB $NTCP^{int}$ taking into account the combined organs irradiation. In this way, given the obtained separate estimates of n_{heart} and n_{lung} reported in Table 1, the ML method provides the following parameter estimates: $\alpha = 0.2$,

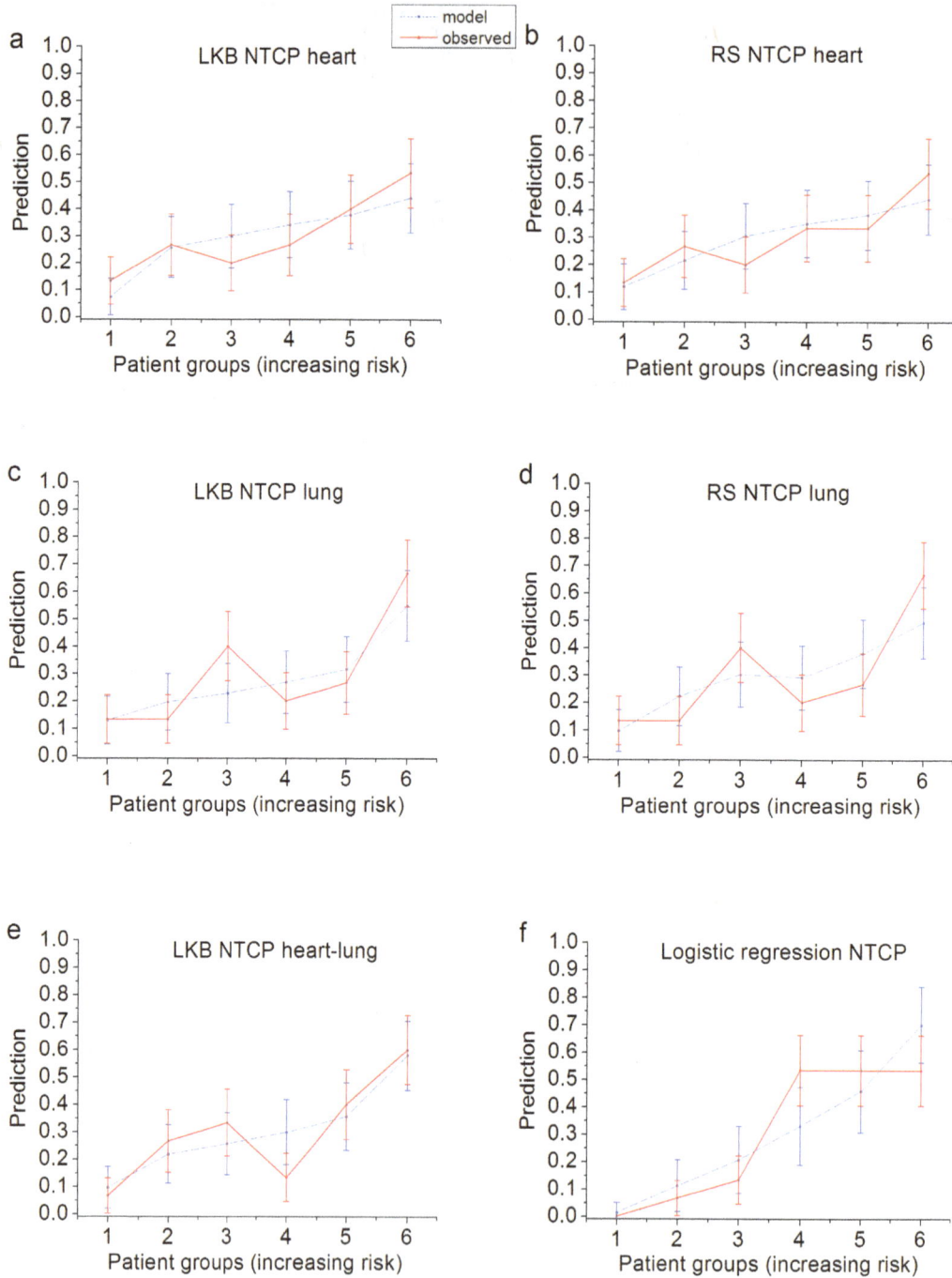

Figure 5. Comparison between the actuarial incidence of radiation-related valvular defects (RVD) in the population and the predicted incidence by each NTCP model. a) heart LKB, b) heart RS, c) lung LKB, d) lung RS, e) three-variable logistic model. Patients were binned according to the considered NTCP model with equal number of patients in each bin. *Abbreviation*- LKB: Lyman-Kutcher-Burman, RS: Relative Seriality, NTCP: Normal Tissue Complication Probability.

$\beta = (2.6 \times 10^5 \text{ Gy})^{-1}$, $D_{50}^{int} = 32.6$ Gy, and $m^{int} = 0.24$. Model prediction performance was only improved slightly, with an AUC of 0.70 (95% CI: 0.59–0.79, discrimination value = 0.34) and an $r_s = 0.31$.

Model comparisons

The logistic NTCP model previously derived using a subset of patients, when applied on the present extended dataset obtained an r_s of 0.50 and an AUC of 0.82 (95% CI: 0.73–0.90, discrimination value = 0.21), thus confirming the good prediction performance of such a model. Of note, the same performance ($r_s = 0.51$ and AUC = 0.82) was obtained refitting the logistic model with the new interaction variable, i.e. $gEUD^{int}$, instead of the heart maximum dose originally included in the logistic regression.

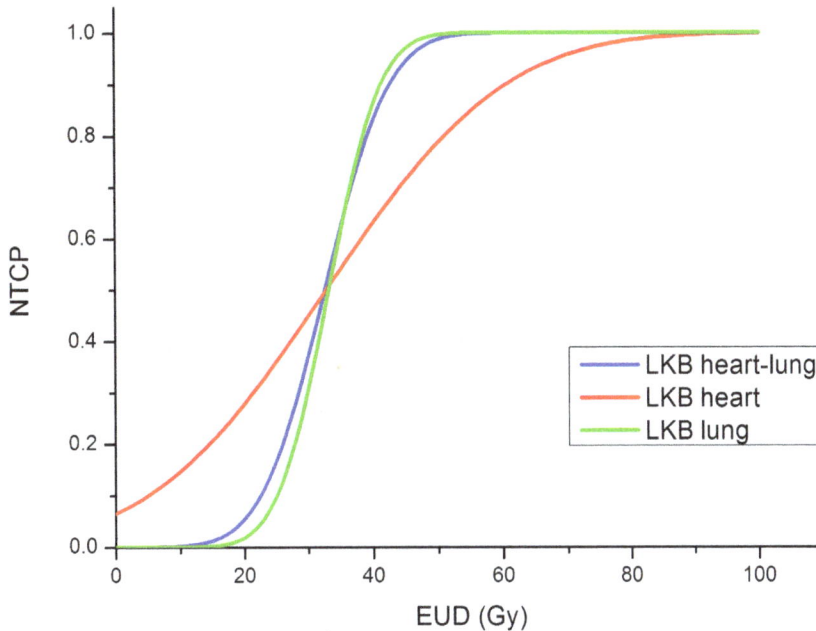

Figure 6. Comparison of different LKB NTCP curves plotted as a function of gEUD. The curve are obtained using parameters estimates by fitting heart (red), lung (green), and combining heart and lung (blue). *Abbreviation-* LKB: Lyman-Kutcher-Burman, NTCP: Normal Tissue Complication Probability, gEUD: generalized Equivalent Uniform Dose.

For the standard NTCP models, including also the combined one, AUC values were considerably lower, and varied in an interval between 0.66 and 0.70. Model comparisons are illustrated by ROC curves in figure 4. There is no difference in prediction performance between LKB and RS models (p>0.5). In addition, independently of the organ chosen as the model input, namely heart DVHs or lung DVHs, we obtain similar prediction performances. The data-driven regression logistic NTCP model, however, applied to the present dataset, resulted in being significantly more predictive (p = 0.03) when compared to heart and lung $NTCP_{LKB}$ and $NTCP_{RS}$ models (figure 4a–b). The logistic regression model outperformed also the combined heart-lung LKB model (figure 4c) although the difference between the AUC values approaches the borderline of statistical significance (p = 0.07).

The comparison between the predicted incidence of RVD by each NTCP model and the actuarial incidence in the population is shown in figure 5.

Discussion

The aim of the present study was to explore alternative options for NTCP modelling for radiation-related heart toxicity. We estimated LKB and RS normal tissue complication probability parameters for radiation induced heart valve dysfunction in order to a) provide a comparator to values reported in the literature [1] for radiation induced heart disease different from RVD; b) consider the possible role of lung irradiation in the development of heart disease [19] and c) understand the benefits of a data-driven approach to NTCP modeling of RVD in contrast to phenomenological models such as LKB or RS models.

The clinical importance of radiation-induced heart disease has been well recognized, including the difficulty in the estimation of related risk due to the long latency time. As pointed out by Trott and coworkers [4] cardiovascular radiation damage may occur insidiously as microvascular ischemic radiation injury leading indirectly to focal myocardial damage and myocardial radiation damage is probably secondary to radiation effects in the myocardial microvascular system. The risk of radiation-induced microvascular disease begins to increase 10 years after irradiation and it is progressive with time and a significant increase of risk has been observed with mean heart doses lower than 10% of the generally accepted tolerance dose to the heart [34]. Data for long-term cardiac mortality were derived from retrospective studies of patients treated with outdated techniques [1] and NTCP parameters were based on the relative seriality model giving a D_{50} of 70 Gy on a Hodgkin's cohort of patients treated between 1972 and 1985. An estimated value of the s parameter equal to one suggested a limited volume dependence. A logistic model [9] has been also applied to dose response in HL in children and adolescents reported in literature [35] estimating a lower D_{50} of 48 Gy for any cardiac morbidity and a D_{50} of 40 Gy for valvular disease.

To date, LKB or RS as an alternative modeling for valvular defects has not been performed, although this type of heart defects has been suggested to be possible candidate as early predictor or surrogate for late cardiac morbidities. In the present work, the parameter estimates obtained from the two NTCP models for RVD data fitted as a function of heart dose were mutually consistent, i.e., both of them confirmed a dependence on the highest-dose volumes of the heart. For both models, the D_{50} value was about 32 Gy. As expected for a mild condition such as valvular disease, we obtained a lower D_{50} value compared to the reported values for cardiac mortality, while it was well within the 95% CI of the results by reported Maraldo et al. [9].

One of the important aspects to consider in modeling radiation induced normal tissue effects such as RVD is that it represents a complex process involving multiple biological pathways and systems. In particular, radiation-induced fibrosis of the lung and its vessels may affect cardiac functions [36] and a heart-lung interaction in radio-induced toxicity to cardiopulmonary system has been reported [19,37,38]. Accordingly, for the first time, a cross modeling exercise was performed: the NTCP models for the radiation induced heart toxicity were also fitted as a function of lung dose. The results of this fitting procedure were comparable or even better (narrower confidence intervals for parameters estimates) than those obtained by heart fitting. For LKB and RS models the D_{50} values ranged in an interval between 24 and 33 Gy. Of note, we observed a serial behavior of the lung when using heart toxicity as endpoint. This result is different from the generally accepted parallel architecture, with a large volume effect, of the lungs when NTCP models were fit to radiation pneumonitis as endpoint. As a consequence, we can hypothesize a different mechanism of damage and a different contribution of lung irradiation to the heart toxicity potentially due to the difference in patho-physiology, although still unknown.

For all models, the spread in ML estimation was assessed using the bootstrap method (Table 2). This gives a measure of how much the different selection of cases might influence the parameters. Interestingly, the more stable results for all three parameters were obtained again for the LKB model applied to the lungs.

Given the good results obtained by applying the LKB model to lung DVHs, we went a step further constructing a combined LKB model based on heart and lung irradiation. The combination parameter α equal to 0.2 reflects a predominant weight of the lung (figure 6) in this analysis, thus confirming the relevance of lung irradiation in the development of RVD. Predictive power, however, was only mildly increased.

The Spearman's correlation coefficients and the ROC analysis gave similar values and thus similar prediction performances for all NTCP models (Table 1), with a higher r_s and only a slightly higher AUC value for the combined LKB model. However, according to figure 5, the combined LKB model is superior as it assigns patients to high or low risk more effectively than all other NTCP models (LKB-heart, LKB-lung, RS-heart, RS-lung). The data-driven logistic regression model (figure 5f) obtained a similar superior behavior. Also, the previously determined logistic regression model applied to the present dataset resulted in a higher prediction performance (AUC = 0.82, r_s = 0.5) compared with all biological NTCP models (AUC values ranging from 0.66 to 0.70).

All together, these results confirm that the heart dose alone cannot be the only critical factor for radiation valvular defects induction. Lung dose may instead contribute significantly, although the mechanism is still to be clarified. In addition, as suggested by the multivariate logistic regression model, the differences in radiation sensitivity between the patients should be also taken into account. Therefore, models based only on critical organ dose may fail to be predictive. In other words, this recalls the concept of biological noise [39] for which all the models are a simplification of more complex biological aspects peculiar to each individual. In the analyzed case, the logistic regression model suggests that the differences in lung and heart volume size may be the key to understand the different individual sensitivity for the development of valvular disease. As already reported in the literature for different radiation-induced toxicity endpoints [40–42], a data-driven and exploratory approach to NTCP modeling emerges as a promising and valuable tool to investigate the radiation induced effects in the cardio-pulmonary system given its multivariate intrinsic nature.

In conclusion, we investigated the application of two traditionally accepted NTCP models, namely Lyman-Kutcher-Burman and Relative Seriality, to clinical data for asymptomatic heart toxicity. Parameter estimates were obtained for RVD data fitted separately as a function of heart dose or lung dose. The performance of each prediction model was assessed. A combined heart and lung LKB model was also proposed, resulting in an increased predictive power. Overall, however, a data-driven regression logistic NTCP model outperformed these simpler NTCP models, validating it as a potentially useful and reliable clinical tool for treatment decision making. It is apparently important to have heart and lung volume parameters as part of the prediction model, although the underlying patho-physiological reasons are not well understood and additional studies will be necessary to further clarify them.

Author Contributions

Conceived and designed the experiments: LC RP. Analyzed the data: LC GP JOD RL RP. Contributed reagents/materials/analysis tools: LC GP JHO VD. Contributed to the writing of the manuscript: LC JOD RP. Data collection: MC NP MP MS.

References

1. Gagliardi G, Constine LS, Moiseenko V, Correa C, Pierce LJ, et al. (2010) Radiation dose-volume effects in the heart. Int J Radiat Oncol Biol Phys 76: S77–85.
2. Kong FM, Pan C, Eisbruch A, Ten Haken RK (2007) Physical models and simpler dosimetric descriptors of radiation late toxicity. Semin Radiat Oncol 17: 108–120.
3. Louwe RJ, Wendling M, van Herk MB, Mijnheer BJ (2007) Three-dimensional heart dose reconstruction to estimate normal tissue complication probability after breast irradiation using portal dosimetry. Med Phys 34: 1354–1363.
4. Trott KR, Doerr W, Facoetti A, Hopewell J, Langendijk J, et al. (2012) Biological mechanisms of normal tissue damage: importance for the design of NTCP models. Radiother Oncol 105: 79–85.
5. Gagliardi G, Lax I, Ottolenghi A, Rutqvist LE (1996) Long-term cardiac mortality after radiotherapy of breast cancer-application of the relative seriality model. Br J Radiol 69: 839–846.
6. Gagliardi G, Lax I, Rutqvist LE (2001) Partial irradiation of the heart. Semin Radiat Oncol 11: 224–233.
7. Eriksson F, Gagliardi G, Liedberg A, Lax I, Lee C, et al. (2000) Long-term cardiac mortality following radiation therapy for Hodgkin's disease: analysis with the relative seriality model. Radiother Oncol 55: 153–162.
8. Maraldo MV, Brodin NP, Aznar MC, Vogelius IR, Munck Af Rosenschold P, et al. (2013) Estimated risk of cardiovascular disease and secondary cancers with

modern highly conformal radiotherapy for early-stage mediastinal Hodgkin lymphoma. Ann Oncol 24: 2113–2118.
9. Maraldo MV, Brodin NP, Vogelius IR, Aznar MC, Munck Af Rosenschold P, et al. (2012) Risk of developing cardiovascular disease after involved node radiotherapy versus mantle field for Hodgkin lymphoma. Int J Radiat Oncol Biol Phys 83: 1232–1237.
10. Cella L, Conson M, Pressello MC, Molinelli S, Schneider U, et al. (2013) Hodgkin's lymphoma emerging radiation treatment techniques: trade-offs between late radio-induced toxicities and secondary malignant neoplasms. Radiat Oncol 8: 22.
11. Heidenreich PA, Hancock SL, Lee BK, Mariscal CS, Schnittger I (2003) Asymptomatic cardiac disease following mediastinal irradiation. J Am Coll Cardiol 42: 743–749.
12. Lancellotti P, Nkomo VT, Badano LP, Bergler-Klein J, Bogaert J, et al. (2013) Expert consensus for multi-modality imaging evaluation of cardiovascular complications of radiotherapy in adults: a report from the European Association of Cardiovascular Imaging and the American Society of Echocardiography. Eur Heart J Cardiovasc Imaging 14: 721–740.
13. Kallman P, Agren A, Brahme A (1992) Tumour and normal tissue responses to fractionated non-uniform dose delivery. Int J Radiat Biol 62: 249–262.
14. Kutcher GJ, Burman C (1989) Calculation of complication probability factors for non-uniform normal tissue irradiation: the effective volume method. Int J Radiat Oncol Biol Phys 16: 1623–1630.

15. El Naqa I, Bradley J, Blanco AI, Lindsay PE, Vicic M, et al. (2006) Multivariable modeling of radiotherapy outcomes, including dose-volume and clinical factors. Int J Radiat Oncol Biol Phys 64: 1275–1286.

16. Cella L, Liuzzi R, Conson M, D'Avino V, Salvatore M, et al. (2013) Multivariate normal tissue complication probability modeling of heart valve dysfunction in Hodgkin lymphoma survivors. Int J Radiat Oncol Biol Phys 87: 304–310.

17. Schultz-Hector S, Sund M, Thames HD (1992) Fractionation response and repair kinetics of radiation-induced heart failure in the rat. Radiother Oncol 23: 33–40.

18. Schultz-Hector S, Trott KR (2007) Radiation-induced cardiovascular diseases: is the epidemiologic evidence compatible with the radiobiologic data? Int J Radiat Oncol Biol Phys 67: 10–18.

19. van Luijk P, Faber H, Meertens H, Schippers JM, Langendijk JA, et al. (2007) The impact of heart irradiation on dose-volume effects in the rat lung. Int J Radiat Oncol Biol Phys 69: 552–559.

20. Di Biase A, Conson M, Cella L, Pugliese N, Picardi M, et al. (2014) Efficacy and toxicity of chemo-radiotherapy in Hodgkin's lymphoma: a single intitution experience. Radiother Oncol 11: 423.

21. Cella L, Conson M, Caterino M, De Rosa N, Liuzzi R, et al. (2012) Thyroid V30 Predicts Radiation-Induced Hypothyroidism in Patients Treated With Sequential Chemo-Radiotherapy for Hodgkin's Lymphoma. Int J Radiat Oncol Biol Phys 82: 1802–1808.

22. Cella L, Liuzzi R, Conson M, Torre G, Caterino M, et al. (2011) Dosimetric predictors of asymptomatic heart valvular dysfunction following mediastinal irradiation for Hodgkin's lymphoma. Radiother Oncol 101: 316–321.

23. Cella L, Liuzzi R, Magliulo M, Conson M, Camera L, et al. (2010) Radiotherapy of large target volumes in Hodgkin's lymphoma: normal tissue sparing capability of forward IMRT versus conventional techniques. Radiat Oncol 5: 33.

24. Feng M, Moran JM, Koelling T, Chughtai A, Chan JL, et al. (2011) Development and validation of a heart atlas to study cardiac exposure to radiation following treatment for breast cancer. Int J Radiat Oncol Biol Phys 79: 10–18.

25. Kong FM, Ritter T, Quint DJ, Senan S, Gaspar LE, et al. (2011) Consideration of dose limits for organs at risk of thoracic radiotherapy: atlas for lung, proximal bronchial tree, esophagus, spinal cord, ribs, and brachial plexus. Int J Radiat Oncol Biol Phys 81: 1442–1457.

26. Deasy JO, Blanco AI, Clark VH (2003) CERR: a computational environment for radiotherapy research. Med Phys 30: 979–985.

27. Marks LB, Yorke ED, Jackson A, Ten Haken RK, Constine LS, et al. (2010) Use of normal tissue complication probability models in the clinic. Int J Radiat Oncol Biol Phys 76: S10–19.

28. Joiner MC, Bentzen SM, Bauman DE (2002) Time-dose relationships: the linear-quadratic approach and the model in clinical practice, Steel GG (ed) Basic clinical radiobiology. 120–146 p.

29. Bentzen SM, Skoczylas JZ, Bernier J (2000) Quantitative clinical radiobiology of early and late lung reactions. Int J Radiat Biol 76: 453–462.

30. Venzon DJ, Moolgavkar SH (1988) A Method for Computing Profile-Likelihood-Based Confidence Intervals. Journal of the Royal Statistical Society Series C (Applied Statistics) 37: 87–94.

31. Semenenko VA, Li XA (2008) Lyman-Kutcher-Burman NTCP model parameters for radiation pneumonitis and xerostomia based on combined analysis of published clinical data. Phys Med Biol 53: 737–755.

32. Deasy JO, Chao KS, Markman J (2001) Uncertainties in model-based outcome predictions for treatment planning. Int J Radiat Oncol Biol Phys 51: 1389–1399.

33. Steyerberg EW, Vickers AJ, Cook NR, Gerds T, Gonen M, et al. (2010) Assessing the performance of prediction models: a framework for traditional and novel measures. Epidemiology 21: 128–138.

34. Andratschke N, Maurer J, Molls M, Trott KR (2010) Late radiation-induced heart disease after radiotherapy. Clinical importance, radiobiological mechanisms and strategies of prevention. Radiother Oncol.

35. Schellong G, Riepenhausen M, Bruch C, Kotthoff S, Vogt J, et al. (2010) Late valvular and other cardiac diseases after different doses of mediastinal radiotherapy for Hodgkin disease in children and adolescents: report from the longitudinal GPOH follow-up project of the German-Austrian DAL-HD studies. Pediatr Blood Cancer 55: 1145–1152.

36. Adams MJ, Hardenbergh PH, Constine LS, Lipshultz SE (2003) Radiation-associated cardiovascular disease. Crit Rev Oncol Hematol 45: 55–75.

37. Ghobadi G, van der Veen S, Bartelds B, de Boer RA, Dickinson MG, et al. (2012) Physiological interaction of heart and lung in thoracic irradiation. Int J Radiat Oncol Biol Phys 84: e639–646.

38. van Luijk P, Novakova-Jiresova A, Faber H, Schippers JM, Kampinga HH, et al. (2005) Radiation damage to the heart enhances early radiation-induced lung function loss. Cancer Res 65: 6509–6511.

39. Bentzen SM (1994) Prediction of radiotherapy response using SF2: why it may work after all. Radiother Oncol 31: 85–86.

40. Cella L, Liuzzi R, Conson M, V DA, Salvatore M, et al. (2012) Development of multivariate NTCP models for radiation-induced hypothyroidism: a comparative analysis. Radiat Oncol 7: 224.

41. Lee TF, Chao PJ, Ting HM, Chang L, Huang YJ, et al. (2014) Using Multivariate Regression Model with Least Absolute Shrinkage and Selection Operator (LASSO) to Predict the Incidence of Xerostomia after Intensity-Modulated Radiotherapy for Head and Neck Cancer. PLoS One 9: e89700.

42. Huang EX, Hope AJ, Lindsay PE, Trovo M, El Naqa I, et al. (2011) Heart irradiation as a risk factor for radiation pneumonitis. Acta Oncol 50: 51–60.

16

A Pragmatic Approach to Assess the Exposure of the Honey Bee (*Apis mellifera*) When Subjected to Pesticide Spray

Yannick Poquet[1], Laurent Bodin[2], Marc Tchamitchian[3], Marion Fusellier[4], Barbara Giroud[5], Florent Lafay[5], Audrey Buleté[5], Sylvie Tchamitchian[1], Marianne Cousin[1], Michel Pélissier[1], Jean-Luc Brunet[1], Luc P. Belzunces[1]*

1 INRA, Laboratoire de Toxicologie Environnementale, UR 406 A&E, CS 40509, 84914 Avignon Cedex 9, France, 2 ANSES, French Agency for Food, Environmental and Occupational Health Safety, 27–31 Avenue du Général Leclerc, 94701 Maisons-Alfort, France, 3 INRA, UR Ecodéveloppement, CS 40509, 84914 Avignon Cedex 9, France, 4 Department of Diagnostic Imaging, CRIP, National Veterinary School (Oniris), Nantes, France, 5 Université de Lyon, Institut des Sciences Analytiques, UMR5280 CNRS Université Lyon 1, ENS-Lyon, 5 rue de la Doua, 69100 Villeurbanne, France

Abstract

Plant protection spray treatments may expose non-target organisms to pesticides. In the pesticide registration procedure, the honey bee represents one of the non-target model species for which the risk posed by pesticides must be assessed on the basis of the hazard quotient (HQ). The HQ is defined as the ratio between environmental exposure and toxicity. For the honey bee, the HQ calculation is not consistent because it corresponds to the ratio between the pesticide field rate (in mass of pesticide/ha) and LD_{50} (in mass of pesticide/bee). Thus, in contrast to all other species, the HQ can only be interpreted empirically because it corresponds to a number of bees/ha. This type of HQ calculation is due to the difficulty in transforming pesticide field rates into doses to which bees are exposed. In this study, we used a pragmatic approach to determine the apparent exposure surface area of honey bees submitted to pesticide treatments by spraying with a Potter-type tower. The doses received by the bees were quantified by very efficient chemical analyses, which enabled us to determine an apparent surface area of 1.05 cm^2/bee. The apparent exposure surface area was used to calculate the exposure levels of bees submitted to pesticide sprays and then to revisit the HQ ratios with a calculation mode similar to that used for all other living species. X-tomography was used to assess the physical surface area of a bee, which was 3.27 cm^2/bee, and showed that the apparent exposure surface was not overestimated. The control experiments showed that the toxicity induced by doses calculated with the exposure surface area was similar to that induced by treatments according to the European testing procedure. This new approach to measure risk is more accurate and could become a tool to aid the decision-making process in the risk assessment of pesticides.

Editor: Eric Jan, University of British Columbia, Canada

Funding: This work was supported in part by the French National Institute for the Agricultural Research (INRA) and by grants from the European Union FEAGA Beekeeping program managed by the INRA–France AgriMer Agreement 11–43 R. YP's doctoral grant was funded by MACIF Foundation (http://www.fondation-macif.org) and Terre d'Abeilles (www.sauvonslesabeilles.com). The funders had no role in study design, data collection and analysis, decision to publish, or preparation of the manuscript.

Competing Interests: The authors have declared that no competing interests exist.

* Email: luc.belzunces@avignon.inra.fr

Introduction

Human activity generates many environmental disruptions and myriads of anthropogenic chemical substances [1]. These substances include plant protection products (PPPs), or pesticides, of which the main families used are herbicides, insecticides and fungicides [2]. As a general feature, chemical substances are subjected to a risk assessment for their effects on human and non-target organisms. The assessment procedure is based on the comparison between the environmental or individual levels of exposure to the substances and the toxicity of these substances, which correspond to the exposure thresholds from which adverse effects can occur in biological organisms exposed through different routes (contact, oral and inhalation) [3,4]. Generally, the exposure

thresholds used in risk assessment for acute effects are toxicological values such as the contact median Lethal Dose or Concentration (LD_{50} or LC_{50}). For long-term studies, and in particular reprotoxic effects, the threshold values used are the No Observed (Adverse) Effect Level or Concentration (NOAEL, NOEL, NOAEC and NOEC), defined as the highest exposure level for which no (adverse) effects were observed. In human risk assessment a more modern approach involves the determination of benchmark doses (BMD) or concentrations, which correspond to the levels of exposure at which a given effect is observed, determined by modeling the entire dose-effect relationship [5,6]. These toxicological values can be lowered by uncertainty or safety factors such as those used to take into account intraspecific variability and extrapolation from model species, which correspond to interspecific variability. From the exposure and toxicological values, a Hazard Quotient (HQ = Exposure/Toxicity) or Toxicity to Exposure Ratio (TER = Toxicity/Exposure) can be derived to assess the risk presented by chemicals or pesticides to human and non-target organisms. Hence, when the exposure level is higher than the toxicological value, the situation is at risk for the considered biological organism, which results in HQ or TER values higher or lower than 1, respectively.

For all organisms including humans, the HQ and TER are calculated on the basis of toxicological data obtained on individuals exposed through the pertinent routes of exposure. In the environment, the honey bee appears as an atypical case because both toxicological methods and risk assessment procedures are not always adapted to the environmental situation. For example, (i) the determination of the LD_{50} is relevant for acute contact during a treatment with the active substance, such as pesticide sprays. Although still performed until now, these data cannot be used to extrapolate the chronic contact toxicity. (ii) For residual contact with contaminated plants, no method exists in the registration procedure of pesticides. In the past, the tarsal contact test was used to assess the toxicity induced by repeated contact with a contaminated surface [7]. However, this test is no longer used today. (iii) No method exists to assess the toxicity elicited by inhalation. (iv) Acute oral LD_{50} values are relevant to assess the toxicity induced by an acute exposure to a pesticide through contaminated food, but are inadequate to determine the chronic oral toxicity [8]. The first laboratory approach to assess the oral chronic toxicity of pesticides was proposed in 2001 [9]. Today, chronic toxicity is being considered for inclusion in the pesticide registration procedure by the French Commission for the Biological Assays (CEB), the European Food Safety Agency (EFSA) and the Society of Environmental Toxicology & Chemistry (SETAC) [10–12]. (v) Up to now, risk assessment in honey bee was only based on acute exposure and not on chronic exposure, as practiced for other organisms, which explains the lack of experimental data [3,4]. (vi) A critical step in the assessment of the risk presented by pesticides to bees is based on the determination of the HQ [11,13]. For the HQ and TER, data of the same nature are compared, namely individual or environmental exposure levels and exposure levels below which no (adverse) effect can be observed, which results in HQ and TER values without units. However, for the honey bee, the contact HQ corresponds to the ratio of the pesticide field rate, expressed in mass/ha (generally g/ha), to LD_{50}, expressed in mass/bee (generally μg/bee). This calculation method for the HQ is used because it is difficult to convert field rates of sprayed pesticides into doses to which honey bees are exposed. This results in the HQ with a unit corresponding to a number of bee per ha, which is not useful to properly assess the risk to bees. Thus, after its introduction by Atkins in 1981 [14], the contact HQ ratio was used empirically to assess the risk of pesticides to the honey bee and the values fluctuated between 25 [13] and 85 as the toxicological threshold [11].

In this study, we used a pragmatic approach to determine the exposure levels of bees subjected to a pesticide treatment in the field. We used experimental sprayings to estimate the apparent exposure surface area of a honey bee that enabled converting pesticide field rates into acute doses received by the bees. In a second step, the accuracy of the exposure surface area was probed by comparing the toxicity induced by spraying at given field rates with the toxicity induced by treatments, achieved according to the procedures of the European and Mediterranean Plant Protection Organization (EPPO) and the Organization for Economic and

Co-operation Development (OECD) [15,16], with doses calculated from field rates and the apparent exposure surface area. Finally, the exposures to which bees can be submitted after pesticide spraying were calculated and the hazard quotients were revisited.

Materials and Methods

Chemicals

Abamectin (Agrimec gold), acetamiprid (Supreme), chlorpyrifos-ethyl (Nelpon 480), cyfluthrin (Baythroïd), cypermethrin (Cyperfor S), deltamethrin (Decis protech), dimethoate (Danadim progress), esfenvalerate (Sumi-alpha), fenoxycarb (Insegar), hexythiazox (Nissorun), imidacloprid (Confidor), iprodione (Rovral WG), lambda-cyhalothrin (Karate xpress), pyriproxyfen (Admiral pro), tau-fluvalinate (Klartan), tebuconazole (Horizon arbo), thiacloprid (Calypso), and thiamethoxam (Flagship pro) were purchased from Escudier Christian SARL (Avignon, France). Clothianidin (Dantop 50 WG) and prochloraz (Octave) were obtained from Coopérative Agricole Provence Languedoc (Châteaurenard, France). Abamectin (97% pure), acetamiprid (98.1% pure), chlorpyrifos-ethyl (98.5% pure), clothianidin (99% pure), cyfluthrin (98% pure), cypermethrin (94% pure), deltamethrin (98% pure), dimethoate (98.5% pure), esfenvalerate (99% pure), imidacloprid (99% pure), lambda-cyhalothrin (98.5% pure), prochloraz (98% pure), tau-fluvalinate (94% pure), thiacloprid (98% pure), and thiamethoxam (98.5% pure) were purchased from TechLab. DMSO (Dimethyl sulfoxide) was obtained from Sigma-Aldrich.

Honey bee collection

Honey bee workers (*Apis mellifera*) were collected from the reserve frames of the hive body from healthy colonies (≥30 000 individuals) that were carefully monitored for their sanitary state in the experimental apiary of the INRA Research Unit *Abeilles* & *Environnement* (*Bees* & *Environment*) of Avignon. After being anesthetized with CO_2, bees were distributed in cages (10.5×7.5×11.5 cm) by groups of 30 individuals and placed in the dark in a thermostated chamber at 28±2°C and 60±10% RH. The ambient temperature of the thermostated chamber was chosen as the temperature preferred by the honeybees during the night [17,18]. Bees were fed *ad libitum* with candy (Apifonda + powdered sugar) and water.

Exposure to pesticide sprays

Bees were exposed by spraying in a Potter-type tower to the 20 different commercial pesticide preparations (Table 1) at application rates chosen to be as close as possible to field conditions. The amounts of active substances sprayed were selected to be less than or equal to the lowest registered dose. Twelve replicates of 30 bees were performed for each pesticide treatment. Bees were first anesthetized and put on a 200 cm^2 Plexiglas disc subjected to rotation at a speed of 23 rpm to ensure a homogeneous deposit of the sprayed solution [19]. The deposit was previously calibrated to obtain a rate of 2.32±0.13 μL/cm^2. In addition to the calibrations, the deposit was controlled just before, during and after each series of 12 replicates (experimental calibration). Immediately after spraying, the bees from 6 replicates were frozen at −80°C to fix the dose of pesticide they received. In parallel, the mortality was followed over time on the remaining 6 replicates by keeping the bees in the thermostated chamber.

Topical exposure to pesticides

Preliminary studies were conducted to assess the mortality rate induced by each pesticide. For each substance, 6 repetitions were

Table 1. Summary of commercial products and their application rates used for the spraying treatment.

Effect	Class	Active substance	Commercial product	Application rate (g a.s./ha)
Fungicide	Dicarboximide	Iprodione	Rovral WG	600
	Imidazole	Prochloraz	Octave	230.5
	Triazole	Tebuconazole	Horizon arbo	75
Growth regulator	Carbamate	Fenoxycarb	Insegar	75
	Carboxamide	Hexythiazox	Nissorun	26
	Pyridine based	Pyriproxyfen	Admiral pro	25
Insecticide	Avermectin	Abamectin	Agrimec gold	2
	Neonicotinoid	Acetamiprid	Supreme	30
		Clothianidin	Dantop 50 WG	3
		Imidacloprid	Confidor	0.2
		Thiacloprid	Calypso	50
		Thiamethoxam	Flagship pro	5
	Organophosphate	Chlorpyrifos-ethyl	Nelpon 480	3
		Dimethoate	Danadim progress	5
	Pyrethroid	Cyfluthrin	Baythroïd	2.5
		Cypermethrin	Cyperfor S	3
		Deltamethrin	Decis protech	1.875
		Esfenvalerate	Sumi-alpha	2
		Lambda-cyhalothrin	Karate xpress	5
		Tau-fluvalinate	Klartan	48

g a.s./ha: gram of active substance per hectare.

systematically performed. However, for the doses inducing a low toxicity, the number of repetitions was increased for an accurate determination of the mortality rates (Table S1). Bees were exposed to 15 out of the 20 active substances because it was not possible to determine a dose-mortality relationship for 5 active substances (fenoxycarb, hexythiazox, iprodione, pyriproxyfen, tebuconazole) that exhibited a very low toxicity ($LD_{50} \geq 100\ 000$ ng a.s./bee). The active substances were diluted in DMSO, and the control groups were treated with pure DMSO. The bees were treated on the thorax according to the EPPO procedure recommended by the European Commission [15,20,21]. Mortality was checked 24, 48, 72 and 96 hours after the exposure, with 96 hours corresponding to the duration at which no significant evolution of mortality was observed for all the tested active substances.

Quantification of 20 pesticides

For each of the 20 pesticides of interest, the active substance was quantified in 3 repetitions. For each repetition, 5 g of frozen honey bees were weighed in a 50 mL centrifuge tube, and 10 mL of acetonitrile, 3 mL of water, 3 mL of heptane, citrate QuEChERS salts and 30 g of steel balls were added for grinding for 4 min at the cadency of 1000 strokes per min using a Geno/Grinder from SPEX Sample Prep (Metuchen, USA). Then, the tube was centrifuged for 2 min at 5000 g, and 6 mL of the lower acetonitrile phase were taken and placed in a pre-prepared 15 mL PSA/C18 tube. This tube was immediately shaken by hand, vortexed for 10 sec and centrifuged for 2 min at 5000 g. Finally, 4 mL of the extract were taken and put in a 10 mL cone-ended glass centrifuge tube for evaporation until 50 µL remained. This remaining extract was kept at −18°C until analysis.

For abamectin, acetamiprid, clothianidin, fenoxycarb, hexythiazox, iprodione, imidacloprid, lambda cyhalothrin, prochloraz,

pyriproxyfen, thiacloprid and thiamethoxam, the analysis was performed on a Waters 2695 series Alliance HPLC (Waters, Milford, MA) coupled to a triple quadrupole mass spectrometer Quattro from Micromass (Manchester, UK) equipped with a Z-spray electrospray interface (ESI). Data were processed with MassLynx 4.1. Electrospray ionization was performed in the positive mode. The chromatographic separations were performed on a Nucleodur Sphinx RP-C18 (50×2 mm, 1.8 µm) column from Macherey-Nagel with in-line filter "krudkatcher" 0.5 µm porosity (Phenomenex). The column oven temperature was set to 40°C; the flow rate was 300 µL/min. Samples were analyzed with the mobile phase (A) water with 0.3 mM of ammonium formate and 0.05% formic acid, and (B) methanol. Ten µL were injected in the 90/10 mobile phase (A)/acetonitrile.

For chlorpyrifos-ethyl, cyfluthrin, cypermethrin, deltamethrin, dimethoate, esfenvalerate, tau-fluvalinate and tebuconazole, the analysis was conducted with a GC-ToF, a 6890 Agilent gas chromatograph coupled to a Time of Flight (ToF) mass spectrometer GCT Premier from Waters. Data were processed with MassLynx 4.1. Chromatographic separation was performed on a 30 m×0.25 mm I.D., with a 0.25 µm film thickness DB-XLB capillary column (Agilent Technologies, Avondale, USA). Helium (purity 99.999%) was used as a carrier gas at a constant flow of 1 mL/min. Injections were performed in the splitless mode, and 1 µL in 90/10 acetonitrile/analyte protectant mix was injected. The mass spectrometer was operated in the electron impact mode (EI, 70 eV). Acquisition was performed in the full scan mode with a scan range of m/z 50–550. Calibration was performed using the calibration wizard, with heptacosa as the reference.

Matrix-matched calibration was used for quantification. In each batch, 6 calibration points were prepared and injected as described

Table 2. Comparison of the commercial and measured concentrations.

Active substance	Commercial concentration	Measured concentration		Difference (%)
		Mean	S.D.	
Abamectin	18 g/L	24.91 g/L	1.27 g/L	+38.4
Acetamiprid	200 g/kg	243.66 g/kg	6.14 g/kg	+21.8
Chlorpyrifos-ethyl	480 g/L	500.20 g/L	0.02 g/L	+4.2
Clothianidin	500 g/kg	453.71 g/kg	23.11 g/kg	−9.3
Cyfluthrin	50 g/L	46.45 g/L	0.09 g/L	−7.1
Cypermethrin	100 g/L	114.25 g/L	0.14 g/L	+14.2
Deltamethrin	15 g/L	14.77 g/L	0.72 g/L	−1.5
Dimethoate	400 g/L	433.35 g/L	0.92 g/L	+8.3
Esfenvalerate	25 g/L	25.10 g/L	0.50 g/L	+0.4
Fenoxycarb	250 g/kg	228.54 g/kg	14.49 g/kg	−8.6
Hexythiazox	104 g/kg	91.24 g/kg	2.94 g/kg	−12.3
Imidacloprid	200 g/L	230.29 g/L	12.24 g/L	+15.1
Iprodione	750 g/kg	794.34 g/kg	7.01 g/kg	+5.9
Lambda-cyhalothrin	50 g/kg	44.85 g/kg	2.47 g/kg	−10.3
Prochloraz	461 g/kg	391.69 g/kg	13.72 g/kg	−15
Pyriproxyfen	100 g/L	97.29 g/L	2.66 g/L	−2.7
Tau-fluvalinate	240 g/L	232.65 g/L	12.80 g/L	−3.1
Tebuconazole	250 g/kg	186.30 g/kg	10.32 g/kg	−25.5
Thiacloprid	480 g/L	448.97 g/L	0.07 g/L	−6.5
Thiamethoxam	10 g/L	10.25 g/L	0.16 g/L	+2.5

S.D.: Standard Deviation.
The concentrations of commercial products are expressed according to their nature, liquid or solid.
The quantification of the active substance was performed in triplicate from the phytopharmaceutical preparation used for the spray application.
The differences were expressed as percentages of the commercial concentrations.

above, with concentrations ranging between 4 and 60 ng/g. Quantification was performed using QuanLynx 4.1.

Physical surface of the honey bee

The surface area of the bees, excluding the wings, was determined by X-ray computed tomography. Imaging was performed on 6 dead bees with a μPET/CT Inveon device (Siemens Preclinical Solutions, Knoxville, TN). The computed tomography (CT) images were acquired with the following settings: X-ray source tube voltage at 40 keV with a constant 500 μA current during 320 ms and 2-degree rotation to generate images with 41 μm of voxel resolution. Three-D reconstructions were performed using COBRA software (Siemens Preclinical Solutions). Using ImageJ, the stacks of images were thresholded, and the regions of interest (ROI) were automatically drawn on binary images. Each ROI was checked, and the surface areas obtained were then summed for each of the resulting 768 slices. The surface area of the wings was measured on 50 bees. The 4 wings were cut at the base of the thorax and placed on a microscope slide and slip covered with soapy water. Pictures of wings were taken under a microscope; ImageJ software was used to delineate the wings and to calculate their surface area.

Data analysis

Statistical analyses were performed with R software (2013). The variations of the deposit distributions were tested using a t-test comparing preliminary and experimental calibrations. Pearson's correlation and a linear regression were used to compare the

Table 3. Comparison of preliminary calibrations and experimental controls of the deposit.

Calibration	Deposit (μL/cm²)		N_c C.I. 95%		Sprayed volume (L/ha)[a]	
	Mean	S.D.			Mean	S.D.
Preliminary	2.32	0.13	90	[2.30, 2.35]	232	13
Experimental	2.32	0.11	60	[2.30, 2.35]	232	11

S.D.: Standard Deviation.
Nc: Number of calibrations.
C.I. 95%: Confidence Interval at 95%.
[a]Sprayed volume corresponds to the deposit in field conditions.

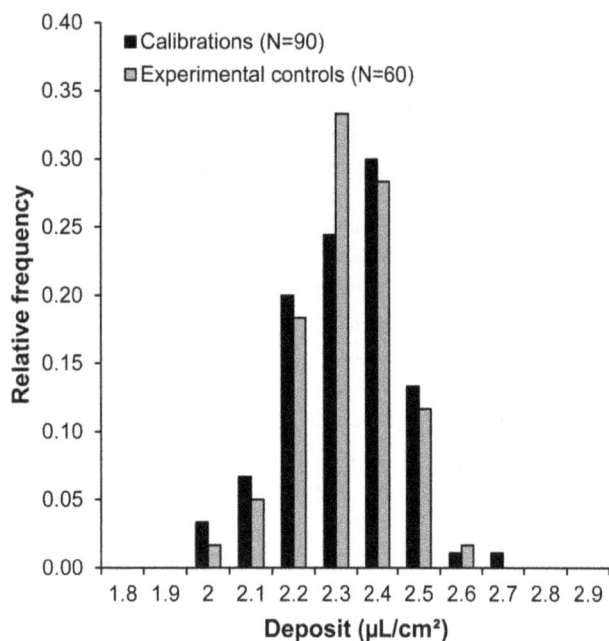

Figure 1. Distribution of the deposit during preliminary calibrations and experimental controls. The preliminary calibrations were performed before the experiment, and the experimental calibrations were performed during the experiment. The deposit was expressed in $\mu L/cm^2$ of the disc. T-test preliminary vs. experimental calibrations; (t = 0.0739, df = 148, p-value = 0.9412).

mortalities obtained by spray contamination and those obtained by the EPPO procedure. For each dose, the stabilization of the dose-mortality response over time was determined with Fisher's exact tests. The mortality was considered stabilized when there were no differences between two consecutive days for all the tested doses.

LD_{50} calculation

The BMD approach consists in the selection of the model that describes the data using appropriate model structures for the type of data (dichotomous or quantal). A mathematical model is applied to the experimental data to produce the dose-response curve with the best fit. Details of the full process on this approach are presented in the BMD Software technical guidance from the US EPA (http://www.epa.gov/ncea/bmds/). For the dichotomous (or quantal) data, the response or effect may be reported as either the presence or absence of an effect. The dose-response models describe how the probability or frequency of a specified response changes with the dose level (50%). The different models were classified by Akaike's Information Criterion (AIC), and the model with the lowest AIC was chosen for the determination of LD_{50} for each active substance.

Results

Control of the active substance concentrations

The concentration of the working solutions of active substances and the 20 commercial pesticide formulations were controlled by chemical analysis (Table 2). The concentration variations of the formulations ranged between −25% (tebuconazole) and +38% (abamectin) of the concentration indicated by the manufacturer. This suggests that the technical process to adjust pesticide concentration is not accurately controlled by the manufacturer.

The measured concentrations were used in all cases to determine the actual exposure levels of the bees after spraying.

Calibration of the deposit in the spraying tower

To check the reliability of the deposit, preliminary calibrations and experimental controls were performed (Figure 1). No differences were found between the deposits performed during the calibration procedure and the experimental controls (t-test; t = 0.0739, df = 148, p-value = 0.9412). The mean values of the deposit for calibrations and experimental controls were $2.32 \pm 0.13 \ \mu L/cm^2$ and $2.32 \pm 0.11 \ \mu L/cm^2$, respectively (Table 3). These volumes corresponded to a field spraying volume of 232 L/ha, which was similar to volumes commonly used in agriculture [22].

Determination of the exposure

Knowing the application rate of pesticides per surface area unit (n g/ha equal to $10 \times n$ ng/cm^2) and the determination of the doses received per bee enabled estimating the apparent exposure surface area of a bee. For each pesticide, the application rate was corrected by the real deposit (see Table 4: Deposit of the experimental control). The dose received by the bees (in ng/g of bee) was determined by chemical analysis of residues. To avoid the degradation of pesticides, *in vivo* biotransformation was stopped by quick freezing of the bees still anesthetized at −80°C immediately after spraying. The mean mass of the bees was determined to calculate the dose received per individual (in ng/bee) (Table 4). The exposure surface area of a bee (in cm^2/bee) is the ratio between the residues (in ng/bee) and the application rate (in ng/cm^2). Considering all the pesticides, the mean apparent exposure surface area was 1.05 ± 0.33 cm^2/bee (n = 20).

Spray toxicity vs. topical toxicity

To check the accuracy and reliability of the estimated mean exposure surface area of a bee for each formulation, the sprayed dose (in g/ha), which was associated with the corresponding mortality rate, was converted into an individual dose (in ng/bee) on the basis of an apparent surface area of 1.05 cm^2/bee. In a second step, this individual dose was topically applied on the thorax according to the EPPO procedure. Then, the mortality rates obtained by spraying and topical application were compared by linear regression analysis (Figure 2). A good linear correlation between mortalities elicited by spraying and topical exposures was found (r^2 = 0.960). It is noteworthy that the slope of the regression was very close to 1 (y = 0.9792x+0.6306), which showed that the mortality induced by topical exposure was not over- or underestimated compared with the response obtained by a spray exposure. The experimental data of the dose-mortality response obtained by topical application are presented in Figures S1, S2, S3, S4, S5, S6, S7, S8, S9, S10, S11, S12, S13, S14 and S15.

Revision of the hazard quotient

The accuracy of the apparent exposure surface area previously estimated enabled calculating a new hazard quotient (HQ) based on the real exposure of the bees. Thus, the current HQ and revisited HQ were compared (Table 5). Currently, in bee toxicology, the HQ of a substance is defined as the ratio between the application rate (in g a.s./ha) and the LD_{50} expressed in μg a.s./bee [13]. The revisited HQ was based on the estimated exposure expressed in ng a.s./bee, calculated from the application rate and the exposure surface area per bee, and the LD_{50} was expressed in ng a.s./bee. This revisited HQ is a relative exposure level corresponding to the number of LD_{50} to which a bee is

Table 4. Determination of the exposure surface area per bee for each active substance.

Active substance	Deposit of the Experimental control (μL/cm²)		Corrected application rate[a] (g a.s./ha)	Residues[b] per bee (ng a.s./g)		Weight per bee (mg/bee)	Residues (ng a.s./bee)	Exposure surface area[c] (cm²/bee)
	Mean	S.D.		Mean	S.D.			
Abamectin	2.35	0.05	2.8	261.1	44	112	29.2	1.04
Acetamiprid	2.43	0.10	38.2	1922.7	152	117	225.0	0.59
Chlorpyrifos-ethyl	2.48	0.10	3.3	263.1	7.1	121	31.8	0.95
Clothianidin	2.24	0.04	2.6	137.5	9.5	125	17.2	0.65
Cyfluthrin	2.20	0.11	2.2	313.5	43.4	113	35.4	1.61
Cypermethrin	2.45	0.04	3.6	335.6	22.5	126	42.3	1.17
Deltamethrin	2.32	0.04	1.8	112.7	4.9	122	13.7	0.75
Dimethoate	2.26	0.14	5.3	451.6	54.4	120	54.2	1.03
Esfenvalerate	2.31	0.08	2.0	186.5	37.8	122	22.8	1.14
Fenoxycarb	2.21	0.20	65.3	4393	40	122	536.0	0.82
Hexythiazox	2.36	0.10	23.2	3143	697	122	383.5	1.66
Imidacloprid	2.33	0.03	0.2	20.2	2	122	2.5	1.07
Iprodione	2.36	0.09	645.1	32980	1058	122	4023.6	0.62
Lambda-cyhalothrin	2.32	0.07	4.5	430	46	122	52.5	1.17
Prochloraz	2.28	0.05	192.7	13990	828	122	1706.8	0.89
Pyriproxyfen	2.24	0.14	23.4	2307	412	122	281.4	1.20
Tau-fluvalinate	2.44	0.09	48.9	5857	483	122	714.5	1.46
Tebuconazole	2.33	0.04	56.1	7370	157	122	899.1	1.60
Thiacloprid	2.32	0.08	46.7	3523.3	417.1	118	415.7	0.89
Thiamethoxam	2.27	0.05	5.0	279.7	14.5	119	33.3	0.66

S.D.: Standard Deviation (n = 3).
g a.s./ha: gram of active substance per hectare.
ng a.s./ha: nanogram of active substance per hectare.
ng a.s./bee: nanogram of active substance per bee.
[a]The application rate was corrected with the measured concentration (Table 3) and the experimental control deposit.
[b]This corresponds to the concentration of active substances found in the bees frozen just after contamination.
[c]The exposure surface area is the ratio between the residues (ng a.s./bee) and the corrected application rate (ng a.s./cm²).
For each treatment, the bees from the 6 replicates were counted, pooled, and weighed; the mean bee weight was determined by dividing the weight of bees by the actual number of bees.

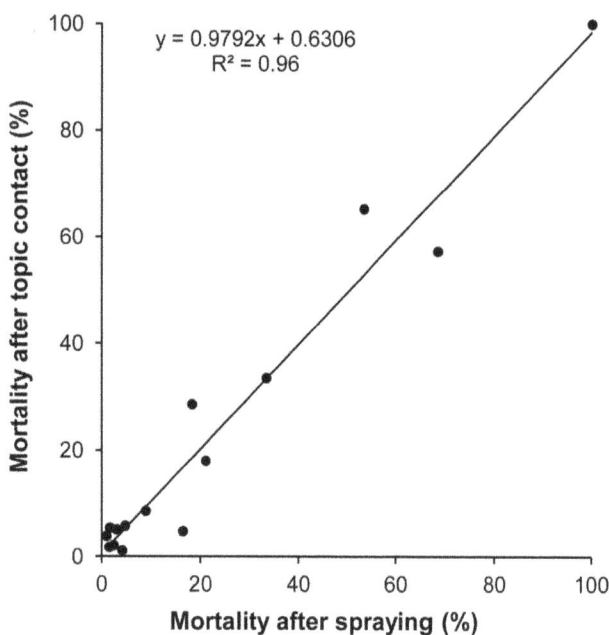

Figure 2. Correlation between mortality induced by spraying and mortality induced by topical treatment. Each dot represents one substance among the 15 tested on bees by thorax topical contact and spraying. The mortality elicited at 48 hours by spraying was given for the chosen field application rate (g a.s./ha) (Table 1). On the basis of the mean exposure surface area (1.05 cm²/bee), the application rate (g a.s./ha) was converted into an individual dose (ng a.s./bee) to treat the bees topically. The dose-mortality relationship at 48 hours was modeled for each of the 15 active substances, which enabled assessing the mortality that could be induced at a given field exposure.

exposed. In addition, based on the dose-mortality relationship determined for each active substance, it was possible to assess the mortality induced at this exposure level (Figures S1, S2, S3, S4, S5, S6, S7, S8, S9, S10, S11, S12, S13, S14 and S15). For each active substance, two scenarios were presented: the most and the least protective that combined the highest LD_{50} and lowest field rate, for the most protective scenario, and the lowest LD_{50} and highest field rate, for the least protective one. The active substances were classified by their revisited HQ as a function of the different values of exposure calculated from the lower and the upper limits of the 95% confidence interval of the exposure surface area (Table S2). No differences in the classification of active substances were found when the lower and upper limits of the confidence interval were used to calculate the revisited HQ.

Determination of the physical surface area of a bee

To investigate the possibility of an overestimation of the exposure surface area of bees, the physical surface area of a bee was determined by X-Ray tomography. The surface areas of the body and the wings were measured separately. The tomographic analyses resulted in 3-D representation of the bees (Figure 3) that enabled calculating the volume (not relevant here) and the surface area of a bee. The exposure surface area was compared to the physical surface area of a bee (Figure 4). The mean body surface area was 2.21 ± 0.20 cm² (n = 6), the mean wing surface area was 1.06 ± 0.03 cm² (n = 50) and the mean total physical surface area of a bee was 3.27 ± 0.23 cm². It was noteworthy that the wings represented almost one third of the total physical surface area of a

bee and that the physical surface area was 3 times higher than the apparent exposure surface area.

Discussion

In this study, we used a pragmatic approach to determine the exposure level of a bee submitted to spraying by an agrochemical at a known field rate. This exposure level enabled assessing the exposure surface area of a honey bee that could be used in the assessment of the risk posed by plant protection products as recommended by the EFSA [11]. The mean apparent exposure surface area was estimated as 1.05 ± 0.33 cm²/bee (n = 20). Various attempts have been made to estimate the apparent exposure surface area of a bee. The first involves the determination of the apparent surface area by projection from photographs, which results in a surface area of approximately 0.5 cm²/bee [23]. We used this method in a previous study to transform field rates into doses received by bees with a good correlation between mortality rates [24]. The second method is more pragmatic and has been performed in an original study by Koch and Weisser, in which caged bees were submitted to a spraying of fluorescein at a field rate of 20 g/ha [25]. With this procedure, exposure levels ranged from 1.62 to 8.51 ng/bee in apple orchards and from 6.34 to 35.77 ng/bee in phacelia. These values correspond to an apparent exposure surface area ranging from 0.0081 to 0.0425 cm²/bee in apple orchards and 0.0317 to 0.1789 cm²/bee in phacelia, which is very different from the surface area determined in the present study. Two phenomena can explain the great discrepancy between these exposure values and those presented here. (i) The fluorescein recovery was achieved by rinsing the bees, which does not enable the extraction of the absorbed fluorescein and leads to important underestimation of fluorescein residues. In our approach, pesticide residues were recovered by an efficient extraction procedure that presents high recovery rates [26]. (ii) In our study, bees were immediately frozen after spraying, which stops the biotransformation of the pesticides. However, in the study of Koch and Weisser, the time elapsed between field exposure and sampling was much higher and close to 20 min. In addition, during the sampling the bees were cooled with dry ice and subsequently frozen in the laboratory. Thus, fluorescein was subjected to biotransformation during the sampling procedure, which can be very rapid; this has been previously observed with pesticides for which *in vivo* half-lives as low as 25 min have been observed [27]. It is noteworthy that the effect of time on fluorescein recovery was described by Koch and Weisser.

For a better assessment, the apparent exposure surface area was estimated with 20 pesticides from several chemical groups. Slight variations in the surface area have been observed from pesticide to pesticide. However, the concentrations of the pesticide solutions were checked analytically, the recovery rates of pesticide extraction were very high and we made sure that the deposit was very constant over time (Table 4). Thus, variations of the apparent exposure surface area were not due to variations in the quantity of the deposited pesticide solution but due to the quantities of the deposited active substance, which depends on their physico-chemical properties and on the components of the pesticide formulations [28].

To test the accuracy of the estimated exposure surface area, the toxicity elicited by sprayings at given field rates was compared with the toxicity induced by the corresponding doses calculated on the basis of the field rates and the exposure surface area. The linear regression analysis showed not only a very good correlation ($r^2 = 0.960$) between mortality induced by field doses and that

Table 5. Determination and comparison of the HQ and the revisited HQ.

Active substance	Time[a] (hours)	Application rate[b] (g a.s./ha)	LD50[c] (μg a.s./bee)	HQ[d]	Exposure[e] (ng a.s./bee)	LD50[f] (ng a.s./bee)	New HQ[g] (revisited)	Expected mortality[h]	LD50 References
Abamectin	24	Min 4.5	Max 0.002	Min 2045	Min 47	Max 2.2	Min 21.48	100%	[34]
	72	Max 22.5	Min 0.001	Max 15709	Max 236	Min 1.43	Max 164.94	100%	E.D. Figure S1
Acetamiprid	72	Min 5	Max 8.090	Min 0.6	Min 53	Max 8090	Min 0.006	2.2%	PED US EPA
	24	Max 100	Min 5.057	Max 20	Max 1050	Min 5057	Max 0.21	10.1%	E.D. Figure S2
Chlorpyrifos-ethyl	96	Min 187.5	Max 0.114	Min 1645	Min 1969	Max 114	Min 17.27	100%	PED US EPA
	96		E.D. 0.060			E.D. 59.52			E.D. Figure S3
Clothianidin	18	Max 1000	Min 0.010	Max 100000	Max 10500	Min 10	Max 1050	100%	PED US EPA
	48	Min 75	Max 0.044	Min 1695	Min 788	Max 44.26	Min 17.79	100%	Agritox Database
	24		E.D. 0.040			E.D. 40.23			E.D. Figure S4
Cyfluthrin	24	Max 75	Min 0.022	Max 3440	Max 788	Min 21.8	Max 36.12	100%	[35]
	48	Min 10	Max 0.037	Min 270	Min 105	Max 37	Min 2.84	99.1%	PED US EPA
	48		E.D. 0.020			E.D. 20.45			E.D. Figure S5
Cypermethrin	48	Max 40	Min 0.001	Max 40000	Max 420	Min 1	Max 420	100%	[36]
	24	Min 15	Max 0.121	Min 124	Min 158	Max 121.25	Min 1.30	71%	E.D. Figure S6
	24	Max 96	Min 0.020	Max 4800	Max 1008	Min 20	Max 50	99.9%	Agritox Database
Deltamethrin	24	Min 4.95	Max 0.108	Min 46	Min 52	Max 107.64	Min 0.48	7.4%	E.D. Figure S7
	48	Max 19.95	Min 0.002	Max 13300	Max 209	Min 1.5	Max 139.65	91.5%	PED US EPA
Dimethoate	24	Max 240	Max 0.454	Min 529	Min 2520	Max 454	Min 5.55	100%	[37]
	96		E.D. 0.163			E.D. 163.33			E.D. Figure S8
Esfenvalerate	48	Max 500	Min 0.001	Max 357143	Max 5250	Min 1.4	Max 3750	100%	[38]
	48	Min 1.5	Max 0.060	Min 25	Min 16	Max 60	Min 0.26	13.0%	[39]
	96		E.D. 0.047			E.D. 47.03			E.D. Figure S9
Fenoxycarb	48	Max 20	Min 0.017	Max 1163	Max 210	Min 17.2	Max 12.21	98.1%	PED US EPA
	48	Min 75	Max >204	Min <0.4	Min 788	Max >204000	Min <0.004	N.C.	[36]
Hexythiazox	48	Max 150	Min >100	Max <2	Max 1575	Min >100000	Max <0.016	N.C.	[40]
	48	Min 25	Max >200	Min <0.1	Min 263	Max >200000	Min <0.001	N.C.	[41]
	48	Max 50	Min >200	Max <0.3	Max 525	Min >200000	Max <0.003	N.C.	[41]
Imidacloprid	48	Min 50	Max 0.230	Min 217	Min 525	Max 230.3	Min 2.28	91.9%	[42]
	96		E.D. 0.096			E.D. 96.21			E.D. Figure S10
Iprodione	48	Max 100	Min 0.007	Max 14925	Max 1050	Min 6.7	Max 156.72	96.8%	[43]
	48	Min 75	Max >200	Min <0.4	Min 788	Max >200000	Min <0.004	N.C.	Agritox Database
	48	Max 1000	Min >25	Max <40	Max 10500	Min >25000	Max <0.42	N.C.	[36]
Lambda-cyhalothrin	48	Min 5	Max 0.098	Min 51	Min 53	Max 98	Min 0.54	23.2%	PED US EPA
	48		E.D. 0.078			E.D. 77.85			E.D. Figure S11

Table 5. Cont.

Active substance	Time[a] (hours)	Application rate[b] (g a.s./ha)	LD50[c] (µg a.s./bee)	HQ[d]	Exposure[e] (ng a.s./bee)	LD50[f] (ng a.s./bee)	New HQ[g] (revisited)	Expected mortality[h]	LD50 References
Prochloraz	48	Max 75	Min 0.038	Max 1974	Max 788	Min 38	Max 20.72	99.9%	PED US EPA
	96	Min 230.5	Max 141.28	Min 2	Min 2420	Max 141280	Min 0.02	40.7%	[44]
Pyriproxyfen	24	Max 598.5	Min 2.657	Max 225	Max 6284	Min 2657	Max 2.37	97.5%	E.D. Figure S12
	48	Min 25	Max >100	Min <0.3	Min 263	Max >100000	Min <0.003	N.C.	[45]
Tau-fluvalinate	48	Max 30	Min 74	Max 0.4	Max 315	Min 74000	Max 0.004	N.C.	PPDB IUPAC
	24	Min 48	Max 13	Min 4	Min 504	Max 12000	Min 0.04	2.1%	[46]
Tebuconazole	48	Max 144	Min 2.532	Max 57	Max 1512	Min 2532	Max 0.60	17.4%	E.D. Figure S13
	48	Min 75	Max >200	Min <0.4	Min 788	Max >200000	Min <0.004	N.C.	[47]
Thiacloprid	48	Max 258	Min >83	Max <3.1	Max 2709	Min >83050	Max <0.033	N.C.	[36]
	48	Min 72	Max 38.820	Min 2	Min 756	Max 38820	Min 0.02	4.1%	Agritox Database
	24		E.D. 19.380			E.D. 19380			E.D. Figure S14
Thiamethoxam	24	Max 180	Min 14.600	Max 12	Max 1890	Min 14600	Max 0.13	9.2%	[35]
	48	Min 50	Max 0.040	Min 1251	Min 525	Max 39.96	Min 13.14	100%	E.D. Figure S15
	24	Max 100	Min 0.024	Max 4167	Max 1050	Min 24	Max 44	100%	Agritox Database

g a.s./ha: mass of active substance per hectare expressed in grams.

µg a.s./bee: mass of active substance per bee expressed in micrograms.

ng a.s./bee: nanogram of active substance per bee.

E.D.: Experimental Data.

LD50: Median Lethal Dose.

HQ: Hazard Quotient (field rate (g/ha)/LD50 (µg/bee)).

Revisited HQ (exposure (ng/bee)/LD50 (µg/bee)).

N.C.: Not Calculated because of the low toxicity of the active substance.

DAR EFSA: Draft Assessment Report of the European Food Safety Authority.

PED US EPA: Pesticides Ecotoxicity Database of the United States Environmental Protection Agency.

[a] Time at which the LD50 was determined. The LD50 values resulting from the experimental data were calculated at the time corresponding to a stabilized mortality.

[b] For each active substance, 2 scenarios of exposure are presented: the lowest and the highest homologated application rate.

[c] For each active substance, the highest and the lowest known LD50 values were compared to the lowest and highest homologated application rates, respectively.

[d] HQ is the ratio between the application rate (g a.s./ha) and the LD50 (µg a.s./bee).

[e] The exposure was calculated from the application rate (ng a.s./cm^2) and the mean exposure surface area determined with the 20 active substances (1.05 cm^2/bee).

[f] The LD50 values from the experimental data were calculated with the BMD software from the US EPA.

[g] The revisited HQ is the ratio between the exposure (ng a.s./bee) and the LD50 (ng a.s./bee).

[h] For each active substance, the dose-mortality relationship was modeled at the time corresponding to a stabilized mortality.

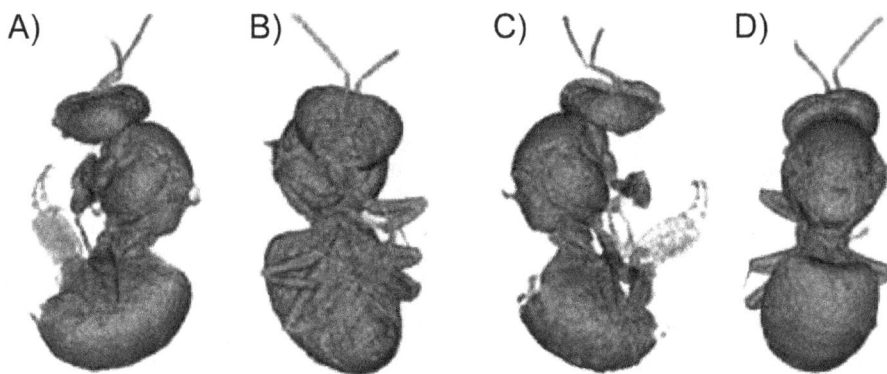

Figure 3. 3D representation of a bee from different angles. Bees were scanned using X-ray tomography. A: Left lateral view; B: Ventral view; C: Right lateral view; D: Dorsal view.

induced by doses calculated with the apparent exposure surface area but also a slope of 0.9792, which is very close to 1. A slope higher or lower than 1 would have revealed an overestimation or underestimation of the apparent exposure surface area, respectively. Thus, a slope of approximately 1 clearly shows that the toxicity induced by spraying at a given field rate can be predicted by the toxicity induced by contact treatment according to the EPPO procedure with the corresponding dose calculated on the basis of the field rate and the apparent exposure surface area of a bee. In other words, this shows that the apparent exposure surface area of a bee can be used in procedures to assess the risk presented by pesticides to bees. Hence, it is possible to derive two formulas that could be used in risk assessment. The first enables calculating the individual dose received by the bees (ID) during the spraying of a pesticide at a given field rate:

$$ID = FR \times 10 \times S$$

where ID is the individual dose expressed in ng/bee; FR is the field rate of the pesticide expressed in g/ha and S is the apparent exposure surface area of 1.05 cm^2/bee. The factor 10 results from the conversion of FR in g/ha into FR in ng/cm^2. It is noteworthy that the standard deviation (0.33 cm^2/bee) or the upper limit of the confidence interval (1.21 cm^2/bee) offers the possibility to consider worse case scenarios of exposure during spraying. The second formula can be used to estimate the field rate that should not be exceeded when a reference value, such as LD$_{50}$ or acute reference dose (ARfD), is available to characterize the toxicity of a pesticide:

$$LFR = \frac{RV}{10 \times S}$$

where LFR is the limit field rate that should not be exceeded expressed in g/ha, RV is the reference value expressed in ng/bee and S is the apparent exposure surface area of 1.05 cm^2/bee.

In this study, we propose a new approach for the determination of the hazard quotient (HQ) in the procedure used for the assessment of the risk presented by pesticides to the honey bee. The HQ is no longer estimated from the field application rates of pesticides (in g/ha) but instead from the exposure to which the bees are subjected (in ng/bee). Thus, the resulting HQ is a value without units because it corresponds to the ratio of coherent exposure and toxicity data. The environmental exposure level to which bees are subjected is expressed in ng/bee. The toxicity, corresponding to the exposure level from which effects may be considered damaging to the bees (or to a bee colony), is also expressed in ng/bee. This approach is used for all living organisms in risk assessment procedures, including humans [3,29]. Until now, the honey bee remained the only organism for which the HQ value was interpreted empirically to manage the risk to bees because it was not based on the ratio of comparable data. This point has also been raised by one agency of the European Union, the DG SANCO [30]. The determination of the exposure surface area of a bee also enables converting previous HQ values into new HQ values (revisited HQ) (new HQ = $1.05 \times 10^{-2} \times$HQ), which in turn enables using the old toxicological data. Moreover, the apparent exposure surface area enables the assessment of the survival probability of bees sprayed by a pesticide at a given field rate on the basis of the dose-mortality relationship. Thus, the

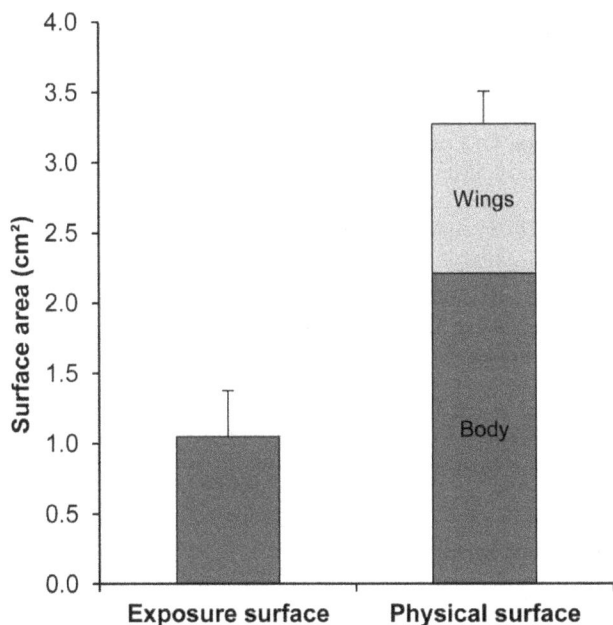

Figure 4. Comparison of the exposure and physical surface area of a bee. Mean exposure surface area (± S.D.) of a bee (average of the 20 commercial products) and mean physical surface area (± S.D.) of a bee (sum of the mean body and wing surface area).

combination of the new HQ with the expected mortality and exposure could be useful tools for decision-making processes in the assessment of pesticide toxicity to the honey bee. However, although the revisited HQ gives a better interpretation of the potential risk presented by a pesticide than the previous HQ, the exposure is still compared to a toxicological value that elicits a mortality rate of 50% in the honey bee risk assessment procedure. For humans and some target organisms (i.e., fish), and for specific toxicity, such as reproductive toxicity, for birds and mammals [31], the risk is based on toxic reference values at which a low mortality or no effect is observed (e.g., NOAEL, NOAEC, ARfD, or Benchmark dose). Consequently, it appears legitimate to reconsider the LD_{50} value as a reference value to assess the risk presented by pesticides to bees.

The apparent exposure surface area of $1.05 \text{ cm}^2/\text{bee}$ does not appear overestimated compared with the physical surface area of $3.27 \text{ cm}^2/\text{bee}$. The physical surface area measured in the present study appears to be higher than that determined in previous studies using graph paper [32,33]. Although X-Ray tomography is not yet sufficiently powerful to take into account the surface hairs on the honeybee thorax, this technique remains more precise than the others described previously. The difference between exposure and physical surface areas can be explained by the fact that the entire surface was not available during the spraying. Indeed, the bees were motionless with their wings folded on the body during the spraying. Then, the exposure surface area does not depend on the total surface area (body + wings = 3.27 cm^2), but is rather a reflection of the body surface area (2.21 cm^2). In this study, the bees were subjected to pesticides on one side, like during a field spraying. Thus, only one half of the body was directly exposed (c.a. 1.11 cm^2), which is close to the apparent exposure surface area (1.05 cm^2).

Supporting Information

Figure S1 **Dose-mortality relationship of honey bees after a single contact contamination of abamectin on the thorax.**

Figure S2 **Dose-mortality relationship of honey bees after a single contact contamination of acetamiprid on the thorax.**

Figure S3 **Dose-mortality relationship of honey bees after a single contact contamination of chlorpyrifos-ethyl on the thorax.**

Figure S4 **Dose-mortality relationship of honey bees after a single contact contamination of clothianidin on the thorax.**

Figure S5 **Dose-mortality relationship of honey bees after a single contact contamination of cyfluthrin on the thorax.**

Figure S6 **Dose-mortality relationship of honey bees after a single contact contamination of cypermethrin on the thorax.**

Figure S7 **Dose-mortality relationship of honey bees after a single contact contamination of deltamethrin on the thorax.**

Figure S8 **Dose-mortality relationship of honey bees after a single contact contamination of dimethoate on the thorax.**

Figure S9 **Dose-mortality relationship of honey bees after a single contact contamination of esfenvalerate on the thorax.**

Figure S10 **Dose-mortality relationship of honey bees after a single contact contamination of imidacloprid on the thorax.**

Figure S11 **Dose-mortality relationship of honey bees after a single contact contamination of lambda-cyhalo-thrin on the thorax.**

Figure S12 **Dose-mortality relationship of honey bees after a single contact contamination of prochloraz on the thorax.**

Figure S13 **Dose-mortality relationship of honey bees after a single contact contamination of tau-fluvalinate on the thorax.**

Figure S14 **Dose-mortality relationship of honey bees after a single contact contamination of thiacloprid on the thorax.**

Figure S15 **Dose-mortality relationship of honey bees after a single contact contamination of thiamethoxam on the thorax.**

Table S1 **Active substances and their doses used for exposures through thoracic topical exposure.** ng a.s./bee: nanogram of active substance per bee. Nr: Number of replicates per dose. ABA = Abamectin, ACE = Acetamiprid, CHL = Chlor-pyrifos-ethyl, CLO = Clothianidin, CYF = Cyfluthrin, CYP = Cypermethrin, DEL = Deltamethrin, DIM = Dimethoate, ESF = Esfenvalerate, IMI = Imidacloprid, LAM = Lambda-cyhalothin, PRO = Prochoraz, TAU = Tau-fluvalinate, THI = Thiacloprid, TMX = Thiamethoxam.

Table S2 **Classification of the 20 active substances by their revisited HQs for different values of exposure surface areas.** An active substance was classified with a HQ≥1 if at least the revisited HQ of one of the two scenarios (Table 5) were equal to or higher than this value. Lower C.I.: Lower limit of the Confidence Interval at 95%. Upper C.I.: Upper limit of the Confidence Interval at 95%.

Acknowledgments

The authors wish to thank Marie Dupré, Jean-Baptiste Philibert and Jacques Sénéchal for their technical help and André Kretzschmar for useful advice in the data analysis.

Author Contributions

Conceived and designed the experiments: LPB YP. Performed the experiments: YP ST MC AB FL BG MF. Analyzed the data: YP LB

MT JLB. Contributed reagents/materials/analysis tools: MP. Contributed to the writing of the manuscript: LPB YP.

References

1. United Nations Environment Programme (UNEP) (2003) Regionally based assessment of persistent toxic substances. Glob Rep: 1–207.
2. United States Environmental Protection Agency (US EPA) (2011) Pesticides Industry Sales and Usage 2006 and 2007 Market Estimates: 1–33.
3. European Chemicals Bureau (2003) Technical Guidance Document (TGD) on Risk Assessment Part I: 1–302.
4. European Chemicals Bureau (2003) Technical Guidance Document (TGD) on Risk Assessment Part II: 1–328.
5. Barnes DG, Daston GP, Evans JS, Jarabek AM, Kavlock RJ, et al. (1995) Benchmark Dose Workshop: Criteria for use of benchmark dose to estimate a reference dose. Regul Toxicol Pharmacol 21: 296–306.
6. EFSA (2009) Guidance of the Scientific Commitee on a request from EFSA on the use of the benchmark dose approach in risk assessment. EFSA J 1150: 1–72.
7. Société Française de Phytiatrie et de Phytopharmacie (SFPP) (1982) Méthode n°95, Méthodes d'essais destinées à connaître les effets des insecticides sur l'abeille domestique (Apis mellifera L.). Comm des Essais Biol: 19.
8. Hatch GE, Kodavanti U, Crissman K, Slade R, Costa D (2001) An "injury-time integral" model for extrapolating from acute to chronic effects of phosgene. Toxicol Ind Health 17: 285–293.
9. Suchail S, Guez D, Belzunces LP (2001) Discrepancy between acute and chronic toxicity induced by imidacloprid and its metabolites in Apis mellifera. Environ Toxicol Chem 20: 2482–2486.
10. Commission des Essais Biologiques (CEB) (2010) Méthode d'évaluation des effets de toxicité aiguë et à court terme des préparations phytopharmaceutiques sur l'abeille domestique (Apis mellifera L.). AFPP method n° 230.
11. European Food Safety Authority (2013) Guidance on the risk assessment of plant protection products on bees (Apis mellifera, Bombus spp. and solitary bees). EFSA J 11: 1–266.
12. Fischer D, Moriarty T (2011) Pesticide Risk Assessment for Pollinators: Summary of a SETAC Pellston Workshop. Pensacola FL (USA). Soc Environ Toxicol ans Chem: 1–43.
13. OEPP/EPPO (2003) EPPO Standards Environmental risk assessment scheme for plant protection products. Bull OEPP/EPPO 33: 141–145.
14. Atkins EL, Kellum D, Atkins KW (1981) Reducing pesticide hazards to honey bees: Mortality prediction techniques and integrated management strategies. Div Agric Sci Univ Calif: 1–20.
15. OEPP/EPPO (2001) Efficacy evaluation of plant protection products, Side-effects on honeybees. Bull OEPP/EPPO 170: 95–99.
16. OECD (1998) OECD guidelines for the testing of chemicals Number 214, Honeybees acute contact toxicity test: 1–7.
17. Schmolz E, Hoffmeister D, Lamprecht I (2002) Calorimetric investigations on metabolic rates and thermoregulation of sleeping honeybees (Apis mellifera carnica). Thermochim Acta 382: 221–227.
18. Grodzicki P, Caputa M (2005) Social versus individual behaviour: a comparative approach to thermal behaviour of the honeybee (Apis mellifera L.) and the American cockroach (Periplaneta americana L.). J Insect Physiol 51: 315–322.
19. Colin ME, Belzunces LP (1992) Evidence of synergy between prochloraz and deltametrin in Apis mellifera L.: A convenient biological approach. Pestic Sci 36: 115–119.
20. European Commission (EC) (2009) Regulation (EC) No 1107/2009 of the european parliament and of the council of 21 october 2009 concerning the placing of protection products on the market and repealing Council Directives 79/117/EEC and 91/414/EEC. Off J Eur Union L 309: 1–50.
21. European Economic Community (EEC) (1991) Council Directive of 15 July 1991 concerning the placing of plant protection products on the market (91/414/EEC). Off J Eur Union L 230: 1–290.
22. Wise JC, Jenkins PE, Schilder AMC, Vandervoort C, Isaacs R (2010) Sprayer type and water volume influence pesticide deposition and control of insect pests and diseases in juice grapes. Crop Prot 29: 378–385.
23. Canton JH, Linders JBHJ, Luttik R, Mensink BJWG, Panman E, et al. (1991) Catch-up operation on old pesticides: an integration. RIVM report 678801002. Natl Inst Public Heal Environ (RIVM), BA Bilthoven, Netherlands: 1–146.
24. Vandame R, Meled M, Colin ME, Belzunces LP (1995) Alteration of the homing-flight in the honey bee Apis mellifera L. exposed to sublethal dose of deltamethrin. Environ Toxicol Chem 14: 855–860.
25. Koch H, Weisser P (1997) Exposure of honey bees during pesticide application under field conditions. Apidologie 28: 439–447.
26. Wiest L, Buleté A, Giroud B, Fratta C, Amic S, et al. (2011) Multi-residue analysis of 80 environmental contaminants in honeys, honeybees and pollens by one extraction procedure followed by liquid and gas chromatography coupled with mass spectrometric detection. J Chromatogr A 1218: 5743–5756.
27. Brunet J-L, Badiou A, Belzunces LP (2005) In vivo metabolic fate of [14C]-acetamiprid in six biological compartments of the honeybee, Apis mellifera L. Pest Manag Sci 61: 742–748.
28. Stevens PJG, Baker EA, Anderson NH (1988) Factors affecting the foliar absorption and redistribution of pesticides. 2. Physicochemical properties of the active ingredient and the role of surfactant. Pestic Sci 24: 31–53.
29. European Chemicals Agency (ECHA) (2013) Guidance for human health risk assessment Volume III, Part B. III: 1–389.
30. SANCO (2002) Guidance document on terrestrial ecotoxicology under council directive 91 /414 /EEC (SANCO/10329/2002 rev 2 final): 1–39.
31. European Food Safety Authority (2009) Guidance document on risk assessment for bird & mammals on request from EFSA. EFSA J 7: 1–139.
32. Johansen CA, Mayer DF, Eves JD, Kious CW (1983) Pesticides and bees. Environ Entomol 12: 1513–1518.
33. Cooper PD, Schaffer WM, Buchmann SL, Cooper BYPD (1985) Temperature regulation of honey bees (Apis mellifera) foraging in the sonoran desert. J Exp Biol 114: 1–15.
34. Draft Assessment Report (DAR) on the active substance Abamectin prepared by the rapporteur Member State The Netherlands in the framework of the Council Directive 91/414/EEC (2006).
35. Iwasa T, Motoyama N, Ambrose JT, Roe RM (2004) Mechanism for the differential toxicity of neonicotinoid insecticides in the honey bee, Apis mellifera. Crop Prot 23: 371–378.
36. University of Hertfordshire (2013) The Pesticide Properties DataBase (PPDB) developed by the Agriculture & Environment Research Unit (AERU). Univ Hertfordsh 2006–2013.
37. Draft Assessment Report (DAR) on the active substance Quizalofop-P-tefuryl prepared by the rapporteur Member State Finland in the framework of the Council Directive 91/414/EEC (2007).
38. Torchio PF (1973) Relative toxicity of insecticides to the honey bee, alkali bee, and alfalfa leafcutting bee (Hymenoptera: Apidae, Halictidae, Megachilidae). J Kansas Entomol Soc 46: 446–453.
39. United Kingdom (1995) Draft Assessment Report (DAR) on the active substance Esfenvalerate prepared by the rapporteur Member State United Kingdom in the framework of the Council Directive 91/414/EEC. 3.
40. Draft Assessment Report (DAR) on the active substance Fenoxycarb prepared by the rapporteur Member State The Netherlands in the framework of the Council Directive 91/414/EEC (2007).
41. Draft Assessment Report (DAR) on the active substance Hexythiazox prepared by the rapporteur Member State Finland in the framework of the Council Directive 91/414/EEC (2006).
42. Schmuck R, Schöning R, Stork A, Schramel O (2001) Risk posed to honeybees (Apis mellifera L, Hymenoptera) by an imidacloprid seed dressing of sunflowers. Pest Manag Sci 57: 225–238.
43. Suchail S, Guez D, Belzunces LP (2000) Characteristics of imidacloprid toxicity in two Apis mellifera subspecies. Environ Toxicol Chem 19: 1901–1905.
44. Draft Assessment Report (DAR) on the active substance Prochloraz prepared by the rapporteur Member State Ireland in the framework of the Council Directive 91/414/EEC (2007).
45. Draft Assessment Report (DAR) on the active substance Pyriproxyfen prepared by the rapporteur Member State The Netherlands in the framework of the Council Directive 91/414/EEC (2005).
46. Draft Assessment Report (DAR) on the active substance Tau-fluvalinate prepared by the rapporteur Member State Denmark in the framework of the Council Directive 91/414/EEC (2007).
47. Draft Assessment Report (DAR) on the active substance Tebuconazole prepared by the rapporteur Member State Denmark in the framework of the Council Directive 91/414/EEC (2007).

17

Evaluation of the Efficacy & Biochemical Mechanism of Cell Death Induction by *Piper longum* Extract Selectively in *In-Vitro* and *In-Vivo* Models of Human Cancer Cells

Pamela Ovadje[1], Dennis Ma[1], Phillip Tremblay[1], Alessia Roma[1], Matthew Steckle[1], Jose-Antonio Guerrero[2], John Thor Arnason[2], Siyaram Pandey[1]*

1 Department of Chemistry & Biochemistry, University of Windsor, Windsor, ON, Canada, 2 Department of Biology, University of Ottawa, Ottawa, ON, Canada

Abstract

Background: Currently chemotherapy is limited mostly to genotoxic drugs that are associated with severe side effects due to non-selective targeting of normal tissue. Natural products play a significant role in the development of most chemotherapeutic agents, with 74.8% of all available chemotherapy being derived from natural products.

Objective: To scientifically assess and validate the anticancer potential of an ethanolic extract of the fruit of the Long pepper (PLX), a plant of the *piperaceae* family that has been used in traditional medicine, especially Ayurveda and investigate the anticancer mechanism of action of PLX against cancer cells.

Materials & Methods: Following treatment with ethanolic long pepper extract, cell viability was assessed using a water-soluble tetrazolium salt; apoptosis induction was observed following nuclear staining by Hoechst, binding of annexin V to the externalized phosphatidyl serine and phase contrast microscopy. Image-based cytometry was used to detect the effect of long pepper extract on the production of reactive oxygen species and the dissipation of the mitochondrial membrane potential following Tetramethylrhodamine or 5,5,6,6'-tetrachloro-1,1',3,3'-tetraethylbenzimidazolylcarbocyanine chloride staining (JC-1). Assessment of PLX *in-vivo* was carried out using Balb/C mice (toxicity) and CD-1 nu/nu immunocompromised mice (efficacy). HPLC analysis enabled detection of some primary compounds present within our long pepper extract.

Results: Our results indicated that an ethanolic long pepper extract selectively induces caspase-independent apoptosis in cancer cells, without affecting non-cancerous cells, by targeting the mitochondria, leading to dissipation of the mitochondrial membrane potential and increase in ROS production. Release of the AIF and endonuclease G from isolated mitochondria confirms the mitochondria as a potential target of long pepper. The efficacy of PLX in *in-vivo* studies indicates that oral administration is able to halt the growth of colon cancer tumors in immunocompromised mice, with no associated toxicity. These results demonstrate the potentially safe and non-toxic alternative that is long pepper extract for cancer therapy.

Editor: Stephanie Filleur, Texas Tech University Health Sciences Center, United States of America

Funding: This study was funded by Windsor & Essex County Cancer Centre Foundation by Seeds4Hope Grant (URL: http://windsorcancerfoundation.org/). The funders had no role in study design, data collection and analysis, decision to publish, or preparation of the manuscript.

* Email: spandey@uwindsor.ca

Introduction

The continuing increase in the incidence of cancer signifies a need for further research into more effective and less toxic alternatives to current treatments. In Canada alone, it was estimated that 267,700 new cases of cancer will arise, with 76,020 deaths occurring in 2012 alone. The global statistics are even more dire, with 12.7 million cancer cases and 7.6 million cancer deaths arising in 2008 [1,2]. The hallmarks of cancer cells uncover the difficulty in targeting cancer cells selectively. Cancer cells are notorious for sustaining proliferative signaling, evading growth suppression, activating invasion and metastasis and resisting cell death among other characteristics [3]. These characteristics pose various challenges in the development of successful anticancer therapies. The ability of cancer cells to evade cell death events has been the center of attention of much research, with focus centered on targeting the various vulnerable aspects of cancer cells to induce different forms of Programmed Cell Death (PCD) in cancer cells, with no associated toxicities to non-cancerous cells.

Apoptosis (PCD type I) has been studied for decades, the understanding of which will enhance the possible development of more effective cancer therapies. This is a form of cell death that is required for regular cell development and homeostasis, as well as a defense mechanism to get rid of damaged cells; cells undergoing apoptosis invest energy in their own demise so as not to become a nuisance [2]. Cancer cells evade apoptosis in order to confer added growth advantage and sustenance, therefore current anticancer therapies endeavour to exploit the various vulnerabilities of cancer cells in order to trigger the activation of apoptosis through either the extrinsic or intrinsic pathways [4,5]. The challenges facing some of the available cancer therapies are their abilities to induce apoptosis in cancer by inducing genomic DNA damage. Although this is initially effective, as they target rapidly dividing cells [6], they are usually accompanied by severe side effects caused by the non-selective targeting of normal non-cancerous cells, suggesting a need for other non-common targets for apoptosis induction without the associated toxicities.

Natural health products (NHPs) have shown great promise in the field of cancer research. The past 70 years have introduced various natural products as the source of many drugs in cancer therapy. Approximately 75% of the approved anticancer therapies have been derived from natural products, an expected statistic considering that more than 80% of the developing world's population is dependent on the natural products for therapy [7]. Plant products especially contain many bioactive chemicals that are able to play specific roles in the treatment of various diseases. Considering the complex mixtures and pharmacological properties of many natural products, it becomes difficult to establish a specific target and mechanism of action of many NHPs. With NHPs gaining momentum, especially in the field of cancer research, there is a lot of new studies on the mechanistic efficacy and safety of NHPs as potential anticancer agents [8].

Long pepper, from the Piperaceae family, has been used for centuries for the treatment of various diseases. Several species of long pepper have been identified, including *Piper longum* (the extract of which is being used in this study), *Piper betle*, *Piper retrofactum*, extracts of which have been used for years in the treatment of various diseases. A long list of uses and benefits are associated with extracts of different *Piper spp*, with reports indicating their effectiveness as good digestive agents and pain and inflammatory suppressants [9]. However, there is little to no scientific validation, only anecdotal evidence, for the benefits associated with the use of long pepper extracts. There are scientific studies have been carried out on several compounds present in extracts of long pepper, including piperines, which has been shown to inhibit many enzymatic drug bio-transforming reactions and plays specific roles in metabolic activation of carcinogens and mitochondrial energy production [10–13], and various piperidine alkaloids, with fungicidal activity [9,14]. Some of these compounds have shown potent anticancer activity [15], suggesting that Long pepper extracts could represent a new NHP, with better selective efficacy against cancer cells.

In this study, we examine the efficacy of an ethanolic extract of Long pepper fruit (PLX) against various cancer cells, as well as attempt to elucidate the mechanism of action, following treatment. Results from this study demonstrate that PLX reduced the viability of various cancer cell types in a dose and time dependent manner, where apoptosis induction was observed, following mitochondrial targeting and the release of pro-apoptotic factors. Due to the low doses of PLX required to induce apoptosis in cancer cell, it was easy to find the therapeutic window of this extract. The induction of apoptosis was found to be caspase-independent, although there was activation of both the extrinsic and intrinsic pathways and the production of ROS was not essential to the mechanism of cell death induction by PLX. The complex polychemical extract of the fruit of the long pepper plant, as a natural health product with unprecedented anticancer activity, provides a way to target multiple vulnerabilities of cancer cells. Even in the presence of certain inhibitors, PLX was efficacious in inducing apoptosis suggesting the potential application of developing PLX as a safe and efficacious cancer therapy.

Materials and Methods

Animal studies were carried out according to the animal care committee protocol approved by the University of Windsor Animal Care Committee; This protocol and project was approved by the animal care committee – Protocol number: AUPP 10–17), in accordance with the Canadian Council of Animal Care (CCAC) guidelines.

Cell Culture

The malignant melanoma cell line G-361, human colorectal cancer cell lines HT-29 and HCT116 (American Type Culture Collection, Manassas, VA, USA Cat. No. CRL-1687, CCL-218 & CCL-247, respectively) were cultured with McCoy's Medium 5a (Gibco BRL, VWR, Mississauga, ON, Canada) supplemented with 10% (v/v) FBS (Thermo Scientific, Waltham, MA, USA) and 40 mg/ml gentamicin (Gibco, BRL, VWR). The ovarian adenocarcinoma cell line OVCAR-3 (American Type Culture Collection, Cat. No. HTB-161) was cultured in RPMI-1640 media (Sigma-Aldrich Canada, Mississauga, ON, Canada) supplemented with 0.01 mg/mL bovine insulin, 20% (v/v) fetal bovine serum (FBS) standard (Thermo Scientific, Waltham, MA, USA) and 10 mg/mL gentamicin. The pancreatic adenocarcinoma cell line BxPC-3 (American Type Culture Collection, Cat. No. CRL-1424) was cultured in RPMI-1640 medium, supplemented with 10% (v/v) fetal bovine serum (FBS) standard and 40 mg/mL gentamicin. Normal-derived colon mucosa NCM460 cell line (INCELL Corporation, LLC., San Antonio, TX, USA) was grown in INCELL's M3Base medium (INCELL Corporation, LLC., Cat. No. M300A500) supplemented with 10% (v/v) FBS and 10 mg/mL gentamicin.

All cells were grown in optimal growth conditions of 37°C and 5% CO_2. Furthermore, all cells were passaged for ≤6 months.

Long Pepper Extraction

Ripe and dried Indian long pepper fruits were obtained from Quality Natural Foods limited, Toronto Ontario. The plant material was ground up and extracted in anhydrous ethanol (100%) in a ratio of 1:10 (1 g plant material to 10 ml ethanol). The extraction was carried out overnight on a shaker at room temperature. The extract was passed through a P8 coarse filter, followed by a 0.45 μm filter. The solvent was evaporated using a RotorVap at 40°C and reconstituted in dimethylsulfoxide (Me_2SO) at a final stock concentration of 450 mg/ml.

Cell Treatment

Cells were plated and grown to 60–70% confluence, before being treated with Long Pepper Extracts (PLX), N-Acetyl-L-cysteine (NAC) (Sigma-Aldrich Canada, Cat. No. A7250), and broad-spectrum caspase inhibitor, Z-VAD-FMK (EMD Chemicals, Gibbstown, NJ, USA) at the indicated doses and durations. NAC was dissolved in sterile water. Z-VAD-FMK was dissolved in dimethylsulfoxide (Me_2SO). PLX was extracted as previously described, reconstituted in Me_2SO. Before treatment, a dilute working concentration of 10 mg/ml in PBS was prepared. Cells were treated with the 10 mg/ml to obtained the final concentrations indicated in the results section.

Table 1. Analysis of five well-known piperamides and crude long pepper extract at a flow rate of 1.0 mL/min with a mobile phase constituted of H_2O and methanol.

Time (mins)	H_2O (%)	MeOH (%)
0.0	37.5	62.5
15.0	35.0	65.0
35.0	0.0	100.0
45.0	0.0	100.0
46.0	37.5	62.5

Assessing the Efficacy of Long Pepper Extract (PLX) In Cancer Cells

WST-1 Assay for Cell Viability. To assess the effect of PLX on cancer cells, a water-soluble tetrazolium salt (WST-1) based colorimetric assay was carried out as per manufacturer's protocol (Roche Applied Science, Indianapolis, IN, USA), to quantify cell viability as a function of cellular metabolism. Equal number of cells were seeded onto 96-well clear bottom tissue culture plates then treated with the indicated treatments at the indicated concentrations and durations. Following treatment, cells were incubated with the WST-1 reagent for 4 hours at 37°C with 5% CO_2. The WST-1 reagent is cleaved to formazan by cellular enzymes in actively metabolizing cells. The formazan product was quantified by taking absorbance readings at 450 nm on a Wallac Victor[3] 1420 Multilabel Counter (PerkinElmer, Woodbridge, ON,

Canada). Cellular viability as a measure of metabolic activity was expressed as percentages of the solvent control groups.

Nuclear Staining. Subsequent to treatment, the nuclei of cells were stained with 10 µM Hoechst 33342 dye (Molecular Probes, Eugene, OR, USA) or 1 mg/ml propidium iodide (PI) (Sigma Aldrich, Mississauga, ON. Canada), to monitor nuclear morphology for apoptosis induction at designated time points and overall cell death. Cells were incubated with 10 µM Hoechst dye and 1 mg/ml PI for 10 minutes and micrographs were taken with a Leica DM IRB inverted fluorescence microscope (Wetzlar, Germany) at 400× magnification. Image-based cytometry was used to quantify the amount of cell death occurring with PI staining.

Annexin V Binding Assay. To confirm the induction of apoptosis, the binding of Annexin V to externalized phosphatidylserine on the outer cellular surface, was assessed. Following

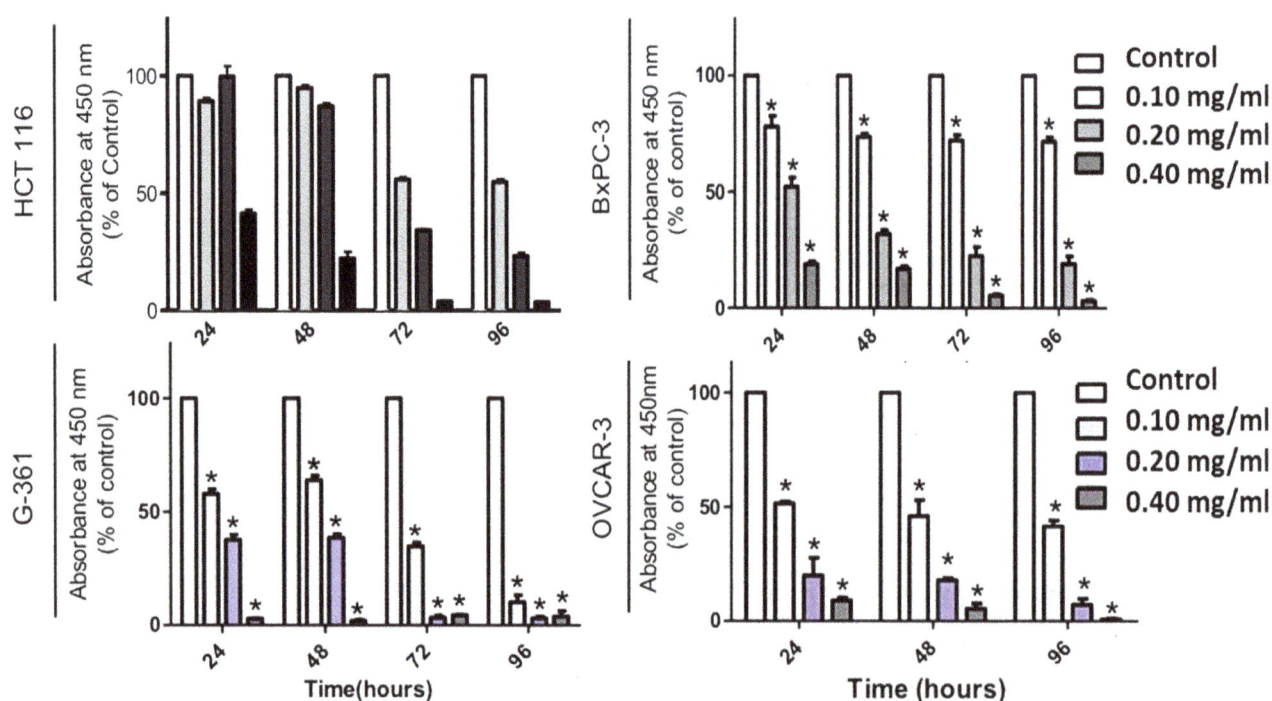

Figure 1. Crude Ethanolic Extract of Long Pepper (PLX) Effectively Reduces the Percentage of Viable Cancer cells in a Dose & Time Dependent Manner. Colon (HCT116), Ovarian (OVCAR-3), Pancreatic (BxPC-3) cancer and Melanoma (G-361) cells were treated with a crude ethanolic extract of long pepper (PLX), following which they were incubated with WST-1 cell viability dye for 4 hours. Absorbance was read at 450 nm and expressed as a percent of the control. Values are expressed as mean ± SD from quadruplicates of 3 independent experiments. **P< 0.0001.

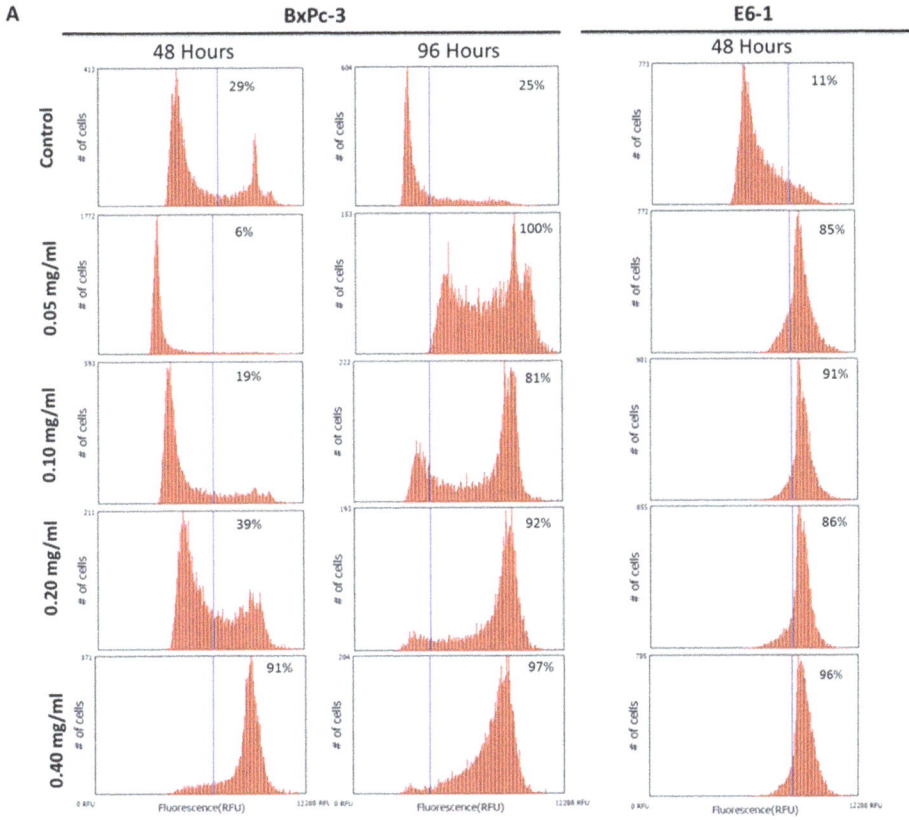

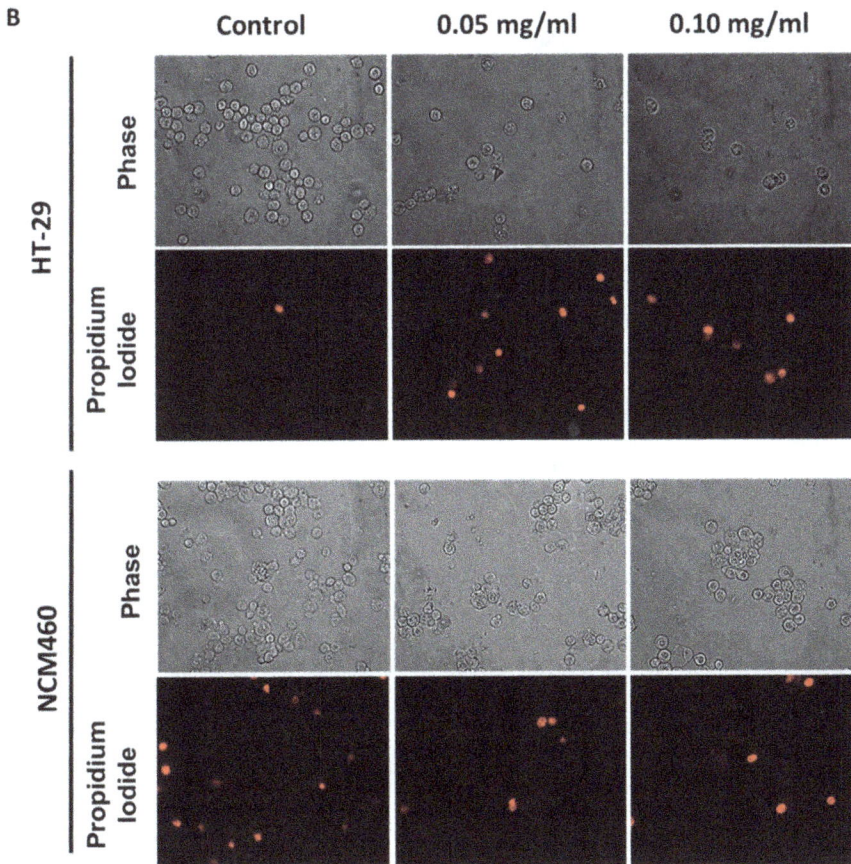

Figure 2. PLX Selectively Induces Cell Death in Human Cancer Cells in a Dose & Time Dependent Manner. (A) Following treatment of Human pancreatic (BxPc-3) cancer and T cell leukemia cells with PLX, at indicated time points, cells were incubated with propidium iodide and assessed for the induction of cell death by image-based cytometry. (B) Similar experiments were carried out in human colon cancer cells (HT-29) and normal colon epithelial cells (NCM460). Fluorescence microscopy was used to assess the induction of cell death as characterized by presence of propidium iodide positive cells. Images were taken at 400× magnification on a fluorescent microscope. Scale bar = 15 μm.

treatment with PLX, cells were washed twice in phosphate buffer saline (PBS). Subsequently, cells were resuspended and incubated in Annexin V binding buffer (10 mM HEPES, 10 mM NaOH, 140 mM NaCl, 1 mM CaCl2, pH 7.6) with Annexin V Alexa-Fluor-488 (1:50) (Invitrogen, Canada, Cat No. A13201) for 15 minutes. In the final 10 minutes of incubation, 10 μM Hoechst and 1 mg/ml propidium iodide were added to the microcentrifuge tube and incubated for the final 10 minutes in the dark. Micrographs were taken at 400× magnification on a Leica DM IRB inverted microscope (Wetzlar, Germany) and image-based cytometry was used to quantify the percentage of programmed cell death (annexin V positive cells) occurring after treatment.

TUNEL Staining to Detect DNA Damage and Quantify Apoptosis. Following PLX treatment, HT-29 cells were labeled with the Terminal deoxynucleotidyl transferase dUTP nick end labeling (TUNEL) assay. The assay was performed according to the manufacturer's protocol (Molecular Probes, Eugene, OR), in order to detect DNA damage. Cells were treated with PLX or VP-16 (as a positive control) at indicated concentrations and time points and analyzed for the fragmentation of DNA. Following treatment, cells were fixed by suspending them in 70% (v/v) ethanol and stored at −20°C overnight. The sample was then incubated with a DNA labeling solution (10 μL reaction buffer, 0.75 μL TdT enzyme, 8 μL BrdUTP, 31.25 μL of dH2O) for 1 hour at 25°C. Each sample was exposed to an antibody solution (5 μL Alexa Fluor 488 labeled anti-BrdU antibody and 95 μL rinse solution). The cells were incubated with the antibody solution for 20 minutes and TUNEL positive cells were quantified by image-based cytometry.

Whole Cell ROS Generation. Following treatment with PLX, cells were incubated with 2′,7′-Dichlorofluorescin diacetate H2DCFDA (Catalog No. D6883, Sigma Aldrich, Mississauga ON. Canada) for 45 minutes. Cells were collected, washed twice in PBS and green fluorescence was observed using a TALI image-based cytometer (Invitrogen, Canada). NAC was used to assess the dependence of PLX on ROS generation and viability.

Assessment of Mitochondrial Function Following PLX Treatment

Tetramethylrhodamine Methyl Ester (TMRM) Staining. To monitor mitochondrial membrane potential (MMP), tetramethylrhodamine methyl ester (TMRM) (Gibco BRL, VWR, Mississauga, ON, Canada) or 5,5,6,6′-tetrachloro-1,1′,3,3′-tetraethylbenzimidazolylcarbocyanine chloride (JC-1) (Invitrogen, Canada) were used. Cells were grown on coverslips, treated with the indicated concentrations of treatments at the indicated time points, and incubated with 200 nM TMRM for 45 minutes at 37°C. Micrographs were obtained at 400× magnification on a Leica DM IRB inverted fluorescence microscope (Wetzlar, Germany). To confirm the results obtained by fluorescence microscopy, image-based cytometry was used to detect red fluorescence. Cells were seeded in 6-well plates and following treatment, cells were incubated with TMRM for 45 minutes, washed twice in PBS and placed in TALI slides. Red fluorescence was obtained using a TALI image-based cytometer (Invitrogen, Canada).

Mitochondrial Isolation to Assess Mitochondrial Targeting. Cells were collected by trypsin, washed once in cold PBS, resuspended in cold hypotonic buffer (1 mM EDTA, 5 mM Tris–HCl, 210 mM mannitol, 70 mM sucrose, 10 μM Leu-pep and Pep-A, 100 μM PMSF), and manually homogenized. The homogenized cell solution was centrifuged at 3000 rpm for 5 minutes at 4°C. The supernatant was centrifuged at 12,000 rpm for 15 minutes at 4°C and the mitochondrial pellet was resuspended in cold reaction buffer (2.5 mM malate, 10 mM succinate, 10 μM Leu-pep and Pep-A, 100 μM PMSF in PBS). The isolated mitochondria were treated with PLX at the indicated concentrations and incubated for 2 hours in cold reaction buffer. The control group was treated with solvent (ethanol). Following 2 hour incubation with extract, mitochondrial samples were vortexed and centrifuged at 12,000 rpm for 15 minutes at 4°C. The resulting supernatant and mitochondrial pellets (resuspended in cold reaction buffer) were subjected to Western Blot analysis to assess for the mitochondrial release/retention of pro-apoptotic factors.

Western Blot Analyses. Protein samples were subjected to SDS-PAGE, transferred onto a nitrocellulose membrane, and blocked with 5% w/v milk TBST (Tris-Buffered Saline Tween-20) solution for 1 hour. Membranes were incubated overnight at 4°C with an anti-endonuclease G (EndoG) antibody (1:1000) raised in rabbits (Abcam, Cat. No. ab9647, Cambridge, MA, USA), an anti-succinate dehydrogenase subunit A (SDHA) antibody (1:1000) raised in mice (Santa Cruz Biotechnology, Inc., sc-59687, Paso Robles, CA, USA), or an anti-apoptosis inducing factor (AIF) antibody raised in rabbits (1:1000) (Abcam, Cat. No. ab1998, Cambridge, MA, USA). After primary antibody incubation, the membrane was washed once for 15 minutes and twice for 5 minutes in TBST. Membranes were incubated for 1 hour at room temperature with an anti-mouse or an anti-rabbit horserad-ish peroxidase-conjugated secondary antibody (1:2000) (Abcam, ab6728, ab6802, Cambridge, MA, USA) followed by three 5-minute washes in TBST. Chemiluminescence reagent (Sigma-Aldrich, CPS160, Mississauga, ON, Canada) was used to visualize protein bands and densitometry analysis was performed using ImageJ software.

In-Vivo Assessment of Long Pepper Extract

Toxicity Assessment. Six week old Balb/C mice were obtained from Charles River Laboratories and housed in constant laboratory conditions of a 12-hour light/dark cycle, in accordance with the animal protocols outlined in the University of Windsor Research Ethics Board- AUPP 10–17). Following acclimatization, mice were divided into three groups (3 animals/control (untreated), 3 animals/gavage control (vehicle treatment) and 4 animals/treatment group). The control untreated group was given plain filtered water, while the second and third group was given 50 mg/kg/day vehicle (Me2SO) or PLX, respectively for 75 days. During the period of study, toxicity was measured by weighing mice twice a week and urine was collected for protein urinalysis by urine dipstick and Bradford assays. Following the duration of study, mice were sacrificed and their organs (livers, kidneys and hearts) were obtained for immunohistochemical and toxicological analysis by Dr. Brooke at the University of Guelph.

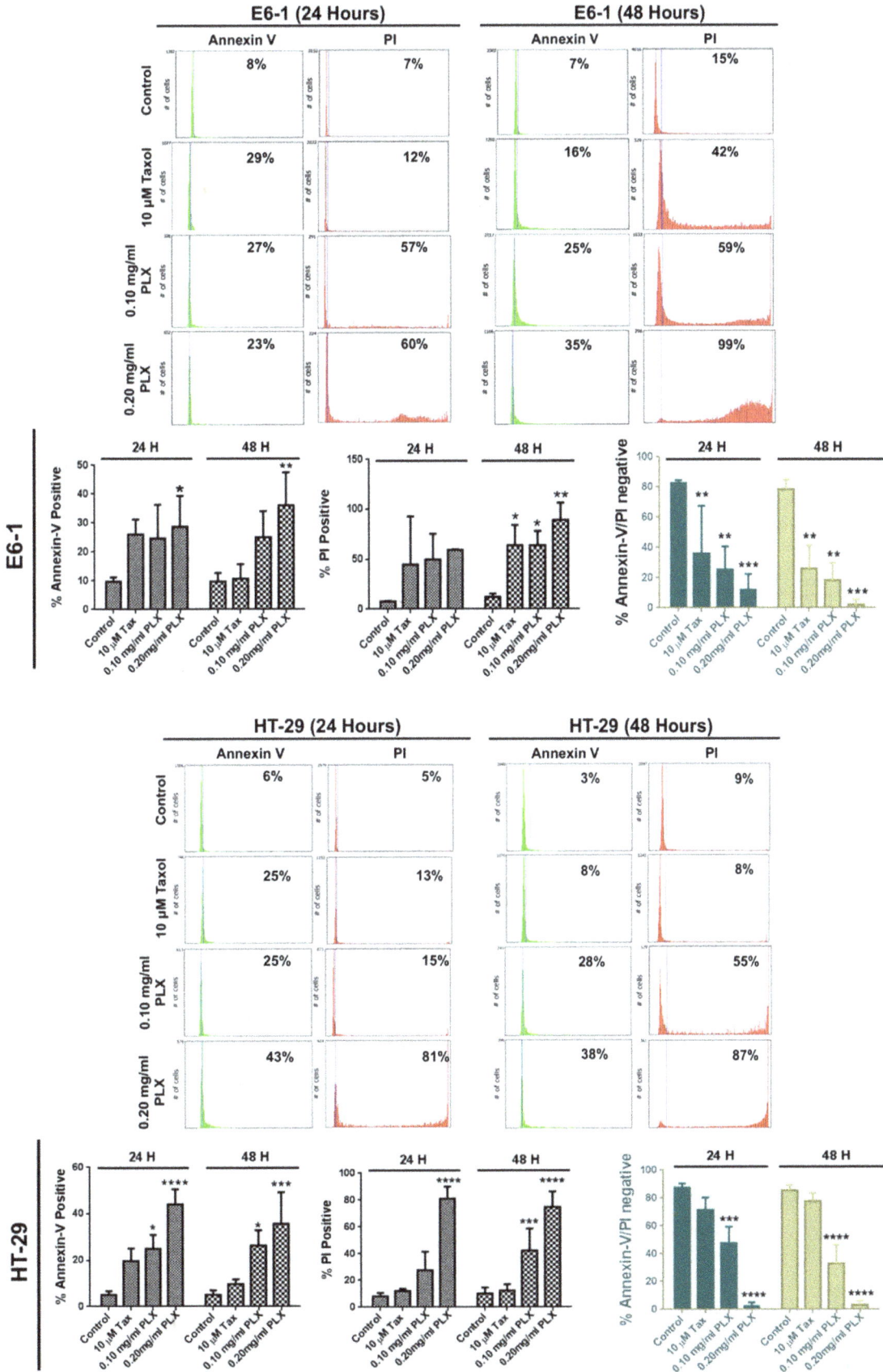

Figure 3. Quantification of Cell Death Induction Following PLX Treatment. Image-Based cytometry was used to quantify apoptotic induction (% Annexin V positive), followed by necrosis (% PI positive) in E6-1 and HT-29 cells following PLX treatment. The lack of annexin V or PI staining was used as an indication of live cells following treatment (%Annexin V/PI negative cells) (*P<0.05, ** P<0.003, ***P<0.0001). (E) To further confirm the induction of apoptosis.

Efficacy of PLX in Tumor Xenograft Models of Immunocompromised Mice. Six week old male CD-1 nu/nu mice were obtained from Charles River Laboratories and housed in constant laboratory conditions of a 12-hour light/dark cycle, in accordance with the animal protocols outlined in the University of Windsor Research Ethics Board- AUPP 10–17). Following acclimatization, the mice were injected subcutaneously in the right and left hind flanks with a colon cancer cell suspension (in Phosphate buffered saline) at a concentration of $2 * 10^6$ cells/mouse (HT-29, $p53^{-/-}$, in the left flank and HCT116, $p53^{+/+}$, in the right flank). Tumors were allowed to develop (approximately a week), following which the animals were randomized into treatment groups of 4 mice per group, a control group, a gavage control group given plain filtered sterile water, as well as gavage regimen of the vehicle (5 μL Me_2SO in PBS) twice a week. The final group was given filtered water supplemented with long pepper extract at a concentration of 100 μg/mL, as well as gavage regimen of long pepper extract (5 μL extract in PBS), twice a week, corresponding to 50 mg/kg/day. The tumors were assessed every other day by measuring the length, width and height, using a standard caliper and the tumor volume was calculated according to the formula π/6*length*width. The mice were also assessed for any weight loss every other day for the duration of the study, which lasted 75 days, following which the animals were sacrificed and their organs and tissues (liver, kidneys, heart and tumors) were obtained and stored in 10% formaldehyde for immunohistochemical and toxicological analysis.

Hematoxylin & Eosin (H & E) Staining. Mice organs were fixed in 10% formaldehyde, following which they were cryosectioned into 10 μm sections and placed on a superfrost/Plus microscope slides (Fisherbrand, Fisher Scientific). Sections of organs were stained according to a standardized H & E protocol [16].

Phytochemical Analysis of Long Pepper Extract by HPLC

HPLC analysis of the long pepper crude extract was carried out at University of Ottawa in the Arnason lab. A total of five well-known piperamides were analyzed and compared to the crude long pepper extract. The extracts and piperamide standards were analyzed on a Luna C18-5u-250×4.6 mm column at 45°C at a flow rate of 1.0 mL/min with a mobile phase constituted of H_2O and methanol as outlined in Table 1. Chromatogram profiles were used to detect the any differences between a sample standard of known piperamides in the crude long pepper extracts.

Statistical Analysis

All experiments were repeated at least three independent times. Representative fluorescence images were shown, where appropriate. Statistical analysis was performed using GraphPad Prism 6.0

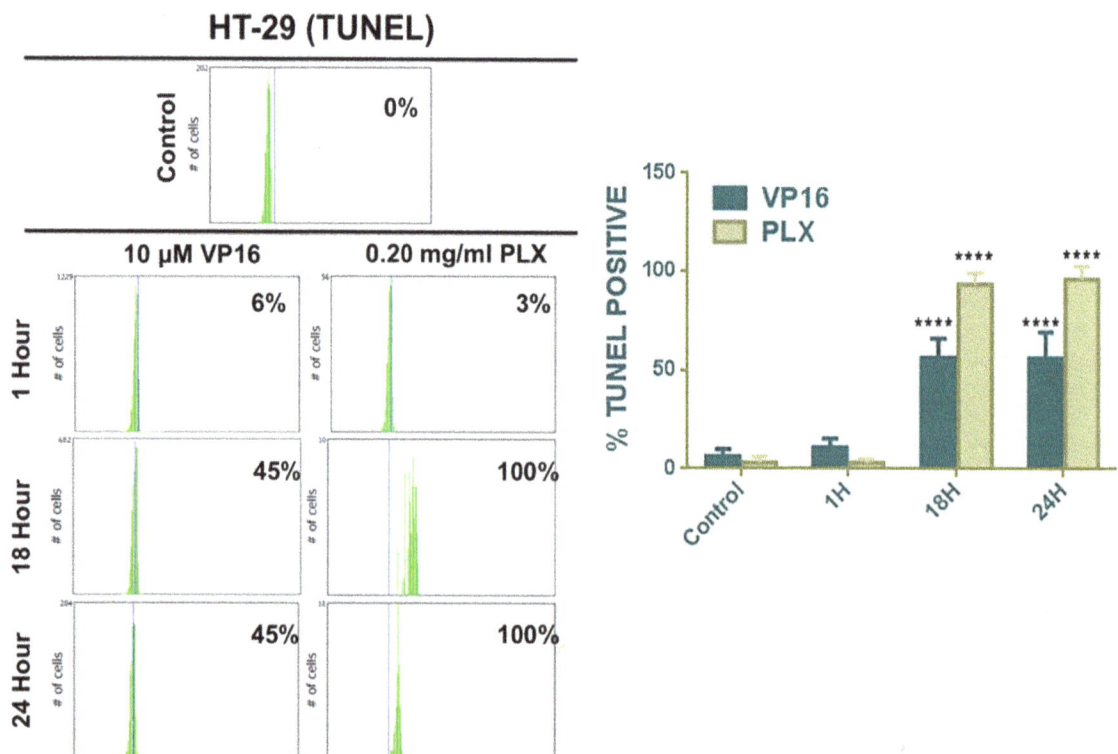

Figure 4. PLX Induces Double-stranded DNA Breaks in Cancer Cells. TUNEL labeling was used to detect DNA fragmentation. Following PLX and VP16 (as a positive control for DNA damage) treatment, cells were labelled with DNA staining solution and quantified by image-based cytometry. Treated cells were compared to the control untreated cell sample. (****P<0.0001).

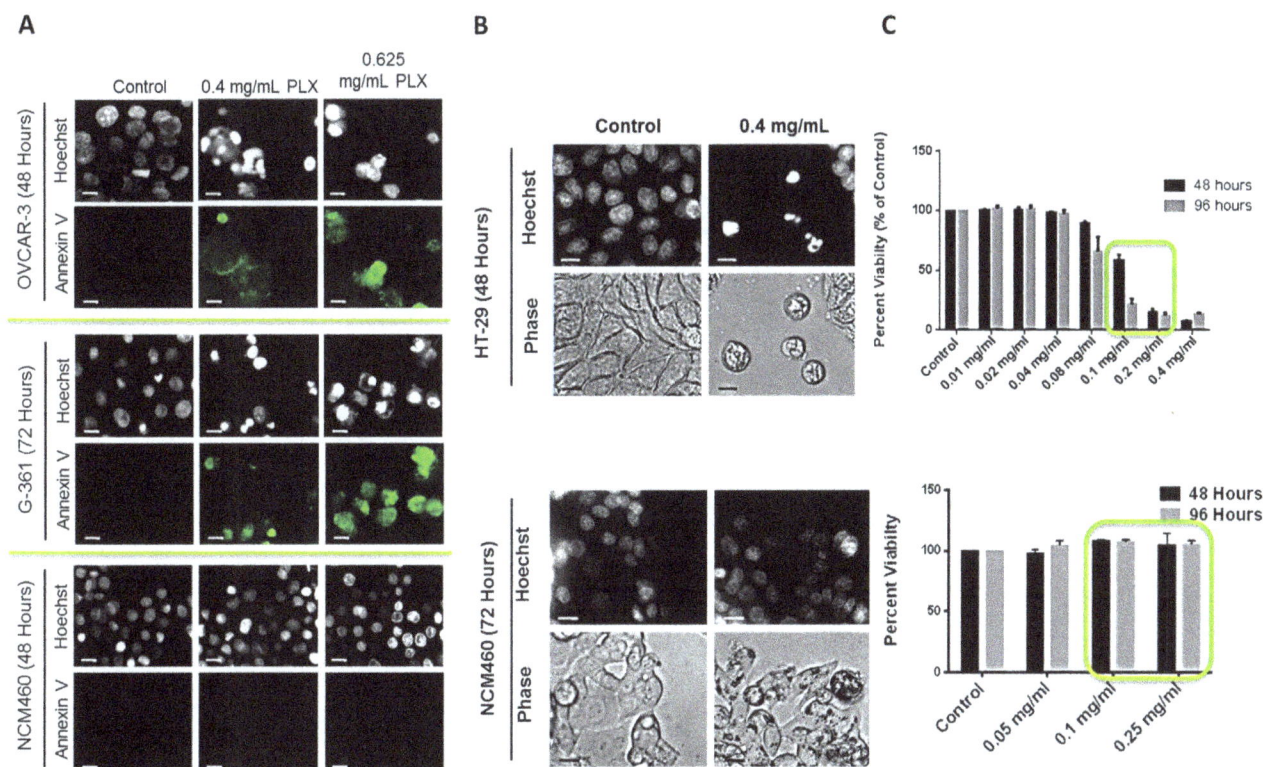

Figure 5. PLX Selectively Targets Cancer Cells for Apoptosis Induction. Subsequent to treatment with PLX, cells (Ovarian; OVCAR-3, Melanoma; G-361 and Normal Colon Epithelia cells (NCM460) were stained with Hoechst to characterize nuclear morphology and Annexin-V to detect apoptotic cells (A) and cellular morphology by phase contrast microscopy (B); Images were taken at 400× magnification on a fluorescent microscope. Scale bar = 15 μm. (C) Following PLX treatment, HT-29 colorectal cancer cells and non-cancerous NCM460 cells were incubated with WST-1 cell viability dye for 4 hours and absorbance was read at 450 nm and expressed as a percent of the control. Values are expressed as mean ± SD of 3 independent experiments. **P<0.0001.

288 software. The mean and standard error of three independent experiments were analyzed for the quantification data. The Student's T-test and two-way Anova were used for statistical analysis.

Results

Ethanolic Extract of Long Pepper (PLX) Effectively and Selectively Reduces the Viability of & Induces Apoptosis in Cancer cells in a Dose & Time Dependent Manner

The first step in understanding the effect of long pepper extract in this study was to assess the effect of PLX on the viability of cancer cells. Following treatment with increasing concentration of PLX at increasing time points, cells were incubated with a water soluble tetrazolium salt, which gets metabolized to a red formazan product by viable cells with active metabolism. This product can then be quantified by absorbance spectrometry. We observed the efficacy of crude PLX in reducing the viability of cancer cells, including colon (HCT116), pancreatic (BxPC-3), ovarian cancer (OVCAR-3) and melanoma cells. This effect was dose and time dependent (Figure 1). To further evaluate the anticancer activity of PLX, we wanted to assess its role in cell death and its selectivity to cancer cells. Our results demonstrate that PLX is able to selectively induce cell death in cancer cells (colon, pancreatic and leukemia) in a dose and time dependent manner, as characterized by the increase in propidium iodide positive cells in cancer cells treated with PLX (Figure 2). Furthermore, this effect was selective, as normal colon epithelial cells remained unaffected by this

treatment, at the same concentrations and time-points (Figure 2B). These results were quantified using image-based cytometry to determine the percentage of cells undergoing apoptosis and total cell death. We observed a 30–40% increase in annexin V positive cells, following PLX treatment and an 80–100% PI positive increase in the same cell samples, confirming the induction of apoptosis, following by necrosis in cultured cancer cells (Figure 3).

DNA fragmentation is a key biochemical feature of apoptosis. To further confirm this induction of apoptosis, TUNEL labelling to detect DNA fragmentation was employed. Quantification results from image-based cytometry show the efficacy of PLX in inducing apoptosis, following DNA fragmentation in HT-29 colon cancer cells in a time dependent manner. VP16, a known chemotherapeutic agent with DNA damaging capabilities, was used as a positive control (Figure 4).

Additionally, apoptosis induction in various cancer cells, melanoma (G-361), ovarian and colon cancer (HT-29) cells, was confirmed by Annexin-V binding assay. This induction of apoptosis was confirmed to be selective to cancer cells, as normal colon cells (NCM460) remained unaffected by PLX treatment. This was indicated by nuclear condensation, cell morphology and externalization of phosphatidyl serine to the outer leaflet of the cell membrane, as indicated by Hoechst staining, phase contrast images and binding of annexin V dye respectively (Figure 5A and B). The selectivity of PLX to cancer cells was further confirmed by the WST-1 cell viability assay that showed that PLX was highly effective at such low doses, a therapeutic window was easily observed (Figure 5C). Treatment of HT-29 with 0.20 mg/ml

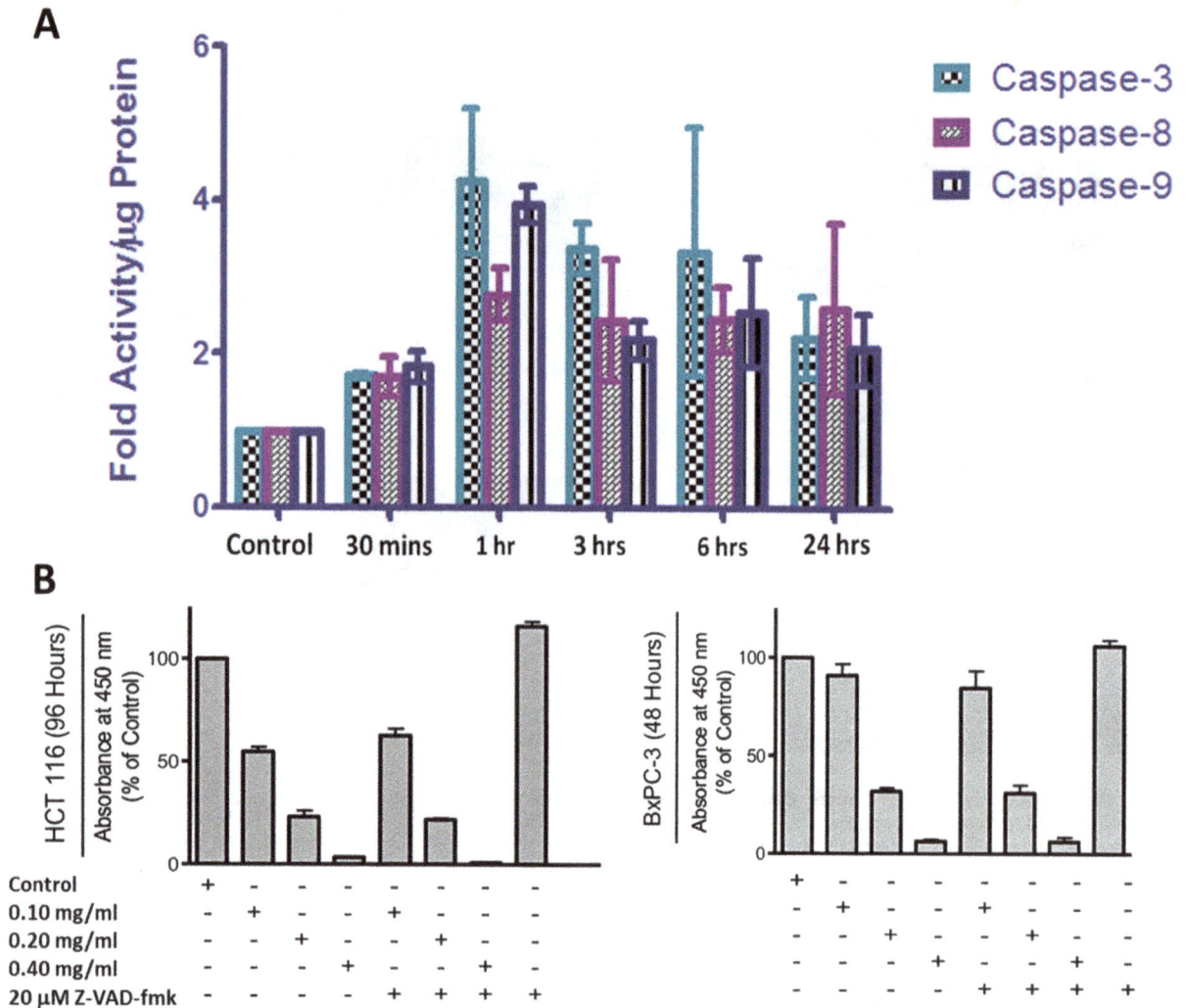

Figure 6. Long Pepper Extract (PLX) Activates the Extrinsic & Intrinsic Pathways of Apoptosis. Following treatment with 0.10 mg/ml PLX, at indicated time points, BxPc-3 cells were collected, washed and incubated with lysis buffer to obtain cell lysate. The cell lysate was incubated with caspase substrates, specific to each caspase (3, 8 and 9) and incubated for an hour. Fluorescence readings were obtained using a spectrofluorometer. An average of 6 readings per well and a minimum of three wells were run per experiment. The results here are reported as activity per μg of protein (in fold) and the average of three independent experiments is shown. (**B**) The reduction in viability was caspase independent, as a pan-caspase inhibitor, Z-VAD-fmk could not prevent the loss of viability induced by PLX treatment in colon and pancreatic cancer cells. Absorbance was read at 450 nm and expressed as a percent of the control. Values are expressed as mean ± SD from quadruplicates of 3 independent experiments. **P< 0.0001.

effectively reduced the viability by approximately 90%, while NCM460 cells remained at 100% viability at the same dose. This indicates that PLX can be more effective at very low doses, further reducing the chances of toxicity associated with treatment.

PLX Induces Caspase-Independent Apoptosis in Human Cancer Cells

Caspases are cysteine aspartic proteases that play a predominant role as death proteases [17]. Their roles in various cell death processes remains controversial, as their activation or inhibition could be essential to the progression of inhibition of cell death pathways [18,19]. To assess the role of caspases in our study, following treatment with 0.10 mg/ml PLX, at indicated time points, BxPc-3 cells were collected, washed and incubated with lysis buffer to obtain cell lysate. The cell lysate was incubated with caspase substrates, specific to each caspase (3, 8 and 9) and

incubated for an hour. Fluorescence readings were obtained using a spectrofluorometer. Our results indicate that PLX is able to activate both pathways (extrinsic and intrinsic apoptosis) in a time dependent manner. This was observed as rapid activation of caspases-3, 8 and 9 were observed as early as an hour, following treatment (Figure 6A).

To determine the importance of these activated caspases to the apoptosis-inducing effect of PLX, colon (HCT116) and pancreatic (BxPc-3) cancer cells were pre-treated with a pan-caspase inhibitor, Z-VAD-fmk (20 μM), for an hour before treatment with PLX. Following treatments, the WST-1 cell viability assay was used to assess for viability and efficacy of PLX. Our results indicate that the inhibition of caspases could not prevent the reduction of viability (Figure 6B), signifying that the effect of PLX in cancer cells is independent of caspase activation.

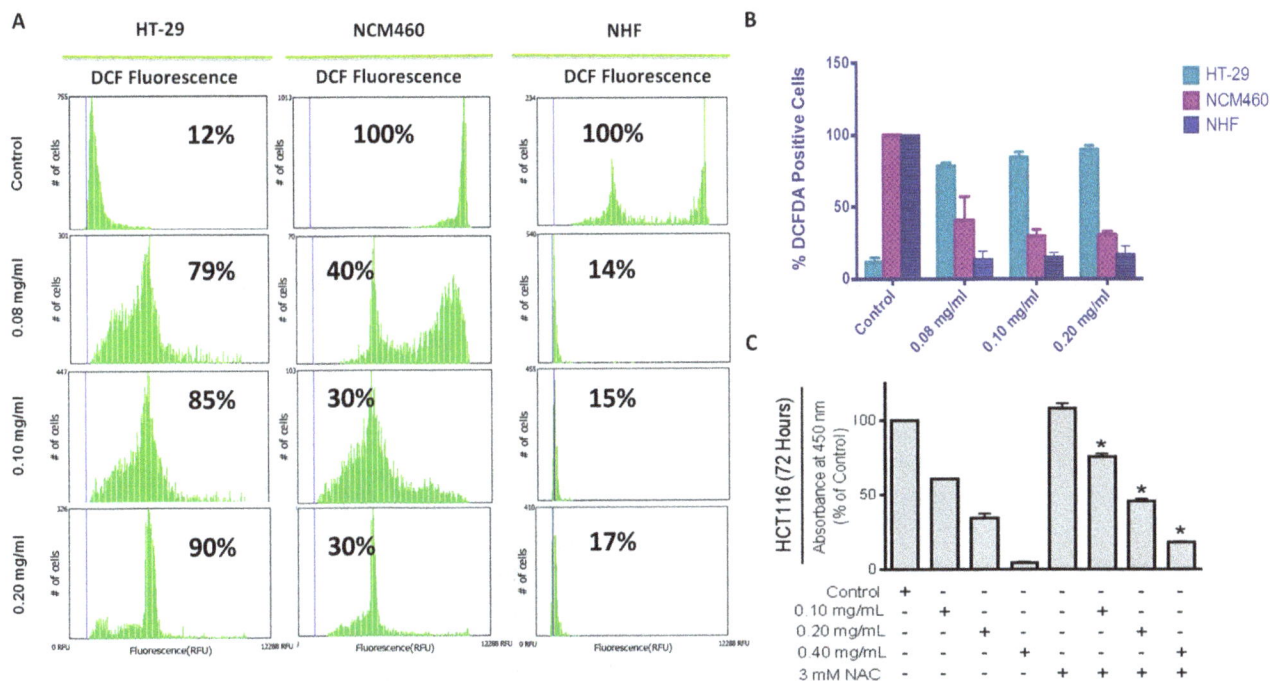

Figure 7. PLX Causes but is Not Dependent on the Production of Reactive Oxygen Species (ROS). (A) Colon cancer (HT-29), Normal Colon Epithelial (NCM460) and Normal Human Fibroblast (NHF) cells were treated with PLX for 48 hours, following which, they were incubated with H₂DCFDA and fluorescence results were obtained using an image based cytometer. Results were quantified using Graphpad prism 6.0 (B). (C) HCT116 colon cancer cells were treated with 3 mM N-acetylcysteine for an hour prior to PLX treatment. Cells were then treated PLX at indicated concentrations for 72 hours, following which the WST-1 assay was performed. Absorbance readings were taken at 450 nm and expressed as a percent of the control. Values are expressed as mean ± SD from quadruplicates of 3 independent experiments. *p<0.05.

Long Pepper Extract Induces Oxidative Stress and Targets the Mitochondria of Cancer Cells

Generation of oxidative stress has been well established as a major player in the induction of several cell death processes, especially apoptosis [20,21]. The next part of our study focused on the role of oxidative stress in PLX induced apoptosis. Following treatment with PLX for 48 hours, cells were incubated with 2′,7′-Dichlorofluorescin diacetate H₂DCFDA for 45 minutes. The resulting green fluorescence histograms were obtained using a TALI image-based cytometer. From the results, it was observed that PLX induced extensive generation of whole cell reactive oxygen species (ROS) in HT-29 colon cancer cells, while acting to suppress any ROS present in the non-cancerous cell lines, NCM460 and normal human fibroblasts (NHF) (Figure 7A & B). This confirms our results of selectivity and indicates that PLX might act as a pro-oxidant in cancer cells in order to induce apoptosis.

To determine if this oxidative stress was essential to PLX activity, HCT116 colon cancer cells were pre-treated with N-acetyl-L-cysteine (NAC), a well-established anti-oxidant, used extensively in vitro studies [22,23], before treatment with PLX. Subsequent to PLX treatment, cells were analyzed for effect of PLX on viability, using the WST-1 viability assay. The results suggest that although PLX acts to induce oxidative stress to cause apoptosis, this oxidative stress is not essential to its activity. Both the cells treated with PLX alone and NAC followed by PLX showed a reduction in their viability (Figure 7C).

The mitochondria have also been shown to play a major role in the progression and execution of apoptosis. The permeabilization of the mitochondrial membrane usually leads to the release of pro-apoptotic factors, including cytochrome c, apoptosis inducing

factor (AIF) and endonuclease G (EndoG) [5,24]. These factors cause a caspase-independent pathway for apoptosis to pass through and could bypass the antioxidant effects of NAC observed in figure 7C.

To assess the efficacy of PLX on the mitochondria of cancer cells, OVCAR-3, HT-29 and NCM460 cells were stained with TMRM, a cationic dye that accumulates in healthy mitochondria. Mitochondrial membrane potential (MMP) dissipation was only observed in OVCAR-3 and HT-29 cells as seen with the dissipation of red TMRM fluorescence, by fluorescence microscopy and image-based cytometry (Figure 8A, B & C). Following mitochondrial membrane collapse, we wanted to determine if there was release of some pro-apoptotic factors. Western blot analysis was used to monitor for the release of AIF and EndoG from isolated OVCAR-3 mitochondria. Results demonstrate that PLX directly caused the release of both AIF and EndoG from the mitochondria of OVCAR-3 cells (Figure 8D). These results provide an insight to the mechanism of PLX action, where the mitochondria appear to be a direct target of PLX for the reduction of viability and the induction of apoptosis.

Long Pepper Extract is Well-Tolerated in Animal Models

Long pepper extracts (mainly water extracts) have been used for centuries and have been associated with various benefits [9]. With all these anecdotal reports of benefits, there have been no reports of toxicities associated with its use. To further scientifically evaluate and validate the safety of PLX, balb/c mice were orally gavaged with 50 mg/kg/day vehicle (DMSO) or PLX for 75 days and the mice were observed for signs of toxicity. To assess for toxicity, mice were weighed twice a week, urine was collected for protein urinalysis studies and following period of treatment, mice

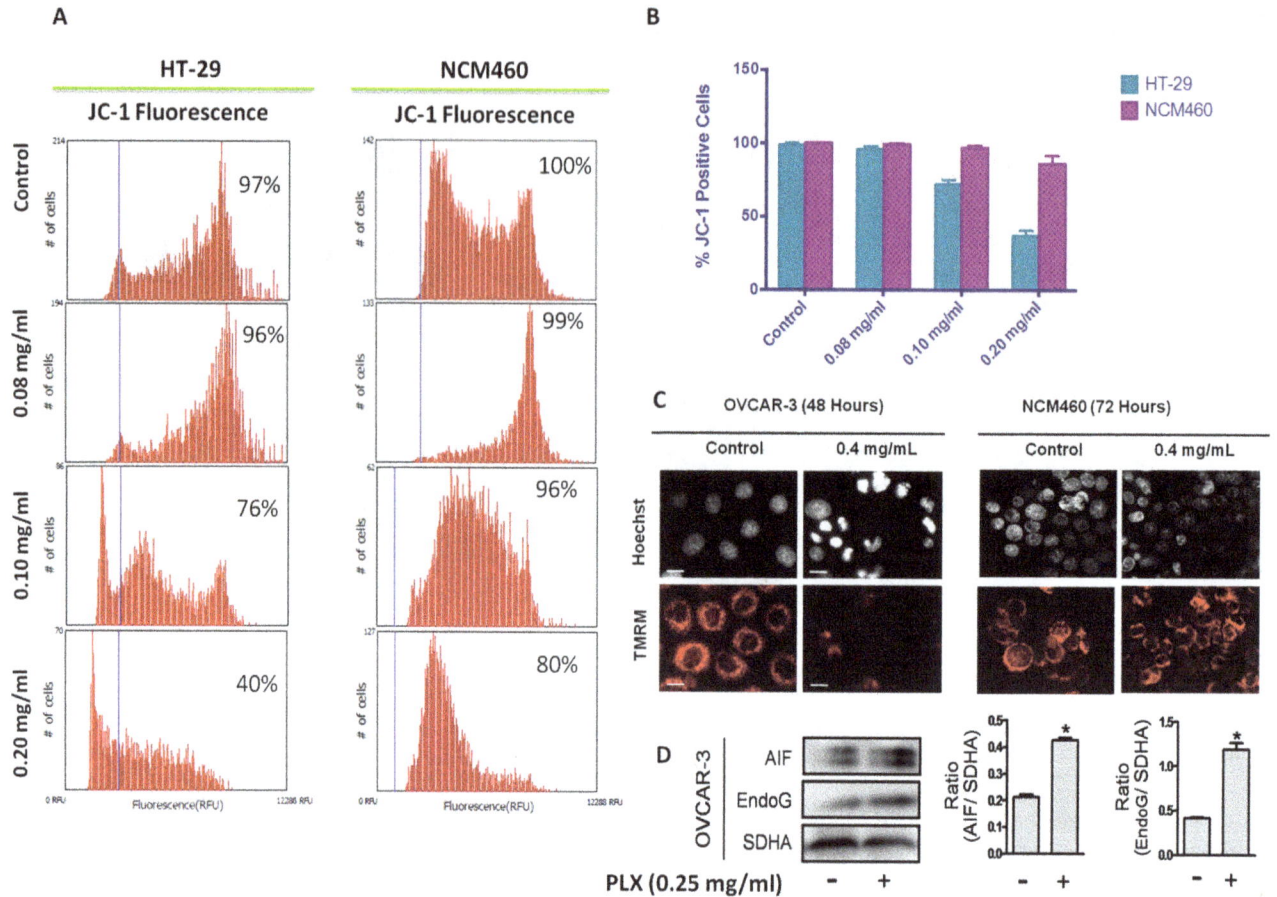

Figure 8. PLX Destabilizes the Mitochondrial Membrane of Cancer Cells. Colon cancer (HT-29), Ovarian cancer (OVCAR-3) and Normal Colon Epithelial (NCM460) cells were treated for 48 hours with PLX, following which, they were incubated with JC-1 (A) or TMRM (C) cationic mitochondrial membrane permeable dyes. Fluorescence readings were obtained using image based cytometry (A) and fluorescence microscopy; corresponding Hoechst dye images are also shown (C). Images were taken at 400× magnification on a fluorescent microscope. Scale bar = 15 μm. (D) Isolated mitochondria of OVCAR-3 cells were treated directly with PLX or solvent control (ethanol) for 2 hours. Following treatment, samples were centrifuged, to obtain mitochondrial supernatants, which were examined for the release of pro-apoptotic factors, AIF and EndoG via western blot analyses, and mitochondrial pellets which were probed for SDHA to serve as loading controls. Image is representative of 3 independent experiments demonstrating similar trends. Values are expressed as mean ± SD of quadruplicates of 1 independent experiment; *$p < 0.01$ versus solvent control (ethanol).

were sacrificed and their organs were obtained for pathological analysis by a certified pathologist at the University of Guelph (Dr. Brooke). Results from this part of the study demonstrate that there was no weight loss overall in mice that were given PLX supplemented water (Figure 9).

To further assess toxicity, urine was collected from mice once a week and protein urinalysis was performed using a urine dipstick and a Bradford protein concentration assay. Protein urinalysis results indicate that there were trace amounts of protein in the urine of mice both from the control and the PLX group, with trace readings corresponding to protein concentrations between 5 and 20 mg/dL. Bradford assays confirm the results obtained by dipstick urinalysis (Figure 9A). There was no major difference between the control group and PLX group, confirming the lack of toxicity associated with oral administration of PLX in drinking water. Furthermore, the hearts, livers and kidneys were obtained following the toxicity study, sliced and stained with hematoxylin and eosin. Results show no gross morphologic difference between the control and the treatment group, confirming the lack of toxicity associated with PLX treatment. Results from the pathologist, indicate that the presence of any lesions in the tissues

are minimal or mild and interpreted as either background or incidental lesions and the lack of lesion type and frequency was enough to conclude no toxicological effect of PLX to the balb/c mice (Table 2).

Oral Administration of Long Pepper Extract Halts the Growth of Human Colon Cancer Xenografts in Immunocompromised Mice

Following efficacy studies, we wanted to further study the efficacy of PLX. For this study, CD-1nu/nu immunocompromised mice were subcutaneously injected with HT-29 cells (left) and HCT116 cells (right). Following the establishment of tumors, mice were separated into three groups, a control group, a vehicle (Me$_2$SO) group and a PLX treated group. Mice were observed for 75 days, with weights and tumor volumes measured twice a week. Results demonstrate that oral administration of PLX could suppress the growth of both p53 WT (HCT116) and p53 mutant (HT-29) tumors *in-vivo*. There were no signs of toxicity, as indicated by increasing weights during the study (Figure 10A & B). Furthermore, H & E staining revealed less nuclei in the PLX

A

	17-May	21-May	30-May	4-Jun	11-Jun	14-Jun
C1	13.697	21.080	27.584		0.977	27.139
C2	21.899	15.543	22.694	31.353		31.478
C3	15.854	17.717	25.700		12.692	24.968
C4	14.027		22.918	32.830	-3.509	33.179
C5		30.405	44.646		6.810	46.738
P1	9.843		22.560		2.273	16.173
P2	30.405	31.913			4.965	34.703
P3	40.077	20.840			4.766	19.105
P4	15.458	34.154				32.123

B

C

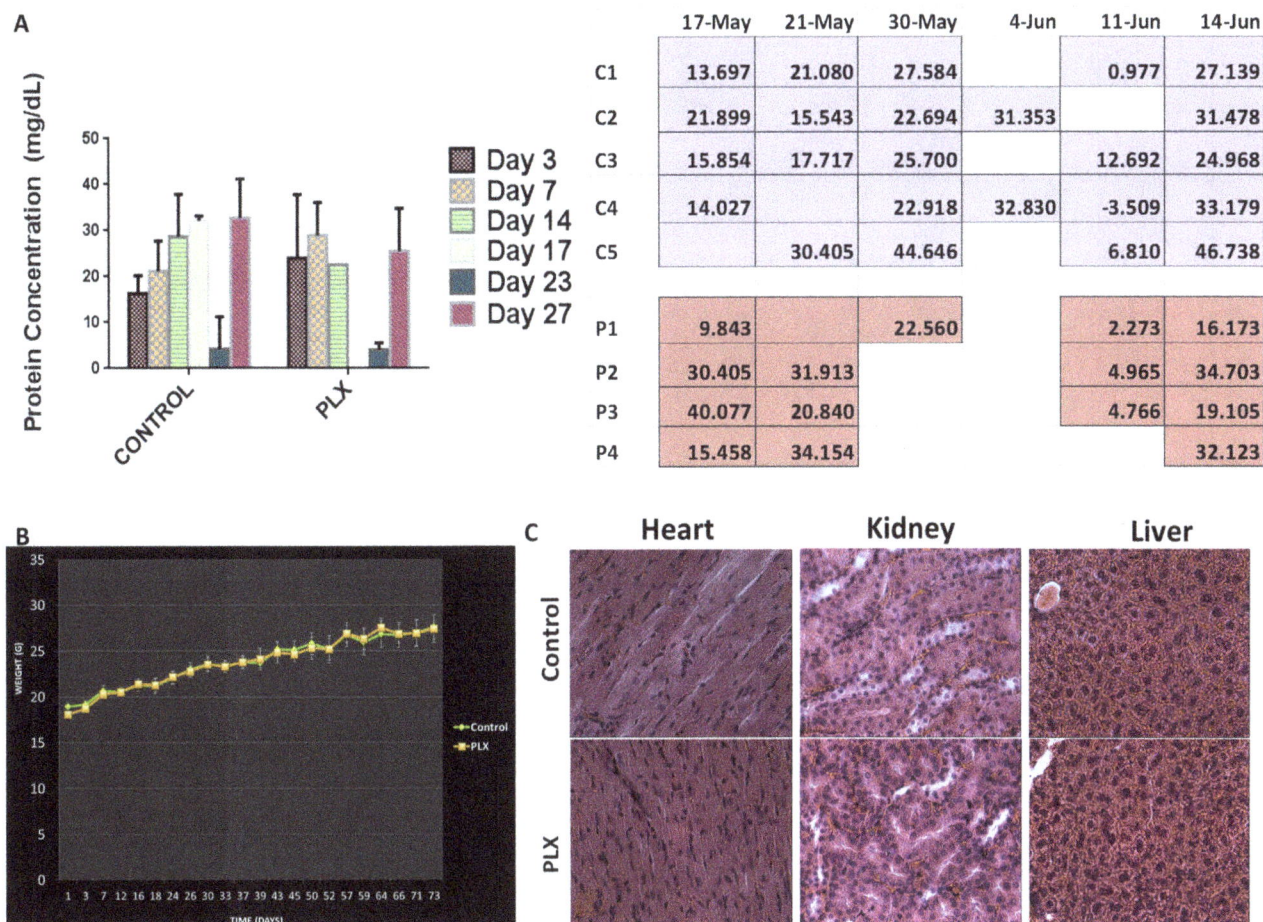

Figure 9. PLX is Well-Tolerated in Mice Models. Balb/C mice were divided into three groups (3 animals/control (untreated), 3 animals/gavage control (vehicle treatment) and 4 animals/treatment group). The control untreated group was given plain filtered water, while the second and third group was given 50 mg/kg/day vehicle (DMSO) or PLX, respectively. Mice were assessed for toxicity with protein urinalysis by Bradford Assay and dipstick analysis (A) and weight changes (B). (C) Hematoxylin and Eosin stained tissue sections of the liver, heart and kidney of control versus PLX treated group. Images were obtained on a bright field microscope at 63× objective.

treated group, compared to the control group, however, as observed in the toxicity studies, there were no gross morphological differences in the livers, kidneys and hearts of the control and PLX groups (Figure 10C).

Analysis of Long Pepper Extract

The availability of several species of long pepper and the host of compounds present within them make it essential to characterize the long pepper extract that has shown potent anticancer activity, both in *in-vitro* and *in-vivo* studies. We ran an HPLC profile study on the crude ethanolic extracts, compared with a piperamide standard mix. The chromatogram profile show that our PLX extract contained several classes of compounds known to be present in piper species, including piperines, piperlongumine and dihydropiperlongumine (Figure 11A & B), suggesting that our extract is a member of the *Piper longum* species.

Discussion

In this report we demonstrate for the first time, the selective anticancer potential of an ethanolic extract of the fruit of long pepper (PLX) in several cancer cell lines. PLX effectively reduced the viability of cancer cells and induced apoptosis in a dose- and

time-dependent manner, at low doses, allowing for a greater therapeutic window in *in-vitro* studies (Figure 1–5). This apoptosis inducing effect was found to be independent of caspases, cysteine aspartic proteases that play a role in the progression and execution of apoptosis (Figure 6B). These results suggest that PLX is not toxic to non-cancerous cells at such low doses, as was observed in the cancer cells. Selectivity and lack of toxicity was confirmed with *in-vivo* toxicological studies.

Damage to the kidneys is a common occurrence during various types to toxic therapies. This damage to the kidney results in large amounts of protein (>3.5 g/day) leaking into the urine [25,26], and this can be measured by various assays. Lack of toxicity was confirmed by the lack of increased protein concentration in the urine samples collected from both the control group and PLX treated group, by two different assays. The urine dipstick method indicated that all urine samples from the control and PLX groups had trace amounts of protein, corresponding to concentrations between 5 mg/dL and 20 mg/dL, well within the acceptable concentration range. Bradford protein assay showed a concentration of approximately 30 mg/dL most days urine was collected (Figure 9A). This is still within the acceptable range of protein concentration in urine. These results confirm anecdotal studies that suggest no associated toxicity or side effects observed with take

Table 2. Summary of Histological Lesions in Balb/C Mice on PLX regimen.

	No Treatment		Vehicle (Gavage Control)			Long Pepper Extract (Treatment group)			
	M1	M2	M1	M2	M3	M1	M2	M3	M4
Liver:									
-Infiltration, leukocyte, predominantly mononuclear, minimal		X	X		X	X			X
-Focal mineralization, minimal									
-Hepatocyte necrosis, minimal									X
-Focus of cellular alteration, eosinophilic, minimal				X				X	
-Hepatocyte vacuolation, lipid type, minimal			X	X			X		
- Hepatocyte vacuolation, lipid type, mild	X			X				X	X
Fibrin thrombus			X						
Heart:									
-Infiltration, leukocyte, predominantly mononuclear, minimal		X				X			X
Myofiber separation and vaculation, minimal (suspect artifact)		X	X						X
Kidney:									
- Infiltration, leukocyte, predominantly mononuclear, minimal	X	X		X		X			
Tubule vacuolation, minimal					X			X	
Fibrin or other extracellular matrix, glomerulus								X	

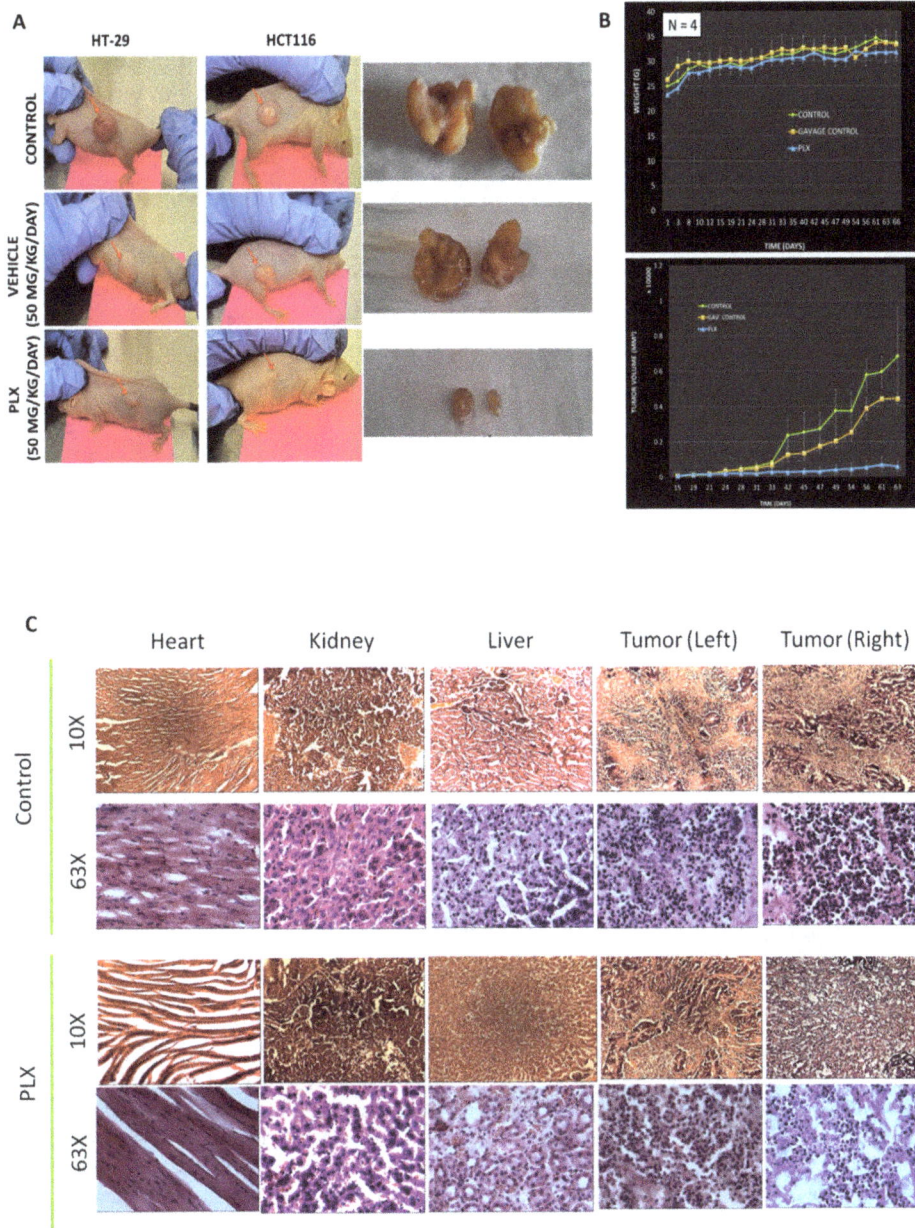

Figure 10. PLX Halts Growth of Colon Tumors in Xenograft Models. CD-1 nu/nu mice were subcutaneously injected with colon cancer cells; HT-29 (p53$^{-/-}$) on the left flank and HCT116 (p53$^{+/+}$) on the right flank. (A) Representative tumor size control mice and 50 mg/kg/day vehicle or PLX treated mice, respectively. PLX halted the growth of both HT-29 and HCT116 tumors *in-vivo*. (B) Average body weights of control and PLX treated mice. The body weights did not vary significantly during the study. Tumor volumes were measured and tumor curve shows the efficacy of 50 mg/kg/day oral administration of PLX. (C) Histopathological analysis of tissue samples obtained from control and PLX-treated animals. Hematoxylin and Eosin stained tissue sections of the livers, hearts, kidneys and tumors. Images were obtained on a bright field microscope at 10× and 63× objective.

long pepper extracts. The efficacy of PLX in *in-vivo* models also showed that not only was PLX well-tolerated, it was also effective at halting the growth of human tumor xenografts of colon cancer in nude mice (Figure 9A and B).

The next step in understanding the effect of PLX on cell death induction in cancer cells was to identify the mechanism of apoptosis induction observed following PLX treatment. The role of oxidative stress in cell death processes has been well characterized. It is well established the reactive oxygen species (ROS) could be the cause or effect of apoptosis induction in cells [20]. Some studies have suggested cancer cells to be more

dependent on cellular response mechanisms against oxidative stress and have exploited this feature to selectively target cancer cells [10]. The role of ROS generation in PLX-induced apoptosis was assessed following treatment. In this study, we found that PLX induced whole cell ROS production in a dose dependent manner, as indicated by the increase in green fluorescence of H$_2$DCFDA dye, cleaved by intracellular esterases and oxidized by ROS present (Figure 7A & B). However, we observed that ROS generation was not completely essential to PLX activity, as the presence of N-acetylcysteine could not entirely hamper the ability of PLX to reduce the viability of colon cancer cells (Figure 7C).

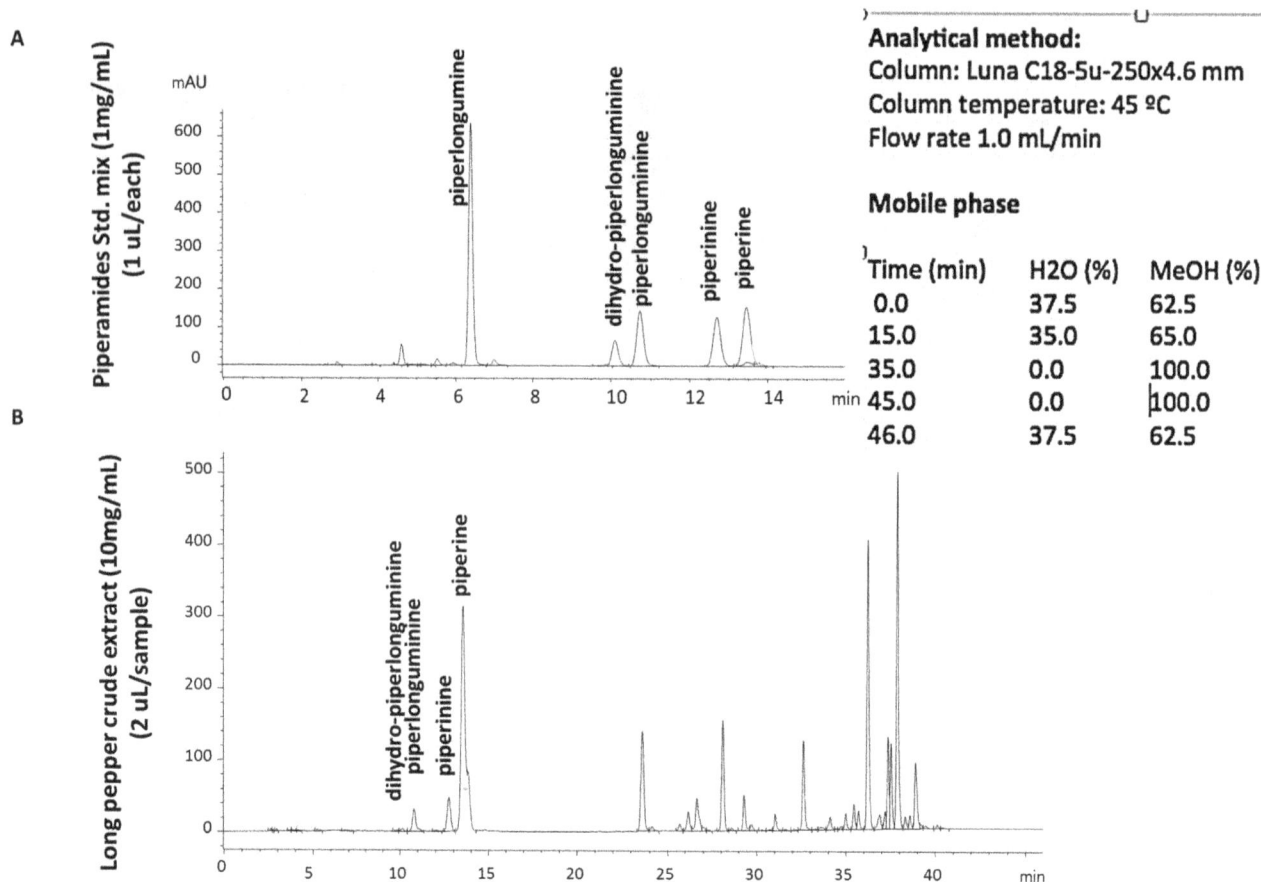

Figure 11. HPLC Analysis of PLX. Chromatograms of *Piper longum* extract (PLX) used for this study (10 mg/mL at 2 μL/Sample) (B) compared to Piperamides Standard mix (1 mg/mL at 1 μL/standard) (A).

The caspase-independence observed in figure 6B, suggest that PLX is acting through pro-apoptotic factors other than caspases. The mitochondria play a major role in the progression and execution of apoptosis. The permeabilization of the mitochondrial membrane usually leads to the release of pro-apoptotic factors, including cytochrome c, apoptosis inducing factor (AIF) and endonuclease G (EndoG) [5,17]. AIF and EndoG execute apoptosis in a caspase-independent possibly leading to the caspase- and partial ROS-independence observed. We show here that PLX caused MMP dissipation in cancer cells, while non-cancerous NCM460 cell mitochondria remained intact following treatment (Figure 8A–C). The dissipation of the mitochondrial membrane led to the release of AIF and EndoG (Figure 8D), allowing for the progression and execution of apoptosis in the absence of caspases and oxidative stress, providing insight to the mechanism of PLX action in cancer cells. Cancer cells differ from non-cancerous cells in variety of ways, which could enhance the selectivity of PLX to cancer cells. The Warburg effect is characterized by the high dependence of cancer cells on glycolysis and low dependence on mitochondria for energy production in cancer cells, therefore creating a more vulnerable target in cancer cell mitochondria [27]. Moreover, various anti-apoptotic proteins associated to the mitochondria have been reported to be highly expressed in cancer cells. Such proteins could serve as targets for selective cancer [28–30].

Unlike isolated natural compounds, there are usually more benefits to using a whole plant extract, with multiple pharmaco-logically active phytochemicals, than a single isolated compound. Multiple components within extracts could have many different intracellular targets, which may act in a synergistic way to enhance specific activities (including anticancer activities), while inhibiting any toxic effects of one compound alone. Additionally, the presence of multiple components may possibly decrease the chances of developing chemoresistance [31]. Moreover, natural extracts can be administered orally to patients, as a safe mode of administration. Some known compounds of the long pepper plants have been isolated and studied for their various activities [9–14].

We now report that the botanical identification of long pepper that was used for this study is *Piper longum* L. (Piperaceae), obtained from India. The phytochemical analysis of our material confirmed that this is the *Piper longum* species. We used the extract of the fruit in this study, since it is the usual part used medicinally and can be harvested sustainably. Although the fruit contains related piperamides, it does not contain piperlongumine, which is mainly present in the root of this plant [32]. The other piperamides present in the fruit such as dihydropiperlongumine likely have similar bioactivity. The small peak of piperlongumine observed in the HPLC chromatogram in Figure 11, as piperlon-gumine may be due to the reduction of piperlongumine to the larger dihyropiperlongumine peak that we observe. The analysis is consistent with *P. longum* fruits, and this is very important and points to the novel findings regarding the anticancer activity of this composition of components.

In a previous study that showed the efficacy of piperlongumine, high concentrations of 10 μM were required for significant cell death induction in cancer cells [10]. In this present study, we report the use of low concentrations of the complex mixture of the ethanolic long pepper extract (containing many bioactive and pharmacologically active compounds) was sufficient in inducing apoptosis in cancer cells selectively. This indicates that the individual bioactive compounds (present in sub micromolar concentrations within the extract) could act synergistically to induce apoptosis in cancer cells at very low concentrations, unlike a single identified compound. These findings highlights that the *Piper spp.* contain novel compounds with potent anticancer activity, in addition to piperlongumine.

In conclusion, our results demonstrate that long pepper extract (PLX), with a long historical use in traditional medicine, is selective in inducing apoptotic cell death in cancer cells by targeting non-genomic targets (e.g. the mitochondria). It is well tolerated in mice models and effective in reducing the growth of human tumor xenotransplants in animal models, when delivered orally. This could open a window of opportunity to develop a novel, safer cancer treatment, using complex natural health products from the Long Pepper.

Author Contributions

Conceived and designed the experiments: PO DM JAG JTA SP. Performed the experiments: PO DM PT AR MS JAG JTA SP. Analyzed the data: PO DM PT AR MS JAG JTA SP. Wrote the paper: PO DM SP.

References

1. Jemal A, Bray F, Ferlay J (2011) Global Cancer Statistics, 61(2): 69–90. doi:10.3322/caac.20107
2. Canadian Cancer Society's Steering Committee on Cancer Statistics (2012) Canadian Cancer Statistics 2012. Toronto, ON: Canadian Cancer Society; 2012.
3. Hanahan D, Weinberg RA (2011) Hallmarks of cancer: the next generation. Cell 144(5): 646–74. doi:10.1016/j.cell.2011.02.013
4. Fadeel B, Orrenius S (2005) Apoptosis: a basic biological phenomenon with wide-ranging implications in human disease. Journal of internal medicine 258(6): 479–517. doi:10.1111/j.1365-2796.2005.01570.x
5. Elmore S (2007) Apoptosis: A review of programmed cell death. Toxicologic pathology 35(4): 495–516. doi:10.1080/01926230701320337
6. Fulda S, Debatin KM (2006) Extrinsic versus intrinsic apoptosis pathways in anticancer chemotherapy. Oncogene 25(34): 4798–811. doi:10.1038/sj.onc.1209608
7. Davidson D, Amrein L, Panasci L, Aloyz R (2013) Small Molecules, Inhibitors of DNA-PK, Targeting DNA Repair, and Beyond. Frontiers in pharmacology 4(January): 5. doi:10.3389/fphar.2013.00005
8. Newman DJ, Cragg GM (2012) Natural products as sources of new drugs over the 30 years from 1981 to 2010. Journal of natural products 75(3): 311–35. doi:10.1021/np200906s
9. Bao N, Ochir S, Sun Z, Borjihan G, Yamagishi T (2013) Occurrence of piperidine alkaloids in Piper species collected in different areas. Journal of natural medicines. doi:10.1007/s11418-013-0773-0
10. Raj L, Ide T, Gurkar AU, Foley M, Schenone M, et al. (2012) Selective killing of cancer cells by a small molecule targeting the stress response to ROS. Nature 481(7382): 534–534. doi:10.1038/nature10789
11. Golovine KV, Makhov PB, Teper E, Kutikov A, Canter D, et al. (2013) Piperlongumine induces rapid depletion of the androgen receptor in human prostate cancer cells. The Prostate 73(1): 23–30. doi:10.1002/pros.22535
12. Jarvius M, Fryknäs M, D'Arcy P, Sun C, Rickardson L, et al. (2013) Piperlongumine induces inhibition of the ubiquitin-proteasome system in cancer cells. Biochemical and biophysical research communications 431(2): 117–23. doi:10.1016/j.bbrc.2013.01.017
13. Meghwal M, Goswami TK (2013) Piper nigrum and Piperine: An Update. Phytotherapy research: PTR, (February). doi:10.1002/ptr.4972
14. Lee SE, Park BS, Kim MK, Choi WS, Kim HT, et al. (2001) Fungicidal activity of pipernonaline, a piperidine alkaloid derived from long pepper, Piper longum L., against phytopathogenic fungi. Crop Protection 20(6): 523–528. doi:10.1016/S0261-2194(00)00172-1
15. Bezerra DP, Militão CG, de Castro FO, et al. (2007) Piplartine induces inhibition of leukemia cell proliferation triggering both apoptosis and necrosis pathways. Toxicol In Vitro vol. 21, no. 1, pp. 1–8
16. Fischer AH, Jacobson KA, Rose J, Zeller R (2008) Hematoxylin and eosin staining of tissue and cell sections. Cold Spring Harbor Protocols 2008(5): pdb-prot4986.
17. Earnshaw WC, Martins LM, Kaufmann SH (1999) Mammalian caspases: structure, activation, substrates, and functions during apoptosis. Annual review of biochemistry 68: 383–424. doi:10.1146/annurev.biochem.68.1.383
18. Thorburn A (2008) Apoptosis and autophagy: regulatory connections between two supposedly different processes. Apoptosis: an international journal on programmed cell death 13(1): 1–9. doi:10.1007/s10495-007-0154-9
19. Zhivotovsky B, Orrenius S (2010) Cell death mechanisms: cross-talk and role in disease. Experimental cell research 316(8): 1374–83. doi:10.1016/j.yexcr.2010.02.037
20. Simon HU, Haj-Yehia A, Levi-Schaffer F (2000) Role of reactive oxygen species (ROS) in apoptosis induction. Apoptosis vol. 5, no. 5, pp. 415–8
21. Madesh M, Hajnóczky G (2001) VDAC-dependent permeabilization of the outer mitochondrial membrane by superoxide induces rapid and massive cytochrome c release. J Cell Biol vol. 155, no. 6, pp. 1003–15.
22. Dekhuijzen P NR (2004) Antioxidant properties of N-acetylcysteine: their relevance in relation to chronic obstructive pulmonary disease. European Respiratory Journal 23(4): 629–636. doi:10.1183/09031936.04.00016804
23. Dodd S, Dean O, Copolov DL, Malhi GS, Berk M (2008) N-acetylcysteine for antioxidant therapy: pharmacology and. Expert Opin Biol Ther 8(12): 1955–1962
24. Earnshaw WC (1999) A cellular poison cupboard. Nature vol. 397, no. 6718, pp. 387–389.
25. Bleske BE, Clark MM, Wu AH, Dorsch MP (2013) The Effect of Continuous Infusion Loop Diuretics in Patients With Acute Decompensated Heart Failure With Hypoalbuminemia. Journal of cardiovascular pharmacology and therapeutics 00(0): 1–4.
26. Fang C, Shen L, Dong L, Liu M, Shi S, et al. (2013) Reduced urinary corin levels in patients with chronic kidney disease. Clinical Science 124(12): 709–717.
27. Warburg O (1956) On the origin of cancer cells. Science vol. 123, no. 3191, pp. 309–14
28. Mathupala SP, Rempel A, Pedersen PL (1997) Aberrant glycolytic metabolism of cancer cells: a remarkable coordination of genetic, transcriptional, post-translational, and mutational events that lead to a critical role for type II hexokinase. J Bioenerg Biomembr vol. 29, no. 4, pp. 339–43
29. Casellas P, Galiegue S, Basile AS (2002) Peripheral benzodiazepine receptors and mitochondrial function. Neurochem Int vol. 40, no, 6, pp. 475–86.
30. Green DR, Kroemer G (2004) The pathophysiology of mitochondrial cell death. Science vol. 305, no. 5684, pp. 626–9.
31. Foster BC, Arnason JT, Briggs CJ (2005) Natural health products and drug disposition. Annual review of pharmacology and toxicology 45: 203–26. doi:10.1146/annurev.pharmtox.45.120403.095950
32. Chandra VB, et al. (2014) Metabolic profiling of Piper species by direct analysis using real time mass spectrometry combined with principal component analysis. Analytical Methods, 4234–4239.

18

Analysis of Non-Typeable *Haemophilous influenzae* VapC1 Mutations Reveals Structural Features Required for Toxicity and Flexibility in the Active Site

Brooke Hamilton[1], Alexander Manzella[1], Karyn Schmidt[2], Victoria DiMarco[1], J. Scott Butler[1,2,3]*

1 Department of Microbiology and Immunology, University of Rochester Medical Center, Rochester, New York, United States of America, 2 Department of Biochemistry and Biophysics, University of Rochester Medical Center, Rochester, New York, United States of America, 3 Center for RNA Biology, University of Rochester Medical Center, Rochester, New York, United States of America

Abstract

Bacteria have evolved mechanisms that allow them to survive in the face of a variety of stresses including nutrient deprivation, antibiotic challenge and engulfment by predator cells. A switch to dormancy represents one strategy that reduces energy utilization and can render cells resistant to compounds that kill growing bacteria. These persister cells pose a problem during treatment of infections with antibiotics, and dormancy mechanisms may contribute to latent infections. Many bacteria encode toxin-antitoxin (TA) gene pairs that play an important role in dormancy and the formation of persisters. VapBC gene pairs comprise the largest of the Type II TA systems in bacteria and they produce a VapC ribonuclease toxin whose activity is inhibited by the VapB antitoxin. Despite the importance of VapBC TA pairs in dormancy and persister formation, little information exists on the structural features of VapC proteins required for their toxic function *in vivo*. Studies reported here identified 17 single mutations that disrupt the function of VapC1 from non-typeable *H. influenzae in vivo*. 3-D modeling suggests that side chains affected by many of these mutations sit near the active site of the toxin protein. Phylogenetic comparisons and secondary mutagenesis indicate that VapC1 toxicity requires an alternative active site motif found in many proteobacteria. Expression of the antitoxin VapB1 counteracts the activity of VapC1 mutants partially defective for toxicity, indicating that the antitoxin binds these mutant proteins *in vivo*. These findings identify critical chemical features required for the biological function of VapC toxins and PIN-domain proteins.

Editor: Manuela Helmer-Citterich, University of Rome Tor Vergata, Italy

Funding: This work was supported by National Institutes of Health Grant GM-099731 to JSB, http://www.nih.gov/. The funders had no role in study design, data collection and analysis, decision to publish, or preparation of the manuscript.

Competing Interests: The authors have declared that no competing interests exist.

* Email: scott_butler@urmc.rochester.edu

Introduction

Type II toxin-antitoxin (TA) systems in bacteria first emerged as a mechanism of post-segregational killing caused by plasmid-borne TA operons [1,2]. Subsequently, the discovery of chromosomally encoded TA systems led to the identification of several apparently distinct mechanisms of action for the encoded toxins [3,4]. These include ribonucleases that hydrolyze mRNA, rRNA and tRNA, DNA gyrase inhibitors and protein kinases that target translation. In nearly all characterized cases, a single operon encodes the toxin and antitoxin genes, often with closely adjacent or overlapping reading frames allowing translational coupling. The Type II TA operons produce protein toxins and antitoxins, which form complexes that inhibit the activity of the toxin. The TA pair also often acts as a transcriptional repressor of the operon, providing a level of feedback regulation upon which various environmental stimuli may act to derepress TA expression. Upon cellular stress, the antitoxin is cleaved by a protease such as Lon, thereby freeing the toxin from the inhibitor and derepressing expression of the TA operon. The free toxin then carries out its primary function, which results in growth inhibition and eventual cell death [5]. Relief of the stress that led to inactivation of the antitoxin allows its

accumulation and inactivation of its cognate toxin, which allows resumption of cell growth. Thus, TA systems have the potential to play a regulatory role in bacterial dormancy, making their study relevant to the problem of pathology caused by bacterial latency. Additionally, stochastic fluctuations in toxin activity within populations of bacteria produce dormant cells resistant to many antibiotics [6,7]. These persisters can contribute to re-establishment of the bacterial population upon discontinuance of the drug. These characteristics make the elucidation of the mechanisms of TA function an important goal for molecular biologists.

VapC toxins comprise the largest family of Type-II toxins in bacteria [8]. They contain a characteristic PIN-domain found in a wide range of bacteria and eukaryotes where they appear to function as endoribonucleases targeted to the process of protein synthesis or ribosome biogenesis [8–10]. Analysis of PIN-domain proteins in bacteria showed that they also exist as single domain proteins (VapC) in TA operons, but their mechanism of action and function remains unclear [9,11]. One of the two VapC proteins (VapC1) from *H. influenzae* inhibits growth when expressed in *E. coli*, an effect countered by co-expression of its associated antitoxin (VapB1) [12]. Recombinant VapC1 caused RNA degradation *in vitro* and addition of VapB1 inhibited this activity. Likewise, VapC proteins from *Pyrobaculum aerophilum*, and *Mycobacterium tuberculosis* demonstrate sequence specific ribonuclease activity *in vitro* [13,14]. Recent findings revealed that VapC toxins from *S. flexneri* and *S. enterica* function as initiator tRNA^{fMet} endonucleases, while toxins from *M. tuberculosis* target RNA structures containing a specific sequence motif, the sarcin-ricin loop of 23S rRNA, or inhibit protein synthesis by binding to mRNAs [15].

Along with questions about the targets of VapC toxins, it remains unclear what aspects of their structure, other than four canonical acidic amino acids, contribute to their activity. We addressed this issue using a novel strategy to identify loss of function mutant alleles of the VapC1 toxin from NTHi and discovered numerous amino acid side chains required for its toxicity. Structural modeling places many of these critical groups in proximity to amino acids predicted to participate in the chemistry of the active site of the enzyme. Our findings also support the conclusion that NTHi VapC1, and possibly many other VapC toxins, use an alternative to the canonical active site found in many VapC toxins and PIN-domain proteins. Finally, our findings indicate that mutations that inhibit VapC toxin activity do not necessarily abrogate binding to its VapB antitoxin *in vivo*. These findings identify critical structural features required for the biological function of this important class of bacterial TA systems.

Materials and Methods

Bacterial strains and growth conditions

All growth assays were conducted in *E. coli* LMG194 (F-ΔlacX74 gal E thi rpsL ΔphoA (Pvu II) Δara714 leu::Tn10) grown in M9 media [16] supplemented with 50 μg/ml ampicillin and 0.2% glycerol. Growth was monitored in 96-well microtiter plates using a Bio-tek Powerwave XS, which measured A_{600} every 15 minutes at 37°C.

Molecular cloning

Plasmids expressing VapC1, or VapC1 and VapB1, were constructed by inserting PCR synthesized DNA between the Nco1 and Xba1 sites of pBAD/*Myc*-His B (Invitrogen), pBAD-eGFP-EcMax or pBAD-sfGFP using standard techniques. PCR primer sequences are available upon request. All inserts were subjected to DNA sequence analysis to verify their identity. pBAD-eGFP-EcMax was constructed by insertion of a chemically synthesized, codon optimized eGFP DNA, digested with Xba1 and Spe1, into the Xba1 site of pBAD/*Myc*-His B. pBAD-sfGFP was constructed by insertion of a PCR product derived from the Super Folder GFP plasmid (Sandia Biotech), digested with Xba1 and Spe1, into the Xba1 site of pBAD/*Myc*-His B. pBAD-eGFP-EcMax and pBAD-sfGFP were constructed with 6x-glycine linkers at the N-termini of GFP and a C-terminal fusion to the *Myc*-6× His coding sequence.

Mutagenesis

VapC1 mutations were created by PCR or oligonucleotide directed site-specific mutagenesis. For PCR mutagenesis, VapC1 was amplified by PCR from pBAD-VapC1 DNA template in five 50 μl reactions containing 20 mM Tris-Cl (pH 8.4), 50 mM KCl, 5 mM Mg₂Cl, 1 mM dNTP, 25 pmoles DNA primers, 1 μg DNA template and 0.1 unit Taq polymerase. Reactions were run at 94°C, 4 mins.; 30×(94°C, 30 sec., 55°C, 30 sec., 72°C, 1 min.); 72°C, 5 mins. Reactions were pooled, and primers and small molecules removed using a PCR purification kit (Qiagen). The DNA was digested with Nco1 and Xba1 and inserted by ligation into the same sites in pBAD-eGFP-EcMax. The ligation mixtures

were transformed into LMG194, plated on Luria Broth agar plates containing 50 μg/ml ampicillin and 0.02% arabinose and incubated for 16 hours at 37°C. Colony GFP fluorescence was analyzed on a Typhoon 9410 imager (GE Biosciences) using the 488 nM blue laser for excitation and the 520BP40 emission filter. Plasmids were recovered from fluorescent colonies and retransformed into LMG194 to confirm phenotypes. The insert portion of the plasmid DNAs from putative mutants were sequenced (Genewiz) before and after transfer of the VapC1 portion into the Nco1 and Xba1 sites of pBAD-sfGFP to verify that only the desired mutations were present.

Oligonucleotide directed site-specific mutagenesis was carried out by a modification of the method of Fisher and Pei [17]. PCR was carried out in a 50 μL reaction containing 10 μL HF iProof Buffer (Bio-Rad), 1 μL forward mutagenic primer (10 nM), 1 μL reverse mutagenic primer (10 nM), 1 μL 10 mM dNTP's, 4.5 μL DMSO, 0.5 μL HF iProof Polymerase (2 units/μL; Bio-Rad) and 10 ng VapC1 DNA template. Reactions were run at 98°C, 3 mins.; 30×(98°C, 30 sec., 65°C, 30 sec., 72°C, 3 min.); 72°C, 5 mins. Twenty units of DpnI (NEB) was added to the reaction and incubated at 37°C for 30 mins. to destroy DNA template strands. Ten μL of the reaction mixture was transformed into Top10 and colonies selected on LB plates containing 50 μg/ml ampicillin at 37°C. The insert portion of the plasmid DNAs from putative mutants was sequenced (Genewiz) to verify that only the desired mutations were present.

Western blot analysis

Cells were grown at 37°C in M9 media supplemented with 50 μg/ml ampicillin and 0.2% glycerol to an A_{600} of 0.3. L-arabinose was added to a final concentration of 0.02% and the incubation continued for 2 hours. Cells were collected by centrifugation and the pellets resuspended in 1× SDS PAGE sample buffer and boiled for five minutes before separation of the proteins by SDS-polyacrylamide gel electrophoresis. Proteins were transferred by electrophoresis to nitrocellulose paper and probed with anti-myc antibody (Invitrogen) or antiGroEL antibody (Sigma) prior to detection with secondary antibodies conjugated with horseradish peroxidase and chemiluminescence reagents.

Results

NTHi VapC1 functions as a GFP fusion protein *in vivo*

VapC toxins, sometimes called PIN-domain proteins, belong to the Pfam database family PF01850, which presently contains 8807 sequences. HMM logo analysis [18] of these proteins reveals significant variation in amino acid sequence, but also several areas of high similarity (Figure 1A). Prominently, the family shares four conserved acidic amino acids that structural analyses indicate coordinate a metal ion in the active sites of the enzymes [10,19]. In several cases, mutations altering each of the four conserved acidic amino acids in the active site of VapC proteins resulted in loss of toxicity *in vivo*, yet the requirement for other amino acids remains unclear [20,21]. Preliminary to mutagenic analysis of a well-characterized VapC1 toxin from NTHi [22], we constructed plasmid vectors that allow conditional expression of the toxin, or both the toxin and antitoxin from the inducible L-arabinose operon promoter (pBAD) and monitored their effects on cell growth (Figure 1). In each case the plasmids express VapC1 as a *myc*-epitope-6× histidine fusion protein and in pBAD-VapBC1, VapB1 and VapC1 are translated as a single transcript that encodes the two open reading frames in their natural arrangement, which allows translational coupling of VapC1 to VapB1 (Figure 1B). As expected, induction of toxin expression with

A

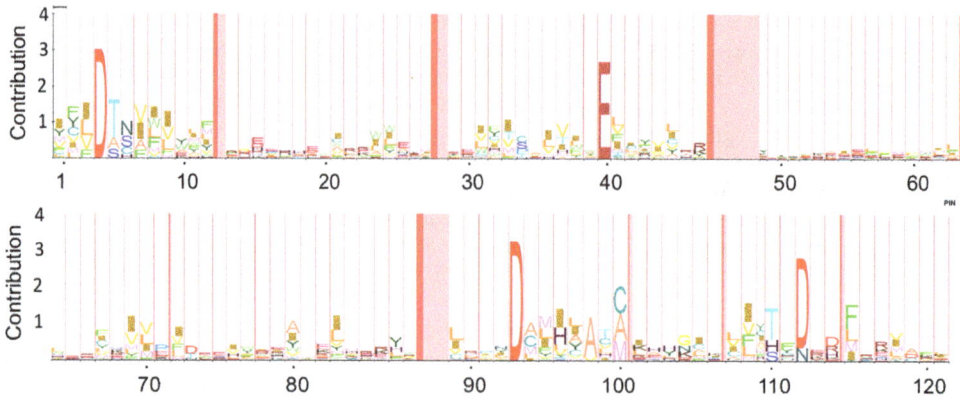

B

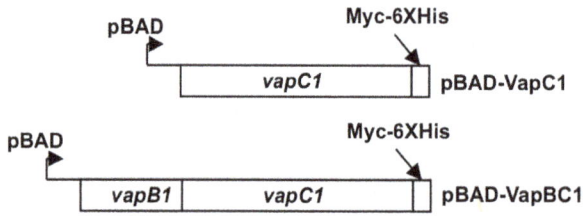

C

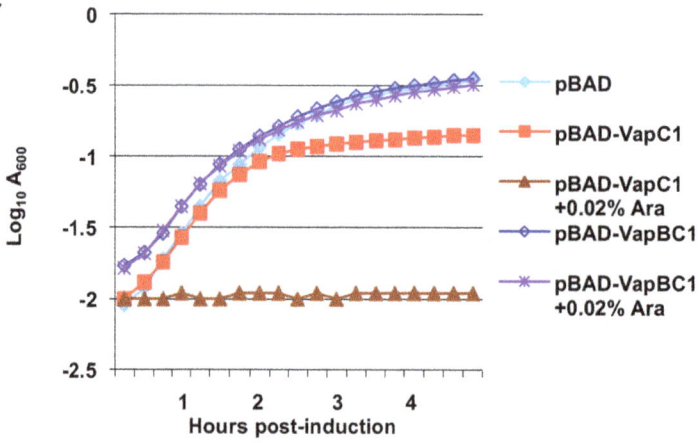

D

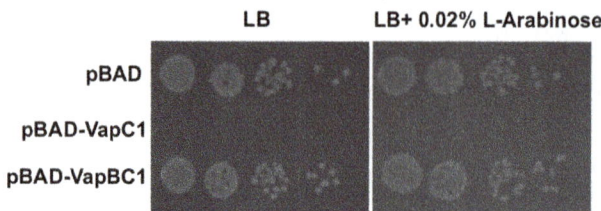

L-arabinose (pBAD-VapC1 +0.02% Ara) leads to growth inhibition in liquid culture (Figure 1C) and on Petri plates (Figure 1D). Because of leaky expression of VapC1, the strain expressing the toxin from the Ara promoter results in poor growth on LB plates even in the absence of the inducer. Expression of the toxin and the antitoxin (pBAD-VapBC1 +0.02% Ara) does not result in significant growth inhibition, indicating that the antitoxin binds to and inactivates the toxin (Figure 1C). Toxicity of VapC1 does not require the presence of *lon*, indicating independence of these phenotypes from Lon-dependent activation of endogenous TA systems (data not shown).

Next, we constructed a C-terminal fusion of VapC1 toxin to eGFP with an intervening 6X-glycine linker (Figure 2A). We asked if the VapC1-eGFP fusion functions as a toxin *in vivo* and found that expression of the fusion protein inhibits cell growth (Figure 2B). We then asked if co-expression of the antitoxin relieves growth inhibition caused by the VapC1-eGFP fusion, and found that cells grow upon co-expression of the antitoxin (Figure 2B) despite expression of the toxin fusion protein in the cells (Figure 2C). These findings show that; (i) the experimental system reflects the known activities of the toxin and antitoxin on cell growth (Figure 1) [12], (ii) the VapC1-eGFP fusion retains its

toxin activity and (iii) VapB1 acts effectively as an antitoxin for the eGFP fusion protein.

Identification of VapC loss of function mutations

To identify amino acids required for VapC toxicity we employed; (i) PCR mutagenesis, (ii) selection for loss of growth inhibition upon induction of expression and (iii) screening for GFP fluorescence to identify mutations that inactivate VapC1-eGFP (Figure 3). Initial attempts at selecting such mutants with VapC lacking the fusion to GFP yielded several mutations (T7P (twice) and E120G), but mostly nonsense mutations. Use of VapC1-eGFP and the screen for GFP fluorescence allowed us to avoid nonsense mutations in VapC1, since these produce truncated VapC1-eGFP polypeptides with background levels of fluorescence (Figure 3). Strains that produce full length, defective VapC1-eGFP grow in the presence of inducer and exhibit substantial fluorescence (arrow, Figure 3). This method yielded 23 isolates with single mutations causing defects in VapC1-eGFP (Table 1). This includes T7P (twice) and E120G, as well as 7 double mutants, two of which contain changes to E120 and one each changing F121, N117 and E43 (Table 1). The fact that the selection yielded the T7P and E120G mutations independently in the *vapC1* and

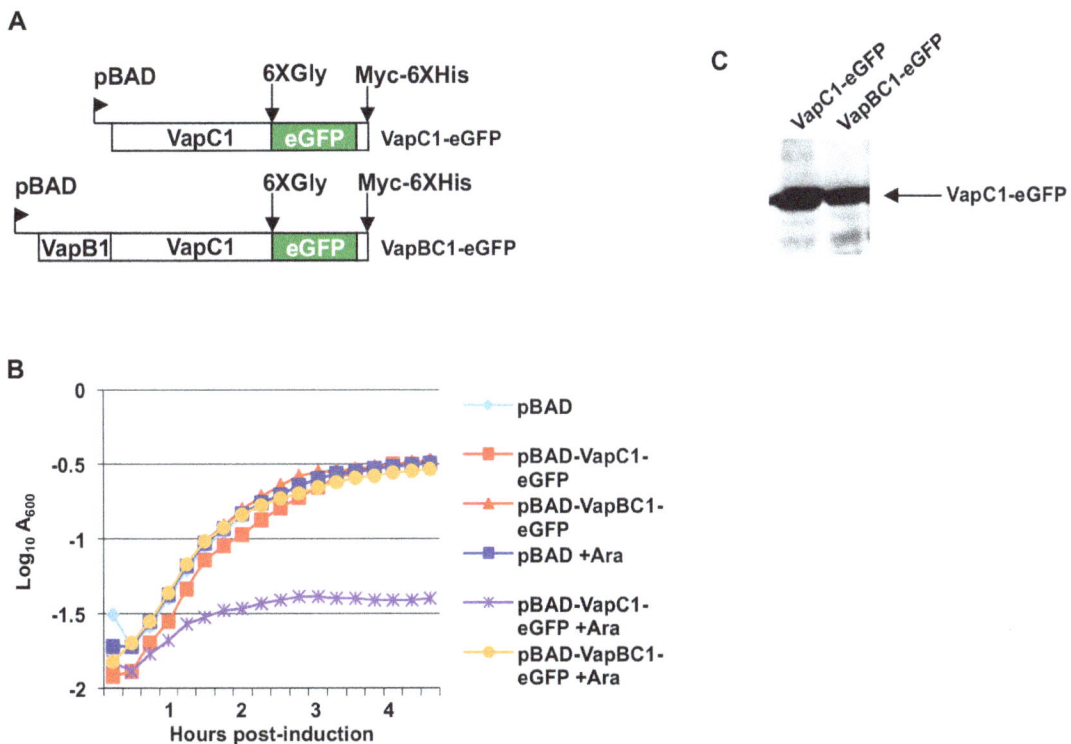

A

pBAD   6XGly   Myc-6XHis

VapC1   eGFP   VapC1-eGFP

pBAD   6XGly   Myc-6XHis

VapB1   VapC1   eGFP   VapBC1-eGFP

C

VapC1-eGFP   VapBC1-eGFP

← VapC1-eGFP

B

Figure 2. Growth characteristics of VapC1-eGFP fusions. *A*. Diagram of *vapC1* or *vapBC1* sequences cloned as *vapC1*-eGFP fusions into pBAD-MychHisB plasmids under control of the L-arabinose inducible pBAD promoter. *B*. Analysis of the growth of LMG194 cells in M9 glycerol with 50 µg/ml ampicillin after induction by addition of L-arabinose to a final concentration of 0.02%. The curves are representative examples of multiple experiments that yielded the same results. *C*. Western blot analysis of VapC1-eGFP from cells grown as in *B* after a 30-minute induction with L-arabinose to a final concentration of 0.02%. Each lane contains lysate from an equal number of cells.

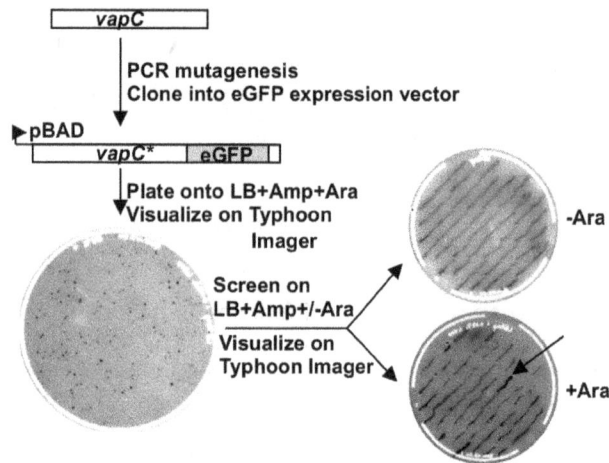

Figure 3. Workflow for isolation of VapC1 loss of function mutations. VapC1 DNA was amplified by PCR with Taq polymerase and inserted in frame with eGFP in pBAD-eGFP-MycHisB using standard DNA cloning techniques. DNA was transformed into Top10 and plated on Luria Broth + ampicillin (50 µg/ml; LBA) plates containing 0.02% L-arabinose. After incubation of the plates at 37°C for 16 hours, colonies were visualized on a Typhoon 9410 imager (excitation at 488 nm; 520BP40 emission filter). Colonies were then screened on LBA plates with and without arabinose, and colonies that grew on both plates and exhibited fluorescence above background were chosen for further analysis.

vapC1-eGFP selections supports the conclusion that the activity of the GFP fusion protein reflects that of the VapC1.

VapC1 mutations cause a range of toxicity defects

Preliminary western blot analysis indicated that cells express each of the mutant proteins at levels similar to wild-type VapC1. However, each of the mutants displayed weak fluorescence compared to the wild type protein co-expressed with VapB1 antitoxin (data not shown). Previous studies showed that mutations in the non-GFP portion of GFP fusion proteins often interfere with the folding of GFP and decrease its fluorescence. The use of superfolder GFP (sfGFP) often solves this problem as it folds more quickly and independently of its fusion partner [23]. Indeed, replacement of GFP with sfGFP in each of the mutants increased their fluorescence about 10-fold. Based on sfGFP fluorescence and western blot analysis, each of the mutant proteins, with the exception of D6A, shows a similar pattern and extent of induction after addition of arabinose (Figure 4A&B). However, varying degrees of toxicity become apparent upon monitoring cell growth, which indicates that the selection/screening scheme identified mutations with a broad range of VapC defects (Figure 4C&D). We also compared how two of the mutations affect the relative toxicity in the context of VapC1 and VapC1-sfGFP to determine whether the sfGFP fusion might attenuate the toxicity of the VapC1 alleles. The results showed that the fusion enhances toxicity of the E120G allele, but has no effect on T7P (data not shown). This finding supports previous observations indicating that sfGFP enhances the activity of its fusion partners by increasing their solubility [23].

Thirteen of the VapC1 mutations result in growth rates similar to the empty plasmid vector upon induction suggesting that the changes cause major defects in toxin activity (Figures 4C&D). The normal side chains of these amino acids lie near the active site of the protein based on modeling VapC1 to the crystal structure of the closely related *S. flexneri* VapC [24] (Figure 5A). Comparison

of NTHi VapC1 with other VapC sequences predicts that three acidic amino acids (D6, D99, E43) should function in the chemical mechanism of toxin activity by coordinating a metal ion in the active site (Figure 1A and 5B). Indeed, modeling of NTHi VapC1 to *S. flexneri* VapC predicts that all three of these side chains sit in close proximity in the structure [25] (Figure 5A). Nevertheless, the selection/screen only identified D99 as essential for activity. So, we created D6A and E43A by site directed mutagenesis and found that although cells express the mutant proteins, they fail to inhibit growth (Figure 4E). Western blot and fluorescence analyses of these mutants indicate comparable levels of E43A, but low expression of D6A relative to the other mutants, suggesting that lack of activity for the D6A mutant may result from instability of protein. Nevertheless, the findings support previous studies indicating that E43 and D99 play a critical role in the activity of VapC and PIN-domain proteins [20,21,26–32]. Importantly, the identification of functional defects caused by mutation of conserved side chains, such as T7, S37, T115, F121 and L127 that are predicted to lie near the active site reveals their requirement for the activity of the toxin.

NTHi VapC toxins utilize a variation of the canonical PIN-domain active site

In VapC proteins, the fourth of four conserved acidic residues is almost always aspartate, which lies in a conserved motif; L/V, X, S/T, X, **D** [33]. However, the sequence in NTHi VapC1 and VapC2, and many other proteobacteria is L, X, S/T, X, **N** (Figure 5B&6A). The polar asparagine cannot participate directly in the inferred coordination of a metal cation required for the chemistry of the active site, and mutation of aspartate at this position in other PIN-domain/VapC proteins inactivates the enzymes [27,28,32]. However, the VapC1 glutamate at position 120 is conserved in bacterial species closely related to NTHi that also lack the canonical aspartate (Figure 5B). Moreover, modeling suggests that the E120 side chain projects into the putative active site in close proximity to D6, E43, and D99 (Figure 5A). Thus, the use of E120 instead of D at position 117 may define an uncharacterized variant active site for VapC-proteins (Figure 5B&6A). In support of this hypothesis, the E120G mutation significantly reduces toxicity of VapC1 (Figures 4C, D&6B). The conservation of N117 in proteobacteria implies its requirement for the activity of the toxin. We tested this by mutating the polar asparagine to a non-polar isoleucine. This mutation inactivates VapC1, consistent with a requirement for a polar side chain at this position (Figure 6A&B). Additionally, the predicted proximity of N117 to the basic amino acids in the active site raised the possibility that its conversion to aspartate might allow it to function in place of E120, as apparently it does in other VapC proteins. Accordingly, we asked whether conversion of N117 to aspartate would restore the activity of the defective E120G toxin. Indeed, the double mutant, VapC1- E120G N117D created by site-directed mutagenesis grows poorly compared to VapC1-E120G, suggesting that it functions effectively as a VapC toxin (Figure 6A&B). In each case, western blot analysis reveals that cells express the mutant proteins upon induction (Figure 6C).

VapC1 mutations that alter toxicity do not abolish interaction with VapB1

Many of the mutations described here abolish the toxin activity of VapC1 *in vitro*. Consistently, many of the mutations we identified occur at highly conserved residues mapping to the modeled active site region of the enzyme (Figure 5), and all but one of the mutant proteins are stably expressed in the cell

Table 1. *VapC1* mutations isolated in this study.

Isolated as *vapC1-GFP*		Isolated as *vapC1*	
Mutant	**Genotype**	**Mutant**	**Genotype**
M1-2-A	S37G	10-M2-9	T7P
M1-2-C	T7P	17-M3-7	L88R
M1-2-D	E120G	9-M2-8	T7P
M1-2-E	E120K, I61V	M4-4	E120G
M1-3-A	A103V		
M1-3-B	A103V		
M1-4-B	N9H, A23V		
M1-4-C	A85P		
M1-4-D	H105R, K19E		
M1-4-E	A103T		
M1-4-I	F121S		
M1-5-B	N110I, I124T		
M1-5-C	S37G		
M1-6-B	E43G, N117Y		
M1-6-C	F121S, I124G		
M1-6-E	S37N		
M1-7-B	D99G		
M1-7-C	T115I		
M1-7-D	C104R		
M1-7-E	R93G, E120G		
M1-7-I	T7P		
M1-7-J	V70A		
M1-8-B	W101C		
M1-8-C	W84R		
M1-8-E	V70A		
M1-8-F	G92V		
M1-8-G	L127H		
M1-8-J	T115A		
M1-1	D6A		
M2-1	E43A		

(Figure 6C). Nevertheless, we cannot eliminate the possibility that the mutations cause some gross protein folding defect. However, antitoxins generally show strong specificity in binding to their cognate toxins [13,34,35]. Analysis of crystal structures of VapB-VapC complexes suggests that the C-terminal third of VapB antitoxins interact directly with VapC toxins [24,36–39]. Interestingly, the most distal portion of VapB binds in the groove of VapC containing the active site of the toxin and VapB side chains appear to interact with VapC amino acids involved in active site chemistry. These considerations strongly suggest that binding of VapB1 to VapC1 requires that the toxin exist in the normally folded state. Accordingly, we tested whether VapB1 could neutralize the toxin activity of several VapC1 mutants *in vivo* by assaying the second activity of the toxins, the ability to specifically bind their antitoxin VapB1. The results show that expression of VapB1 counteracts the toxicity of the A103V, W84R, E120G and E120G N117D VapC1 mutants (Figure 7). These findings reveal that these mutations do not have a major effect on the antitoxin binding activity of VapC1 and support our

conclusion that the mutations do not have a major negative effect on the structure of the toxin *in vivo*.

Discussion

VapC proteins comprise the largest family of toxins in the Type II TA systems of bacteria. Recent studies revealed the function of three members of this family as endonucleases that cleave initiator tRNA^{fMet} in *S. flexneri* and *S. typhimurium*, or the sarcin-ricin loop of 23S rRNA in *M. tuberculosis* [15,21]. Although the activities of this important class of proteins and their eukaryotic relatives depends critically on four conserved acidic side chains, little functional evidence exists on the importance of other amino acids in prokaryotes, nor the related PIN-domains in eukaryotes. The findings presented here identify critical structural requirements for the biological function of VapC toxins and provide evidence for a conserved, alternative configuration of the active site in the VapC toxins of many bacteria.

Many of the VapC1 mutations identified here eliminate toxicity *in vivo* thereby identifying novel structural requirements for the

A

B

C

D

E

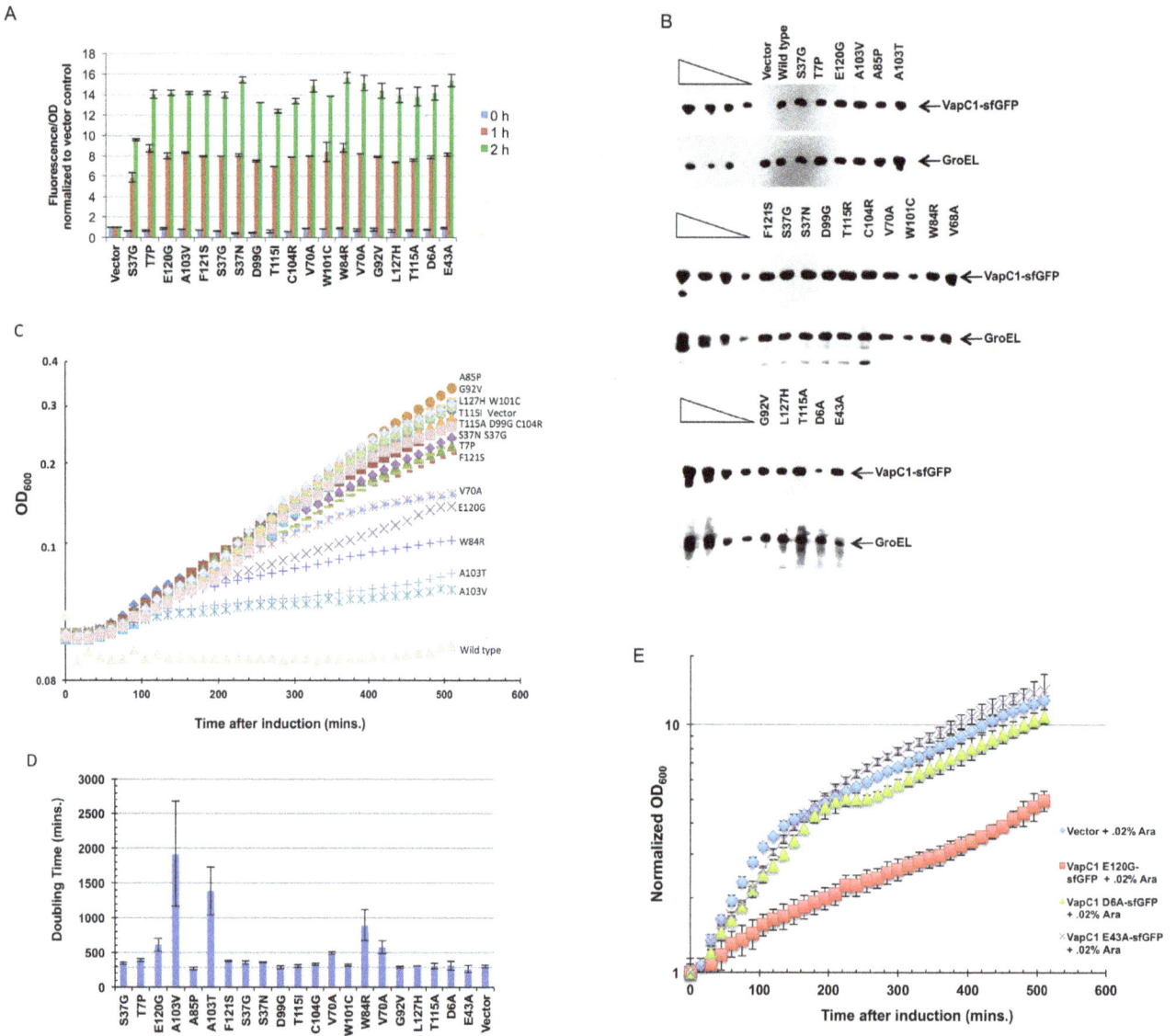

Figure 4. VapC1 mutations cause a spectrum of toxicity defects. *A.* Fluorescence yield from LMG194 cells carrying VapC1 mutants grown in M9 glycerol with 50 μg/ml ampicillin as a function of time after induction with arabinose at a final concentration of 0.02%. Fluorescence was measure in triplicate in a Typhoon 9410 Imager and normalized to the OD$_{600}$ of the culture. *B.* Western blot analysis of VapC1 mutant proteins isolated 60 minutes after induction with arabinose at a final concentration of 0.02%. Blots were probed with anti-myc antibody for VapC1 proteins and anti-GroEL as a loading control. The first four lanes in each panel show a two-fold dilution series of VapC1-sfGFP as a control for signal linearity. *C.* Analysis of the growth of LMG194 cells expressing the indicated VapC1 mutants in M9 glycerol with 50 μg/ml ampicillin after induction by addition of L-arabinose to a final concentration of 0.02%. The curves are one set of examples of two biological replicates whose average doubling time and standard error is shown in (D). *D.* Doubling times for cells expressing VapC1 mutants. Values represent the doubling times calculated for the first 510 minutes of growth and are the average of two independent biological replicates, shown with error bars representing the standard error. *E.* Analysis of the growth of LMG194 cells expressing the indicated VapC1 mutants in M9 glycerol with 50 μg/ml ampicillin after induction by addition of L-arabinose to a final concentration of 0.02%. Time points on the curves are the average of three biological replicates with error bars representing the standard deviation.

activity of VapC and PIN-domain proteins [24,36–39]. Arcus et al. suggested that the conserved T7 stabilizes the conformation of metal cation binding side chain D6 by H-bonding interactions. Our results indicate that VapC activity requires T7, consistent with their proposal, as well as the side chain's conservation in most VapC toxins and the PIN-domains of eukaryotic nucleases such as SMG6 and EST1 [28,40]. We also find a requirement for T115, which is conserved as T or S, typically two residues from the fourth conserved aspartate in VapC toxins (Figure 1A). This amino acid is also conserved in eukaryotic PIN-domain proteins and the

structure of SMG6 presented by Glavan et al. indicates that it participates in a H-bond network with acidic amino acids that co-ordinate the essential metal cation in the active site [28]. Thus, T115 likely plays an essential role in stabilizing the configuration of these side chains in the active site, or it may contribute to activation of water for phosphodiester bond hydrolysis [8,28,41].

NTHi VapC1 toxicity and the activity of eukaryotic relatives also require some combination of counterparts of D6, E43 and D99, the acidic side chains predicted to co-ordinate the active site metal based on structures of VapC and PIN-domain proteins

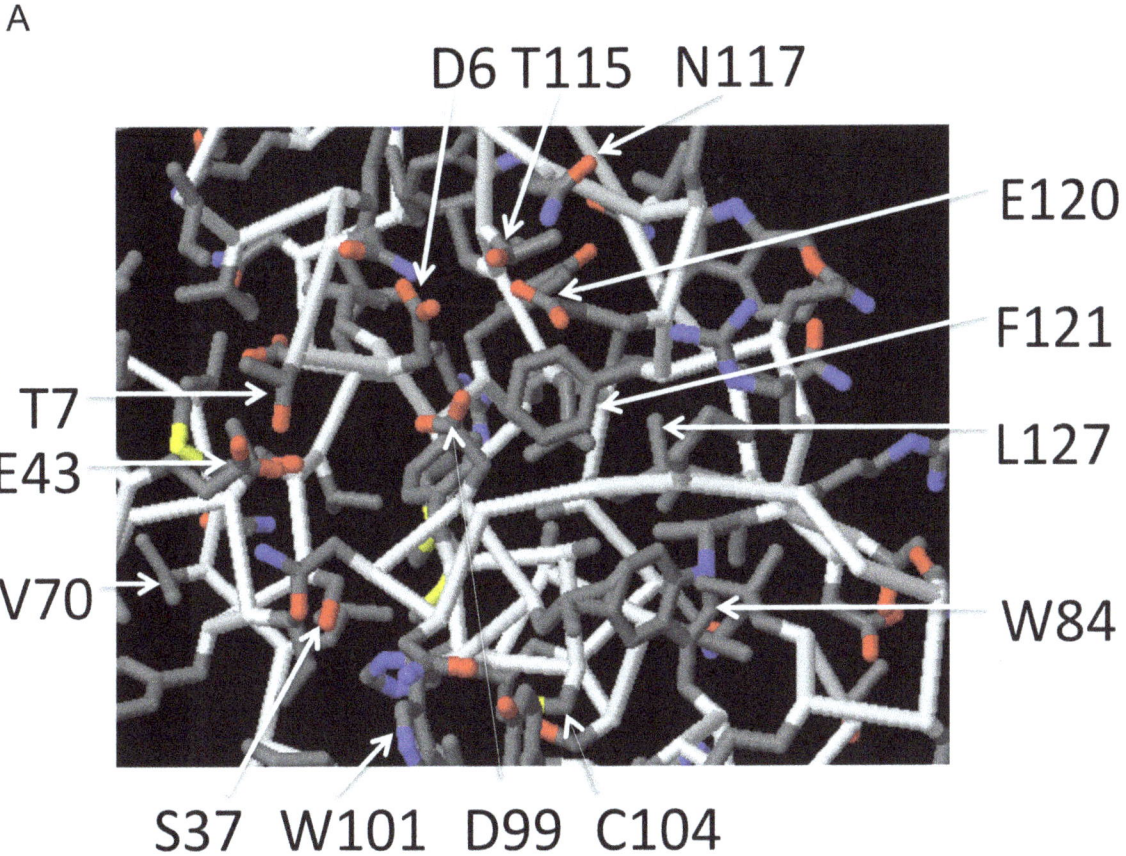

A

B

Figure 5. Structural analysis of VapC1 mutations. *A.* Position of mutations affecting activity of NTHi VapC1. NTHi VapC1 was modeled to *Shigella flexneri* VapBC (MMDB ID: 94821; PDB ID: 3TND) using Phyre [25]. Modeling confidence was 100% for 98% of the VapC1 sequence. Arrows indicate mutated NTHi VapC1 side chains. Colors correspond to; white (peptide backbone), grey (amino acid side chains), blue (nitrogen), yellow (sulfur) and red (oxygen). *B.* Comparison of NTHi VapC proteins with several VapC proteins from the listed species. Asterisks indicate the position of NTHi VapC1 mutations described herein. Black boxes indicate identity in at least four of seven species and gray boxes indicate similarity in at least four of seven species.

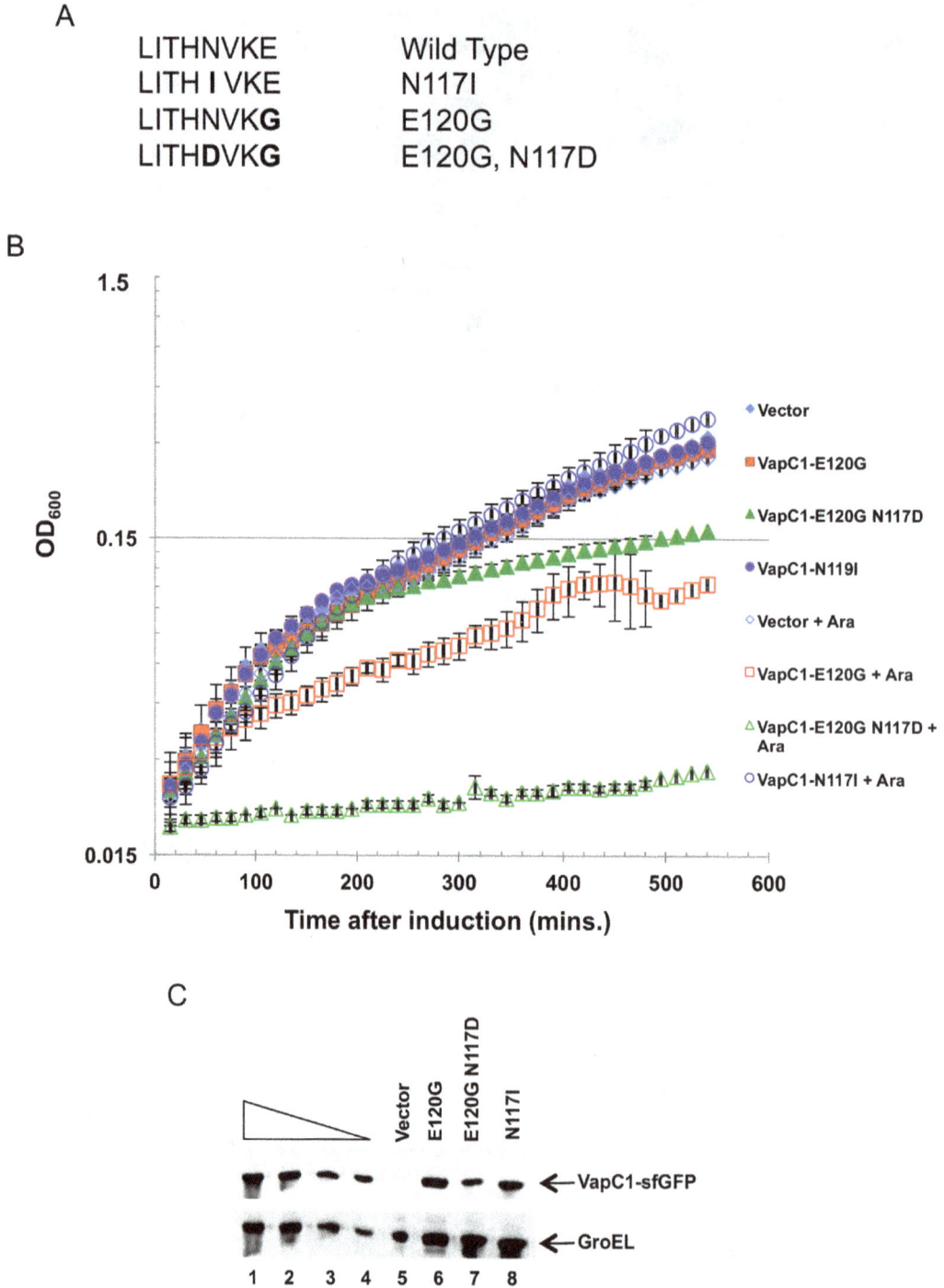

A

LITHNVKE	Wild Type
LITH I VKE	N117I
LITHNVK**G**	E120G
LITH**D**VK**G**	E120G, N117D

B

C

Figure 6. N117D suppresses the E120G defect. *A.* Comparison of the amino acid sequence of VapC1 and mutants from positions 113 to 120. Mutations are indicated in bold. *B.* Analysis of the growth of LMG194 cells expressing the indicated alleles of VapC1 in M9 glycerol with 50 µg/ml ampicillin after induction by addition of L-arabinose to a final concentration of 0.02%. Time points on the curves are the average of three biological replicates with error bars representing the standard deviation. *C.* Western blot analysis of VapC1 mutant proteins isolated 60 minutes after induction with arabinose at a final concentration of 0.02%. Blots were probed with anti-myc antibody for VapC1 proteins and anti-GroEL as a loading control. The first four lanes in the panel show a two-fold dilution series of VapC1-sfGFP as a control for signal linearity.

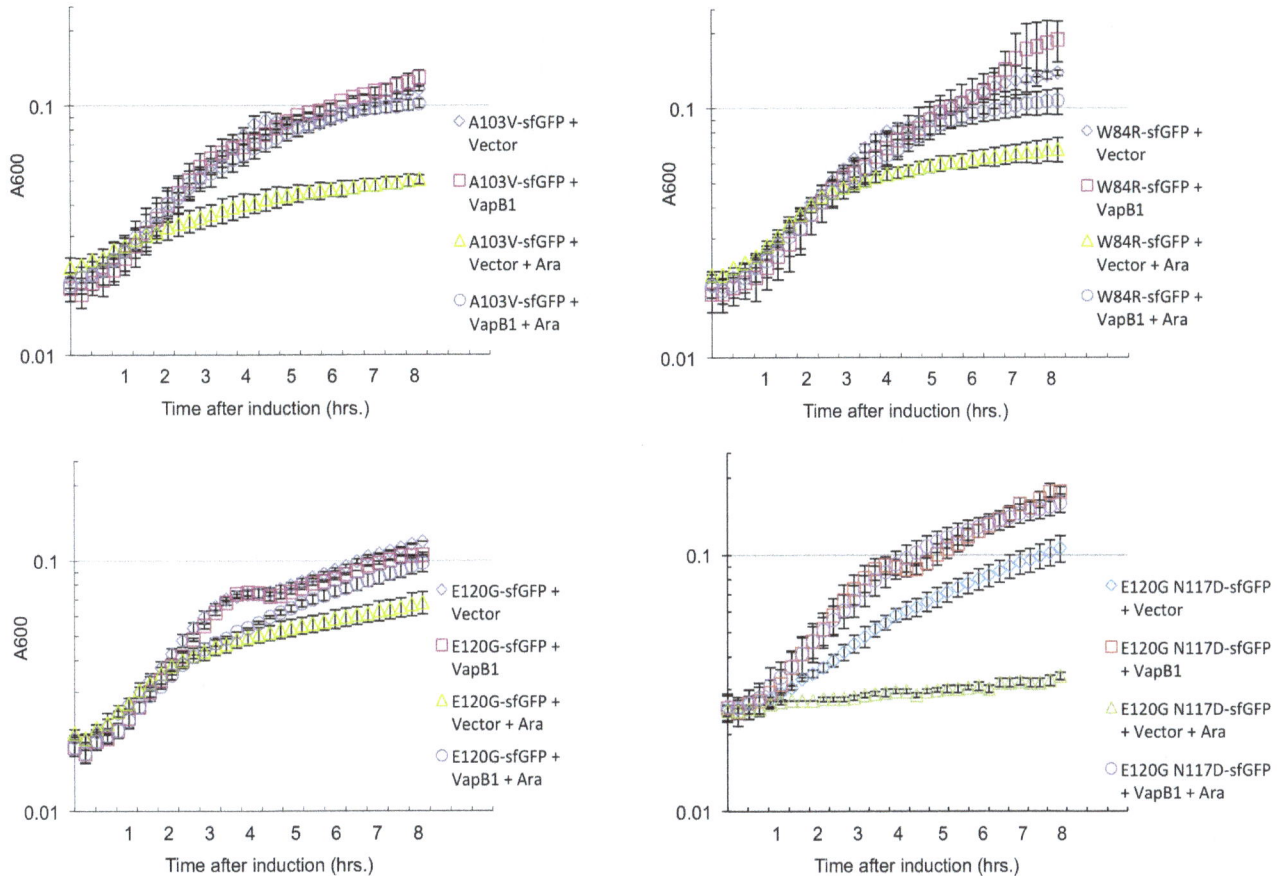

Figure 7. Ability of antitoxin VapB1 to relieve toxicity of VapC1 mutants. *A.* Analysis of the growth of LMG194 cells expressing the indicated alleles of VapC1 in M9 glycerol with 50 µg/ml ampicillin after induction by addition of L-arabinose and/or IPTG to a final concentration of 0.02% and 0.5 mM, respectively. Time points on the curves are the average of two biological replicates with error bars representing the standard error.

[21,26–28] (Figure 1A). Our finding of a requirement for D99 is consistent with the results of Cline et al. who found that VapC1 with a D99N mutation no longer functioned as a toxin, but could interact with VapB1 to form a complex that binds the VapBC1 promoter [42]. Interestingly, our findings indicate that VapC1 from NTHi employs E120 rather than the aspartate conserved in many other VapC toxins at position 117, the fourth canonical acidic side chain thought to play a role in stabilizing the catalytic metal ion via a water bridge [33]. E120 also exists in NTHi VapC2 as well as the VapC toxins from *R. felis* and *S. flexneri*, and VapC toxins from many species of proteobacteria lacking the counterpart of D117 (Figure 5B). As in the modeling to the *S flexnerii* VapC, E120 of NTHi VapC1 projects into the active site of the structure, modeled by Phyre2 to the *R. felis* VapC, consistent with evidence suggesting that it makes hydrogen bond contacts with the conserved equivalents of N8 and T115 in *R. felis* VapC [36]. These observations support the conclusion that this alternative acidic side chain plays an essential role in the function of VapC toxins in a wide variety of bacteria. Indeed, we found that mutation of asparagine at 117 to aspartate largely compensates for loss of E120 in VapC1, suggesting a certain degree of flexibility in the active site of these toxins. The fact that expression of VapB1 inhibits the toxicity of VapC1 E120G and E120G, N117D suggests that these mutations do not cause major alterations in the structure of the toxin. Interestingly, *M. tuberculosis* VapB20 has the canonical aspartate in a position similar to canonical VapC

proteins, while *S. flexneri* and *S. typhimurium* have the alternative equivalent of E120. It remains unknown whether this difference governs the substrate specificity of VapC20 for 23S rRNA and the VapC toxins from *S. flexneri* and *S. typhimurium* for initiator tRNA^{fMet}.

Our analysis also revealed a dependence of VapC1 on several other side chains not previously predicted to play an essential role in the activity of VapC toxins. These include the aromatic amino acids W84, W101 and F121. Structural modeling predicts that these side chains lie near the active site suggesting that they could play a role in RNA substrate binding via stacking interactions with nucleobases (Figure 5A). Indeed, the model positions the conserved F121 facing into the active site consistent with a role in positioning RNA for hydrolysis.

Crystal structures of VapB-VapC complexes indicate that the C-terminal third of VapB antitoxins interact with a cleft in the VapC toxins that includes the active site [24,36-39]. Analysis of the structures suggests that interaction between VapC and VapB partners requires side chains necessary for VapC toxin activity. Despite the critical nature of these contacts for the biological fuction of VapBC pairs, no functional evidence exists to support this model. We tested this in the cases where VapC1 mutations diminished, but did not eliminate toxicity *in vivo*. The results indicate that none of these mutations has a measurable effect on the ability of the VapB1 to block the toxicity of the VapC mutants *in vivo*. In the case of, A103V, W84R, E120G, and the double mutant E120G N117D, expression of VapB1 fully counteracts VapC1 toxicity. The ability of VapB1 to interact functionally with these mutant toxins suggests that, despite their important roles in VapC1 toxicity, these amino acids do not play an essential role in the interaction with the antitoxin. Moreover, the fact that VapB antitoxins make specific contacts in and around the active site of their cognate toxins supports our conclusion that the ability of VapB1 to recognize and suppress the toxicity of mutant VapC1 *in vivo* indicates that these mutations do not cause significant misfolding of the toxin.

In summary, the findings reported here reveal critical structural features required for the biological function VapC toxins, and PIN-domain proteins in general. The results support the conclusion that the activity NTHi VapC1 requires a novel, alternative active site motif that is likely employed by many other members of this toxin family. This raises the intriguing possibility that VapC target specificity may be governed by small differences in the enzymes' active sites.

Acknowledgments

We dedicate this work to the memory of our late friend and colleague Rebekka Sprouse. This work would not have been possible without her cheerful and excellent assistance. We are grateful to members of the Butler Lab for helpful discussions and comments on the manuscript.

Author Contributions

Conceived and designed the experiments: JSB. Performed the experiments: BH AM KS VD. Analyzed the data: BH AM KS VD. Wrote the paper: BH AM KS VD JSB.

References

1. Gerdes K, Rasmussen PB, Molin S (1986) Unique type of plasmid maintenance function: postsegregational killing of plasmid-free cells. Proc Natl Acad Sci U S A 83: 3116–3120.
2. Jaffe A, Ogura T, Hiraga S (1985) Effects of the ccd function of the F plasmid on bacterial growth. J Bacteriol 163: 841–849.
3. Gerdes K (2000) Toxin-antitoxin modules may regulate synthesis of macromolecules during nutritional stress. J Bacteriol 182: 561–572.
4. Hayes F (2003) Toxins-antitoxins: plasmid maintenance, programmed cell death, and cell cycle arrest. Science 301: 1496–1499.
5. van Kessel JC, Hatfull GF (2008) Mycobacterial recombineering. Methods Mol Biol 435: 203–215.
6. Fasani RA, Savageau MA (2013) Molecular mechanisms of multiple toxin-antitoxin systems are coordinated to govern the persister phenotype. Proc Natl Acad Sci U S A 110: E2528–2537.
7. Maisonneuve E, Shakespeare LJ, Jorgensen MG, Gerdes K (2011) Bacterial persistence by RNA endonucleases. Proc Natl Acad Sci U S A 108: 13206–13211.
8. Arcus VL, McKenzie JL, Robson J, Cook GM (2011) The PIN-domain ribonucleases and the prokaryotic VapBC toxin-antitoxin array. Protein Eng Des Sel 24: 33–40.
9. Anantharaman V, Aravind L (2003) New connections in the prokaryotic toxin-antitoxin network: relationship with the eukaryotic nonsense-mediated RNA decay system. Genome Biol 4: R81.
10. Clissold PM, Ponting CP (2000) PIN domains in nonsense-mediated mRNA decay and RNAi. Curr Biol 10: R888–890.
11. Arcus VL, Rainey PB, Turner SJ (2005) The PIN-domain toxin-antitoxin array in mycobacteria. Trends Microbiol 13: 360–365.
12. Daines DA, Wu MH, Yuan SY (2007) VapC-1 of nontypeable Haemophilus influenzae is a ribonuclease. J Bacteriol 189: 5041–5048.
13. Ahidjo BA, Kuhnert D, McKenzie JL, Machowski EE, Gordhan BG, et al. (2011) VapC toxins from Mycobacterium tuberculosis are ribonucleases that differentially inhibit growth and are neutralized by cognate VapB antitoxins. PLoS One 6: e21738.
14. McKenzie JL, Duyvestyn JM, Smith T, Bendak K, Mackay J, et al. (2012) Determination of ribonuclease sequence-specificity using Pentaprobes and mass spectrometry. Rna 18: 1267–1278.
15. Winther KS, Brodersen DE, Brown AK, Gerdes K (2013) VapC20 of Mycobacterium tuberculosis cleaves the Sarcin-Ricin loop of 23S rRNA. Nat Commun 4: 2796.
16. Miller JH (1972) Experiments in molecular genetics. Cold Spring Harbor, N.Y.: Cold Spring Harbor Laboratory. xvi, 466 p. p.
17. Fisher CL, Pei GK (1997) Modification of a PCR-based site-directed mutagenesis method. Biotechniques 23: 570–571, 574.
18. Schuster-Bockler B, Schultz J, Rahmann S (2004) HMM Logos for visualization of protein families. BMC Bioinformatics 5: 7.
19. Bunker RD, McKenzie JL, Baker EN, Arcus VL (2008) Crystal structure of PAE0151 from Pyrobaculum aerophilum, a PIN-domain (VapC) protein from a toxin-antitoxin operon. Proteins 72: 510–518.
20. Sharp JD, Cruz JW, Raman S, Inouye M, Husson RN, et al. (2012) Growth and translation inhibition through sequence specific RNA binding by a mycobacterium tuberculosis VAPC toxin. J Biol Chem.
21. Winther KS, Gerdes K (2011) Enteric virulence associated protein VapC inhibits translation by cleavage of initiator tRNA. Proc Natl Acad Sci U S A 108: 7403–7407.
22. Daines DA, Wu MH, Yuan SY (2007) VapC-1 of nontypeable Haemophilus influenzae is a ribonuclease. J Bacteriol 189: 5041–5048.
23. Pedelacq JD, Cabantous S, Tran T, Terwilliger TC, Waldo GS (2006) Engineering and characterization of a superfolder green fluorescent protein. Nat Biotechnol 24: 79–88.
24. Dienemann C, Boggild A, Winther KS, Gerdes K, Brodersen DE (2011) Crystal structure of the VapBC toxin-antitoxin complex from Shigella flexneri reveals a hetero-octameric DNA-binding assembly. J Mol Biol 414: 713–722.
25. Kelley LA, Sternberg MJ (2009) Protein structure prediction on the Web: a case study using the Phyre server. Nat Protoc 4: 363–371.
26. Bleichert F, Granneman S, Osheim YN, Beyer AL, Baserga SJ (2006) The PINc domain protein Utp24, a putative nuclease, is required for the early cleavage steps in 18S rRNA maturation. Proc Natl Acad Sci U S A 103: 9464–9469.
27. Fatica A, Tollervey D, Dlakic M (2004) PIN domain of Nob1p is required for D-site cleavage in 20S pre-rRNA. Rna 10: 1698–1701.
28. Glavan F, Behm-Ansmant I, Izaurralde E, Conti E (2006) Structures of the PIN domains of SMG6 and SMG5 reveal a nuclease within the mRNA surveillance complex. Embo J 25: 5117–5125.
29. Huntzinger E, Kashima I, Fauser M, Sauliere J, Izaurralde E (2008) SMG6 is the catalytic endonuclease that cleaves mRNAs containing nonsense codons in metazoan. Rna 14: 2609–2617.
30. Lamanna AC, Karbstein K (2009) Nob1 binds the single-stranded cleavage site D at the 3'-end of 18S rRNA with its PIN domain. Proc Natl Acad Sci U S A 106: 14259–14264.
31. Lebreton A, Tomecki R, Dziembowski A, Seraphin B (2008) Endonucleolytic RNA cleavage by a eukaryotic exosome. Nature 456: 993–996.
32. Schneider C, Leung E, Brown J, Tollervey D (2009) The N-terminal PIN domain of the exosome subunit Rrp44 harbors endonuclease activity and tethers Rrp44 to the yeast core exosome. Nucleic Acids Res 37: 1127–1140.
33. Anantharaman V, Aravind L (2006) The NYN domains: novel predicted RNAses with a PIN domain-like fold. RNA Biol 3: 18–27.
34. Ramage HR, Connolly LE, Cox JS (2009) Comprehensive functional analysis of Mycobacterium tuberculosis toxin-antitoxin systems: implications for pathogenesis, stress responses, and evolution. PLoS Genet 5: e1000767.
35. Zhu L, Sharp JD, Kobayashi H, Woychik NA, Inouye M (2010) Noncognate Mycobacterium tuberculosis toxin-antitoxins can physically and functionally interact. J Biol Chem 285: 39732–39738.
36. Mate MJ, Vincentelli R, Foos N, Raoult D, Cambillau C, et al. (2012) Crystal structure of the DNA-bound VapBC2 antitoxin/toxin pair from Rickettsia felis. Nucleic acids research 40: 3245–3258.
37. Mattison K, Wilbur JS, So M, Brennan RG (2006) Structure of FitAB from Neisseria gonorrhoeae bound to DNA reveals a tetramer of toxin-antitoxin heterodimers containing pin domains and ribbon-helix-helix motifs. J Biol Chem 281: 37942–37951.
38. Miallau L, Faller M, Chiang J, Arbing M, Guo F, et al. (2009) Structure and proposed activity of a member of the VapBC family of toxin-antitoxin systems. VapBC-5 from Mycobacterium tuberculosis. J Biol Chem 284: 276–283.
39. Min AB, Miallau L, Sawaya MR, Habel J, Cascio D, et al. (2012) The crystal structure of the Rv0301-Rv0300 VapBC-3 toxin-antitoxin complex from M. tuberculosis reveals a Mg(2)(+) ion in the active site and a putative RNA-binding site. Protein Sci 21: 1754–1767.
40. Takeshita D, Zenno S, Lee WC, Saigo K, Tanokura M (2006) Crystallization and preliminary X-ray analysis of the PIN domain of human EST1A. Acta crystallographica Section F, Structural biology and crystallization communications 62: 656–658.
41. Takeshita D, Zenno S, Lee WC, Saigo K, Tanokura M (2007) Crystal structure of the PIN domain of human telomerase-associated protein EST1A. Proteins 68: 980–989.
42. Cline SD, Saleem S, Daines DA (2012) Regulation of the vapBC-1 toxin-antitoxin locus in nontypeable Haemophilus influenzae. PLoS One 7: e32199.

19

The Efficacy of the Ribonucleotide Reductase Inhibitor Didox in Preclinical Models of AML

Guerry J. Cook[1], David L. Caudell[2], Howard L. Elford[3], Timothy S. Pardee[1,4]*

1 Wake Forest University Health Sciences, Department of Internal Medicine, Section on Hematology and Oncology, Winston-Salem, North Carolina, United States of America, **2** Department of Pathology, Section of Comparative Medicine, Wake Forest University Health Sciences, Winston-Salem, North Carolina, United States of America, **3** Molecules for Health, Richmond, Virginia, United States of America, **4** Wake Forest University Comprehensive Cancer Center, Winston-Salem, North Carolina, United States of America

Abstract

Acute Myeloid Leukemia (AML) is an aggressive malignancy which leads to marrow failure, and ultimately death. There is a desperate need for new therapeutics for these patients. Ribonucleotide reductase (RR) is the rate limiting enzyme in DNA synthesis. Didox (3,4-Dihydroxybenzohydroxamic acid) is a novel RR inhibitor noted to be more potent than hydroxyurea. In this report we detail the activity and toxicity of Didox in preclinical models of AML. RR was present in all AML cell lines and primary patient samples tested. Didox was active against all human and murine AML lines tested with IC_{50} values in the low micromolar range (mean IC_{50} 37 μM [range 25.89–52.70 μM]). It was active against primary patient samples at concentrations that did not affect normal hematopoietic stem cells (HSCs). Didox exposure resulted in DNA damage and p53 induction culminating in apoptosis. In syngeneic, therapy-resistant AML models, single agent Didox treatment resulted in a significant reduction in leukemia burden and a survival benefit. Didox was well tolerated, as marrow from treated animals was morphologically indistinguishable from controls. Didox exposure at levels that impaired leukemia growth did not inhibit normal HSC engraftment. In summary, Didox was well tolerated and effective against preclinical models of AML.

Editor: Francesco Bertolini, European Institute of Oncology, Italy

Funding: This work was supported by the Doug Coley Foundation for Leukemia Research, the Frances P. Tutwiler Fund, and the National Cancer Institute (award P30CA012197, 1K08CA169809-01; TSP). The funders had no role in study design, data collection and analysis, decision to publish, or preparation of the manuscript.

Competing Interests: HLE is President and a shareholder of Molecules for Health and has a financial interest in therapeutic potential. All other authors declare that they have no competing interests.

* Email: tspardee@wakehealth.edu

Introduction

Acute Myeloid Leukemia (AML) is an aggressive, genetically heterogeneous malignancy of the marrow wherein neoplastic myeloid progenitors suppress healthy HSCs leading to marrow failure, and ultimately death. Each year in the US there are approximately 12,000 new cases and 9,000 deaths from AML [1]. This malignancy has a dismal overall five year survival rate of 30–40%, but for those over 60 overall survival drops to less than 10% [2–4]. AML is a disease of the elderly, with a median onset age of 70 and more than 70% of patients are over the age of 60 at diagnosis [2]. For this population the incidence of AML has slowly been climbing over the past several decades; however, the one year survival rate remains virtually unchanged [5]. These patients desperately need new treatment strategies.

The standard treatment of AML has remained unchanged for decades despite intense research [6,7]. For those patients fortunate enough to achieve a remission most will relapse, often with chemoresistant disease [8]. Many frail and elderly patients are not candidates for additional intensive chemotherapy [9]. This highlights the need for the development of new therapeutic targets.

AML is genetically heterogenous with several distinct recurring genetic abnormalities [10]. In the last decade there have been many advances in understanding the different driving mutations in this disease. Despite this increased understanding therapies designed to target these mutations have led to only transient responses as genetically distinct subclones with decreased reliance on the target are selected for and relapse occurs. An alternative approach would be to target a "final common pathway" (i.e. a pathway that all leukemia cells, regardless of driving mutations, will need to accomplish in order to generate additional leukemia cells). One such pathway is DNA synthesis. Ribonucleotide Reductase (RR) catalyses the rate limiting step in DNA synthesis converting ribonucleotides into deoxyribonucleotides. Hydroxyurea (HU), a RR catalytic subunit inhibitor, has clinical activity in AML as a cytoreductive agent and in the palliative setting where other agents have been deemed too intensive [11]. Its effectiveness is hindered by a low affinity for RR as well as gastro-intestinal and myelosuppressive toxicities. Clinical trials in elderly and unfit AML patients have shown that HU treatment has a minimal marrow response rate [11]. Since HU has limited clinical activity in AML, RR has been an underutilized target in AML treatment. Recently, there has been a resurgence of interest in RR as a target in AML. RR has been identified as a target of 5-azacitidine, an azanucleoside used to treat AML and myelodysplastic syndromes [12]. Additionally, a phase I trial of an 20-mer antisense oligonucleotide targeting RR combined with high dose cytarabine led to a number of complete remissions in a group of poor risk patients [13]. These studies suggest that RR is a valuable target for AML treatment.

Didox is a RR inhibitor developed from HU. It has replaced the amino group with 3, 4-dihydroxyphenol. Didox displays a 20 fold more potent inhibition of RR than HU [14]. Additionally, Didox reduces both purine and pyrimidine nucleotide pools compared to purine only inhibition seen with HU [14]. Previous groups have shown Didox to have a favorable toxicity in various preclinical models compared to HU [15–17]. A phase I trial in metastatic carcinoma determined the maximum tolerated dose (MTD) of 6 g/m^2 with peak plasma levels of 300 μM [18]. Didox has been shown to have activity against two AML cell lines *in vitro* with significant variability [19]. However, the efficacy of Didox in AML has not been extensively evaluated. In these studies we have examined the cellular effects and efficacy of Didox in preclinical models of AML.

Materials and Methods

All primary samples were collected under an IRB approved protocol by Stony Brook University Medical Center or the Comprehensive Cancer Center of Wake Forest University. All patients gave written consent using an IRB approved consent form. Primary samples were obtained during clinically indicated procedures. The Comprehensive Cancer Center of Wake Forest University Institutional Animal Care and Use Committee approved all mouse experiments.

Reagents

Didox was a gift from Howard Elford, Ph.D. at Molecules for Health, Inc. (Richmond, VA). Didox for animal studies was freshly made each time by dissolving in 5% dextrose water, with the animals receiving 425 mg/kg. For the *in vitro* studies Didox was dissolved in phosphate buffered saline (PBS) at concentrations of 10 mM and 1 mM and stored at −20°C until use. It was then diluted in the culture medium to the final concentration.

Cell Culture Aad Viability Assays

Human lines were maintained in RPMI media (Gibco) supplemented with 10% FBS, penicillin and streptomycin. All murine lines were derived from fetal liver cells infected with MLL-ENL and NRas^{G12D} or Flt3 ITD expressing vectors [20]. Murine lines were maintained in stem cell media (40% IMDM, 40% DMEM, 20% FBS, with or without murine SCF 10 ng/mL, murine IL-6 2 ng/mL, and murine IL-3 0.4 ng/mL). Viability assays were carried out according to the manufacturer's protocols with the Cell Titer-Glo system (Promega).

Primary Samples

All primary samples were collected under an IRB approved protocol by Stony Brook University Medical Center or the Comprehensive Cancer Center of Wake Forest University. Primary samples were obtained during clinical procedures. Cells were collected by centrifugation, resuspended in ACK lysis buffer (150 mM NH$_4$Cl, 10 mM KHCO$_3$, 0.1 mM EDTA) at room temperature for 5 minutes, centrifuged again, washed with PBS, and stored at −80°C until use. Normal hematopoietic stem cells were obtained from healthy allogeneic stem cell transplant donors. As an alternate method, cells were obtained by Ficoll-gradient centrifugation, and stored at −80°C until use.

H2AX Assays

Cells were fixed in 4% neutral buffered formalin, permeabilised in PBS with 0.2% Triton-X 100. To visualize phosphorylated γH2AX, we used anti-pH2AX (#2577, 1:100; Cell Signalling Technologies) with an Alexa Fluor 594-conjugated donkey anti-rabbit antibody (1:1000, A-21207; Invitrogen). Cells were visualized with fluorescence microscopy.

Western Blot

Cells were lysed in Laemmli buffer(1.6 mL 10% SDS, 500 μL 1 M Tris-HCl [pH 6.8], 800 μL glycerol, 400 2-mercaptoethanol, 4.7 mL H$_2$O), and samples separated by SDS-PAGE before transfer to an Immobilon polyvinylidene difluoride membrane (Millipore). Primary antibodies against p53 (IMX25, 1:1000; Leica Microsystems), actin (AC-15, 1:5000; Abcam), anti-pH2AX (#2577, 1:1000; Cell Signaling Technologies) and a secondary antibody anti-mouse (#7076, 1:5000; Cell Signaling) or anti-rabbit (#7074, 1:5000; Cell Signaling) were used. For RR detection, a primary antibody against the M2 subunit of RR (1:1000; sc-10846, Santa Cruz Biotechnology) was used followed by secondary anti-goat antibody (1:1000; ab98826, AbCam).

Table 1. Primary patient sample characteristics.

Patient	Sex	Age	Diagnosis	Karyotype
A1	M	33	AML	Del 7, inv 3
A2	M	53	AML	Normal, Flt3+
A3	F	89	AML	Trisomy 8, der(4)add(4)
A4	F	59	AML	Normal, Flt3-
A5	M	69	AML	Normal, Flt3+
C1	M	74	AML	Del 7q
C2	F	82	AML	Not obtained
C3	M	66	AML w/monocytic differentiation	Complex karyotype:
				trisomy 13, trisomy 19, t(11; 19)
M1	F	60	Acute monocytic leukemia	Trisomy 8, trisomy 9
M2	F	68	AML	Normal
M3	F	80	AML	Normal

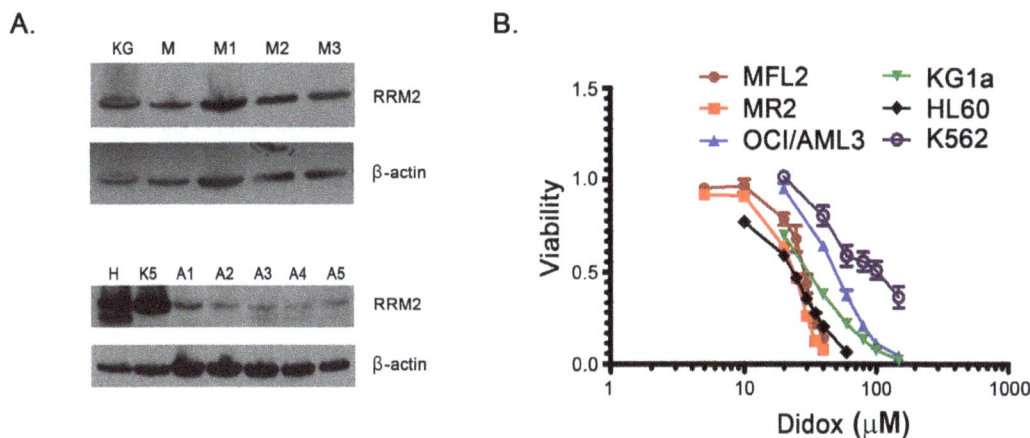

Figure 1. RR is expressed in AML. A. Western blots performed for RR small subunit. AML patient samples (bone marrow, M1–M3, leukopheresis A1–A5), and cell lines (K – KG1a, M – MFL2, H – HL-60, K5 – K562). B. Growth curves. Cell lines were treated with Didox for 72 hours. Viability was assessed and normalized to untreated controls.

Annexin V/PI Assays

Human and murine cells were plated at 100,000 cells/mL and 50,000 cells/mL respectively and treated with the indicated drugs for 48 or 72 hours. The cells were then washed in PBS and stained with propidium iodide (PI) (Sigma-Aldrich) and allophycocyanin (APC)-conjugated annexin V in a binding buffer (0.1 M HEPES [pH 7.4], 1.4 NaCl, and 25 nM CaCl2 solution; BD PharMingen) according the manufacturer's protocol. All flow cytometric analysis was carried out on the BD Accuri C6 cytometer (BD Biosciences).

Colony Formation Studies

Primary patient samples and normal human hematopoietic stem cells (HSCs) were thawed and incubated in hematopoietic progenitor media (C-28020, PromoCell, Heidelberg, Germany) for 24 hours with a titration of Didox. Human lines were incubated as indicated above for 24 hours with a titration of Didox. Cells were washed with PBS and resuspended in IMDM supplemented with 20% FBS, and placed in ColonyGel High Cytokine Formulation media (ReachBio). Experiments were performed in triplicate. Colonies were counted on or after day 7. Colonies of 8 or more cells were counted as established in Shankar et al. [21].

In vivo Efficacy Studies

The Comprehensive Cancer Center of Wake Forest University Institutional Animal Care and Use Committee approved all mouse experiments. Luciferase-tagged leukemia cells were transplanted into 8- week old, sublethally irradiated (4.5 Gy) C57Bl/6 mice by tail vein injection of 1.0×10^6 cells per mouse. Mice were injected with 150 mg/kg D-Luciferin (Gold Biotechnology), anesthetised with isoflurane, and imaged using the IVIS 100 imaging system (Caliper LifeSciences). Mice began treatment with Didox upon detection of clear signal. The animals were treated with daily administrations of Didox at 425 mg/kg Didox (Molecules for Health) by intraperitoneal injection (IP) for 5 days. Control animals received 5% dextrose water by IP injection. Repeat imaging was performed on the day following the final treatment.

Toxicology and Murine BM Engraftment Studies

Normal, age-matched C57Bl/6 mice were given an identical treatment regimen as the efficacy studies. Seventy-two hours following the last dose, the animals were sacrificed, bilateral femur cells harvested, and organs fixed in 10% neutral-buffered formalin followed by routine tissue processing and sectioning, and hematoxylin and eosin staining. In a blinded analysis, a veterinary pathologist reviewed the slides with a Nikon Eclipse 50i light microscope. Photographs of the tissue sections were taken with a NIS Elements D3.10 camera and software system. For the transplant assay, Ly5.1+ C57/Bl6 mice received 8 Gy of irradiation and injected with 1.0×10^6 Ly5.2+ bone marrow cells from the Didox or control treated donors by tail vein injection. Three weeks post injection the mice were sacrificed, and bilateral femur cells harvested. The cells were stained with APC-conjugated anti-Ly5.2 Ab (BD PharMingen) and analyzed by flow cytometry.

Table 2. Inhibitory concentrations of murine and human AML.

Cell Line	IC$_{50}$ (µM)	CI 95%
OCI/AML3	49.26	46.56, 52.10
KG1a	32.45	30.26, 34.79
HL-60	30.83	23.51, 40.43
K562	52.70	39.91, 69.59
MFL2	30.85	24.10, 39.49
MR2	25.89	23.75, 28.23

A.

B.

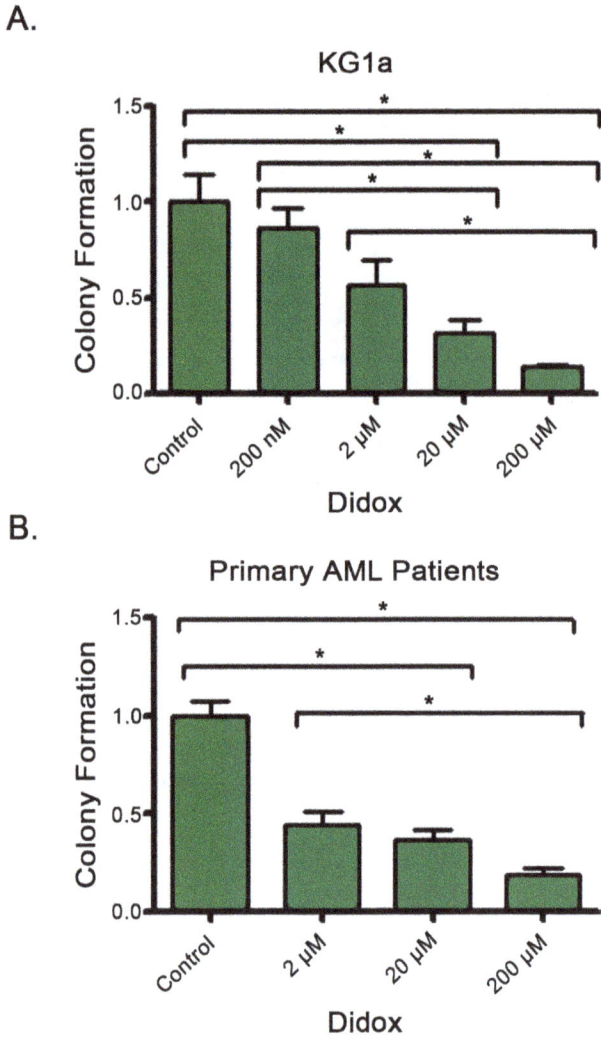

Figure 2. Didox has activity against AML in colony formation assays. A. Didox reduced colony formation in KG1a cells. Cells were exposed to titration of Didox for 24 hours before incubation in methylcellulose (7–8 days). Mean colony formation was assessed in triplicate in 3 experiments and normalized to untreated controls. B. Didox exposure reduced colony formation in primary AML samples. Primary samples (C1–C3) were exposed to a titration of Didox for 24 hours before incubation in methylcellulose (12–14 days). Mean colony formation was assessed in triplicate in 3 experiments and normalized to untreated controls. * = p value less than 0.05.

Statistical Analysis

Groups of 3 or more were analyzed using a one way ANOVA. All means were compared by a student's 2-tailed t test. The *in vivo* survival graphs were generated with the Kaplan-Meier method, with p values determined by the log-rank test. All analyses were performed using GraphPad Prism Version 5.02 (GraphPad Software). A p value ≤ 0.05 was considered significant.

Results

Didox is active against AML *in vitro*

RR has previously been shown to be upregulated in a variety of malignancies. To confirm expression of RR in AML we subjected cell lines and patient samples to western blot using an anti-RR antibody (clinical data from patient samples is shown in Table 1).

Despite multiple distinct genetic abnormalities in the patient samples and cell lines we found detectable levels of RR in all samples tested (Figure 1A) consistent with RR being a final common pathway target. Having confirmed expression we sought to determine the activity of Didox in AML. We performed 72 hour viability assays with titrations of Didox (0–200 μM) in a panel of human and murine AML lines. Didox was active against all lines tested, with IC_{50}'s in the low micromolar range (mean 37 μM [range 25.89–52.70 μM], Figure 1B, Table 2). These data demonstrate ubiquitous expression of RR in AML and that Didox has activity against AML cell lines at clinically achievable concentrations.

Didox has activity against primary AML samples

As cell lines represent only a small subset of AML patients and have been kept in culture for many years, we sought to determine if Didox had any activity against primary patient samples. We performed colony formation assays on 3 primary AML samples, as well as KG1a cells. Cells were exposed to clinically achievable concentrations of Didox (0–200 μM) for 24 hours before incubation in methylcellulose (7–14 days). Consistent with our cell line data Didox, in a dose dependent fashion, significantly reduced colony formation in all samples tested (Figure 2 A–B). Didox demonstrated activity against colony forming progenitor cells from both primary patient samples and cell lines.

Didox induces DNA damage and apoptosis

Previously, Didox has been shown to induce cell death via apoptosis [19,22]. In order to determine if this occurred in our models we exposed a murine AML cell line expressing the MLL-ENL fusion protein and an internal tandem duplication mutation in the Flt3 receptor (MFL2) to a titration of Didox (0–60 μM) and collected samples at 48 hours. Samples were assessed for annexin V binding and PI staining. Didox exposure led to apoptosis in a dose dependent fashion (Figure 3A). Didox exposure results of a depletion of deoxyribonucleotides (dNTPs) leading to double strand breaks in the DNA [14]. To assess for the induction of DNA strand breaks we probed for γH2AX foci in KG1a cells exposed to increasing concentrations of Didox for 24 hours. We found an increase in positive foci with Didox exposure (Figure 3B). To confirm the induction of DNA damage we exposed MFL2 cells to a titration of Didox and performed a western blot for γH2AX. Consitent with our previous result we saw a dose dependent increase in γH2AX (Figure 3C). To evaluate the effect of Didox on DNA damage response proteins we examined p53 induction. We used the p53 sufficient cell line, OCI/AML3, which recapitulates the p53 status most often seen in AML patients [23]. Didox exposure resulted in increased p53 levels over a 24 hour period (Figure 3D). These experiments have shown that Didox exposure leads to DNA damage and subsequent p53 response, ultimately culminating in apoptosis *in vitro*.

Didox acts through the p53 damage response pathway in p53 sufficient AMLs *in vitro*

In AML, p53 mutations affect 10–15% of patients leading to chemoresistance and overall poorer prognosis [24]. Given this clinical relevance and the above data that suggested Didox acted through p53, we next formally tested this by knocking down p53 in a murine AML by western blot (Figure 4A). We observed an increase in resistance to Didox in our p53 knock down compared to our controls in 3 independent viability experiments, each done in triplicate (Figure 4B). This resistance was confirmed in a second knock down of p53 in a separate murine AML (Figure 4C).

A.

B.

DAPI Blue
γH2AX Red

C.

D. OCI/AML3

MFL2

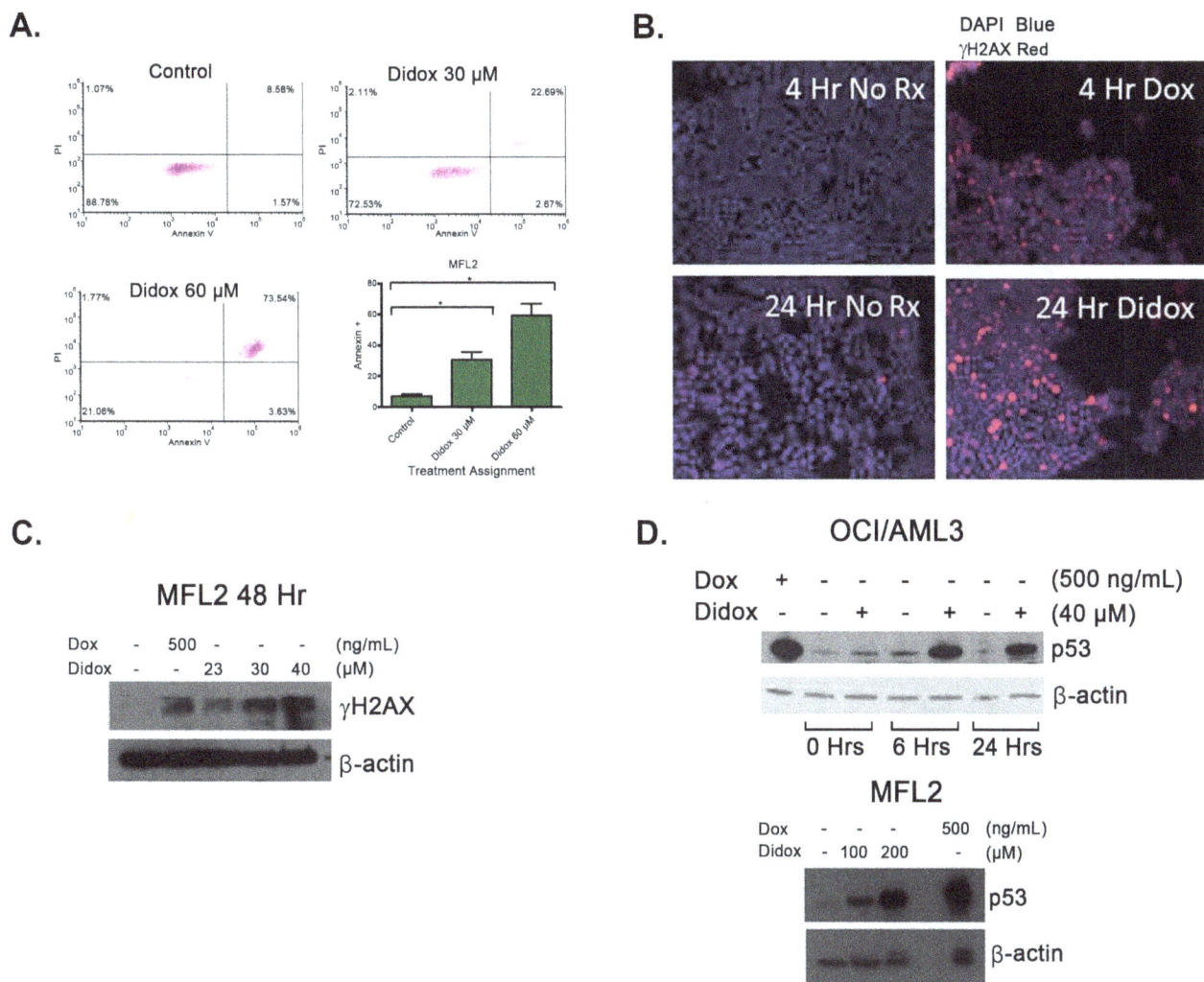

Figure 3. Didox induces DNA damage and apoptosis *in vitro*. A. Didox induced apoptosis at 48 hours. MFL2 cells were exposed to 30 μM, or 60 μM Didox, or a vehicle control and assessed for annexin V binding and PI staining by flow cytometry. B. KG1a cells were exposed to 20 μM Didox for 24 hours or 500 ng/mL doxorubicin for 4 hours and evaluated for γH2AX staining. C. MFL2 cells were exposed to the indicated drug for 48 hours. The cells were collected and lysed before western blot assessment for γH2AX. D. OCI/AML3 cells were exposed to Didox for 48 hours. MFL2 cells were exposed to Didox for 6 hours. The cells were collected and lysed before western blot assessment for p53. Doxorubicin at 500 ng/ml was used as a positive control. * = p of value less than 0.05.

Deletion of p53 is rare in AML; however, there are other clinically relevant alterations which lead to p53 suppression. Our lab has shown that p53 suppression occurs in meningioma-1 (MN1) overexpressing AML [25], along with decreased apoptosis, and chemoresistance [26]. MN1+ murine AML cells demonstrated resistance to Didox compared to GFP controls in 3 viability experiments, each done in triplicate (Figure 4D). This highlights the importance of patient selection in future clinical trials.

Didox reduces leukemic burden and provides a survival benefit in chemoresistant models of AML *in vivo*.

In order to evaluate Didox in a more clinically relevant setting, we moved to an *in vivo* model which has been shown to recapitulate many of the features of human AML [20]. This syngeneic model has genetic lesions associated with human disease and displays many of the histopathologic features of human AML. Additionally, as an immune competent, syngeneic model, it recapitulates important immune and microenvironment interactions.

Both *in vivo* models express the poor prognostic fusion protein MLL-ENL. The second genetic alteration needed for leukemogenesis was provided by either the Nras^{G12D} (MR2) or the Flt3 internal tandem duplication (Flt3 ITD). Luciferase tagged AML cells were injected into sublethally irradiated (4.5 Gy) recipients and allowed to engraft. Once engraftment was established by bioluminescent imaging, the animals received daily administrations of Didox at 425 mg/kg via IP injection (Figure 5A) over 5 days. Didox treatment significantly reduced leukemic burden compared to vehicle treated controls (Figure 5 B–C, p = 0.0026 and p = 0.0342). More importantly, Didox provided a significant survival benefit (Figure 5D, p<0.0001 and p = 0.0094). This data demonstrates that Didox has activity against syngeneic AML models *in vivo*.

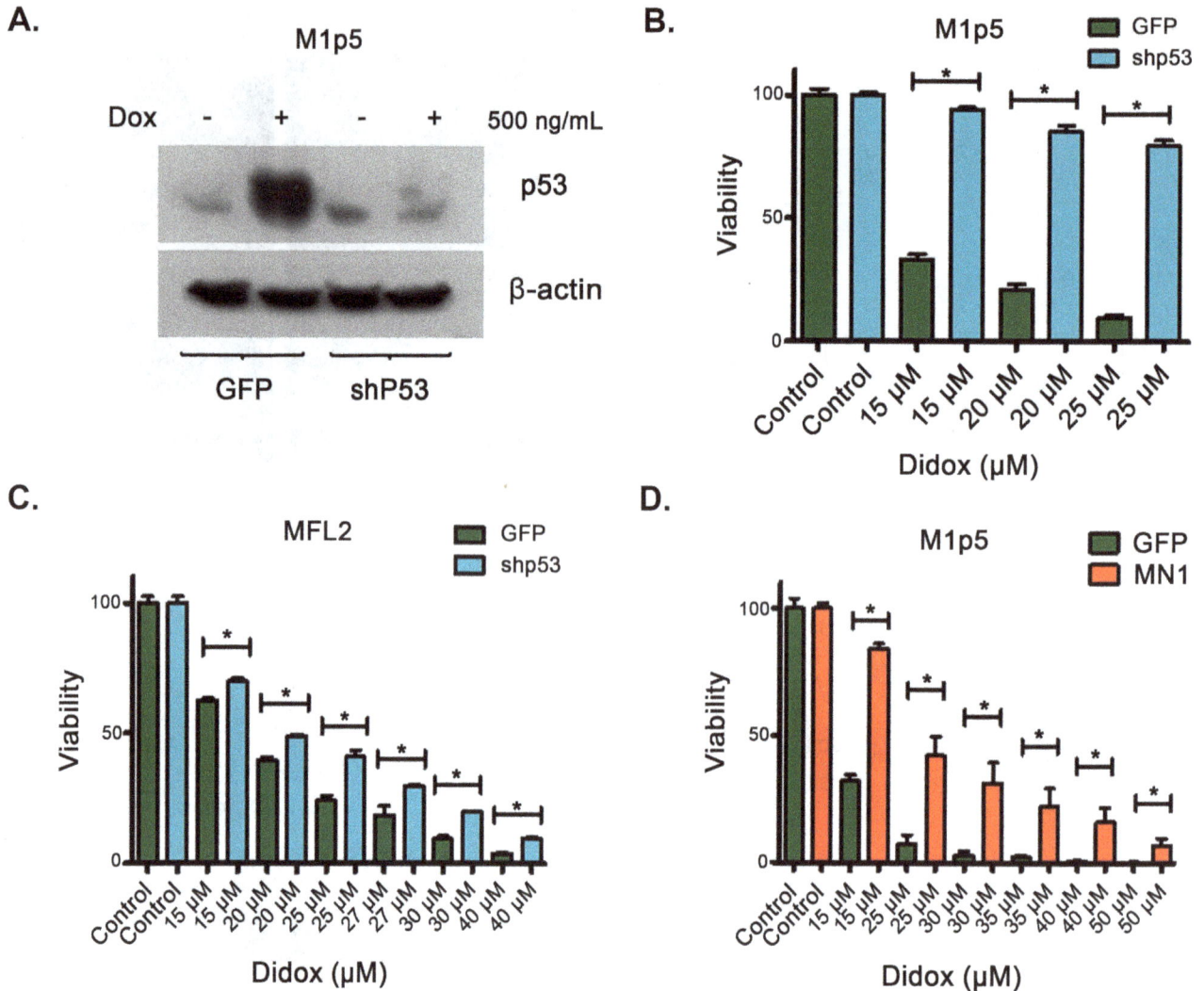

Figure 4. MN1 overexpression and p53 knockdown induce resistance in AML *in vitro.* A. Confirmation of KD in M1p5 cells. B. M1p5 shP53 or GFP cells were exposed to a titration of Didox (0–25 µM) for 72 hours and viability assays performed. C. MFL2 shP53 or GFP cells were exposed to a titration of Didox (0–40 µM) for 72 hours and viability assays performed. D. 3 independent 72 hour viability assays with MN1 and GFP controls, in triplicate with titrations of Didox (0–50 µM).* = p of value less than 0.05.

Didox is well tolerated in normal C57Bl/6 mice, and does not harm hematopoietic stem cells

Since we have shown that Didox treatment reduced leukaemic burden compared to controls *in vivo*, we wanted to interrogate its effects on normal tissues at the dose and schedule used in the survival studies. Normal C57Bl/6 mice received the same Didox regimen as the efficacy study mice and were sacrificed 72 hours following the final treatment. In a blinded analysis, a veterinary pathologist was unable to distinguish morphological differences between the two groups (Figure 6A). This demonstrates that Didox has minimal effect on normal tissue morphology. However, this does not tell us the consequences of Didox treatment on the function of normal HSCs. To determine the effects of Didox on normal human hematopoietic progenitors we performed colony formation assays on 3 normal samples. In contrast to our results with primary patient samples Didox treatment lead to only a modest and non-significant reduction in colony formation of normal progenitors, even at the highest dose tested (Figure 6B). In order to determine the effect of Didox on normal HSCs we

determined the ability of Didox treated marrow cells to engraft in syngeneic recipients. Normal C57Bl/6 mice (Ly5.2+) were treated as in the AML efficacy studies and their marrow harvested 72 hours following last treatment and transplanted into lethally irradiated Ly5.1+ recipients. After 3 weeks recipients were sacrificed and engraftment was determined by flow cytometry (Figure S1). Didox treated marrow engrafted at least as well as the control marrow (Figure 6C). These data demonstrate that Didox does not cause gross tissue toxicity at the effective dose in C57Bl/6 mice, nor does it harm the function of normal progenitors or HSCs. These data suggest a large therapeutic window.

Discussion

AML is an aggressive malignancy that primarily effects the elderly population. It is characterised by high genetic heterogeneity and poor overall 5 year survival [2]. The frontline treatments in AML have remained virtually unchanged for decades, and while many patients may have a transient response to chemotherapy, most will relapse with chemoresistant disease [8]. This

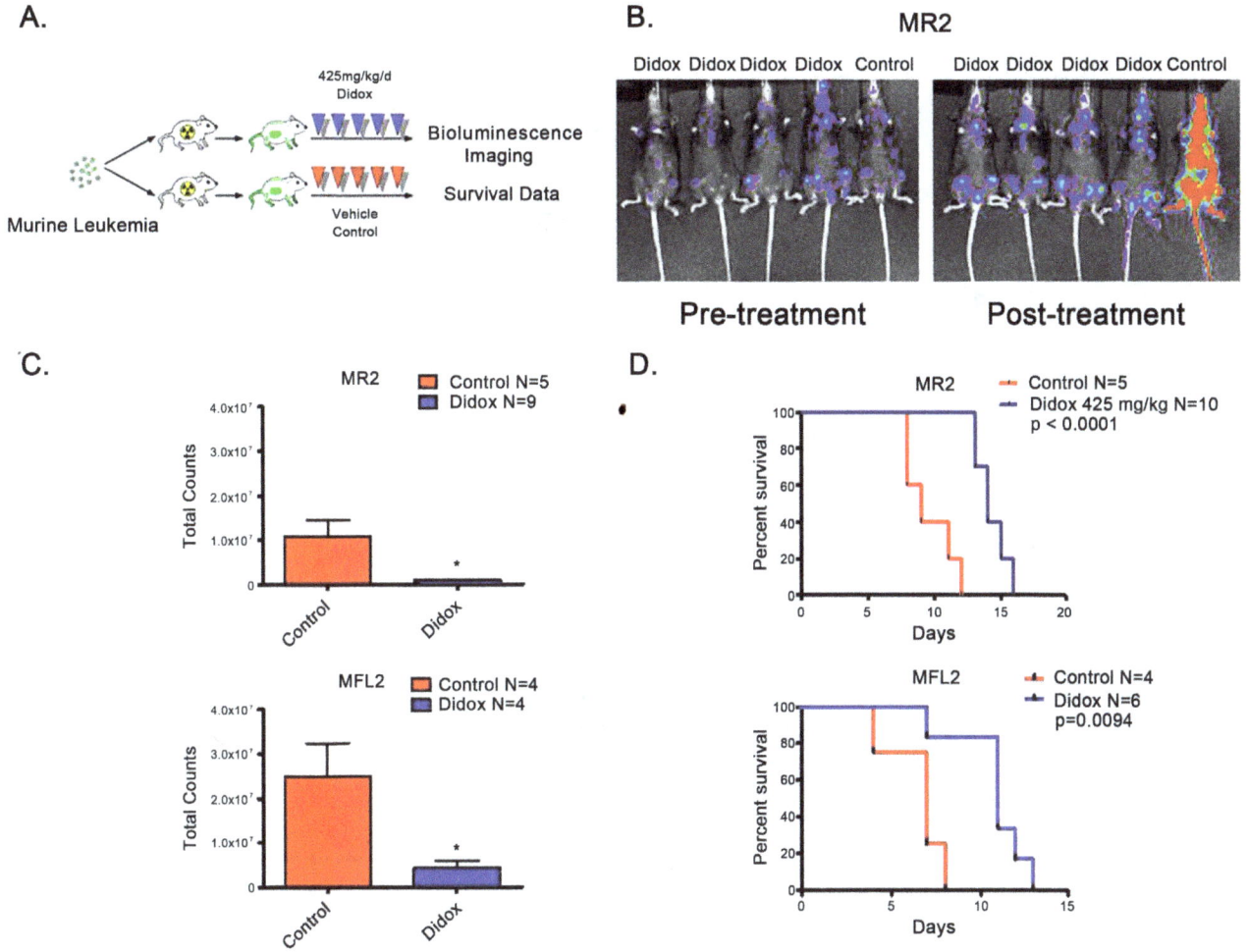

Figure 5. Didox has activity in AML models *in vivo*. A. Schema. 1.0×10^6 luciferase tagged AML cells were injected into sublethally irradiated (4.5 Gy) recipients and allowed to engraft. Engraftment was monitored by bioluminescent imaging (IVIS 100 imager). Animals received 5 days of Didox at 425 mg/kg or D5 water control via intraperitoneal injection (IP). Animals were followed for survival. B. Representative bioluminescent images from Nras[G12D] (MR2) mice pre- and post-treatment. C. Quantitation of bioluminescence post-treatment. D. Kaplan-Meier survival curves of Didox *in vivo* studies from start of treatment. * =p of value less than 0.05.

highlights both the dearth of progress in AML treatment and the desperate need for the development of new therapies.

A strategy that targets a metabolic pathway required by all leukemia cells regardless of driving mutation has the potential to be effective even in a genetically heterogenous disease like AML. One such pathway is DNA synthesis. The rate limiting reaction of DNA synthesis is catalysed by RR and has been shown to be upregulated in many malignancies [27–30]. The classical inhibitor, HU, has had limited use in the clinic due to poor affinity to RR, lack of durable responses and associated toxicities. However, there has been a resurgence of interest in RR inhibition in AML.

Didox was developed from HU and displays 20 fold more potent affinity for RR than its predecessor. It reduces both purine and pyrimidine pools. Moreover, it has been shown to have a more favorable toxicity profile compared to HU in preclinical models [15,31]. The MTD was determined from a phase I trial, but it has not yet been extensively studied in AML.

We have investigated the efficacy of Didox, a novel RR inhibitor, *in vitro* and *in vivo* in preclinical models of AML. We made several key observations: 1. RR was ubiquitously expressed in all samples and cell lines tested. 2. Didox had activity in all cell lines and patient samples tested with IC_{50} values in the low micromolar range. 3. Didox exposure led to DNA damage, p53 induction, and apoptosis. 4. Didox was effective against two *in vivo* models of AML. 5. Didox treatment did not cause gross tissue toxicity in non-leukemic animals. And finally, Didox did not harm normal haematopoietic progenitors or stem cells.

Didox had activity across a panel of cell lines and primary patient samples with diverse cytogenetic characteristics, suggesting inhibition of RR is effective regardless of their driving mutations. This is supported by our finding that RR is expressed in all cell lines and patient samples. The IC_{50} values for all lines tested clustered in the low micromolar range with a mean value of 37 μM (range 25.89–52.70 μM) despite the wide variety of driving mutations in the lines tested. Importantly, all IC_{50} values were well below the peak plasma levels achieved at the MTD of Didox in a phase I clinical trial [18]. In addition, primary patient samples were also impaired in their ability to form colonies following Didox exposure at levels below those achieved in clinical trials. This is the first data, to our knowledge, that demonstrates Didox efficacy against primary patient derived AML cells. These results

A.

Control Treated, Small Intestine

Didox Treated, Small Intestine

Control Treated, Bone Marrow

Didox Treated, Bone Marrow

B.

C.

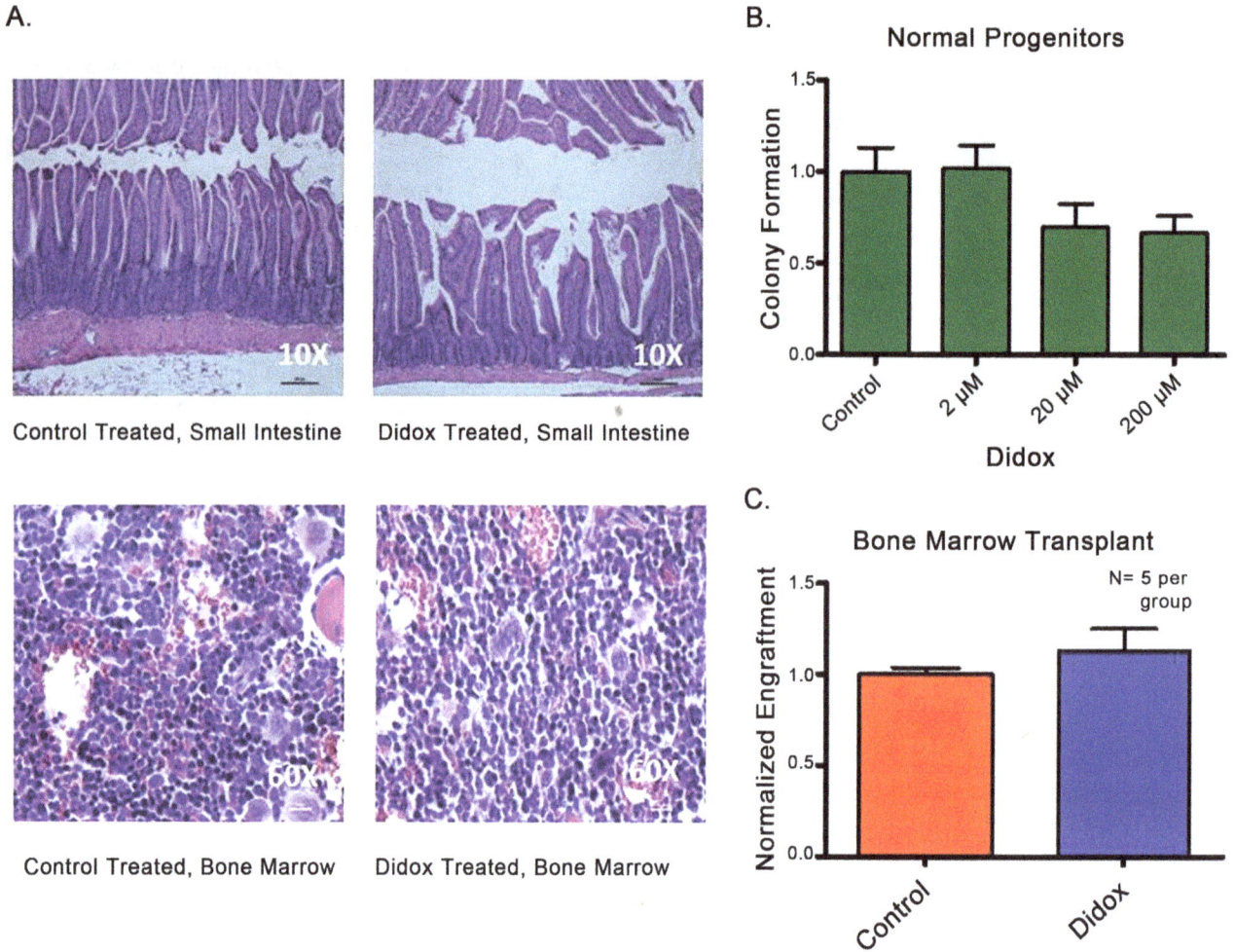

Figure 6. Didox is well tolerated. A. Didox treated C57Bl/6 mice showed no difference in tissue morphology compared to vehicle treated controls as read by a veterinary pathologist blinded to treatment assignment. Representative H&E sections of gastrointestinal tract (Small Intestine) and bone marrow from Didox (n = 3) and control treated animals (n = 3). B. Colony formation assays performed on normal HSCs following 24 hour Didox exposure (0–200 µM), p = 0.09. C. Didox treatment does not harm normal HSCs. C57Bl/6 mice were treated for 5 days with 425 mg/kg Didox or a vehicle control via IP injection. 72 hours post treatment the animals were sacrificed and their marrow harvested. Marrow was then transplanted into lethally irradiated (8 Gy) Ly5.1+ recipients and allowed to engraft. Post-engraftment the animals were sacrificed, marrow harvested, and analyzed for Ly5.2+ by flow cytometry. Engraftment values were normalized to vehicle controls. N = 5 per group.

suggest that Didox is effective at doses that are achievable in a clinical setting.

Didox has been shown to cause reductions and imbalances in the dNTP pools in multiple cancer cell lines including leukaemia cells [19,32]. This dNTP imbalance can lead to several consequences including nucleotide misincorporation and stalled replication forks (reviewed in [33]). Didox treatment also suppresses RAD51 expression, a key DNA repair enzyme in myeloma cells [22] and inhibits the upregulation of other DNA repair proteins in gliosarcoma cells [32]. This simultaneous induction of DNA damage and inhibition of repair results in apoptosis. This mechanism is attractive for the treatment of AML as patient samples have shown impairments in DNA damage response [34]. Consistent with this we have demonstrated Didox induces DNA damage and increased p53 levels followed by apoptosis in our models.

In previous studies, this laboratory has examined the effects of MN1 in AML. MN1 overexpression is associated with a poor prognosis in patients. Its overexpression led to accelerated

leukemic growth, chemoresistance, suppression of p53, and decreased apoptosis in preclinical models. This increase in resistance seen with MN1 overexpression may be due to the previously described p53 suppression in these cells.

Our *in vitro* results demonstrate that Didox, when present throughout a 24 or 72 hour period at clinically achievable concentrations efficiently induce leukemia cell death. However, they do not address the ability Didox to induce leukemia cell death when given as a daily bolus with leukemia cells in their appropriate microenvironment. Several studies have demonstrated the protective effect of the marrow microenvironment in AML [35–37]. Our *in vivo* studies using a syngeneic, immunocompetent AML model demonstrate a reduction in leukemic burden and a significant increase in survival following 5 daily doses of Didox. These data show that Didox can induce leukemia cell death even in the marrow microenvironment and further suggest it will be an effective agent in the treatment of AML patients.

In previous reports Didox has been shown to be less toxic to the hematopoietic system than HU [38]. Suppression of normal hematopoiesis by current AML therapies is a major cause of treatment related mortality in these patients. Our studies have confirmed the low toxicity of Didox on normal hematopoietic progenitors *in vitro* and for the first time on HSCs *in vivo*. The reasons for this large therapeutic window are not clear, but there are several possible contributing factors. Leukemia cells are likely to have a high reliance on RR for proliferation as RR activity has been shown to correlate with proliferation and to be elevated in cancer cells [39]. Furthermore, oncogenic transformation is an inherently stressful process and renders cells more susceptible to DNA damage [40].

In summary, our results highlight an underutilized target in AML treatment through the use of a novel inhibitor. We demonstrated the activity of Didox both *in vitro* and *in vivo* in preclinical models of AML. Consistent with previous studies in other models Didox was well tolerated, with limited toxicities,

suggesting that this is a promising therapeutic for combination regimens with both targeted and standard therapies [15,31]. Such studies are currently underway.

Supporting Information

Figure S1 Facs analysis of engrafted Didox treated marrow. Shown is a representative dot plot and histogram analysis of femur samples collected from Ly5.1+ C57Bl/6 mice following injection with Didox treated Ly5.2 treated marrow cells.

Author Contributions

Conceived and designed the experiments: GJC TSP. Performed the experiments: GJC. Analyzed the data: GJC TSP DLC. Contributed reagents/materials/analysis tools: HLE. Wrote the paper: JGC TSP.

References

1. Howlader NA, Krapcho M, Neyman N, Aminou R, Waldron W, et al., eds. (2011) SEER Cancer Statistics Review, 1975–2008. Bethesda, MD: National Cancer Institute.
2. Farag SS, Archer KJ, Mrozek K, Ruppert AS, Carroll AJ, et al. (2006) Pretreatment cytogenetics add to other prognostic factors predicting complete remission and long-term outcome in patients 60 years of age or older with acute myeloid leukemia: results from Cancer and Leukemia Group B 8461. Blood 108: 63–73.
3. Dohner H, Estey EH, Amadori S, Appelbaum FR, Buchner T, et al. (2010) Diagnosis and management of acute myeloid leukemia in adults: recommendations from an international expert panel, on behalf of the European LeukemiaNet. Blood 115: 453–474.
4. Rollig C, Thiede C, Gramatzki M, Aulitzky W, Bodenstein H, et al. (2010) A novel prognostic model in elderly patients with acute myeloid leukemia: results of 909 patients entered into the prospective AML96 trial. Blood 116: 971–978.
5. Alibhai SM, Leach M, Minden MD, Brandwein J (2009) Outcomes and quality of care in acute myeloid leukemia over 40 years. Cancer 115: 2903–2911.
6. Estey E, Dohner H (2006) Acute myeloid leukaemia. Lancet 368: 1894–1907.
7. Longo DL (2012) Harrison's principles of internal medicine. New York: McGraw-Hill.
8. Kantarjian HM, Keating MJ, Walters RS, McCredie KB, Freireich EJ (1988) The characteristics and outcome of patients with late relapse acute myelogenous leukemia. J Clin Oncol 6: 232–238.
9. Ferrara F, Palmieri S, Mele G (2004) Prognostic factors and therapeutic options for relapsed or refractory acute myeloid leukemia. Haematologica 89: 998–1008.
10. Gilliland DG, Jordan CT, Felix CA (2004) The molecular basis of leukemia. Hematology Am Soc Hematol Educ Program: 80–97.
11. Burnett AK, Milligan D, Prentice AG, Goldstone AH, McMullin MF, et al. (2007) A comparison of low-dose cytarabine and hydroxyurea with or without all-trans retinoic acid for acute myeloid leukemia and high-risk myelodysplastic syndrome in patients not considered fit for intensive treatment. Cancer 109: 1114–1124.
12. Aimiuwu J, Wang H, Chen P, Xie Z, Wang J, et al. (2012) RNA-dependent inhibition of ribonucleotide reductase is a major pathway for 5-azacytidine activity in acute myeloid leukemia. Blood 119: 5229–5238.
13. Klisovic RB, Blum W, Wei X, Liu S, Liu Z, et al. (2008) Phase I study of GTI-2040, an antisense to ribonucleotide reductase, in combination with high-dose cytarabine in patients with acute myeloid leukemia. Clin Cancer Res 14: 3889–3895.
14. Cory JG, Cory AH (1989) Inhibitors of ribonucleoside diphosphate reductase activity. New York: Pergamon Press. ix, 273 p. p.
15. Mayhew CN, Mampuru LJ, Chendil D, Ahmed MM, Phillips JD, et al. (2002) Suppression of retrovirus-induced immunodeficiency disease (murine AIDS) by trimidox and didox: novel ribonucleotide reductase inhibitors with less bone marrow toxicity than hydroxyurea. Antiviral Res 56: 167–181.
16. Kaul DK, Kollander R, Mahaseth H, Liu XD, Solovey A, et al. (2006) Robust vascular protective effect of hydroxamic acid derivatives in a sickle mouse model of inflammation. Microcirculation 13: 489–497.
17. Gallaugher LD, Henry JC, Kearns PN, Elford HL, Bergdall VK, et al. (2009) Ribonucleotide reductase inhibitors reduce atherosclerosis in a double-injury rabbit model. Comp Med 59: 567–572.
18. Veale D, Carmichael J, Cantwell BM, Elford HL, Blackie R, et al. (1988) A phase 1 and pharmacokinetic study of didox: a ribonucleotide reductase inhibitor. Br J Cancer 58: 70–72.
19. Grusch M, Fritzer-Szekeres M, Fuhrmann G, Rosenberger G, Luxbacher C, et al. (2001) Activation of caspases and induction of apoptosis by novel ribonucleotide reductase inhibitors amidox and didox. Exp Hematol 29: 623–632.

20. Zuber J, Radtke I, Pardee TS, Zhao Z, Rappaport AR, et al. (2009) Mouse models of human AML accurately predict chemotherapy response. Genes Dev 23: 877–889.
21. Shankar DB, Li J, Tapang P, Owen McCall J, Pease LJ, et al. (2007) ABT-869, a multitargeted receptor tyrosine kinase inhibitor: inhibition of FLT3 phosphorylation and signaling in acute myeloid leukemia. Blood 109: 3400–3408.
22. Raje N, Kumar S, Hideshima T, Ishitsuka K, Yasui H, et al. (2006) Didox, a ribonucleotide reductase inhibitor, induces apoptosis and inhibits DNA repair in multiple myeloma cells. Br J Haematol 135: 52–61.
23. Nakano Y, Naoe T, Kiyoi H, Kitamura K, Minami S, et al. (2000) Prognostic value of p53 gene mutations and the product expression in de novo acute myeloid leukemia. Eur J Haematol 65: 23–31.
24. Wattel E, Preudhomme C, Hecquet B, Vanrumbeke M, Quesnel B, et al. (1994) p53 mutations are associated with resistance to chemotherapy and short survival in hematologic malignancies. Blood 84: 3148–3157.
25. Pardee TS (2012) Overexpression of MN1 confers resistance to chemotherapy, accelerates leukemia onset, and suppresses p53 and Bim induction. PLOS One 7: e43185.
26. Heuser M, Beutel G, Krauter J, Dohner K, von Neuhoff N, et al. (2006) High meningioma 1 (MN1) expression as a predictor for poor outcome in acute myeloid leukemia with normal cytogenetics. Blood 108: 3898–3905.
27. Elford HL, Wampler GL, van't Riet B (1979) New ribonucleotide reductase inhibitors with antineoplastic activity. Cancer Res 39: 844–851.
28. Wang LM, Lu FF, Zhang SY, Yao RY, Xing XM, et al. (2012) Overexpression of catalytic subunit M2 in patients with ovarian cancer. Chin Med J (Engl) 125: 2151–2156.
29. Matsusaka S, Yamasaki H, Fukushima M, Wakabayashi I (2007) Upregulation of enzymes metabolizing 5-fluorouracil in colorectal cancer. Chemotherapy 53: 36–41.
30. Okamura H, Kamei T, Sakuma N, Hanai N, Ishihara T (2003) Ribonucleotide reductase immunoreactivity in adenocarcinoma cells and malignant or reactive mesothelial cells in serous effusions. Acta Cytol 47: 209–215.
31. Inayat MS, El-Amouri IS, Bani-Ahmad M, Elford HL, Gallicchio VS, et al. (2010) Inhibition of allogeneic inflammatory responses by the Ribonucleotide Reductase Inhibitors, Didox and Trimidox. Journal of Inflammation-London 7.
32. Horvath Z, Hochtl T, Bauer W, Fritzer-Szekeres M, Elford HL, et al. (2004) Synergistic cytotoxicity of the ribonucleotide reductase inhibitor didox (3,4-dihydroxy-benzohydroxamic acid) and the alkylating agent carmustine (BCNU) in 9L rat gliosarcoma cells and DAOY human medulloblastoma cells. Cancer Chemother Pharmacol 54: 139–145.
33. Mathews CK (2006) DNA precursor metabolism and genomic stability. FASEB J 20: 1300–1314.
34. Rosen DB, Putta S, Covey T, Huang YW, Nolan GP, et al. (2010) Distinct patterns of DNA damage response and apoptosis correlate with Jak/Stat and PI3kinase response profiles in human acute myelogenous leukemia. PLOS One 5: e12405.
35. Garrido SM, Appelbaum FR, Willman CL, Banker DE (2001) Acute myeloid leukemia cells are protected from spontaneous and drug-induced apoptosis by direct contact with a human bone marrow stromal cell line (HS-5). Exp Hematol 29: 448–457.
36. Macanas-Pirard P, Leisewitz A, Broekhuizen R, Cautivo K, Barriga FM, et al. (2012) Bone marrow stromal cells modulate mouse ENT1 activity and protect leukemia cells from cytarabine induced apoptosis. PLOS One 7: e37203.
37. Garrido SM, Appelbaum FR, Willman CL, Banker DE (2001) Acute myeloid leukemia cells are protected from spontaneous and drug-induced apoptosis by direct contact with a human bone marrow stromal cell line (HS-5). Experimental Hematology 29: 448–457.
38. Mayhew CN, Phillips JD, Greenberg RN, Birch NJ, Elford HL, et al. (1999) In vivo and in vitro comparison of the short-term hematopoietic toxicity between

hydroxyurea and trimidox or didox, novel ribonucleotide reductase inhibitors with potential anti-HIV-1 activity. Stem Cells 17: 345–356.

39. Takeda E, Weber G (1981) Role of Ribonucleotide Reductase in Expression of the Neoplastic Program. Life Sciences 28: 1007–1014.

40. Benhar M, Dalyot I, Engelberg D, Levitzki A (2001) Enhanced ROS production in oncogenically transformed cells potentiates c-Jun N-terminal kinase and p38 mitogen-activated protein kinase activation and sensitization to genotoxic stress. Molecular and Cellular Biology 21: 6913–6926.

20

Assessment of Toxic Effects of the Methanol Extract of *Citrus macroptera* Montr. Fruit via Biochemical and Hematological Evaluation in Female Sprague-Dawley Rats

Nizam Uddin*, Md. Rakib Hasan, Md. Mahadi Hasan, Md. Monir Hossain, Md. Robiul Alam, Mohammad Raquibul Hasan, A. F. M. Mahmudul Islam, Tasmina Rahman, Md. Sohel Rana

Department of Pharmacy, Jahangirnagar University, Savar, Dhaka, 1342, Bangladesh

Abstract

Citrus macroptera Montr. (*C. macroptera*) is locally known as Satkara. The fruit of this plant is used as appetite stimulant and in the treatment of fever. This study therefore aimed to evaluate the toxic effects of the fruit extract using some biochemical and hematological parameters in rat model. The effects of methanol extract of *Citrus macroptera* Montr. fruit administered at 250, 500 and 1000 mg/kg body weight were investigated on hematological and biochemical parameters in Sprague-Dawley female rats. Moreover, histopathological study was performed to observe the presence of pathological lesions in primary body organs. The extract presented no significant effect on body weight, percent water content, relative organ weight and hematological parameters in rat. Significant decrease from control group was observed in the levels of triglyceride, total cholesterol, low density lipoprotein and very low density lipoprotein; thus leading to significant decrease of cardiac risk ratio, castelli's risk index-2, atherogenic coefficient and atherogenic index of plasma at all doses. 500 mg/kg dose significantly decreased alkaline phosphatase ($P<0.05$), 1000 mg/kg dose significantly increased high density lipoprotein cholesterol ($P<0.05$) and 250 mg/kg dose significantly decreased the level of glycated hemoglobin ($P<0.05$) from the control group. There were no significant alterations observed with other serum biochemical parameters. Histopathological study confirmed the absence of inflammatory and necrotic features in the primary body organs. Study results indicate that methanolic fruit extract is unlikely to have significant toxicity. Moreover, these findings justified the cardio-protective, moderate hepato-protective and glucose controlling activities of the fruit extract.

Editor: Michael Bader, Max-Delbrück Center for Molecular Medicine (MDC), Germany

Funding: This study was supported with funding from Jahangirnagar University Annual Research Grant (Grant no: JU-ARG-2012-005). The funder had no role in study design, data collection and analysis, decision to publish, or preparation of the manuscript.

Competing Interests: The authors have declared that no competing interests exist.

* Email: sami.pharm22@gmail.com

Introduction

Medicinal plants were and are still one of the major sources of modern medicine. Interest in medicinal plant's pharmacognosy has increased due to using trend of phytotherapy as alternative medicine [1,2]. Plants produce bioactive compounds that act as defense mechanism against predators and at the same time may be toxic in nature for our health. With the increased interest in the pharmacological activities of the medicinal plants, there is a surge for thorough scientific investigations of these medicinal plants for efficacy and potential toxicity. Proper scientific evidence is necessary to establish the use of plants for medicinal purposes as safe, non-toxic and pharmacologically active.

Citrus macroptera Montr., a semi wild species of citrus genus, is known as 'Satkara' in Bangladesh. It may be mentioned here that the English meaning of Satkara is 'Wild orange'. The maximum height of the tree of this fruit is 5 meter. The diameter of the fruit is 6–7 cm. The fruit becomes yellow when it ripens and its rind is

thick. As the pulp of this fruit is somewhat dry, it does not have enough juice, which is very sour and a bit bitter [3]. Chowdhury et al. (2008) reported the antioxidant activities of crude extracts of the stem bark of ***Citrus macroptera*** **and isolated** lupeol and stigmasterol [4]. Waikedre et al. (2010) reported the anti-microbial activity of essential oil of ***Citrus macroptera*** **a**gainst five bacteria and five fungi strains. Besides, the author found the presence of beta-pinene as major component [5]. Rana et al. (2012) reported that essential oils obtained by hydro-distillation from the fresh peels of *Citrus macroptera* contained limonene, beta-caryophyllene and geranial as main compounds [6]. Gaillard et al. (1995) isolated edulinine, ribalinine and isoplatydesmine and five aromatic compounds [7]. The people of Bangladesh eat this fruit as a vegetable. The fruit is used as ingredient in cooking different kinds of meat and chicken. Nowadays many Bangladeshi and Indian restaurants offer meat and chicken curries cooked with Satkara. Traditionally, this fruit is used as appetite stimulant and in treatment of fever [8]. In spite of the diverse uses of this fruit, there seems to be a dearth of information about the toxicity of this fruit. Therefore, we have designed our study protocol to evaluate the possible toxicity of the methanolic fruit extract via biochemical and hematological assessment as well as histopathological study in rat model. In addition, the results of the study can provide researchers with the safe levels of the doses of methanolic fruit extract. In this study we used methanol solvent for extraction because this solvent can dissolve various polar bioactive compounds as well as lipophilic compounds. Moreover, it is easy to evaporate this solvent and we get maximum bioactive compounds of the extract by minimizing the loss of compounds due to excessive heat [9].

Materials and Methods

Chemicals and reagents

Methanol was bought from SIGMA (Sigma-Aldrich, St Louis, USA). Ketamine inj. was obtained from ACI Pharmaceuticals Ltd., Bangladesh. All clinical diagnostic kits were purchased from Human Laboratories, Germany. All other chemicals and reagents used were of analytical grade.

Plant material

Fruits of *Citrus macroptera* were collected from Sylhet, Bangladesh and authenticated by an expert Taxonomist. A voucher specimen (Acc. No. 38619) was deposited in Bangladesh National Herbarium for future reference. No field studies were carried out in this study as the fruits were purchased from some local markets of Sylhet, Bangladesh. No specific permissions were required.

Preparation of plant extract

At first peels were removed. Then the pulp were cut into pieces and then dried in a hot air oven (Size 1, Gallen kamp) at reduced temperature (not more than 50°C) to make suitable for extraction process. Then the dried fruit materials (500 gm) were treated with sufficient amount of pure methanol (1000 ml) for one week at room temperature with occasional shaking (solvent to fruit ratio was 2:1). The extract was filtered through a cotton plug followed by Whatman No. 1 filter paper. The filtrate was then evaporated under reduced pressure to give a dark green viscous mass and stored at 4°C until it was used. The yield value for the methanol extract was 29.02%.

Animals and experimental set-up

Sprague-Dawley female rats weighing between 170–230 g were collected from Pharmacology Laboratory, Department of Pharmacy, Jahangirnagar University and were acclimatized to normal laboratory conditions for one week prior to study and were assessed to pellet diet and water *ad libitum*. Temperature of facility was (22 ± 3) °C and light/darkness alternated 12 h apart. The research activities were conducted in accordance with the internationally accepted principles of the US guidelines (NIH publication #85-23, revised in 1985) and following the approval by the Biosafety, Biosecurity and Ethical Committee [Approval Number: BBECJU/N2013(21)] of Faculty of Biological Sciences of Jahangirnagar University, Savar, Dhaka, Bangladesh. The study was carried out in the Department of Pharmacy, Jahangirnagar University.

Experimental procedure

The animals were assigned to four groups of five animals each. Group-1 was treated as control and group-2, 3 and 4 were treated with 250 mg/kg, 500 mg/kg and 1000 mg/kg doses of methanol

extract of *C. macroptera* fruit respectively for 21 days. Different doses of the extract of *C. macroptera* were administered orally by stomach tube. Rats were weighed weekly and observed for behavioral changes, feeding and drinking habits, and general morphological changes. At the end of the 21-day treatment period, after 18 hours fasting, rats from each group were anaesthetized by administration (i.p) of ketamine (500 mg/kg body weight) [10]. Blood samples were collected from post vena cava of rats into EDTA (Ethylene diamine tetra acetic acid) sample tubes for hematological analysis and plain sample tubes for serum generation for biochemical analysis. Serum was obtained after allowing blood to coagulate for 30 minutes and centrifuged at 4000 g for 10 min using bench top centrifuge (MSE Minor, England). The supernatant serum samples were collected using dry Pasteur pipette and stored in the refrigerator for further analysis. All analyses were completed within 24 hours of sample collection [11].

Hematological analysis

Blood samples were analyzed using established procedures and automated Sysmex KX-21 hematology analyzer. Parameters that were recorded included Hemoglobin (Hb), Red blood cells (RBC), White blood cells (WBC), Platelets, Erythrocyte Sedimentation Rate (ESR), Packed cell Volume (PCV), Mean corpuscular volume (MCV), Mean corpuscular hemoglobin (MCH), Mean corpuscular hemoglobin concentration (MCHC), Pro-calcitonin (PCT), Packed cell volume (PCV), Red cell distribution width - standard deviation (RDW –SD), Red cell distribution width - coefficient of variation (RDW-CV), Platelet larger cell ratio (P-LCR), Platelet distribution width (PDW), Mean platelet volume (MPV), Neutrophils, Basophils, Lymphocytes, Monocytes and Eosinophils.

Biochemical analysis

Serum samples were analyzed for urea, albumin, total protein, total cholesterol (TC), high density lipoprotein (HDL) cholesterol, triglycerides (TG), uric acid, alkaline phosphatase (ALP), aspartate transaminase (AST) and alanine transaminase (ALT) using Human commercial kits and Humalyzer 3500. Moreover, glycated hemoglobin (HbA1c) test was performed to find out the amount of glycated hemoglobin (HbA1c) using Bio Rad D-10 analyzer. Very low density lipoprotein (VLDL) cholesterol and Low density lipoprotein (LDL) cholesterol concentrations were calculated using the following Friedewald equations [12]:

i. LDL cholesterol (mg/dL) =

(Total cholesterol − HDL cholesterol − Triglyceride / 5)

ii. VLDL cholesterol (mg/dL) = Triglyceride / 5.

The atherogenic indices were calculated as follows:

Cardiac Risk Ratio (CRR) = TC/HDL − C [13]
Atherogenic Coefficient (AC) = (TC − HDL − C)/HDL − C [14]
Atherogenic Index of Plasma (AIP) = log (TG/HDL − C) [15]
Castelli's Risk Index − 2 (CRI − 2) = LDL − C/HDL − C [16]

Histopathology

After the collection of blood, all the animals were euthanized for gross pathological examinations of the major organs. The organs such as: hearts, kidneys, lungs, livers, spleens, fallopian tubes, thymuses and ovaries were collected from all the animals for histopathology. The weights of the organs were determined. The relative organ weights were calculated by dividing the individual weight of each organ with the final body weight of each rat. The percent water content was determined by subtracting the dry weight of each organ from the respective weight of each wet organ. Then it was planned to perform histo-pathological examination for the control and high dose group initially. If any histopatholgical findings were observed with high dose group, the mid and low dose groups were to be studied. The selected organs were fixed in 10% neutral buffered formalin, trimmed and a 4–5 μm thickness of tissue sections were stained with hematoxylin and eosin for histopathological investigation using established protocols [17]. The photomicrographs were taken with Olympus DP 72 microscope.

Data analysis

Data were expressed as mean ± SEM (Standard Error of Mean). Repeated measures ANOVA and One-way ANOVA followed by Dunnett's multiple comparison was performed to analyze data sets. $P < 0.05$ was considered significant. Statistical programs used were SPSS (version 16, IBM software Inc, USA) and GRAPHPAD PRISM (version 6.02; GraphPad Software Inc., San Diego, CA, USA).

Result

Effect of the extract on the body weight, % water content and relative organ weight of rats

There were no signs and symptoms of toxicity and death recorded after three week treatment period. From the figure 1 it is ascertained that body weight did not gradually increase at all doses in comparison with control. There was no significant deviation in weight gain from control at any doses in this three- week treatment period. Table-1 and 2 present effects of different doses of methanol

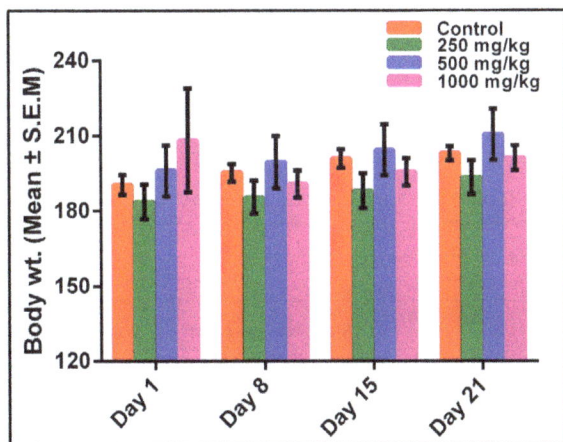

Figure 1. Effect of methanol extract of *C. macroptera* fruit on body weights (g) of Sprague-Dawley female rats in 21 days treatment period. RM ANOVA with Dunnett's multiple comparison was performed to analyze this weight variation in different days. No significant different was found when compared to control group. Time effect was found not significant ($P > 0.05$).

extract on % water content and relative weight of different body organs of rats. No significant difference was noticed in % water content and relative organ weight of primary body organs (Table 1 and 2).

Effect of extract on the hematological parameters

The effects of different doses of the extract on the hematological parameters are tabulated in table 3. No significant difference was found with all hematological parameters.

Effect of extract on the biochemical parameters

Treatment with different doses of methanol extract did not have any significant adverse effect on hepatic biomarker enzymes ALT and AST while 500 mg/kg dose significantly decreased the activity of ALP enzyme. Moreover, three different doses of the extract did not alter the level of total protein and albumin which are major tests to assess liver damage (Table 4). Besides, methanol extract significantly reduced the level of LDL, VLDL, TG, TC, CRR, CRI-2, AC and AIP which are the imperative assays for cardiovascular diseases. Furthermore, 1000 mg/kg dose significantly ($P < 0.05$) increased the level of HDL. The determination of uric acid and urea is the biomarker of the normal function of kidney. Insignificant ($P > 0.05$) changes were found in the level of these two renal biomarkers. Moreover, 250 mg/kg dose significantly reduced HbA1c ($P < 0.05$) whereas in high doses the fruit extract failed to show positive response (Table 4).

Histopathological observations

There were no overt pathological lesions observed both at high and low doses of the methanol extract in histopathological study. In the figure 2 photomicrograph of histopathological study of 1000 mg/kg dose and control were presented. No abnormal signs of toxicity were found in the high dose. Histopathological observations confirmed the normal cellular architecture of the tested organs.

Discussion

Daily oral doses of the methanol extract up to 1000 mg/kg did not cause any physical abnormalities or death after three week treatment period. In a previous study Uddin et al (2014) performed the acute toxicity of this fruit extract. Administration of doses up to 4000 mg/kg (the highest dose) produced no mortality which was accompanied by normal physical activity of the tested animals [18]. This study strengthens the safety of the extract.

The body of a human being manages a large number of complicated interactions with a view to maintaining balance within a usual range. These interactions make compensatory changes easier which support normal physical and psychological functions. This process is indispensable to the survival of humans and other species. This process is essential to the survival of the person and to our species [19]. 75% weight of the body of an infant and 55% weight of the body of an elderly person are water. It is vital for maintaining cellular homeostasis. Dehydration can cause several physiological disorders [20]. In our study we found no significant alteration in % water content of primary organs from control group which buttresses the claim that the fruit extract does not have toxic effects on normal fluid content and role of body fluid in maintaining homeostasis system. Alteration in the normal weight of the body indicates impairment of normal function of different body organs. Methanol extract did not show any significant alteration on the body weight of the rats compared to control group in 3-week treatment period (Figure 1). It can be

Table 1. % Water content of different organs treated with different doses of methanol extract of *C. macroptera* fruit.

Organ	Control	250 mg/kg	500 mg/kg	1000 mg/kg
Heart	34.04±1.867	36.121±1.523	34.973±3.011	36.262±2.262
Kidney	47.008±1.458	48.565±1.043	48.403±1.011	48.276±2.007
Lung	42.271±4.066	51.637±0.481	49.128±2.862	42.75±4.877
Liver	58.263±1.185	62.147±1.817	60.882±1.688	61.082±2.068
Spleen	38.909±0.820	43.386±2.043	34.971±1.291	34.202±0.887

Values are presented as mean±S.E.M (n = 5). No significant result was found when compared against control. One way ANOVA followed by Dunnett's multiple comparison was performed to analyze this data set.

suggested that this extract has no negative impact on the body weight of rats treated with three different doses. Relative organ weight may serve as indication of pathological and physiological status in man and animals. Toxic substances induce abnormal metabolic reactions that affect primary organs such as heart, liver, spleen, kidney and lung [21]. Our findings suggest that three doses of the methanol extract of fruit are non-toxic on all vital organs tested in this study. Furthermore, three doses of the fruit extract showed no toxicity on reproductive organs such as fallopian tube and ovary. Therefore, this fruit extract is considered safe for maintaining the normal function of the organs.

Hematological assessment is useful to determine the extent of toxic effects of plant extracts on the blood constituents of an animal [22]. The analysis of blood parameters is closely related to risk evaluation because when tests involve rodents, the hematological system has a higher predictive value of any abnormal toxicity signs and symbols in humans [23]. We found no noticeable hemolytic changes on RBC, Hb, PCV, MCH, MCV, MCHC, RDW-SD and RDW-CV. These findings exclude the possibility of occurrence of anemic condition and other erythrocyte cells related disorders (thalassemia, polycythemia, liver disease, hypothyroidism etc.). Increase in the production of WBC and it's differentials is generally considered to be a marker of stress and a defence mechanism triggered by immune system against various inflammatory conditions (Polymyalgia rheumatica, bacterial infections, hemorrhage, leukemia etc.). The non-significant changes in the level of WBC and differentials including platelet and its indices, neutrophils, lymphocytes, monocytes and eosinophils observed in this study at three doses level suggest the non-toxicity of the fruit extract. Platelet indices are important biomarkers for the early diagnosis of thromboembolic diseases.

MPV and PDW are simple platelet indices which are increased during platelet activation [24]. Besides, P-LCR is also considered as an indicator of risk factor associated with thromboembolic ischemic events [25]. A high ESR and PCT indicates that inflammation (Bacterial infections, sepsis, arthritis, etc.) occurs somewhere in the body. Therefore, non-significant impact on the ESR, PCT, WBC and differential counts posits that the fruit extract has no contribution to the induction of infectious diseases and thromboembolic disorders. Moreover, it is safe for hematopoietic system of the body.

Urea and uric acid are the biomarkers of kidney function and retention of these products in the body indicates renal damage [26–28]. In this present study, there was no significant increase ($P>0.05$) in the amount of urea and uric acid when compared with the control group. Hence this fruit extract is considered safe and has no destructive effect on normal kidney functions. Elevation in the level of serum transaminase enzymes activities is highly indicative of hepatic impairment in animals [29]. The insignificant change in plasma ALT activity with AST at the doses of 250, 500 and 1000 mg/kg indicates that the extract caused no changes in the liver. ALT is a kind of cytoplasmic enzyme that increases in plasma which is an indication of injuries caused by toxic agents to the liver. Liver injury is characterized by predominant elevation of the ALT and increased activity of mitochondrial enzyme AST in plasma reflects severe tissue injuries [30]. However, 500 mg/kg dose significantly ($P<0.05$) reduced ALP level (table 4) which may account for protective effect on liver disorders. But in 1000 mg/kg the extract did not present significant result. It would indicate selective activity in the median dose and non-selective activity in the highest dose. That is why further research work should be conducted to verify this reason.

Table 2. Relative Organ weight profile of rats treated with different doses of methanol extract of *C. macroptera*.

Organ	Control	250 mg/kg	500 mg/kg	1000 mg/kg
Heart	0.2245±0.002	0.2428±0.007	0.227±0.003	0.243±0.009
Kidney	0.2246±0.004	0.2484±0.016	0.231±0.009	0.215±0.020
Lung	0.5019±0.067	0.457±0.009	0.4±0.024	0.481±0.041
Liver	2.025±0.100	2.387±0.121	2.04±0.08	2.3±0.078
Spleen	0.2749±0.008	0.313±0.005	0.314±0.02	0.304±0.013
Ovary	0.0235±0.002	0.026±0.001	0.024±0.001	0.025±0.001
Fallopian tube	0.2122±0.016	0.2127±0.016	0.204±0.03	0.2±0.026
Thymus	0.127±0.007	0.1078±0.011	0.120±0.004	0.110±0.004

Values are presented as mean±S.E.M (n = 5). No significant result was found when compared against control. One way ANOVA followed by Dunnett's multiple comparison was performed to analyze this data set.

Table 3. Effect of different doses of methanol extract of *C. macroptera* fruit on the hematological parameters of rats.

Hematological parameters	Control	250 mg/kg	500 mg/kg	1000 mg/kg
ESR(mm)	5.4±0.748	8±0.836	5.2±1.012	6.6±1.077
RBC($\times 10^{12}$/L)	7.016±0.192	6.532±0.245	7.402±0.241	7.388±0.088
WBC ($\times 10^9$/L	5.32±0.5	4.95±0.76	4.944±0.421	3.538±0.530
PLT($\times 10^9$/L)	417.2±43.787	412.8±11.425	468.2±51.361	417±40.707
Hb(g/dl)	13.4±0.448	14.125±0.125	13.74±0.430	14.04±0.252
HCT/PCV(%)	48.04±1.403	47.56±1.307	47.18±1.383	47.78±1.012
MCV(fL)	67.84±1.525	73.62±3.103	63.76±0.78	64.66±0.951
MCHC (g/dl)	27.86±0.235	25.72±1.437	29.1±0.23	29.42±0.284
MCH (pg)	19.12±0.385	18.86±1.084	18.58±0.162	19.02±0.172
RDW-SD (fL)	43.72±1.184	49.275±4.636	38.76±0.62	40.52±1.66
RDW-CV (%)	19.66±0.250	21.5±1.662	19.36±0.097	19.46±0.764
PDW (μm)	13.56±0.892	14.55±1.12	12.44±0.242	13.04±0.654
MPV (fL)	10.3±0.3	11.175±0.45	10.22±0.156	10.24±0.273
P-LCR	28.62±2.383	34.275±3.456	27.92±1.151	28.46±1.92
PCT (μg/L)	0.432±0.050	0.67±0.106	0.506±0.064	0.428±0.042
N (%)	39.48±4.233	39.92±3.222	34.92±0.421	31.725±3.164
L (%)	57.84±4.212	53.84±4.84	58.16±2.13	60.06±3.504
M (%)	1.66±0.13	4.86±2.345	2.94±0.271	2.94±0.842
E (%)	1.02±0.351	1.38±0.871	1.32±0.554	3.675±1.575
N/L	0.7218±0.137	0.7892±0.134	0.603±0.017	0.416±0.061

Here N = Neutrophils, L = Lymphocyte, M = Monocyte, E = Eosinophils, PLT = Platelet and N/L = Neutrophil/Lymphocyte ratio. Values are presented as mean±S.E.M (n = 5). No significant result was found when compared against control. One way ANOVA followed by Dunnett's multiple comparison was performed to analyze this data set.

Table 4. Effect of different doses of methanol extract of *C. macroptera* fruit on biochemical safety parameters in rats.

Biochemical parameters	Control	250 mg/kg	500 mg/kg	1000 mg/kg
TP(g/dl)	5.096±0.077	4.544±0.214	5.194±0.156	5.188±0.21
ALB(g/dl)	3.82±0.216	3.4±0.124	3.5234±0.090	3.7142±0.186
GLB(g/dl)	1.276±0.251	1.1442±0.27	1.671±.150	1.4744±0.144
A/G	3.620±0.907	3.9837±1.20	2.1732±0.181	2.6292±0.308
TG (mg/dl)	67.222±1.195	46.854±2.928*	36.84±1.501*	34.22±4.94*
TC (mg/dl)	75.946±1.964	69.326±0.267*	68.608±0.515*	66.102±0.896*
HDL (mg/dl)	56.9498±1.802	59.674±0.6	60.609±0.34	62.17±0.636*
LDL (mg/dl)	5.5518±1.097	0.2812±0.134*	0.631±0.301*	0.388±0.061*
VLDL (mg/dl)	13.4444±0.241	9.3708±0.585*	7.368±0.3*	6.844±0.987*
ALT(IU/L)	49.136±1.634	45.95±0.735	49.48±1.43	46.42±0.852
AST(IU/L)	94.54±1.740	90.8±1.870	90.058±0.48	90.248±0.472
ALP(IU/L)	361.62±7.891	353.86±15.523	314.63±2.826*	363.5±4.193
U (mg/dl)	34.684±2.316	34.716±1.258	38.528±2.647	39.83±2.342
UA (mg/dl)	2.0824±0.283	3.0162±0.331	1.7098±0.236	1.4068±0.143
HbA1c (%)	2.74±0.16	1.92±0.115*	2.92±0.243	2.72±0.213
CRR	1.3353±0.022	1.1622±0.011*	1.132±0.008*	1.0638±0.02*
CRI-2	0.097±0.012	0.004±0.002*	0.010±0.005*	0.006±0.001*
AC	0.3353±0.022	0.1622±0.011*	0.132±0.007*	0.0638±0.02*
AIP	1.042±0.012	0.941±0.017*	0.878±0.009*	0.845±0.033*

TP = Total protein, ALB = Albumin, GLB = Globulin, U = Urea and UA = Uric Acid. Values are presented as mean±S.E.M (n = 5). One way ANOVA followed by Dunnett's multiple comparison was performed to analyze this data set. * $P<0.05$ when compared against control.

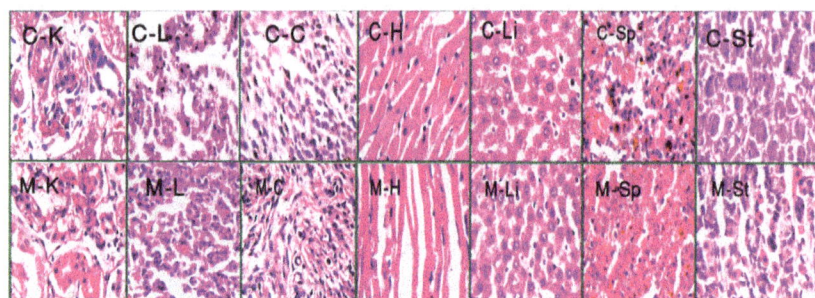

Figure 2. Histopathological photomicrographs of control group and 1000 mg/kg dose group of *C. macroptera* **(×100 magnification).** No presence of discernible lesions including inflammation and necrosis were observed. Here, C-K= Control-Kidney, C-L= Control-Lung, C-C= Control-Cecum, C-H= Control-Heart, C-Li= Control-Liver, C-Sp= Control-Spleen, C-St= Control-Stomach, M-K=1000 mg/kg dose-Kidney, M-L=1000 mg/kg dose-Lung, M-C=1000 mg/kg dose-Cecum, M-H=1000 mg/kg dose-Heart, M-Li=1000 mg/kg dose-Liver, M-Sp=1000 mg/kg dose-Spleen and M-St=1000 mg/kg dose-Stomach.

The level of plasma albumin decreases in response to inflammation [31]. Recent studies have shown that not only albumin concentration but also albumin function are reduced in liver disorders such as liver cirrhosis [32]. The non-significant variation in the level of TP, albumin, globulin and albumin-globulin ratio provides logistic support behind the non-toxic effect of this fruit extract on liver and no link with liver dysfunction.

A high plasma triglyceride level is both an independent and synergistic risk factor for cardiovascular diseases [33] and is often related to hypertension [34], obesity and diabetes mellitus [35]. Elevated total cholesterol level is a familiar and well-known risk factor for developing atherosclerosis and other cardiovascular diseases [36]. High levels of plasma LDL and VLDL cholesterol are responsible for cardiovascular diseases [37] which are accompanied with hypertension and obesity [38]. In this study a very significant decrease was observed in the levels of TC, TG, LDL and VLDL cholesterol which strengthen the lipid lowering activity and represents cardio-protective effect of the fruit extract. Low plasma HDL cholesterol is also a major predictor for cardiovascular diseases [37]. High plasma HDL cholesterol exerts a protective effect by enhancing reverse cholesterol transport through scavenging excess cholesterol from peripheral tissues in our body. 1000 mg/kg dose exhibited very good activity ($P<0.05$) by increasing the level of HDL. This finding further gives strong support for cardio-protective effect of the extract. With these findings (discussed above) in hand we evaluated atherogenic indices which are powerful indicators of the risk of cardiovascular diseases. The higher the values of atherogenic indices the higher the risk of developing cardiovascular disease and vice versa [36]. Methanolic fruit extract reduced three atherogenic indices with significant value $P<0.05$. Moreover. three doses of the fruit extract significantly lowered the value of AIP ($P<0.05$). Hematological parameters MPV and P-LCR are also related to cardiovascular disorders. Higher levels of these parameters coupled with neutrophil/lymphocyte ratio can serve as indication of coronary heart disease [25,39,40]. In this study non-significant variation of these parameters from control group provides vital evidences in favor of reduced atherogenic indices and protective effect of the methanolic fruit extract against cardiovascular disorders. Moreover, at low dose fruit extract prevented significant increase in HbA1c in blood. In diabetic condition the level of HbA1c is enhanced due to the production of excessive glucose in blood which further react with blood hemoglobin and creates glycated hemoglobin [41]. Uddin et al (2014) found hypoglycemic activity of the same fruit extract via both *in-vivo* OGTT (Oral Glucose Tolerance Test) model and *in-vitro* α- amylase inhibitory assay, which further substantiated blood glucose level controlling activity [18]. In high doses we did not find any significant HbA1c reduction activity. This may have happened due to the loss of selective activity. That is why further study is required to find out the exact reason. Lipid metabolism abnormality in diabetes is characterized by increase in TC, TG, LDL cholesterol and fall in HDL cholesterol [34]. We recorded significant decrease in the serum levels of these biomarkers which is discussed previously. Moderate activity in decreasing glycated hemoglobin coupled with the reduction of lipid profile proved the efficacy of the fruit extract as moderate hypoglycemic agent and it can control blood glucose level.

Furthermore, up to 1000 mg/kg no discernible lesions including inflammation and necrosis were found. That is why it is logical to infer that methanol extract has no toxic effect on primary body organs when administered at 250, 500 and 1000 mg/kg doses for 3 weeks in rats. Uddin et al, (2014) detected the presence of saponins, steroids and terpenoids in the fruit extract. Therefore, these phytochemicals may exert the non-toxic effect as well as afore-mentioned therapeutic potentials [18].

Conclusions

In a nutshell, the non-toxic effect evaluated by biochemical and hematological assessment suggests a wide margin of safety for therapeutic doses. The extract has no significant toxic effect on biological parameters. Besides the medicinal uses, we recorded significant cardio-protective effect with moderate hepato-protective and hypoglycemic activities exerted by this fruit extract. These findings justify the therapeutic potential of the fruit. Further research projects should be launched to isolate and characterize active principles and elucidate molecular structures with precise pharmacology.

Acknowledgments

The authors are greatly thankful to Wazed Miah Science Research Center (WMSRC), Jahangirnagar University for taking photomicrographs of histopathological slides to complete this research work.

Author Contributions

Conceived and designed the experiments: NU M. Rakib Hasan. Performed the experiments: NU M. Rakib Hasan M. M. Hasan M. M. Hossain MRA M. Raquibul Hasan. Analyzed the data: NU M. Rakib Hasan. Contributed reagents/materials/analysis tools: TR MSR. Wrote the paper: NU MSR. Managed Literature search: AFMMI.

References

1. Gupta SS (1994) Propects and perpectives of normal plants products in medicine. Indian J Pharmacol 26: 1–12.
2. Das SS, Das S, Pal S, Mujib A, Dey S (1999) Biotechnology of medicinal plants-Recent advances and potential. UK 992 Publications: Hyderabad. pp.126–139.
3. Elevitch CR (2006) Traditional Trees of Pacific Islands: Their Culture, Environment, and Use. Hawaii: Permanent Agriculture Resources. pp.243–276.
4. Chowdhury SA, Sohrab MH, Datta BK, Hasan CM (2008) Chemical and Antioxidant Studies of *Citrus macroptera*. Bang J Sci Ind Res 43: 449–454.
5. Waikedre J, Dugay A, Barrachina I, Herrenknecht C, Cabalion P, et al. (2010) Chemical composition and antimicrobial activity of the essential oils from New Caledonian *Citrus macroptera* and *Citrus hystrix*. Chem Biodivers 7: 871–877.
6. Rana VS, Blazquez MA (2012) Compositions of the volatile oils of *Citrus macroptera* and *C. maxima*. Nat Prod Commun 7: 1371–1372.
7. Gaillard E, Muyard F, Bevalot F, Regnier A, Vaquette J (1995) [Rutacea from New Caledonia. Chemical composition of stem bark of *Citrus macroptera* Montr]. Ann Pharm Fr 53: 75–78.
8. Rahmatullah M, Afsana K, Morshed N, Prashanta KN, Sadar UK, et al. (2010) A Randomized Survey of Medicinal Plants used by Folk Medicinal Healers of Sylhet Division, Bangladesh. Adv in Nat App Sci 4: 52–62.
9. Jaroszynska J (2003) The Influence of Solvent Choice on the Recovery of Phytogenic Phenolic Compounds Extracted from Plant Material. Pol J Environ Stud 12: 481–484.
10. Ringer DH, Dabich L (1979) Hematology and clinical biochemistry. In: Baker HJ, Lindsey JR, Weisbroth SH, editors. The laboratory Rat, volume 1, Biology and diseases. San Diego: Academic Press. pp.105–121.
11. Wolford ST, Schroer RA, Gohs FX, Gallo PP, Brodeck M, et al. (1986) Reference range data base for serum chemistry and hematology values in laboratory animals. J Toxicol Environ Health 18: 161–188.
12. Friedewald WT, Levy RI, Fredrickson DS (1972) Estimation of the concentration of low-density lipoprotein cholesterol in plasma, without use of the preparative ultracentrifuge. Clin Chem 18: 499–502.
13. Martirosyan DM, Miroshnichenko LA, Kulakova SN, Pogojeva AV, Zoloedov VI (2007) Amaranth oil application for coronary heart disease and hypertension. Lipids Health Dis 6: 1.
14. Brehm A, Pfeiler G, Pacini G, Vierhapper H, Roden M (2004) Relationship between serum lipoprotein ratios and insulin resistance in obesity. Clin Chem 50: 2316–2322.
15. Dobiasova M (2004) Atherogenic index of plasma [log(triglycerides/HDL-cholesterol)]: theoretical and practical implications. Clin Chem 50: 1113–1115.
16. Castelli WP, Abbott RD, McNamara PM (1983) Summary estimates of cholesterol used to predict coronary heart disease. Circulation 67: 730–734.
17. Carleton H (1980) Carleton's Histological techniques. London: Oxford University Press.
18. Uddin N, Hasan MR, Hossain MM, Sarker A, Hasan AH, et al. (2014) *In vitro* alpha-amylase inhibitory activity and *in vivo* hypoglycemic effect of methanol extract of Citrus macroptera Montr. fruit. Asian Pac J Trop Biomed 4: 473–479.
19. Guyton CA (1986) Textbook of Medical Physiology. Philadelphia: W.B Saunders Company. pp.2–7.
20. Popkin BM, D'Anci KE, Rosenberg IH (2010) Water, hydration, and health. Nutr Rev 68: 439–458.
21. Dybing E, Doe J, Groten J, Kleiner J, O'Brien J, et al. (2002) Hazard characterisation of chemicals in food and diet. dose response, mechanisms and extrapolation issues. Food Chem Toxicol 40: 237–282.
22. Ashafa AOT, Yakubu MT, Grierson DS, Afolayan AJ (2009) Effects of aqueous leaf extract from the leaves of *Chrysocoma ciliate* L. on some biochemical parameters of Wistar rats. Afr J Biotechnol 8: 1425–1430.
23. Olson H, Betton G, Robinson D, Thomas K, Monro A, et al. (2000) Concordance of the toxicity of pharmaceuticals in humans and in animals. Regul Toxicol Pharmacol 32: 56–67.
24. Vagdatli E, Gounari E, Lazaridou E, Katsibourlia E, Tsikopoulou F, et al. (2010) Platelet distribution width: a simple, practical and specific marker of activation of coagulation. Hippokratia 14: 28–32.
25. Grotto HZ, Noronha JF (2004) Platelet larger cell ratio (P-LCR) in patients with dyslipidemia. Clin Lab Haematol 26: 347–349.
26. Newman DJ, Price C (1998) Renal function and nitrogen metabolites. In: Burtis CA, Ashwood ER, editors. Tietz Texbook of Clinical Chemistry. Philadelphia: W.B. Saunders; 1998. pp.1204–1270.
27. Odutola AA A, Co Zaria S (1992) Rapid Interpretation of Routine Clinical Laboratory Test. Nigeria: Asekome, S and Company, Zaria. pp.1–30.
28. Johnson RJ, Nakagawa T, Jalal D, Sanchez-Lozada LG, Kang DH, et al. (2013) Uric acid and chronic kidney disease: which is chasing which? Nephrol Dial Transplant 28: 2221–2228.
29. Tennant BC (1997) Hepatic function. In: Kaneko JJ, Harvey JW, Bruss ML, editors. Clinical Biochemistry of Domestic Animals. Singapore: Harcourt Brace and Company Asia PTE. Limited. pp.327–52.
30. Martins AC (2006) Clinical chemistry and metabolic medicine. UK: Edward Arnold Ltd. pp.7–15.
31. Ruot B, Breuille D, Rambourdin F, Bayle G, Capitan P, et al. (2000) Synthesis rate of plasma albumin is a good indicator of liver albumin synthesis in sepsis. Am J Physiol Endocrinol Metab 279: E244–251.
32. Garcia-Martinez R, Caraceni P, Bernardi M, Gines P, Arroyo V, et al. (2013) Albumin: pathophysiologic basis of its role in the treatment of cirrhosis and its complications. Hepatology 58: 1836–1846.
33. McBride P (2008) Triglycerides and risk for coronary artery disease. Curr Atheroscler Rep 10: 386–390.
34. Zicha J, Kunes J, Devynck MA (1999) Abnormalities of membrane function and lipid metabolism in hypertension: a review. Am J Hypertens 12: 315–331.
35. Shen GX (2007) Lipid disorders in diabetes mellitus and current management. Curr Pharm Anal 3: 17–24.
36. Ademuyiwa O, Ugbaja RN, Idumebor F, Adebawo O (2005) Plasma lipid profiles and risk of cardiovascular disease in occupational lead exposure in Abeokuta, Nigeria. Lipids Health Dis 4: 19.
37. Lichtenstein AH, Appel LJ, Brands M, Carnethon M, Daniels S, et al. (2006) Diet and lifestyle recommendations revision 2006: a scientific statement from the American Heart Association Nutrition Committee. Circulation 114: 82–96.
38. Shepherd J (1998) Identifying patients at risk for coronary heart disease: treatment implications. Eur Heart J 19: 1776–1783.
39. Ayhan S, Ozturk S, Erdem A, Ozlu MF, Memioglu T, et al. (2013) Hematological parameters and coronary collateral circulation in patients with stable coronary artery disease. Exp Clin Cardiol 18: e12–15.
40. Endler G, Klimesch A, Sunder-Plassmann H, Schillinger M, Exner M, et al. (2002) Mean platelet volume is an independent risk factor for myocardial infarction but not for coronary artery disease. Br J Haematol 117: 399–404.
41. Pari L, Saravanan R (2004) Antidiabetic effect of diasulin, a herbal drug, on blood glucose, plasma insulin and hepatic enzymes of glucose metabolism in hyperglycaemic rats. Diabetes Obes Metab 6: 286–292.

Permissions

The contributors of this book come from diverse backgrounds, making this book a truly international effort. This book will bring forth new frontiers with its revolutionizing research information and detailed analysis of the nascent developments around the world.

We would like to thank all the contributing authors for lending their expertise to make the book truly unique. They have played a crucial role in the development of this book. Without their invaluable contributions this book wouldn't have been possible. They have made vital efforts to compile up to date information on the varied aspects of this subject to make this book a valuable addition to the collection of many professionals and students.

This book was conceptualized with the vision of imparting up-to-date information and advanced data in this field. To ensure the same, a matchless editorial board was set up. Every individual on the board went through rigorous rounds of assessment to prove their worth. After which they invested a large part of their time researching and compiling the most relevant data for our readers.

The editorial board has been involved in producing this book since its inception. They have spent rigorous hours researching and exploring the diverse topics which have resulted in the successful publishing of this book. They have passed on their knowledge of decades through this book. To expedite this challenging task, the publisher supported the team at every step. A small team of assistant editors was also appointed to further simplify the editing procedure and attain best results for the readers.

Apart from the editorial board, the designing team has also invested a significant amount of their time in understanding the subject and creating the most relevant covers. They scrutinized every image to scout for the most suitable representation of the subject and create an appropriate cover for the book.

The publishing team has been an ardent support to the editorial, designing and production team. Their endless efforts to recruit the best for this project, has resulted in the accomplishment of this book. They are a veteran in the field of academics and their pool of knowledge is as vast as their experience in printing. Their expertise and guidance has proved useful at every step. Their uncompromising quality standards have made this book an exceptional effort. Their encouragement from time to time has been an inspiration for everyone.

The publisher and the editorial board hope that this book will prove to be a valuable piece of knowledge for researchers, students, practitioners and scholars across the globe.

List of Contributors

Keya Shah, Kelly Lien, Henry Lam and Yoo-Joung Ko
Sunnybrook Odette Cancer Centre, University of Toronto, Toronto, ON, Canada

Kelvin Chan
Sunnybrook Odette Cancer Centre, University of Toronto, Toronto, ON, Canada
Division of Biostatistics, Dalla Lana School of Public Health, University of Toronto, Toronto, ON, Canada

Doug Coyle
University of Ottawa, Ottawa, ON, Canada

Diana Mora-Obando, Julián Fernández, José María Gutiérrez and Bruno Lomonte
Instituto Clodomiro Picado, Facultad de Microbiología, Universidad de Costa Rica, San José, Costa Rica

Cesare Montecucco
Department of Biomedical Sciences, University of Padova, Padova, Italy

Irene Wuethrich, Janneke G. C. Peeters, Annet E. M. Blom, Christopher S. Theile, Zeyang Li, Eric Spooner, Hidde L. Ploegh and Carla P. Guimaraes
Whitehead Institute for Biomedical Research, Department of Biology, Massachusetts Institute of Technology, Cambridge, Massachusetts, United States of America

Szilamér Ferenczi and Krisztina J. Kovács
Institute of Experimental Medicine, Laboratory of Molecular Neuroendocrinology, Budapest, Hungary

Mátyás Cserháti, Csilla Krifaton, Sándor Szoboszlay and Balázs Kriszt
Szent István University, Department of Environmental Protection and Safety, Gödöllő, Hungary

József Kukolya
Central Environmental and Food Science Research Institute, Department of Microbiology, Budapest, Hungary

Zsuzsanna Szőke and Balá zs Kőszegi
Soft Flow Hungary R&D Ltd., Pécs, Hungary

Mihá ly Albert
CEVA Phylaxia Ltd, Budapest, Hungary

Teréz Barna
University of Debrecen, Department of Genetics and Applied Microbiology, Debrecen, Hungary

Miklós Mézes
Szent István University, Department of Nutrition, Gödöllő, Hungary

Daniel R. Swale
Department of Anesthesiology, Vanderbilt University Medical Center, Nashville, TN, United States of America

Rene Raphemot
Department of Anesthesiology, Vanderbilt University Medical Center, Nashville, TN, United States of America
Department of Pharmacology, Vanderbilt University School of Medicine, Nashville, TN, United States of America

Jerod S. Denton
Department of Anesthesiology, Vanderbilt University Medical Center, Nashville, TN, United States of America
Department of Pharmacology, Vanderbilt University School of Medicine, Nashville, TN, United States of America
Institute of Chemical Biology, Vanderbilt University School of Medicine, Nashville, TN, United States of America
Institute for Global Health, Vanderbilt University, Nashville, TN, United States of America

Matthew F. Rouhier and Peter M. Piermarini
Department of Entomology, Ohio Agricultural Research and Development Center, The Ohio State University, Wooster, OH, United States of America

Emily Days
Institute of Chemical Biology, Vanderbilt University School of Medicine, Nashville, TN, United States of America

C. David Weaver
Department of Pharmacology, Vanderbilt University School of Medicine, Nashville, TN, United States of America
Institute of Chemical Biology, Vanderbilt University School of Medicine, Nashville, TN, United States of America

Kimberly M. Lovell, Leah C. Konkel, Darren W. Engers and Sean F. Bollinger
Department of Pharmacology, Vanderbilt University School of Medicine, Nashville, TN, United States of America
Department of Chemistry, Vanderbilt University School of Medicine, Nashville TN, United States of America

Corey Hopkins
Department of Pharmacology, Vanderbilt University School of Medicine, Nashville, TN, United States of America
Institute for Global Health, Vanderbilt University, Nashville, TN, United States of America
Department of Chemistry, Vanderbilt University School of Medicine, Nashville TN, United States of America

Sara L. Montgomery, Daria Vorojeikina and Matthew D. Rand
Department of Environmental Medicine, University of Rochester School of Medicine and Dentistry, Rochester, New York, United States of America

Wen Huang, Trudy F. C. Mackay and Robert R. H. Anholt
Department of Biological Sciences, Genetics Program, and W. M. Keck Center for Behavioral Biology, North Carolina State University, Raleigh, North Carolina, United States of America

Duan Gui, Yong Sun, Qin Tu and Yuping Wu
Guangdong Provincial Key Laboratory of Marine Resources and Coastal Engineering, School of Marine Sciences, Sun Yat-Sen University, Guangzhou, China

Ri-Qing Yu
Department of Biology, University of Texas at Tyler, Tyler, Texas, United States of America

Laiguo Chen
Urban Environment and Ecology Research Center, South China Institute of Environmental Sciences (SCIES), Ministry of Environmental Protection, Guangzhou, China

Hui Mo
South China Botanical Garden, Chinese Academy of Sciences, Guangzhou, China

Mayankbhai Patel, Santhosh Palani, Arijit Chakravarty, Johnny Yang, Wen Chyi Shyu and Jerome T. Mettetal
Drug Metabolism and Pharmacokinetics, Takeda Pharmaceuticals International Co., Cambridge, Massachusetts, United States of America

Komal Kalani and Santosh Kumar Srivastava
Medicinal Chemistry Department, CSIR-Central Institute of Medicinal and Aromatic Plants, Lucknow, 226015 (U.P.) India
Academy of Scientific and Innovative Research (AcSIR), Anusandhan Bhawan, New Delhi, 110 001, India

Vikas Kushwaha, Richa Verma and P. K. Murthy
Division of Parasitology, CSIR-Central Drug Research Institute, Lucknow, 226001, UP, India

Pooja Sharma
Metabolic & Structural Biology Department, CSIR-Central Institute of Medicinal and Aromatic Plants, Lucknow, 226015 (U.P.) India

Mukesh Srivastava
Clinical and Experimental Medicine, Biometry section, CSIR-Central Drug Research Institute, Lucknow, 226001, UP, India

Feroz Khan
Metabolic & Structural Biology Department, CSIR-Central Institute of Medicinal and Aromatic Plants, Lucknow, 226015 (U.P.) India
Academy of Scientific and Innovative Research (AcSIR), Anusandhan Bhawan, New Delhi, 110 001, India

Stephenie D. Prokopec and John D. Watson
Informatics and Bio-computing Program, Ontario Institute for Cancer Research, Toronto, Ontario, Canada

Raimo Pohjanvirta
Laboratory of Toxicology, National Institute for Health and Welfare, Kuopio, Finland
Department of Food Hygiene and Environmental Health, University of Helsinki, Helsinki, Finland

Paul C. Boutros
Informatics and Bio-computing Program, Ontario Institute for Cancer Research, Toronto, Ontario, Canada
Department of Medical Biophysics, University of Toronto, Toronto, Ontario, Canada
Department of Pharmacology & Toxicology, University of Toronto, Toronto, Ontario, Canada

Jasmine L. Hamilton and Muhammad Imran ul-haq
The Centre for Blood Research, Department of Pathology and Laboratory Medicine, Life Sciences Institute, The University of British Columbia, Vancouver, British Columbia, Canada

Neelima Nair, Suraj Unniappan and Azadeh Hatef
Veterinary Biomedical Sciences, Laboratory of Integrative Neuroendocrinology, Western College of Veterinary Medicine, University of Saskatchewan, Saskatoon, Saskatchewan, Canada

Jayachandran N. Kizhakkedathu
The Centre for Blood Research, Department of Pathology and Laboratory Medicine, Life Sciences Institute, The University of British Columbia, Vancouver, British Columbia, Canada
Department of Chemistry, The University of British Columbia, Vancouver, British Columbia, Canada

Rukhsanda Aziz, Xiaoe Yang, Wendan Xiao and Tingqiang Li
Ministry of Education Key Laboratory of Environmental Remediation and Ecological Health, College of Environmental and Resource Sciences, Zhejiang University, Hangzhou, China

Muhammad Tariq Rafiq
Ministry of Education Key Laboratory of Environmental Remediation and Ecological Health, College of Environmental and Resource Sciences, Zhejiang University, Hangzhou, China
Department of Environmental Science, International Islamic University, Islamabad, Pakistan

Peter J. Stoffella
Indian River Research and Education Center, Institute of Food and Agricultural Sciences, University of Florida, Fort Pierce, Florida, United States of America

Aamir Saghir
Institute of Statistics, Zhejiang University, Hangzhou, China

Muhammad Azam
College of Agriculture and Biotechnology, Zhejiang University, Hangzhou, China

Maame Anima Sarfo and Betty Norman
Komfo Anokye Teaching Hospital, Kumasi, Ghana

Fred Stephen Sarfo, Richard Phillips and George Bedu-Addo
Komfo Anokye Teaching Hospital, Kumasi, Ghana
Kwame Nkrumah University of Science and Technology, Kumasi, Ghana

David Chadwick
The James Cook University Hospital, Middlesbrough, United Kingdom

John Paul Ekwaru and Paul J. Veugelers
School of Public Health, University of Alberta, Edmonton, Alberta, Canada

Jennifer D. Zwicker
School of Public Policy, University of Calgary, Calgary, Alberta, Canada

Michael F. Holick
Section of Endocrinology, Nutrition and Diabetes, Department of Medicine, Boston University School of Medicine, Boston, Massachusetts, United States of America

Edward Giovannucci
Harvard School of Public Health, Departments of Nutrition and Epidemiology, Boston, Massachusetts, United States of America

Giuseppe Palma and Vittoria D'Avino
Institute of Biostructure and Bioimaging, National Council of Research (CNR), Naples, Italy

Marco Salvatore
Department of Advanced Biomedical Sciences, Federico II University School of Medicine, Naples, Italy

Laura Cella, Raffaele Liuzzi, Manuel Conson and Roberto Pacelli
Institute of Biostructure and Bioimaging, National Council of Research (CNR), Naples, Italy
Department of Advanced Biomedical Sciences, Federico II University School of Medicine, Naples, Italy

Joseph O. Deasy and Jung Hun Oh
Department of Medical Physics, Memorial Sloan Kettering Cancer Center, New York, New York, United States of America

Novella Pugliese and Marco Picardi
Department of Clinical Medicine and Surgery, Federico II University School of Medicine, Naples, Italy

Yannick Poquet, Sylvie Tchamitchian, Marianne Cousin, Michel Pélissier, Jean-Luc Brunet and Luc P. Belzunces
INRA, Laboratoire de Toxicologie Environnementale, UR 406 A&E, CS 40509, 84914 Avignon Cedex 9, France

Laurent Bodin
ANSES, French Agency for Food, Environmental and Occupational Health Safety, 27–31 Avenue du Général Leclerc, 94701 Maisons-Alfort, France

Marc Tchamitchian
INRA, UR Ecodéveloppement, CS 40509, 84914 Avignon Cedex 9, France

Marion Fusellier
Department of Diagnostic Imaging, CRIP, National Veterinary School (Oniris), Nantes, France

Barbara Giroud, Florent Lafay and Audrey Buleté
Université de Lyon, Institut des Sciences Analytiques, UMR5280 CNRS Université Lyon1, ENS-Lyon, 5 rue de la Doua, 69100 Villeurbanne, France

Pamela Ovadje, Dennis Ma, Phillip Tremblay, Alessia Roma, Matthew Steckle and Siyaram Pandey
Department of Chemistry & Biochemistry, University of Windsor, Windsor, ON, Canada

Jose-Antonio Guerrero and John Thor Arnason
Department of Biology, University of Ottawa, Ottawa, ON, Canada

Brooke Hamilton, Alexander Manzella and Victoria DiMarco
Department of Microbiology and Immunology, University of Rochester Medical Center, Rochester, New York, United States of America

Karyn Schmidt
Department of Biochemistry and Biophysics, University of Rochester Medical Center, Rochester, New York, United States of America

J. Scott Butler
Department of Microbiology and Immunology, University of Rochester Medical Center, Rochester, New York, United States of America
Department of Biochemistry and Biophysics, University of Rochester Medical Center, Rochester, New York, United States of America
Center for RNA Biology, University of Rochester Medical Center, Rochester, New York, United States of America

Guerry J. Cook
Wake Forest University Health Sciences, Department of Internal Medicine, Section on Hematology and Oncology, Winston-Salem, North Carolina, United States of America

David L. Caudell
Department of Pathology, Section of Comparative Medicine, Wake Forest University Health Sciences, Winston-Salem, North Carolina, United States of America

Howard L. Elford
Molecules for Health, Richmond, Virginia, United States of America

Timothy S. Pardee
Wake Forest University Health Sciences, Department of Internal Medicine, Section on Hematology and Oncology, Winston-Salem, North Carolina, United States of America
Wake Forest University Comprehensive Cancer Center, Winston-Salem, North Carolina, United States of America

Nizam Uddin, Md. Rakib Hasan, Md. Mahadi Hasan, Md. Monir Hossain, Md. Robiul Alam, Mohammad Raquibul Hasan, A. F. M. Mahmudul Islam, Tasmina Rahman and Md. Sohel Rana
Department of Pharmacy, Jahangirnagar University, Savar, Dhaka, 1342, Bangladesh

Index